KU-227-335

Contents

GENETICS

PSYCHOLOGY

SOCIAL PROCESSES

THE SCIENTIFIC BASIS OF PSYCHIATRY
Second Edition

Edited by

Malcolm P.
MA (Cantab),
Consultant Psychia
Lecturer, Royal Fre

and

Michael W.
BA, PhD
Professor of Psycho
Egham, Surrey

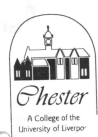
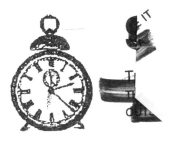
W.B. SAUNDERS COMPANY LTD
London · Philadelphia · Toronto · Sydney · Tokyo

This book is printed on acid free paper

W.B. Saunders Company Ltd   24–28 Oval Road
London NW1 7DX

The Curtis Center
Independence Square West
Philadelphia, PA 19106–3399

55 Horner Avenue
Toronto, Ontario M8Z 4X6, Canada

Harcourt Brace Jovanovich (Australia) Pty Ltd,
30–52 Smidmore St
Marrickville, NSW 2204, Australia

Harcourt Brace Jovanovich Japan Inc.
Ichibancho Central Building, 22-1 Ichibancho
Chiyoda-ku, Tokyo 102, Japan

First published 1983
Second edition 1992

A catalogue record for this book is available from the British Library.

ISBN 0-7020-1448-6

Typeset by Alden Multimedia Ltd
Printed and bound in Great Britain by Hartnolls Ltd., Bodmin, Cornwall

Contributors

C.R. Brewin PhD, FBPsS
Senior Scientist, MRC Social and Community Psychiatry Unit, Institute of Psychiatry, De Crespigny Park, London SE5 8AF, UK

A.C. Carr MA (Cantab), AKC, MB BS, MRCS, MRCP, MRCPsych, MPhil
Chief Consultant Psychiatrist, Department of Psychiatry, Hamilton Civic Hospitals, 237 Barton Street, East Hamilton, Ontario L8L 2X2, Canada

J.L. Cox MA, DM, FRCPsych, DPM, FRCP (Edin)
Professor of Psychiatry, School of Postgraduate Medicine and Biological Sciences, Keele University, Thornburrow Drive, Hartshill, Stoke-on-Trent, ST4 7QB, UK

M.D. Craggs BSC, PhD
Senior Scientific Staff, MRC Neurological Prostheses Unit; Senior Lecturer, Department of Neurology, Institute of Psychiatry, De Crespigny Park, London SE5 8AF, UK

F. Creed MA, MD, FRCP, FRCPsych
Senior Lecturer and Honorary Consultant Psychiatrist, University Department of Psychiatry, Rawnsley Building, Manchester Royal Infirmary, Oxford Road, Manchester M13 9WL, UK

A.N. Davison BSC, BPharm, PhD, DSc, FRCPath
Past Professor of Neurochemistry, Institute of Neurology; *Present* Professor (Emeritus), Department of Pathology, Hunterian Institute, Royal College of Surgeons, Lincolns Inn Fields, London WC2A 3PN, UK

J.M. Elliott MA, DPhil
Lecturer in Neuropharmacology, St Mary's Hospital Medical School, Norfolk Place, London W2 1PG, UK

M.W. Eysenck BA, PhD
Professor of Psychology, Royal Holloway and Bedford New College, University of London, Egham, Surrey TW20 0EX, UK

P.B.C. Fenwick MB BChir(Cantab), DPM, FRCPsych
Consultant Neuropsychiatrist, Maudsley Hospital; Senior Lecturer, Institute of Psychiatry, De Crespigny Park, Denmark Hill, London SE5 8AF; Clinical Neuro-physiologist, Radcliffe Infirmary, Oxford, UK

J. Freeman BSc, MEd, PhD, FBPsS
President, European Council for High Ability, 21 Montagu Square, London W1H 1RE, UK

C.D. Frith MA, Dip Psych, PhD
CRC Division of Psychiatry, Northwick Park Hospital, Watford Road, Harrow HA1 3UJ; MRC Cyclotron Unit, RPMS, Hammersmith Hospital, Ducane Road, London, UK

T. Fundudis PhD, MA, Dip Psychother, CPsychol, FBPsS
Consultant in Clinical Psychology, Fleming Nuffield Unit, Newcastle-upon-Tyne Health Authority, Jesmond, Newcastle-upon-Tyne NE2 3AE; Associate Teacher in Child and Adolescent Psychology, Department of Child Health, University of Newcastle-upon-Tyne NE1, UK

M.J. Gawel MB BCh, MA, MRCP (UK), FRCP (C)
Assistant Professor Medicine (Neurology), University of Toronto, Sunnybrook Health Science Centre, 2075 Bayview Avenue, Toronto, M4N 3M5; Staff Neurologist, Scarborough Centenary Hospital, Scarborough, Ontario, Canada

M. Gill MD, MRCPsych
Wellcome Research Fellow, Genetics Section, Institute of Psychiatry, De Crespigny Park, London SE5 8AF, UK

S.R. Hirsch BA, MD, MPhil, FRCP, FRCPsych
Professor of Psychiatry, Charing Cross and Westminster Medical School, St Dunstan's Road, London W6 8RP, UK

L.L. Iversen MA, PhD, FRS
Director, Neuroscience Research Centre, Merck Sharp & Dohme Research Laboratories, Terlings Park, Eastwick Road, Harlow, Essex CM20 2QR, UK

M.S. Jorsh MB BCh, MRCPsych
Lecturer, University of Keele, School of Postgraduate Medicine and Biological Sciences, North Staffordshire Hospital Centre, Thornburrow Drive, Hartshill, Stoke-on-Trent ST4 7QB; Senior Registrar, St Edwards' Hospital, Cheadle Road, Cheddleton, Staffordshire ST13 7ED, UK

S. Kindler MD
Department of Psychiatry, Herzog Hospital, PO Box 140, Jerusalem, Israel

I. Kolvin BA, MD, FRCPsych, DipPsych
Professor of Child and Family Mental Health, The Royal Free Hospital School of
Medicine and The Tavistock Centre, London, UK

B.T. Kugler BSc, PhD
Director, Harper House Children's Service, North-West Thames Regional Health
Authority; Honorary Senior Lecturer, Department of Paediatrics, University
College and Middlesex School of Medicine, London, UK

B. Lerer MD
Associate Professor, Department of Psychiatry, Hebrew University, Hadassah
Medical School, PO Box 12000, Jerusalem 91120, Israel

G. Lewis MSc, MRCPsych
Lecturer, Institute of Psychiatry, De Crespigny Park, London SE5 8AF; Honorary
Senior Registrar, Maudsley Hospital, Denmark Hill, London SE5 8AZ, UK

A. M. Macdonald BSc
Research Worker, Genetics Section, Institute of Psychiatry, De Crespigny Park,
London SE5 8AF, UK

A.V.P. Mackay MA, BSc, PhD (Cantab), MB ChB, FRCP (Edin), FRCPsych
Physician Superintendent, Argyll and Bute Hospital, Lochgilphead, Argyll,
PA31 8LD; McIntosh Lecturer in Psychological Medicine, University of
Glasgow, UK

D. Mackay BA, MSc, AFBPsS
Medical Directorate Manager and Honorary Clinical Psychologist, Weston Area
Health Trust, Weston General Hospital, Grange Road, Weston-Super-Mare
BS23 4TQ, UK

K.D. MacRae MA, PhD, FIS
Reader in Medical Statistics, Charing Cross and Westminster Medical School,
St Dunstan's Road, London W6 8RP, UK

I.C. McManus MA, MD, PhD
Senior Lecturer in Psychology, St Mary's Hospital Medical School, Praed Street,
London W2 1NY; University College London, Gower Street, London WC1E 6BT,
UK

A. Mann MD, MPhil, FRCP, FRCPsych
Professor of Epidemiological Psychiatry, Institute of Psychiatry, De Crespigny
Park, London SE5 8AF; Royal Free Hospital School of Medicine, London, UK

R.M. Murray MPhil, MD, DSC, FRCP, FRCPsych
Professor of Psychological Medicine, King's College Hospital and Institute of
Psychiatry, De Crespigny Park, Denmark Hill, London SE5 8AF, UK

W. Ll. Parry-Jones MA, MD, FRCPsych, FRCP (Glasg), DPM
Professor of Child and Adolescent Psychiatry, University of Glasgow, Royal Hospital for Sick Children, Yorkhill, Glasgow G3 8SJ, UK

D.F. Peck BA, DipPsych
Area Clinical Psychologist, Craig Phadrig Hospital, Inverness IV3 6PJ, UK

P. Pichot
President, World Psychiatric Association; Professor, Faculté de Médecine, Université René Descartes, Centre Hospitalier Saint-Anne, 100 Rue de la Santé, 75674 Paris Cedex 14, France

R.G. Priest MD, FRCP (Edin), FRCPsych
Professor of Psychiatry, St Mary's Hospital Medical School, South Wharf Road, London W2 1PG, UK

B. Shapira MD
Lecturer, Department of Psychiatry, Hebrew University, Hadassah Medical School, PO Box 12000, Jerusalem 91120; Department of Psychiatry, Herzog Hospital, PO Box 140, Jerusalem, Israel

P. Sham MA, MSc, MRCPsych
Wellcome Training Fellow, Genetics Section, Institute of Psychiatry, De Crespigny Park, London SE5 8AF, UK

A. Steptoe MA, DPhil
Professor of Psychology, Psychology Department, St George's Hospital Medical School, Cranmer Terrace, London SW17 0RE, UK

A.B. Summerfield MA, PhD, CPsychol, FBPsS
Senior Lecturer in Psychology, United Medical and Dental School of Guy's and St Thomas's Hospitals, London, UK

C.J.A. Taylor BSc, MB BS, MRCPsych
Research Psychiatrist and Honorary Senior Registrar, Institute of Psychiatry (Genetics Section), De Crespigny Park, London SE5 8AF, UK

C. Vögele Dip Psych, PhD
Lecturer in Health Psychology and Psychophysiology, School of Psychology, University of Birmingham, Edgbaston, Birmingham B13 9EH, UK

J.A. Weinman BA, PhD
Professor, Unit of Psychology, Medical School, Guy's Hospital, London Bridge, London SE1 9RT, UK

M.P.I. Weller MA (Cantab), CPsychol, FBPsS, MB BS, FRCPsych
Consultant Psychiatrist, Friern, Whittington and Royal Northern Hospitals; Honorary Senior Lecturer, Royal Free Hospital School of Medicine, Friern Barnet Road, London N11 3BQ, UK

Preface

Numerous scientific disciplines underpin and inform the practice of psychiatry. Physiology and psychology are obvious examples, but pharmacology, biochemistry, epidemiology, genetics and statistics are equally relevant. The purpose of this book is to present a concise survey of the principal contributions made by these disciplines. Within so vast a field of study the aim has been to emphasize core concepts and interconnections.

The pressing need for a work of this kind was brought home to Malcolm Weller when preparing a course for students studying for the membership examination of the Royal College of Psychiatrists. No textbook was available which brought together, even in outline, the corpus of basic scientific knowledge that is a prerequisite to clinical psychiatric practice. The task of creating such a work was facilitated by the widespread encouragement and by the ready, enthusiastic response to requests for contributions from distinguished scientists in many fields of medicine, sociology and psychology.

In this second edition we have deepened the content and extended the range of subject matter as well as updating the text. We hope this single volume now covers the major areas of importance.

Each chapter is intended to explore an important topic, providing an overview of sufficient depth to act as an introduction to further reading. To preserve this approach, references are often to review articles or a single, recent reference. Papers of historical importance, or which cover possibily contentious issues, are also cited. In one or two instances, such as the chapter by Professor Davison, it was thought worthwhile to explore an important and developing field more fully.

Most medical practitioners have little contact with psychology during their training. Generous space has therefore been devoted to this discipline in order to provide a broader basic coverage, and contact points with psychiatry have been stressed whenever possible. Clinical psychology has taken two paths; psychometric testing and personal therapy, using both behavioural and psychotherapeutic procedures. Despite a considerable literature on learning theory, much in personal therapy remains to be clarified and has only recently come under critical examination. The development of the psychotherapies has been included to illustrate the different lines of approach and the chapters on learning and personality discuss some of the conceptual issues in behaviour therapy. Some appreciation of the construction and limitations of psychometric tests was felt desirable and a chapter has been devoted to rating scales. Practising psychiatrists particularly need instruction in this area in order to appreciate better the assistance they can obtain from their highly trained colleagues, and at the same time to recognize the limitations of their test instruments.

Malcolm Weller
Michael Eysenck

Acknowledgements

We have been helped in many ways by a large number of people in the preparation of this book and are grateful to the following for discussion: Dr Sean Baumann, Dr Peter Cooksey, Dr Tim Corn, Professor Valerie Cowie, Dr Tim Crow, Dr Martin Elliot, Dr Paul Flower, Dr Elliot Gershon, Dr Michael Jacobs, Professor Daniel van Kammen, Professor Robert Kendall, Professor Malcolm Laider, Professor Julian Leff, Professor Anthony Mann, Dr Angus Mackay, Dr Christopher Mountjoy, Dr John Pilgrim and Dr David Wright.

We also thank Mrs Carol Dawson and Miss Ruth Norton for secretarial assistance, Glaxo Research Laboratories for secretarial finance, and the librarians at the Royal Society of Medicine, the Royal Free Hospital and particularly Friern Hospital.

Finally, we are grateful to those individuals and institutions that have provided material for the illustrations.

Introduction

— 1

Changing Frontiers

M.P.I. Weller and M.W. Eysenck

In this introductory chapter attention is drawn to a number of experimental findings from different scientific disciplines which constitute areas of interest to psychiatric concepts and practice. The connections between these findings and psychiatry are developed and when possible the abnormal is related to the normal. Some knotty areas of disagreement, which seem to contain clues for progress, are mentioned. Homeostasis, adaptation and plasticity are afforded special consideration as central properties of biological functioning.

Of necessity, the discussion is selective and limited to a few broad areas. The reader is referred throughout to the appropriate sections of the book for fuller treatments and a comprehensive background. Some of the findings mentioned in this chapter are comparatively old but still seem innovative and provide a useful conceptual framework to contemporary thought; however, many are recent and have not yet been fully incorporated into traditional views, but offer fruitful opportunities for further exploration.

Brain Organization

Living things have evolved ways of dealing with environmental hazards. Sensory data are received from surface receptors, enabling the organism to protect itself from noxious contacts. In the more evolved and mobile life forms of the Animal Kingdom, sensory data are also received from the eyes, ears and nose, thus enabling the animal to scan the more distant environment for potential hazards. Information is also fed back from joints and muscles, indicating position and movement (proprioception) and allowing the fine tuning of responses. The internal environment is governed by homeostatic processes, which also depend on feedback systems. Appetites, too, are a form of self-detection, governed by the survival needs of the organism.

Like the homeostatic processes in the body, the activities of the brain can be compared to the operation of a complex feedback system. Various models have been proposed which help our understanding. Machines exhibiting quasi-purposive and adaptive behaviour have been devised, based on servo-mechanisms embodying automatic control principles. Norbert Weiner founded the multi-disciplinary science of Cybernetics (a term meaning steersman in Greek) as a discipline for exploring these characteristics and data processing has become a central theme.

Complex systems are often described as 'temperamental' and animate characteristics attributed, as when the term 'she' is used for ships and aeroplanes.
Increasing complexity is accompanied by the potential for complex aberrations.
The behaviour of feedback systems is predictable if the variables are known.
However, the behaviour seldom coincides with common sense expectations, even
when the system is comparatively simple. Transitions from one output state to
another may be discontinuous. Just as calm flowing water breaks up into increasing turbulence when moving, first to rapids and then to waterfalls, so many
natural phenomena are governed by processes that have varying degrees of
turbulence. At certain stages a process of non-linear oscillations sets in. The
unpredictability of the system at these stages is known by the self-explanatory
term of a 'chaotic region' (Bauer *et al.*, 1975). At critical junctures, very small
changes in the initial conditions can lead to very different outcomes. Because of
these chaotic regions, interactions in complex systems, such as meteorological,
ecological and economic systems, often cannot be fully anticipated.

The mathematics describing such systems has developed from fluid dynamics
in which deterministic motion, such as convection currents, breaks down into
very brief epochs of 'deterministic chaos' in which the outcome is exquisitely
dependent on the initial conditions. It is likely that such episodes occur in a wide
variety of phenomena and they have been demonstrated in the growth of
populations, the weather and physiological processes, such as the electroencephalogram and the electrocardiogram.

Analogies between the brain and electronic systems can be misleading and the
corresponding constraints on their interactions. Brain mechanisms are characterized by redundancy and plasticity. Pasamanick and Knobloch (1961) postulated
a continuum of reproductive casualty, from conception to the perinatal period, so
that we all fall short of our original potential, and compensatory mechanisms,
repair and adaptability are essential. Neural tissue has the capacity to establish
connections during early development and to strengthen those connections, as
well as allowing others to decay (Perry and Cowey, 1982). Compensation occurs
and functions are maintained in the event of injury (Lashley, 1929). Such a system
is robust and adaptable, being unaffected by the failure of any one particular
component—'Adaptability is probably the most distinctive characteristic of life'
(Selye, 1950). In electronic equipment, such as the digital computer, each pathway
is critical and all the components must be highly reliable.

Networks of units in which the components are linked in excitatory or
inhibitory ways have shown remarkable learning capacity if the strength of the
linkages can be modified according to output criteria for given inputs. The
mechanism, known as parallel distributed processing, has many analogies with
brain mechanisms. It is fast in operation, robust and relatively impervious to the
failure of some components (Clark, 1989). The system is well suited to detecting
a signal embedded in noise (Servan-Schrieber *et al.*, 1990) and for speedy
processing, such as sensory perception, and could run in conjunction with a serial
symbol processing system, suited for logico-deductive reasoning.

Machines can be considered in terms both of their behaviour and of their
components: 'The machine as a whole works under the control of two distinct

principles. The higher one is the principle of the machine's design, and this harnesses the lower one, which consists in the physical and chemical processes on which the machine relies.' (Polanyi, 1962) (see Chapters 8, 9 and 11, this volume).

A variety of techniques have demonstrated that mammalian cortical neurones are organized in columns running from the pial surface to the white matter. These columns operate as functional units. Information from the sense organs is relayed and transformed many times before it reaches dedicated receptor areas in the brain that detect specific features—such as form, colour, depth and motion in the visual cortex—which are then segregated into separate pathways and structures (e.g. Ts'o *et al.*, 1990). Adjacent columns and regions are insulated from one another, enabling them to operate as largely autonomous regions, although this insulation partially breaks down in epileptic seizures (see Chapter 10, this volume). The insulation between adjacent channels is also seen in the corticopetal receptor pathways in which lateral inhibition sharpens sensory discrimination.

Wilder Penfield and his colleagues applied direct stimulation to the brains of human subjects during operations for the removal of epileptic foci, and mapped out the functional motor and sensory organization (Penfield and Rasmussen, 1950). Stimulation of the temporal lobe produced experiences akin to 'made' thoughts and feelings, in accord with temporal lobe epileptic aura and psychotic experiences.

The regional cerebral autonomy led Norman Geschwind (1965) to conceptualize the brain as a collection of interlocking subsystems. He investigated stroke patients, some of whom demonstrated sensory inattention and neglect. Geschwind emphasized that connections between brain regions could be interrupted, and used the term 'disconnection syndrome', first proposed by Dejerine and Leipman, for this group of disorders (see Chapters 8 and 19, this volume).

If specific functional areas are disturbed, alternative strategies are adopted, resulting in abnormal functioning as remarkable as deep dyslexia, in which the sense but not the actual words can be read (e.g. reading 'vacation' for the word 'holiday'). Agnosia is a striking example to contrast with deep dyslexia. In this condition the elements can be registered but cannot be organized into wholes (Gestalten). These phenomena relate to the ordinary observation that a melody is recognizable when all the notes are changed when the key is altered. The converse also applies and the same notes can be part of different melodies. These complementary observations are central to the Gestalt school of psychology, founded by Wertheimer and developed by his pupils Koffka and Köhler, which stressed that the whole (Gestalt) could be recognized as an entity, even when the parts were changed, as in all familial resemblances.

Sperry and his colleagues (1969) investigated epileptic patients in whom the major interhemispheric pathway, the corpus collosum, was surgically divided, in a final attempt to control otherwise intractable seizures. The work of these researchers and that of Geschwind suggest that consciousness, or self-awareness, is dependent on the functional integrity of particular subsystems and their access to left hemisphere speech centres. By injecting sodium amytal into the right carotid artery the whole right hemisphere can be selectively anaesthetized. Before the anaesthetic passes through the circle of Willis to the left hemisphere the subject is often unaware that anything has happened (Hommes and Panhuysen, 1970).

Specific areas of the brain are dedicated to particular functions (see Chapter 8), but adaptations to brain damage indicate that vicarious use can be made of alternative areas (Lashley, 1950) and that the entire brain operates as an integrated system with a widespread and diffuse representation of learned behaviour. Exploration of these polarized concepts has been advanced by the application of standardized psychological tests to brain-damaged humans (see Chapter 8, this volume).

There was a surprising delay between the development of psychometric tests and their application to brain-damaged patients, which first occurred as late as 1940. Attitudes in psychology and neurology may have contributed to the delay. The philosophical approach to psychology adopted in many centres was combined with the climate of opinion created by the views of the eminent neurologist Henry Head (1926), who held that the approach of Broca and Wernicke was creating an almost phrenological approach to neurology (see Chapter 8, this volume).

Until the pioneering work of the psychologist Donald Hebb, the frontal lobe has been considered the centre for the highest organization of intellectual activity. However, the researchers found that lesions to this area did not decrease the IQ score (Hebb and Penfield, 1940). Hudson (1966) has shown that motivation and persistence (impaired by frontal lobe damage) are as important for achievement as intellectual ability. Similarly, Douglas Savage, working with medical students at Newcastle University, found that work study habits were more important than IQ in determining final examination success.

Regional Specialization and Mass Action

The functions of particular brain areas can be undertaken by other areas. This adaptation is facilitated by the temporary retention of part of the system. Lashley (1950) showed that recovery of function occurred after brain damage produced in two successive stages to bilateral homologous cortical areas. Perhaps similar adaptations operate in insidious brain damage in childhood, such as occurs in hydrocephalus, which is compatible with high intelligence, even when the cortex has been reduced to a thin rim of tissue (Lewin, 1981). Adaptation continues even in the senium and dendritic growth is still evident in late life (Buell and Coleman, 1979; see Chapter 9, this volume).

Earlier Sherrington (1906) had electrically stimulated the brains of animals and described the organization of the motor cortex. The brain lesion experiments of Lashley (1929) pointed in a different direction for higher cognitive functions, but some of Lashley's work is complementary to Sherrington's findings. Sherrington had described an 'instability of the motor point', whereby repeated stimulation of a single region in the motor cortex led to a change in the motor response.

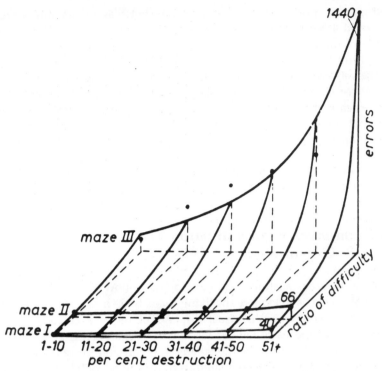

FIG. 1.1 Errors in maze-learning increase both with the difficulty of the maze and proportionally to the amount of destruction of the cerebral cortex (from Lashley, 1929).

Lashley had observed that specific functions could be preserved when a large proportion of the functional cortical area undertaking the function was destroyed.

Lashley expressed the view that the entire brain has a role in maze-learning ability and that it was the amount, and not the site, of brain tissue destruction that interfered with performance on this task. Similar results have been obtained by other workers (Maier, 1932). Glees and Cole (1950) showed that skilled motor movements were restored after a succession of small cerebral lesions in monkeys, each lesion extending the earlier lesion and invading a progressively larger area surrounding it. The effects could be demonstrated most sensitively by requiring novel responses of the lesioned animal, but once again it was the extent and not the site of the lesion that determined the outcome. This finding of a diffuse organization of learned behaviour is described as 'mass action' or 'equipotentiality' and remains a useful model for dementia.

Early dementia may be masked successfully in intelligent people. The problem can be exposed by applying tasks of insufficient difficulty. The smooth exponential curves found in Lashley's rat experiments, in which maze-running errors are related to the extent of cortical destruction (see Fig. 1.1), are more plausible than the discontinuous model proposed by Blessed *et al.* (1968). These workers suggested that humans have a reserve capacity of about 10% of their cerebral tissue, and suggest that brain lesions are tolerated without a perceptible decline in performance if destruction is less than this, but that a dementing process can be detected if these reserves are invaded.

Some of the clearest evidence of the complexities of brain organization has emerged from the research of cognitive neuropsychologists. Their central focus is on the various patterns of cognitive impairment to be found in brain-damaged patients (see Ellis and Young, 1988). The major finding that has emerged from this research is that there are often highly specific impairments (e.g. words can be read but not non-words, or vice versa). This high degree of specificity suggests that the brain is organized in the form of numerous specialized processing modules. These modules allegedly function relatively independently of each other. As a consequence, the partial or total destruction of a module through brain damage may not affect the functioning of other modules.

Some Non-invasive Investigation Techniques and Brain Organization

In addition to gross anatomy and histology, we now have non-invasive techniques that enable us to explore the living brain. Brain functioning can be literally illuminated by computerized visual displays of regional cerebral blood flow, demonstrated by means of radioactive xenon. Weinberger *et al.* (1986) showed that blood flow rates in the dorsolateral pre-frontal cortex were lower in schizophrenic patients when compared to flow in non-frontal areas. The reduced blood flow remained unaffected when the schizophrenic patients performed the Wisconsin Card Sorting Test, which normally activates this region, while the control subjects showed the expected increase. Gustafson and Hagberg (1975a) had earlier shown that the pattern of personality and cognitive changes in pre-senile dementia could be related to the relative reduction and preservation of blood flow to certain cerebral regions. Frontal lobe blood flow reduction was associated with apathy and indifference, and temporal lobe reduction, combined with frontal preservation, with obsessive characteristics.

When the electroencephalogram (EEG) is analysed mathematically, a greater than normal degree of synchrony between temporal areas is found in schizophrenia (Flor-Henry and Yeudall, 1979; Weller and Montagu, 1979; see Chapter 10, this volume), suggesting a partial failure of localized cerebral autonomy.

The dynamics of neural events can be traced with radioactive glucose derivatives which, when suitably structured, are caught in metabolic pathways, highlighting the most active sites. Initially the positron-emitting tracer carbon-14 deoxyglucose was used for this quantitative autoradiography of positron emission tomography (PET) and then fluorine-18 deoxyglucose. The technique has allowed exciting insights into normal and abnormal brain functioning with a resolution of about 8 mm. A second technique uses radioactive compounds that have longer half-lives and are thus cheaper to produce, not needing a nearby cyclotron. This single photon computed tomography (SPECT) is somewhat less sensitive but reduces radiation risks, permitting repeated tomograms, and is more readily available.

PET studies have clarified normal physiological functioning, particularly in the sensory modalities. In macaques and normal human subjects there are changes in the regional cerebral blood flow in the visual cortex as the subjects discriminate between different attributes (shape, colour and velocity) of the same set of visual stimuli. Discrimination sensitivity to subtle changes was improved in humans by selective attention to specific attributes, rather than having attention divided between them, illustrating a cognitive control of neurophysiological processes. This performance enhancement was accompanied by an increased activity of different regions of the extrastriate visual cortex (Corbetta *et al.*, 1990).

There is a pre-frontal reward circuit, possibly by projections to the cingulate and entorhinal area from dopamine-containing neurones in the medial and sulcal subdivisions (see Phillips and Fiberger, 1989). Most PET studies in schizophrenia have shown a decrease in frontal lobe metabolic activity, consonant with a decrease in regional cerebral blood flow in the frontal area, but there are discrepant studies, including one showing the contrary effect (Cleghorn *et al.*, 1990; Paulman *et al.*, 1990; see Buchsbaum and Haier, 1987). The studies may be reconciled on the basis of the neuropsychological profiles, the lowered frontal activity being associated with deficit symptoms and impairment on complex cognitive tasks requiring sustained attention and abstraction (e.g. Paulman *et al.*, 1990; Liddle, 1990).

PET has produced contradictory findings in depression, depending in part on which glucose compound was used, whether patients were tested with their eyes open or closed, and whether or not painful stimuli were applied, as a means of activating the frontal lobes. Post *et al.* (1987) found that glucose utilization was reduced in the right temporal lobe compared to the left.

Nuclear magnetic resonance (NMR) has demonstrated longer proton T_1 relaxation times (a measure of the average mobility of water protons in membranes and fluids) in brain tissue of bipolar depressives, which were normalized after lithium therapy, but were unchanged in controls given lithium (Rangel-Guerra *et al.*, 1983). Similar results were found in red blood cells (Rosenthal *et al.*, 1986).

It has been widely supposed that pain perception is essentially a subcortical phenomenon, based on the painless procedure of cortical stimulation. Nevertheless, cognitive strategies for ameliorating intractable pain suggests otherwise and a frontal component has been implicated by virtue of an increase in frontal cerebral blood flow after noxious stimuli. A combination of the functional information from PET with the anatomical information from NMR has mapped out active areas of the brain, including cortical regions in response to painful pulses of heat to the forearm. There is contralateral activation of the anterior cingulate, a part of the limbic system that probably influences emotional and affective responses (and which is the site of neurosurgical procedures for relieving intractable pain). In addition both the primary and secondary somatosensory cortices are also activated, whereas vibration causes activation of the primary somatosensory cortex alone (Talbot *et al.*, 1991).

Development

Certain experiences, which must occur at critical times, are essential if development is to proceed normally. Conversely, exposure to adverse experiences at certain stages of development are likely to undermine the effectiveness of particular functions or experiences of behaviour. Various forms of sensory deprivation lead to perceptual anomalies, accompanied by functional morphological changes in neurones. Cats deprived of normal visual experience from birth have an absent or reduced responsiveness to those visual features which were specifically excluded from their experience, such as horizontal or vertical stripes, but normal development depends on more than appropriate visual stimulation. Integrated experience, including proprioceptive reinforcement, is necessary. If one kitten walks around its environment, its vision develops normally, whereas if it pulls another kitten around the same environment in a yoked trolley, the visual perception of the kitten which is passively taken around does not develop normally (Held and Hein, 1963).

Complex motor control depends as much, or more, on maturation than on practice. In a classic experiment Carmichael (1926) showed that amblystoma reared in an anaesthetic solution swam as effectively as practised controls in 30 min, a period compatible with the clearance of the anaesthetic. Maturation was similarly found to be more important than practice when comparing identical twins. One twin was given stair-climbing practice denied the other, but the practised twin did not seem to have benefited by the experience (Gesell and Thompson, 1929).

Sex Hormones

Rudimentary behaviour is often inherited but subsequently modified by social influences. For example, courtship behaviour seems pre-programmed but careful observation shows that environmental influences shape the details, as with bird song (see Chapter 25, this volume). Appropriately for courtship song, the song centre which, like speech, is lateralized to the left hemisphere in birds (see Chapter 8, this volume), is influenced by testosterone (Arnold and Saltiel, 1979) and has input connections with the auditory cortex. In the female brain the corresponding neural nuclei and network essential for male song production are also present, albeit of smaller size, and are necessary for conspecific song recognition (Brenowitz, 1991).

Sexual dimorphism has been observed in the brains of many species, including 23 measurements in man accounting for gender-related variance in brain weight (de Lacoste et al., 1990). Animal experiments have shown that sex hormones control this divergence, which probably occurs in utero and shortly after birth (Raisman and Field, 1973; Gorski and Harlan, 1977). A transient sexual responsiveness followed by the disappearance of the population of oestrogen receptors has been demonstrated in the cerebral cortex of rats during the first 14 days of life (McEwen, 1979). Just as female embryogenesis is modified by endogenous androgens to produce the male phenotype, exposure to exogenous androgens modifies mature sexual preferences and behaviour. Such exposure can occur through a shared placental circulation with a male twin (Gandelman *et al.*, 1977), or through the adrenogenital syndrome, with an excessive adrenal production of androgens (Ehrhardt and Baker, 1974).

The bonding of a mother to her child is usually as intense as that of the child to its mother—'just as much as the calf wants to suckle, the cow wants to give suck'. The bonding may be facilitated by those same factors which lead to the state of emotional lability, known as 'the blues', about four days after parturition.

In primates a rise in prolactin is associated with maternal (Tindall, 1978) and paternal (Dixson and George, 1982) behaviour. In rats maternal behaviour is regulated by progesterone and oestradiol (Bridges and Russell, 1981); oestradiol lowers brain β-endorphin (Shaikh *et al.*, 1978), and subcutaneous morphine disrupts maternal behaviour (Bridges and Grimm, 1982). Direct brain application of morphine suggests that the effect may be mediated by the medial preoptic area, an area involved in the oestrogen-stimulated onset of maternal behaviour (Numan *et al.*, 1977). (As Bridges and Grimm point out, human opiate addiction may distort maternal responsiveness.)

Physical changes that affect mental functioning occur throughout life. Some of these are clearly evident, while others may be masked and attributed to other mechanisms. The maturation of the nervous system during infancy and the endocrine alterations at puberty are striking. So too are the typical onset of schizophrenia in the late teens and early twenties, and the increased frequency of depression (see Chapter 30, this volume) and neurotic disorders with age in people of previously stable personality (Bergman, 1971). Emotional stability is dependent on the integrity of the right hemisphere and there seems to be a specific vulnerability of this hemisphere to ageing (Weller and Latimer-Sayer, 1985).

Neurophysiological and Genetic Considerations in Mental Illnesses

Freud believed that our understanding of mental illness, including the functional illnesses, will ultimately be clarified by neurophysiology and biochemistry, and his belief is being vindicated. Perhaps the most exciting field is in the affective illnesses, where a variety of biochemical and endocrinological changes have been demonstrated with some consistency (see Chapter 30, this volume). Post-traumatic, post-encephaleptic and epileptic psychoses have increased our awareness of organic factors in mental illness, as have psychotic manifestations in certain metabolic disturbances, such as Wilson's disease and porphyria. The possibilities of perinatal damage, particularly in relation to schizophrenia, are discussed in Chapter 21, this volume.

Each of us is innately equipped to react to sudden changes. The startle response is potent and irresistible. Less obviously, minor physiological changes occur in response to any sudden change in the perceptual field; the heart rate, pupillary diameter, respiratory rate and sweating, all alter. This so-called orienting response is dependent on the integrity of the limbic system, which also controls attentional mechanisms and emotional responses. The orienting response is disordered in schizophrenia (Gruzelier et al., 1981), as is the ability to focus attention and to modulate between focused and extensive or scanning attention. Similar abnormalities can be induced in primates by damage to the limbic system, and an abnormal cellular arrangement has been described in the hippocampus of post-mortem schizophrenic brains (Falkai et al., 1988; see Roberts, 1991), with a thinner parahippocampal gyrus on the left (Young et al., 1991), findings with neurodevelopmental implications. A compact cellular arrangement would predispose to synchronous firing (McBain et al., 1990), as found in electroencephalographic coherence analysis from this region (Flor-Henry and Yeudall, 1979; Weller and Montagu, 1979).

There has been a failure to find a correlation between duration of illness and enlarged ventricular brain ratios in schizophrenia (see Weinberger et al., 1983; Young et al., 1991), suggesting that the observed brain changes may precede the onset of symptoms. The pre-morbid characteristics, including impaired educational attainment, are consistent with this view.

Evidence of the inheritance of intelligence as well as its modification by environmental factors can be found in both animals and man (Skodak and Skeels, 1949; Honzik, 1957) (see Chapter 19, this volume). Two strains of rats were selectively bred, one of which was made up of rats which were adept at maze running, while the other consisted of rats poor in this ability (Tyron, 1963). Testing the progeny of both groups many generations later, the same divergence in ability was noted (Rosenzweig, 1969).

Genetic factors have been demonstrated in disorders which lead to devastating subnormality and shortened life expectancy (see Chapter 13, this volume). Until now, treatment and management have been aimed at amelioration of the effects of these disorders. The exciting possibility of treating genetically transmitted disorders at source has acquired a new dimension in the work on enzyme replacement in lysosomal-storage diseases (Grabowski and Desnick, 1981), leucocyte adhesion deficiency (Wilson et al., 1990), and severe combined immunodeficiency (Ferrari et al., 1991).

A genetic component is apparent too in neuroses, although it is weaker than in manic-depressive psychosis and schizophrenia, and a predisposition to alcoholism has been found by some researchers (Goodwin, 1976). Predisposition is a useful term that describes a tendency, leaving open the opportunity for environmental modification. This notion has precedents in the work of Ivan Pavlov, with his concept of strong and weak nervous systems in relation to the difficulty or ease with which some dogs were seriously perturbed. These concepts continue to resonate in current thinking.

The frustration of expectation, as well as actual loss, can lead to mental illness. The ability to adapt to change is important for emotional poise and diminishes with age. Disappointment illustrates the relevance of attitudes and the difficulties caused by excessive aspirations. Uncertainty distresses animals as well as human beings. Pavlov made an ellipse progressively approximate to a circle, rewarding the recognition of the latter but not the former. As the discrimination became more difficult, his experimental dogs became disturbed. This experiment is sometimes misunderstood, and it is worth stressing that neither stimulus was paired with punishment.

Amongst the neurotic disorders, it is particularly difficult to empathize with those suffering from obsessional-compulsive neurosis. Of all the neurotic disorders the genetic component is greatest in this disorder and the favourable response to selective leucotomy suggests an organic basis. In regional blood-flow experiments with demented patients obsessional traits were associated with reduced temporal blood flow and a relatively preserved frontal blood flow (Gustafson and Hagberg, 1975b). Reduced frontal blood flow in schizophrenia (Ingvar and Franzen, 1974) is paralleled by reduced metabolic activity (Buchsbaum and Haier, 1987), and neuropsychological findings (Scarone *et al.*, 1982). The apathy and lack of volition which characterize the negative features of schizophrenia relate to these findings (Liddle, 1990).

Some aspects of personality seem to have a biological substrate (see Chapter 22, this volume) and character seems to be set very early in life, if not *in utero*, and certain behavioural dimensions measured by separate, independent raters have been shown to persist from shortly after birth to school age (Rutter *et al.*, 1964). The susceptibility of most mental illnesses has a genetic component, which implies biological correlates. Recent animal work has shown modification of an important behavioural index of depression by a novel means. Neural implants from serotonin-containing pineal tissue and catecholamine-containing adrenal medullary tissue were successfully implanted into the frontal cortex of adult rats. These implanted animals were resistant to the development of learned helplessness under stressful conditions, while implants of muscle tissue had no discernible effect on a control population (Sagen *et al.*, 1990).

Cognition and Psychopathology

It is generally acknowledged that several different factors play a part in the aetiology of most forms of psychopathology. So far as depression and the anxiety disorders are concerned, there is increasing evidence that the cognitive system is involved in their genesis and maintenance. An important reason why it is only comparatively recently that cognitive factors have been studied systematically is because cognitive psychology itself only became firmly established during the 1960s. Many of the paradigms and theoretical ideas used in recent studies of psychopathology are based on work carried out by cognitive psychologists during the 1980s (see Chapter 17, this volume).

Much of the initial impetus for a cognitive approach to anxiety and depression comes from the theoretical writings of Beck, who has consistently argued for the importance of schemas (sets of organized expectations). According to Beck and Clark (1988):

> The schematic organisation of the clinically depressed individual is dominated by an overwhelming negativity . . . . As a result of . . . negative maladaptive schemas, the

depressed person views himself as inadequate, deprived and worthless, the world as presenting insurmountable obstacles, and the future as utterly bleak and hopeless.   (p. 26)

With respect to the anxiety disorders:

The maladaptive schemas in the anxious patient involve perceived physical or psychological threat to one's personal domain as well as an exaggerated sense of vulnerability.   (p. 26)

While anxious and depressed patients differ from normal individuals in terms of cognitive structures such as schemas, they also differ from normals with respect to cognitive processes. As Brewin (Chapter 14, this volume) points out, there is an important theoretical distinction between conscious or controlled cognitive processes on the one hand and non-conscious or automatic processes on the other. It is probably the case that both kinds of cognitive processes need to be considered in order to achieve a full understanding of the role played by cognitive functioning in clinical anxiety and depression.

In terms of biological utility, the function of anxiety is presumably to facilitate the rapid detection of threatening stimuli. From this perspective, anxious patients can be regarded as having over-developed the ability to detect threat to a point where they are hypervigilant and treat even innocuous stimuli as threatening. Pre-attentive and attentional processes are involved in threat detection, and anxious patients differ from normals in the functioning of these processes in the presence of threat (Eysenck, 1991, see Chapter 14, this volume).

Thus, a cognitive approach to clinical anxiety and depression is proving of value, even though it obviously needs to be complemented by other approaches (e.g. genetic and life-events). It is no coincidence that cognitive therapy is being used increasingly for the treatment of anxiety and depression (Brewin, 1988). The expertise of cognitive psychologists in identifying abnormalities in cognitive processes and structures, combined with the clinical experience of cognitive therapists, may well prove extremely fruitful.

Cyclical and Physiological Changes

Internal bodily changes alter mood and cognitive functioning. These changes can result from disease or normal physiology. Around the fourth day after childbirth many women endure an episode of emotional lability, which George Stein has shown to be associated with weight changes. Changes in cognitive function also occur at this time (Yalom et al., 1968). Post-puerperal psychosis runs in families and tends to be repeated in the same individual, suggesting a particular pattern of disturbance to the endocrine changes. Dr A. Metz of Littlemore Hospital, Oxford (Metz, 1983) has shown that those women who suffer maternity blues initially have more platelet α2-adrenoreceptors, which remain elevated during the blue episode, when compared to women who escape this experience (see Chapter 30, this volume, for a discussion on the inhibitory α2-adrenoreceptors which regulate the release of noradrenaline in the CNS. The density and sensitivity is increased in depression and are decreased with a variety of antidepressants).

Endocrine disorders, particularly those affecting thyroid and adrenal functioning, frequently produce mental changes which include anxiety, depression, euphoria and psychosis. Marked endocrine changes occur throughout the 24-hour cycle of sleep and waking which are accompanied by subtle changes in performance. Perturbations of these diurnal variations are induced by flights that cross time zones, and may trigger affective illness in vulnerable persons (Jauhar and Weller, 1982).

Aquatic creatures follow a tidal lunar cycle, which dictates behaviour such as breeding. This is apparent even if they have been born in an aquarium. In the mature female, monthly alterations in endocrine levels cause discernible changes in emotional poise. In Western countries it is unusual for the menarche to occur in the months of March and October, being particularly unusual in March (Valsik, 1965). Seasonal sex hormone changes also occur in males (Reinberg *et al.*, 1978), which may relate to seasonal increases in suicide and depression, with a spring excess for both sexes and a secondary autumn peak for females (Meares *et al.*, 1981). The spring excess of affective illness occurs in many parts of the world (e.g. Jauhar and Weller, 1982). Spring is, of course, the time of competition for mates and breeding territory, and a persisting reduction in competitiveness following defeat reduces needless repetition of contests and confers an advantage on the species, if not on the defeated competitor (see Chapter 25, this volume).

Sex hormones subtly modulate sensitivity to neurotransmitters and may account, in part, for the increasing incidence of depression with age (see Chapter 30, this volume), as well as the seasonal pattern of affective illness.

Infections and Mental Illness

The relationship between season and affective illness can also be seen in schizophrenia. Winter birth has been related to this illness—the colder the winter the stronger the association—suggesting a possible infective aetiology. The effect is robust and apparent in both hemispheres (Hare, 1979; Templer and Veleber, 1982). It is much more apparent in patients without a family history of psychiatric disorder (O'Callaghan *et al.*, 1991).

The number of cases of acute psychoses increased during the influenza epidemic of 1918 (Menninger, 1928) and an association has been found between schizophrenia and the pandemic of influenza A2 in pregnant women during the second trimester in Helsinki and Denmark (Mednick *et al.*, 1988, 1990). There has been partial confirmation and partial refutation in data from Scotland, over the epidemic years of 1918, 1919 and 1957, with an increase noted in mothers infected during the child's sixth month of gestation. There is considerable methodological controversy between the two research groups (e.g. the diagnosis in the second study was based on the most recent admission, while the first was a diagnosis of schizophrenia on any occasion (Kendell and Kemp, 1989)).

There is an undoubted genetic component in schizophrenia (see Chapter 13, this volume), but the genetics are obscure, being neither dominant nor recessive. The possibility of an infection contracted *in utero* or perinatally has been linked to neurodevelopmental brain abnormalities in schizophrenia (see Roberts, 1991). Infection is not always easy to distinguish from familial linkage and a genetic mechanism may be assumed when an infective process is actually responsible. A particular strain of mice is prone to develop cancer of the mammary glands in maturity. Although this suggests a genetic propensity, it has been shown that the cancers do not develop if the mice are suckled by a foster mother from a different strain. They are then protected from what is now considered an infective agent known as Bittner's milk factor (Bittner, 1939). Similarly, Wood and Darling (1961) have reported human mammary carcinoma occurring over four generations. As with the mice in the third generation, the cancer occurred only in those women breast-fed by their mothers.

Many of the chronic schizophrenic patients in British psychiatric hospitals were the victims of a pandemic of encephalitis lethargica (Ravenholt and Foege, 1982), while antibody titres, particularly to herpes simplex, have suggested recurrent subclinical encephalitis in some fluctuating psychoses (Fields and Blattner, 1958; Shearer and Finch, 1964). The antigen to herpes simplex is concentrated in the temporal lobes and limbic structures, and is often asymmetrical between the two hemispheres (Esiri, 1982). These findings are compatible with the lateralized deficits seen in schizophrenia (see Gruzelier, 1979 for a review, and discussion in Chapter 13, this volume). Two studies with some overlap of researchers, firstly with a total of 60 schizophrenic patients and later with 178, have shown raised antibody to cytomegalovirus in the cerebrospinal fluid (Torrey et al., 1982).

The possibility of an infective agent being responsible for some cases of schizophrenia is based on circumstantial evidence and supposition. However, both Kuru and Creutzfeldt-Jacob dementia seem to be caused by a transmissible agent (see Roos and Johnson, 1977, for review).

Mental illness can be precipitated by stress in both the *milieu extérieur* and the *milieu intérieur*. Almost any debilitating physical illness predisposes to mental illness. Mononucleosis (Cadie et al., 1976) and occult cancer (Fras et al., 1967), for example, are associated with depression.

Toxins

The resilience of living organisms depends to some extent on their ability to detoxify potentially harmful substances. Pharmacologists devise compounds which bypass mechanisms that have evolved to render innocuous commonly encountered natural substances, and these compounds may lead to toxic psychoses (see Davison, 1981 for review). Chemicals that have not existed previously on earth are being produced for various purposes and are creating hazards not previously encountered by living organisms. The very precise conditions of the *milieu intérieur*, which are necessary for normal functionings, may be disturbed by some of these agents, particularly in vulnerable groups. For example, hyperactive children have been shown to become more disturbed when exposed to dyes commonly used in manufactured foods (Weiss et al., 1980).

A substance in American street drugs, MPTP (1-methyl-4-phenyl-1,2,3,6-tetrahydropyridine), produced severe irreversible Parkinson's disease. Chemists working with the compound, which seems to be toxic to nigrostriatal neurones, were also affected (Ballard *et al.*, 1985). These observations suggest the possibility of a natural toxin that may be responsible for some idiopathic cases, while the monoamine oxidase inhibitor, deprenyl, seems to retard the progression of Parkinson's disease (Tetrud and Langston, 1989, 1990). A neurotoxin that targets a specific dopaminergic pathway opens the possibility of other system-specific toxins, and the action of deprenyl encourages hope for wider prophylactic benefit from this and other agents. For example, prophylaxis seems possible after denervation, the usual atrophy and neuronal death being inhibited *in vitro* and *in vivo* by the calcium ion blocking agent flunarizine (Rich and Hollowell, 1990), and some success in retarding the progress of Alzheimer's type dementia has been claimed for the calcium ion blocking drug nimodipine (Tollefson, 1990).

Naturally-occurring substances can also be neurotoxic. One hypothesis for the unique dementia on the island of Guam, called Guam ALS Parkinson's dementia, for its resemblance to amyotrophic lateral sclerosis (ALS) and Parkinson's disease, is a neuronal excitatory substance present in a seed, β-methylamino-alanine (BMAA). In 1987 Canadians suffered hippocampal damage and permanent memory impairment reminiscent of Alzheimer's disease after eating mussels that were later found to have a high concentration of a glutamate analogue, domoic acid. Glutamate acts as a potent excitatory neurotransmitter which can induce cell death, and glutamates are widely used as flavour enhancers in foodstuffs, including baby foods.

Aluminium has been associated with dementia that sometimes occurs during renal dialysis and has also been found in excessive concentrations in the plaques of some patients dying with Alzheimer's dementia (Duckett, 1976), and the Parkinsonism dementia of Guam (Perl *et al.*, 1982). One is concerned at the common use of aluminium for cooking utensils and the ingestion of large amounts of aluminium salts for dyspeptic conditions.

The amount of lead in children's teeth correlates negatively with classroom behaviour and scholastic achievement (Needleman *et al.*, 1979). Manganese intoxication has resulted in psychoses in Chilean miners (Cotzias, 1958). Arsenic, copper, mercury and thallium intoxication are not unusual. Less commonly, antimony, barium, bismuth, boron, gallium, gold, magnesium, molybdenum, rubidium, nickel, selenium, tellurium, tin, vanadium, zinc and, of course, lithium, have shown animal and/or human neurotoxicity. Interactions between metals cause lower amounts to be toxic in conditions of dietary imbalance (Perl *et al.*, 1982). This extensive list raises concern that repeated injections may inadvertently introduce cumulative amounts of noxious substances. Injections, commonly used in the maintenance treatment of schizophrenia, circumvent gastrointestinal mucosal processes, which are known to regulate absorption of some metals.

Plasticity and Cellular Memory

Calcium-dependent neurophysiological changes have been described with implications for arousal mechanisms, learning and memory. Calcium is both a carrier of positive charge, contributing to cell excitability, and a second messenger within the cell for various cellular responses. There are at least three types of voltage-dependent calcium channels; an L-type that inactivates slowly, an N-type, activated by strong depolarization, and a T-type activated by weak depolarization. These channels contribute to synaptic plasticity (see Edmonds et al., 1990).

The extrusion of neurotransmitter from the pre-synaptic bottom is modulated by Ca^{2+}, which in turn causes an increase in efflux of K^+ and two neurotrans-mitters, the excitatory amino acid glutamate and noradrenaline (Nichols et al., 1990). Ca^{2+} seems to have a role in mobilizing synaptic vesicles for exocytosis, and gradually accumulates in cells, providing a basis for facilitation and represent-ing a potential repository of memory and learning. This process is one of the possible mechanisms for the 'kindling' of epilepsy, particularly in the hippocampal area, where the small extracellular volume and tortuous diffusion pathways set constraints on the diffusion of ions in the mammalian brain (McBain et al., 1990; see Chapter 10, this volume). The repeated stimulation from damaged cells will lead to an increased excitability in intact cells exposed to the stimulation, including interconnected homotopic areas of the contralateral cortex. The toxic effect of glutamate, discussed previously, may be responsible for destructive changes, and the association between temporal lobe epilepsy and the emergence of psychosis some 14 years later, first described by Slater et al. (1963).

There is a reciprocal interaction between a subtype of the glutamate receptor, N-methyl-aspartate (NMDA), which may be particularly sensitive to excitation during development. It has been hypothesized that this interaction and the neurodestructive effects of excessive glutamate activity could be a model for schizophrenia and tardive dyskinesia (Olney, 1990).

Noradrenaline blocks the Ca^{2+}-activated K^+ conductance subsequent to the entry of Ca^{2+} into the neurone, thereby greatly increasing the number of spike discharges elicited by a depolarizing stimulus (Madison and Nicoll, 1982). Even when noradrenaline hyperpolarizes the cell membrane and depresses the response to threshold current pulses, the adaptation to stimulation is still reduced. Noradrenaline thus produces the combined effect of suppressing weak inputs and enhancing strong ones. In information theory terms this would be described as increasing the signal-to-noise ratio in the central nervous system during arousal. There are obvious implications for our concepts of vigilance and attention (see Chapter 15, this volume).

Experiments on vertebrates have shown that long-term memory can be disrupted by inhibiting protein synthesis (Barondes, 1975) and sensitivity to disruption is maximal within an hour of training. This observation, inter alia, has led Goelet et al. (1986) to suggest a model whereby short-term memory is achieved by modifications to existing cellular proteins, whereas long-term memory is subserved by proteins under the control of genes in the cell, which are influenced by the same factor, or factors, that are involved in short-term memory.

This model is consistent with the phenomena of imprinting, first described in birds, in which the bird is peculiarly sensitive to visual stimuli at a critical age (see

Chapter 25, this volume). Whatever stimulus is presented at this time exerts a persistent, irresistible attraction. Fortunately it is the mother that is usually imprinted in this manner. Following stimulation, radioactively labelled amino acids (the building blocks of protein) are incorporated into specific brain regions, and if this incorporation is chemically prevented, the phenomenon does not occur and the imprinting does not take place (Horn, 1979).

Psychosomatic Illness

The term psychosomatic implies that the psyche (including mental set and attitude) influences bodily processes. The corollary, that bodily dysfunction is associated with mental symptoms, is well known in endocrine and other illnesses (e.g. Cadie *et al.*, 1976; Fras *et al.*, 1967). Despite an unfortunate dualism implicit in the term psychosomatic, the outcome of many chronic diseases is probably influenced by early experience, coping strategies and psychological defences, cognitive style and the perception of threat, the social context in which threat occurs, and the presence or absence of an opportunity to react. This is sufficiently widely believed for extreme claims sometimes to be made by practitioners of 'alternative' medicine, for successful intervention by modifying some of these factors, particularly for incurable conditions.

In the face of threat the flight-or-fight response involves physiological changes. If these responses are prolonged they are likely to exert a toll (Selye, 1950). Observations on patients with gastric fistulae—the celebrated cases of Alexis St Martin (Beaumont, 1833) and Tom (Wolf and Wolff, 1947)—demonstrated prolonged engorgement of the gastric blood supply following even transient anger, and reduced gastric secretion, motility and vascularity accompanying sadness or fear. The vascular changes in the gastric mucosa are paralleled by readily observable changes in the perfusion of the skin, changes which signal our emotional state to others, and emphasize a connection between psychological states and dermatological conditions, such as rosacea and atopic eczema.

The detrimental effect of stress on the sexual attractiveness, fecundity and life expectancy of animals are factors that limit breeding and survival, balancing population size to resources. For example, mortality is increased some seven to nine times in grouse that fail to obtain breeding territory (Jenkins *et al.*, 1963). The strong effect is probably mediated through immunological systems, since it is disease, rather than predation or starvation, which is largely responsible for the sharply increased mortality. We may suffer some stress-related diseases as the inheritors of such population control mechanisms.

Lymphocyte responsiveness is reduced in rats in direct relationship to graded stressors (Keller *et al.*, 1981), and is decreased in humans after distressing experiences (Irwin *et al.*, 1990), such as bereavement (Bartrop *et al.*, 1977), when non-suicidal mortality is increased (Parkes *et al.*, 1969). Depressed subjects had significantly poorer damage repair to DNA in lymphocytes exposed to X-ray radiation than other, non-medicated, psychiatric patients with lower levels of depression on the MMPI scale (Kiecolt-Glaser and Glaser, 1987).

In accord with these observations, the proliferative potential of lymphocytes (blastogenesis) to a mitogen was reduced in 15 bereaved men (Kiecolt-Glaser and Glaser, 1986), and major depressive disorder and threatening life-events are independently associated with a 50% reduction of natural killer cell cytotoxicity, independent of age, alcohol consumption or tobacco smoking (Irwin et al., 1990). However, the relationship is clouded by methodological pitfalls and the need to control for diagnosis, illness severity, medication status, assay technique, and appropriate matching of controls for age, sex and ethnic background (see Stein et al., 1991). Nevertheless, despite some negative findings, in one of the most rigorously controlled trials (Schleifer et al., 1989), severity of depression, measured by the Hamilton Depression Rating Scale, was significantly associated with suppression of mitogen proliferative responses, independently of age, and there was a significant age-related difference between depressed patients and controls in the mitogen responses and the number of T4 lymphocytes.

The lymphocytopenia associated with stress has been attributed to increased levels of corticosteroids (Ahmed et al., 1974), which are often raised in depression. This is probably only one of the mediating mechanisms since there are more generalized disturbances of the hypothalamic—hypophyseal axis in depression, apparent in disturbances of growth hormone, luteinizing hormone and thyroid stimulating hormone, all of which modify immune function (Holsboer, 1987), as do neuropeptides (Maclean and Reichlin, 1981), which too are disturbed under stressful conditions (Risch, 1982; Janowsky et al., 1983).

Not surprisingly, with so many putative mechanisms of mediation, mortality is increased in depression from numerous causes, as well as accidental injury and suicide (see Stein et al., 1991). Galen in 'De Tumoribus' claimed to have observed that melancholic women are more prone to carcinoma than are sanguine women. Since then many researchers, including Carl Rokitansky, have made similar assertions (e.g. Schmale, 1958, Bahnson and Bahnson, 1966).

Two specific examples out of many will suffice to emphasize this point.

(1) As predicted in advance, a two-fold increase in the odds of death from cancer was associated with depression in 2020 middle-aged employed men ($P < 0.001$) during 17 years of follow-up (Shekelle et al., 1981).
(2) In a series of 16 men and 32 women with leukaemia or lymphoma, the symptoms developed in the wake of experiences interpreted as personal losses in all but two of the cases, both of whom were women (Greene, 1966).

Despite such strong findings, similar studies have not always found a positive association (see Stein et al., 1991). Malaise and discomfort might have been endured more readily before the loss, but became the source of medical complaints during a period of distress. Similar arguments may apply to early, often cited studies. Hinckle and Wolff (1958) demonstrated an apparent clustering of diseases in a susceptible group, work which was extended by Holmes and Rahe (1967) who developed a schedule of recent experiences and demonstrated a relationship between these and illness. However, the relationship may be spurious, a stressful accumulation of events may prompt help seeking, rather than being initiated by the illness itself, a supposition with experimental backing (Mechanic, 1975).

A further source of variability in the links between life-events and illness is the difference in coping strategies, which seem both to predispose to certain diseases and to influence prognosis. Ineffective psychological defences lead to higher cortisol excretion during psychosocial stress (Vickers, 1988). In contrast to the assumptions of psychoanalysis, denial of illness was one of the successful strategies in favouring recurrence-free survival from treated breast cancer (Greer et al., 1979) perhaps by limiting anxiety, since high anxiety has been related to a poor prognosis in established diseases (Derogatis et al., 1976). As would be expected, it is early-stage, non-metastatic cancers which seem to be most suscept-ible to psychological set (Greer, 1991) and Greer proposes that the term denial could be restated advantageously as 'positive avoidance'.

Habitual styles of behaviour too play a part. Thomas and Greenstreet (1973) showed that emotional expression was excessively restricted in the nine doctors who developed cancer from a cohort of 1130 white male medical students interviewed prospectively and followed-up annually. This tumour group also had consistently low scores on a family attitude questionnaire for demonstrating their feelings, matriarchal dominance and closeness. We do not know if the similarity in behaviour of the patients and the family members indicates a learnt or inherited model of behaviour patterns. Thomas's results are in accord with a longitudinal Swedish study which showed that personality changes precede the onset of cancer (Hagnell, 1966), and with Bahnson and Bahnson's (1966) findings that cancer patients tend to deny and repress conflictual impulses and emotions to a higher degree than do other people. Similarly, and in contrast to Mechanic's arguments regarding the propensity to seek help, Henderson (1966) calls atten-tion to the blatant denial in 50 cancer patients associated with delay in seeking help.

In addition to associations with cancer, Thomas and Greenstreet (1973) also found distinctive psychological attributes preceding hypertension and coronary artery occlusion, as well as suicide and mental illness, with well-marked inter-group differentiation. Lloyd and Cawley (1978) similarly have shown that psychopathology predates myocardial infarction in a substantial group of patients and hostility and inner directed anger were related to the extent and severity of coronary artery disease in another study (Nunes et al., 1987).

The question naturally arises as to whether personality is in some way linked to psychosomatic disorders, either causally or through common genetic factors, or whether particular personality attributes lead to certain behaviours, such as smoking, which themselves cause the disorder. The answer is probably both. Kissen (1966), for example, has shown that the poorer the outlet for ventilating emotions, the less the exposure to cigarette smoke required to induce lung cancer.

Psychosomatic disorders are related to the degree of control that can be exercised over the environment. In experiments with yoked monkeys, the executive monkey, which could prevent shocks by taking suitable evasive action, developed stomach ulcers while the other monkey did not (Brady et al., 1958). In different experiments, the executive monkey developed hypertension (Herd et al., 1969). In the first experiment the executive monkey was selected on the basis of initially quicker responses, thus introducing a bias that might have favoured the more physiologically reactive monkey. The intervals between stress and the adequacy of feedback are probably important. In these experiments evasive action had to be taken frequently. In similar experiments with yoked rats, the warning occurred at well-spaced intervals, allowing feedback on the adequacy of evasive responses. Under these conditions, the yoked rat, rather than the executive rat, developed ulcers (Weiss, 1972).

In yoked human experiments, subjects who could control the duration of exposure to distressing photographs showed less autonomic disturbance, as measured by galvanic skin resistance, than their helplessly yoked companions (Geer and Maisel, 1972). Similarly, cognitive performance was more disrupted by uncontrollable loud sounds than by equally loud controllable ones. In this experiment the controlling groups did not in fact exercise their option to terminate the annoying sound, but performed better nevertheless (Glass and Singer, 1972), indicating that the belief in having control is itself pacificatory, a fact well known to politicians!

Control over the environment has recently been related to low basal cortisol levels among wild, dominant baboons, as, too, are outlets for ventilating their aggression on subordinate members of the troup, high levels of social skill, predictability, and social affiliations. The baboons with low basal cortisol levels are perceptive and adopt successful styles of dominance behaviour (Sapolsky, 1990) picking fights that they generally win, thus maintaining their dominant positions over long periods.

These findings accord with human experience. In now classic experiments, the awful stress of helplessly watching their children die of cancer led to increased cortisol metabolites in the parents' urine (Friedman et al., 1963; Wolff et al., 1964). Coping style influenced the outcome, with lower cortisol metabolite levels amongst those who applied religious rationalizations, denied the facts of the illness, and who lost themselves in the details of the management. In a less harrowing experiment, salivary cortisol was raised in a group with little control over a demanding cognitive task administered over a four hour period. In accord with the observations on the parents of moribund children, the rise was attenuated in those subjects who adopted a cognitive strategy of reframing the experimental situation in a positive and self-encouraging way (Bohnen et al., 1991).

Professional and managerial workers, who it is presumed have a degree of control over their work schedules, have substantially lower mortality from ischaemic heart disease than those they manage, even when allowance is made for known risk factors (Lancet editorial, 1981; see also Strole et al., 1962; Segal, 1966).

Loss or abrogation of control over the environment can be seen with other bodily systems, particularly if there is psychological and organ susceptibility. Inevitably some newly inducted American army recruits exposed to the highly controlled military environment develop duodenal ulcers. These occurred in recruits with 'evidence of major unresolved and persistent conflicts', who were also hypersecretors of pepsinogen. An interaction between high serum pepsinogen and coping ability was also found (Weiner *et al.*, 1957). This is reinforced by the observation that just as with Thomas and Greenstreet's (1973) and Bahnson and Bahnson's (1966) cancer sufferers, and in the hypersecretors of cortisol amongst some wild dominant baboons, and all subordinate baboons (Sapolsky, 1990), failure to express anger and hostility were evident in the ulcer prone group: 'they went out of their way to rationalize, deny and displace such feeling. The need to please and placate authority figures as potential sources of affection was particularly striking.'

Excessive emotional control might form a constellation with fatalism, helplessness and psychological morbidity. Such a clustering was found, which adversely affected the outcome of breast cancer (see Watson *et al.*, 1991). Similarly, self-reported childhood unhappiness, suppression of behaviour that might cause offence and avoidance of conflict were positively associated with colorectal cancer in 637 cases, independently of dietary risk factors, family history of colorectal cancer, socioeconomic and marital status, religion and country of birth (Kune *et al.*, 1991).

Methods that have been claimed to reduce the physiological changes induced by stress include relaxation, meditation, autogenic training and biofeedback (Budzynski *et al.*, 1970; Brener and Kleinman, 1970; Knapp, 1967; Sterman, 1982). All of these techniques share the common property of emphasizing that the 'locus of control' lies with the sufferer, which may help to counter the undesirable effects of a perception of excessive external control.

Attitude, personality and control, real or imagined, seem to affect the incidence of certain illnesses and the outcome of others. Social relationships too are undoubtedly important, affecting such things as survival on home dialysis (Wai *et al.*, 1981). Disasters seem to reinforce altruism and shared deprivations seem to make them easier to bear. The increased social cohesion at times of war is thought to be the reason for the reduction in suicide at such testing times.

Social Interactions

The bonding forces of the flock and herd (Lorenz, 1963) are evident in man (see Chapter 25, this volume). Poor integration of the individual in society and anomic social cohesion are conducive to illness (e.g. Fernando, 1975; Fenig and Levav, 1991), affect treatment and merit a consideration of social factors. Social factors can alter our perceptions and moods. Our behaviour to others and theirs to us is modified by a host of subtle indications given unconsciously in a number of non-verbal ways (see Chapters 25 and 26, this volume), including autonomic changes. Our position in society is partially dependent on this signalling system, which may act to limit intraspecies aggression by indicating dominance and submission.

As stressed by Farr (1987), Mead's (1938) contribution was to set language and human communication in an evolutionary context, to regard language as an inherently social phenomenon and to interpolate the notion of 'self' between those of 'mind' and 'society'.

Emotions and reactions conjured by the shared meanings of the 'significant symbols' of language extend the range, subtlety and complexity of the emotions elicited by the 'releaser stimuli' (see Chapter 25, this volume) of expressive gesture and the tone of animal communications, which are inextricably interwoven with the need for agonistic and placatory signals.

In childhood the development of the concept of other selves is imperfect and fragile. Feral children, who develop apart from human kind, are intellectually retarded with a distorted identity (Itard, 1801) and 'never recapture(d) that pristine surge of growth which is the charm and the distinction of infancy.' (Gesel, 1942, p. 88). The problems were illustrated in the film of Kaspar Hauser, who had been woefully neglected and kept in isolation as a child. A similar case, but of a young girl, was described by Curtiss (1977), in whom the normal lateralization of language to the left cerebral hemisphere did not seem to take place, judged on the basis of a variety of dichotic, tachistoscopic and psychometric tests. This anomalous lateralization was also described in another female case investigated at Oxford University.

The hunger of the infant for interaction and play are prerequisites for learning and the acquisition of skills, but also for the concept of self. The first use of the words 'I' and 'me' start to appear in the vocabulary of blind children when they begin to play with dolls (Fraiberg and Adelson, 1973) and they are more intellectually handicapped than deaf children (Furth, 1966), (it is important to exclude blindness and deafness consequential on brain damage from such a comparison). Socially inculcated or amplified characteristics, such as achievement drive, coupled with fear of failure, can powerfully influence adult behaviour (McClelland et al., 1953) and increase the likelihood of neuroses (Price, 1969). Cultural factors, too, affect stress and pain tolerance (Sanua, 1960; Lambert et al., 1960) and sex role stereotypes (Buss, 1981; Stevenson-Hinde and Hinde, 1986), manifest in such areas as cognitive style and attitudes.

In his analysis of significant life-events, George Brown detected a tendency for adverse events to cluster in time (see Chapter 27, this volume). Verbal and non-verbal signals of distress and defeat (see Chapters 25 and 26, this volume) can be counter-productive, evoking a spurning, unhelpful response as a corollary to 'nothing succeeds like success'. The erect bearing, steady, level gaze, relaxed manner and mild, even tones of the unthreatened are difficult to sustain by the humbled and the dejected (cf. painted relief from the Temple of Ptah at Memphis, XIXth Dynasty, Fig. 25.1, this volume).

The effects of social pressure are open to experimental investigation and the results are sometimes surprising. A stationary spot of light, lacking a frame of reference in a dark room, appears to move. The experience is influenced by social factors and typically a group of observers reaches a concordant view on the changes of direction of this illusory motion (Sherif and Sherif, 1956). Using stooges to give deliberately false opinions, Solomon Asch (1956) was able to induce many subjects to declare that a line of obviously different length was the same length as a standard line. Those who yielded quickly to the social pressure tended to continue yielding. Other experiments have demonstrated that views declared in public, even if they were not held initially, are thereafter defended with conviction. The experiment consisted of requiring subjects to give political speeches from outlined scripts contrary to their political views. The audience was little moved but the speaker was much influenced by the experience.

Perceptions are shaped by over-optimism. People in a long queue perceive their position in the queue accurately up to the point where the available number of places has been announced. If they occupy a position beyond this point, they underestimate the number of people in front of them (Mann and Taylor, 1969). Assessments of qualities are affected in a similar manner, so that once commitments are made there is a tendency to overestimate the virtues of one's choice and underestimate the faults. Festinger (1951) described this tendency as arising from a desire to reduce what he termed 'cognitive inconsistency or dissonance'. Festinger has proposed that people will shape their concepts to try and make things that are not psychologically consistent seem more consistent. The term 'cognitive' emphasizes that the theory deals with relations among items of information which may be about feelings, opinions, things in the environment and so on.

The effects of reducing cognitive dissonance applies to spouses as well as motor cars, which have been selected from amongst many competing alternatives. Loyalty to one's family, clan and nation is dependent on a corresponding negative attitude to non-members. Konrad Lorenz (1963) has argued that the cohesive forces of the pack, flock and herd take their origin from aggressive behaviour patterns that are turned outwards. Likewise, courtship behaviour and pair bonding are modifications of aggressive behaviour (see Chapter 25, this volume).

Hierarchical systems are often ambiguous. In a triad, an individual may be doubly dominant (A), doubly subordinate (C) or intermediate (B).

Model 1

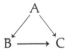

or the relationship may be indecisive

Model 2

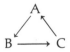

The same ambiguous positioning can, of course, be expanded into larger groupings. An individual in the second model has no clear linear relationship to other members of the group. A person's status and identity are generated by the groups of which he is a member. In a complex society, where people fulfil diverse roles, the second model often operates and unexpectedly steep and discontinuous shifts in status may occur following some reversal or decline in fortune.

Social support in many forms militates against becoming ill (Segal and Phillips, 1967). Integration into the cultural matrix and the possession of a confidante protects against the despondency produced by adversity (see Chapter 27, this volume). Reassurance is the next best thing to actual safety and security, if the reassurance is credible. This is particularly true if the threat is imaginary and may at the very least convert uncertainty, which is often even more unsettling than bad news, into an acceptable, even if unpalatable, reality. The ability to accept reassurance depends on trust. This in turn hinges on the experience of 'good enough' parenting by the threatened person and probably the status and authority of the person providing the assurance. This formulation explains why doctors sometimes have greater success in providing reassurance than do their paramedical colleagues. Paradoxically, the untrusting may be constantly seeking reassurance because their need for reassurance cannot be satisfied.

Provided the family environment is satisfactory, the well-known Isle of Wight study demonstrated that brain damage in children was not accompanied by behavioural disturbance. If the home environment was unsatisfactory, a child with some degree of damage was less robust in dealing with life's difficulties (Rutter *et al.*, 1970). These social findings may not only accord with our expectations, but also sharpen our appreciation of social therapy. Many patients improve on entering hospital, but the precise determining factors remain to be clarified.

Overriding Factors

Science is self-purifying. What cannot be confirmed is quickly forgotten, while replicable research results allow us to distinguish between fact and opinion, and creates a foundation for sound clinical practice. An experiment is sometimes described as a 'question put to nature'. A successful scientific experiment results in a clear answer. According to G.W. Allpert, the aims of science are 'understanding, prediction and control above levels achieved by unaided commonsense'. Scientific knowledge is public knowledge, unaffected by fashion and potentially replicable by all with sufficient training.

Models of the world, or paradigms, as they have been called, can be maintained only as long as our observations about the world fit the models. There are always some discrepant findings and in the end one paradigm gives way to another. These epoch-making paradigm-shifts (Kuhn, 1961) are presaged by difficulties which can be either ignored or examined minutely. It is easier to ignore the difficulties, but it is also fruitful to focus on them. Charles Darwin remarked that if he came across an opinion with which he disagreed, he made a special point of noting it down, as otherwise he felt sure that he would forget it.

The priorities of health-care professionals arise out of the prevailing social attitudes. Mental health has never been a fashionable field. The priorities of physical, technological and cultural well-being are often in rivalry: the evidence favours a causal link between such social factors as unemployment and ill health, including mortality (Brenner, 1981).

Psychiatric beds are available on a capitation basis, although the social deprivation of particular areas generates additional burdens on psychiatric services (Hirsch, 1988). Many psychiatrically unwell gravitate to London (Royal College of General Practitioners, 1981), which has been particularly deprived of funding, initially under the Resource Allocation Working Party (RAWP) formula, now, despite a national scarcity of nurses, because of 'overmanning' in hospital trusts! Psychiatric hospitals are closing in England and Wales but there has not been an increase in 'community' provisions to correspond to the persistent reduction in beds. Facilities such as day centres and supervised hostel accommodation are provided at the discretion of the Local Authorities. These resources, like the health services themselves, are unevenly distributed so that none of the 35 London boroughs are providing day care to the minimal guidelines of the Government White Paper. Local Authorities are obliged to provide accommodation for the vulnerable homeless but this obligation is easily circumvented (Brahams and Weller, 1986). Reprovision hostels are selective and publish criteria which reject typical chronic psychotic patients.

The gravitation of the seriously mentally unwell to the anomic, decaying city areas, documented in a classic study in Chicago (Faris and Dunham, 1939) is evident today in Britain (Inter-Register Technical Committee, 1982). Despite earnest attempts to guard against such a situation, the Westminster Association of Mental Health recently reported that 28% of long-stay psychiatric patients discharged into this central London Borough were homeless on follow-up.

In several surveys, almost half those sleeping on the streets in London were or had been hallucinated or deluded, figures which do not include alcoholic or drug-induced states. Physical illness is common and many fail to apply for their benefit entitlements (Weller, 1989).

Kraepelin emphasized that the early features of schizophrenia often 'made the patient a habitual criminal and vagrant'. Many of the destitute recently interviewed in London had been to prison, mostly for a string of minor offences, but sometimes for murder and attempted murder. The frequency of current or previous psychosis was significantly increased in this group (Weller, 1989). In support of these observations recent reports describe a history of *previous* psychiatric disturbance in 20% of prisoners in the United Kingdom, which earlier surveys suggest is probably an underestimate amongst recidivists (West, 1977).

These problems are international. The conditions inside prison are likely to aggravate existing problems and highlight serious new ones. Warner (1985) points out that around 6–8% of prisoners in local jails in the United States are psychotic, but that they account for only 2–5% of jail admissions (Swank and Winer, 1976; Petrich, 1976; Lamb and Grant, 1982). Homelessness and unemployment create an understandable reluctance to grant bail in the United States (Lamb and Grant, 1982; Swank and Winer, 1976; Service *et al.*, 1981; Petrich, 1976), so that three-quarters of a random sample in Bryce Hospital in Alabama had been confined to prison while waiting for psychiatric hospital admission, with similar problems here in the United Kingdom (Research and Planning Paper 46, Home Office, 1988).

Despite undoubted advances in our understanding of psychiatric illness, there are obvious defects in our system of care. In devising more flexible and comprehensive systems of treatment and management to deal with the many different levels of incapacity and illness, adequate resources must be allocated for the needs of the most seriously ill.

References

Ahmed, A., Herman, C.M., Knudsen, R.C., Sode, J., Strong, D.M. and Sell, K.W. (1974). Effect of exogenous and endogenous glucocorticosteroids on the *in vitro* stimulation of lymphocytes from sedated and awake restrained healthy baboons. *J. Surg. Res.* **161**, 172–182.

Arnold, A.P. and Saltiel, A. (1979). Sexual difference in pattern of hormone accumulation in the brain of a songbird. *Science (NY)* **205**, 702–705.

Asch, S.E. (1956). Studies of independence and submission to group pressure: 1. A minority of one against a unanimous majority. *Psychol. Monogr.* **70** (no. 416).

Atkins, P.T., Surmeier, D.J. and Kitai, S.T. (1990). Muscarinic modulation of a transient H^+ conductance in rat neostriatal neurons. *Nature* **344**, 240–242.

Bahnson, C.B. and Bahnson, M.B. (1966). Role of the ego defenses: denial and repression in the etiology of malignant neoplasm. *Ann. NY Acad. Sci.* **125**, 827–845.

Ballard, P.A., Tetrud, J.W. and Langston, J.W. (1985). Permanent human Parkinsonism due to 1-4-methyl-4-phenyl-1,2,3,6-tetrahydropyridine (MOTP): 7 cases. *Neurology* **35**, 949–956.

Barondes, S.H. (1975). In: D. Deutch and J.A. Deutch (eds) *Short Term Memory*, pp. 379–390. New York: Academic Press.

Bartrop, R.W., Luckhurst, E., Lazarus, L., Kiloh, L.G. and Penny, R. (1977). Depressed lymphatic function after bereavement. *Lancet* **ii**, 834–836.

Bauer, L., Keller, H.B. and Reiss, E.L. (1975). Multiple eigenvalues lead to secondary bifurcation. *Siam Rev.* **17**, 101–122.

Beaumont, W. (1833). In: A. Combe (ed.) *Experiments and Observations on the Gastric Juice and the Physiology of Digestion*. Edinburgh: Maclachlan and Stewart.

Beck, A.T. and Clark, D.A. (1988). Anxiety and depression: an information processing perspective. *Anxiety Res.* **1**, 23–36.

Bergman, K. (1971). The neuroses of old age. In: D.W.K. Kay and A. Walk (eds) *Recent Developments in Psychogeriatrics* (*Br. J. Psychiat.* Special Publication No. 6), pp. 39–50. London: Gaskell.

Bittner, J.J. (1939). Relation of nursing to extra-chromosomal theory of breast cancer in mice. *Am. J. Cancer* **35**, 90–97.

Blessed, G., Tomlinson, B.E. and Roth, M. (1968). The association between quantitative measures of dementia and of degenerative changes in the cerebral grey matter of elderly subjects. *Br. J. Psychiat.* **114**, 797–811.

Bohnen, N., Nicolson, N., Sulon, J. and Jolles, J. (1991). Coping style, trait anxiety and cortisol reactivity during mental stress. *J. Psychosomat. Res.* **35**, 141–147.

Brady, J.V., Porter, R.W., Conrad, D.G. and Mason, J.W. (1958). Avoidance behaviour and the development of gastroduodenal ulcers. *J. Exp. Analysis Behav.* **1**, 69–73.

Brahams, D. and Weller, M.P.I. (1986). Crime and homelessness among the mentally ill. *Medico-legal J.* **54**, 42–53.

Brener, J. and Kleinman, R. (1970). Learned control of decreases in systolic blood pressure. *Nature (Lond.)* **226**, 1063–1064.

Brenner, M.H. (1981). Unemployment and health (letter). *Lancet* **ii**, 874–875.

Brenowitz, E.A. (1991). Altered perception of species-specific song by female birds after lesions of a forebrain nucleus. *Science* **251**, 303–305.

Brewin, C.R. (1988). *Cognitive Foundations of Clinical Psychology*. London: Lawrence Erlbaum Associates Ltd.

Bridges, R.S. and Grimm, C.T. (1982). Reversal of morphine disruption of maternal behaviour by concurrent treatment with the opiate antagonist naloxone. *Science (NY)* **218**, 166–168.

Bridges, R.S. and Russell, D.W. (1981). Steroidal interactions in the regulation of maternal behaviour in virgin female rats: effects of testosterone, dihydrotestosterone, oestradiol, progesterone and the aromatase inhibitor 1,4,6-androstatriene-3,17-dione. *J. Endocr.* **90**, 31–40.

Brown, T.M. and McAfee, D.A. (1982). Long-term synaptic potentiation in the superior cervical ganglion. *Science (NY)* **215**, 1411–1413.

Buchsbaum, M.S. and Haier, R.J. (1987). Functional and anatomical imaging: Impact on schizophrenia research. *Schizophrenia Bull.* **13**, 115–132.

Budzynski, T.H., Stoyva, J.M. and Adler, C. (1970). Feedback induced muscle relaxation: application to tension headache. *J. Behav. Ther. Exp. Psychiat.* **1**, 205–211.

Buell, S.J. and Coleman, P.D. (1979). Dendritic growth in the aged human brain and failure of growth in senile dementia. *Science (NY)* **206**, 854–856.

Buss, D.M. (1981). Predicting parent–child interactions from children's activity level. *Dev. Psychol.* **17**, 59–65.

Cadie, M., Nye, R.J. and Storey, P. (1976). Anxiety and depression after infective mononucleosis. *Br. J. Psychiat.* **128**, 559–561.

Carmichael, L. (1926). The development of behaviour in vertebrates experimentally removed from the influence of external stimulation. *Psychol. Rev.* **34**, 34–47.

Chung, S.H. (1977). Synaptic memory in the hippocampus. *Nature (Lond.)* **266**, 677–678.

Clark, A. (1989). *Microrecognition: Philosophy, Cognitive Science and Parallel Distributed Processing*. Cambridge, MA: MIT Press.

Cleghorn, F.M., Garnett, E.S., Nahmias, C. *et al.* (1990). Increased frontal and reduced parietal glucose metabolism in acute untreated schizophrenia. *Psychiat. Res.* (in press).

Corbetta, M., Miezin, F.M., Dobeyer, S., Shulman, G.L. and Petersen, S.E. (1990). Attentional modulation of neural processing of shape, color, and velocity in humans. *Science* **248**, 1556–1558.

Cotzias, G.C. (1958). Manganese in health and disease. *Physiol. Rev.* **38**, 502–503.

Curtiss, S. (1977). *Genie: A psycholinguistic study of a modern day 'wild child'*. New York: Academic Press.

Davison, K. (1981). Diagnoses not to be missed: toxic psychosis. *Br. J. Hosp. Med.* **26**, 530–537.

de Lacoste, M.-C., Adesanya, T. and Woodward, D.J. (1990). Measurement of gender differences in the human brain and their relationship to brain weight. *Biol. Psychiat.* **28**, 931–942.

Derogatis, L.R., Abeloff, M.D. and McBeth, C.D. (1976). Cancer patients and their physicians in the perception of psychological symptoms. *Psychosomatics* **17**(4), 197–201.

Dixson, A.F. and George, L. (1982). Prolactin and parental behaviour in a male New World primate. *Nature (Lond.)* **299**, 551–553.

Duckett, S. (1976). Aluminium and Alzheimer's disease (letter). *Arch. Neurol.* **33**, 730–731.

Edmonds, B., Klein, M., Dale, N. and Kandel, E.R. (1990). Contributions of two types of calcium channels to synaptic transmission and plasticity. *Science* **250**, 1142–1147.

Ehrhardt, A.A. and Baker, S.W. (1974). Fetal androgens, human central nervous system differentiation, and behaviour sex differences. In: R.C. Friedman, R.M. Richart and R.L. Vande Wiele (eds) *Sex Differences in Behaviour.* New York: Wiley.

Ellis, A.W. and Young, A. (1988). *Human Cognitive Neuropsychology.* London: Lawrence Erlbaum Associates Ltd.

Esiri, M.M. (1982). Herpes simplex encephalitis: an immunohistological study of the distribution of viral antigen within the brain. *J. Neurol. Sci.* **54**, 209–226.

Eysenck, M.W. (1991). *Anxiety: The Cognitive Perspective.* London: Lawrence Erlbaum Associates Ltd (in press).

Falkai, P., Bogerts, B., Roberts, G.W. and Crow, T.J. (1988). Measurement of the alpha-cell-migration in the entorhinal region: a market for the developmental disturbances in schizophrenia? *Schizophrenia Res.* **1**, 157–158.

Faris, R.E.L. and Dunham, H.W. (1939). *Mental Disorders in Urban Areas.* Chicago: University of Chicago Press.

Farr, R. (1987). The science of mental life: A social perspective. Presidential address to the British Psychological Society, 6 April 1986. *Bull. Br. Psychol. Soc.* **40**, 1–17.

Fenig, S. and Levav, I. (1991) Demoralization and supports among holocaust survivors. *J. Nerv. Ment. Dis.* **179**, 167–172.

Fernando, S.J.M. (1975). A cross-cultural study of some familial and social factors in depressive illness. *Br. J. Psychiat.* **127**, 46–53.

Ferrari, G., Rossini, S., Giavazzi, R. *et al.* (1991). An *in vivo* model of somatic cell gene therapy for human severe combined immunodeficiency. *Science* **251**, 1363–1370.

Festinger, L. (1951). *A Theory of Cognitive Dissonance.* Stanford: University Press; London: Tavistock.

Fields, W.S. and Blattner, R.J. (1958). *Viral Encephalitis.* Symposium of the Fifth Annual meeting of the Houston Neurological Society, pp. 118–162. Springfield, Illinois: Thomas.

Flor-Henry, P. and Yeudall, L.T. (1979). Neuropsychological investigation of schizo-phrenia and manic-depressive psychosis. In: J. Gruzelier and P. Flor-Henry (eds) *Hemisphere Asymmetries of Function and Psychopathology,* pp. 341–362. Amsterdam, New York and London: Elsevier.

Fraiberg, S. and Adelson, E. (1973). Self-representation in language and play: observations on blind children. *Psychoanal. Q.* **42**, 539–562.

Fras, I., Litin, E.M. and Pearson, J.S. (1967). Comparison of psychiatric symptoms in carcinoma of the pancreas with those in some other intra-abdominal neoplasms. *Am. J. Psychiat.* **123**, 1553–1562.

Friedman, S., Mason, J. and Hamburg, D. (1963). Urinary 17-hydroxycorticosteroid levels in parents of children with neoplastic diseases: a study of chronic psychological stress. *Psychosomat. Med.* **25**, 364–378.

Furth, H.G. (1966). *Thinking Without Language: Psychological Implications of Deafness.* Free Press.

Gandelman, R., Von Saal, F.S. and Reinisch, J.M. (1977). Continuity to male fetuses affects morphology and behaviour of female mice. *Nature (Lond.)* **266**, 722–724.

Geer, J. and Maisel, E. (1972). Evaluating the effects on the prediction–control confound. *J. Personality Social Psychol.* **23**, 314–319.

Geschwind, N. (1965). Disconnexion syndromes in animals and man. *Brain* **88**, 237–294; 585–644.

Gesel, A. (1942) *Wolf Child and Human Child.* London: The Scientific Book Club.

Gesell, A. and Thompson, H. (1929). Learning and growth in identical infant twins: an experimental study on the method of co-twin control. *Genet. Psychol. Monogr.* **6**, 1–24.

Glass, D.C. and Singer, J.E. (1972). *Urban Stress: Experiments on Noise and Social Stressors.* New York: Academic Press.

Glees, P. and Cole, J. (1950). Recovery of skilled motor functions after small repeated lesions of motor cortex in macaque. *J. Neurophysiol.* **13**, 137–148.

Goelet, P., Castellucci, V.F., Schacher, S. and Kandel, E.R. (1986). The long and short of long-term memory—a molecular framework. *Nature* **322**, 419–422.

Goodwin, D. (1976). *Is Alcoholism Hereditary?* Oxford: University Press.

Gorski, R. and Harlan, R. (1977). Perinatal hormone exposure and the development of neuro-endocrine regulatory processes. *J. Toxicol. Envir. Health* **3**, 97–121.

Grabowski, G.A. and Desnick, R.J. (1981). Enzyme replacement in genetic diseases. In: J.S. Holcenberg and J. Roberts (eds) *Enzymes as Drug*, pp. 167–208. Chichester, Wiley.

Greene, W.A. (1966). The psychosocial setting of the development of leukemia and lymphoma. *Ann NY Acad. Sci.* **125**, 794–801.

Greer, S. (1991). Psychological response to cancer and survival. *Psychol. Med.* **12**, 43–50.

Greer, S., Morris, T. and Pettingale, K.W. (1979). Psychological response to breast cancer: effect on outcome. *Lancet* **ii**, 785–787.

Gruzelier, J. (1979). Synthesis and critical review of the evidence for hemisphere asymmetries of function in psychopathology. In: J. Gruzelier and P. Flor-Henry *Hemisphere Asymmetries of Function in Psychopathology*, pp. 647–672. Amsterdam: Elsevier/North-Holland Biomedical.

Gruzelier, J., Connolly, J., Eves, F., Hirsch, S., Zaki, S., Weller, M.P.I. and Yorkston, N. (1981). Effects of propranolol and phenothiazines on electrodermal orienting and habituation in schizophrenia. *Psychol. Med.* **11**, 93–108.

Gustafson, L. and Hagberg, B. (1975a). Emotional behaviour, personality changes and cognitive reduction in pre-senile dementia: related to regional cerebral blood flow. *Acta Psychiat. Scand. (Suppl.)* **257**, 37–71.

Gustafson, L. and Hagberg, B. (1975b). Dementia onset in the presenile period. A cross-sectional study. *Acta Psychiat. Scand. (Suppl.)*, 251.

Hagnell, O. (1966). The premorbid of persons who develop cancer in a total population investigated in 1947 and 1957. *Ann. NY Acad. Sci.* **125**, 846–85.

Hare, E.H. (1979). Schizophrenia as an infectious disease. *Br. J. Psychiat.* **135**, 468–470.

Head, H. (1926). *Aphasia and Kindred Disorders of Speech.* Cambridge: University Press.

Hebb, D.O. and Penfield, W. (1940). Human behaviour after extensive bilateral removals from the frontal lobes. *Arch. Neurol. Psychiat.* **44**, 421–438.

Held, R. and Hein, A. (1963). Movement-produced stimulation in the development of visually guided behaviour. *J. Comp. Physiol. Psychol.* **56**, 872–876.

Henderson, J.G. (1966). Denial and repression as factors in the delay of patients with cancer presenting themselves to the physician. *Ann. NY Acad. Sci.* **125**, 856–864.

Herd, J.A., Morse, W.H., Kelleher, R.T. and Jones, L.G. (1969). Arterial hypertension in the squirrel monkey during behavioural experiments. *Am. J. Physiol.* **217**, 24–29.

Hinckle, L.E. and Wolff, H.G. (1958). Ecological investigations of the relationship between illness, life experiences and the social environment. *Ann. Intern. Med.* **49**, 137–138.

Hirsch, S.R. (1988). *Psychiatric Beds Use and Service Planning* (Gaskell Psychiatry Series). London: Royal College of Psychiatrists.

Hislop, G.T., Waxler, N.E., Coldman, A.J., Elwood, J.M. and Kan, L. (1987). The prognostic significance of psychosocial factors in women with breast cancer. *J. Chronic Dis.* **40**, 729–735.

Holmes, T.H. and Rahe, R.H. (1967). The social readjustment rating scale. *J. Psychosom. Res.* **11**, 213–218.

Holsboer, F. (1987). Psychoneuroendocrine strategies. In: G.A. Fava and T.N. Wise (eds) *Research Paradigms in Psychosomatic Medicine*, pp. 185–233. Basel, London, New York: Karger.

Hommes, O.R. and Panhuysen, L.H.H.M. (1970). Bilateral intracarotid amytal injection. A study of dysphasia, disturbance of consciousness and paresis. *Psychiatr. Neurol. Neurochir. (Amst.)* **73**, 447–459.

Honzik, M.P. (1957). Developmental studies of parent–child resemblance in intelligence. *Child Dev.* **28**, 215–228.

Horn, G. (1979). Imprinting in search of neural mechanisms. *Trend. Neurosci.* **2**, 219–222.

Horn, J.P. and McAfee, D.A. (1980). Alpha-adrenergic inhibition of calcium-dependent potentials in rat sympathetic neurones. *J. Psysiol. (Lond.)* **301**, 191–204.

Hudson, L. (1966). *Contrary Imaginations*. London: Methuen. (Also Harmondsworth. Middx: Penguin—1968 edn.)

Hughes, S. (1990). Inside madness. *Br. Med. J.* **301**, 1476–1477.

Ingvar, D.H. and Franzen, G. (1974). Abnormalities of cerebral blood flow distribution in patients with chronic schizophrenia. *Acta Psychiat. Scand.* **50**, 425–462.

Inter-Register Technical Committee (1982). *Psychiatric Care in Eight Register Areas. Statistics from Eight Psychiatric Case Registers in Great Britain 1976–1981*. Southampton: University of Southampton.

Irwin, M., Patterson, T., Smith, T.L. *et al.* (1990). Reduction of immune function in life stress and depression. *Biol. Psychiat.* **27**, 23–30.

Itard, E.M. (1801). *De L'éducation d'un Homme Sauvage, ou Des Premiers Développements Physiques et Moraux du Jeune Sauvage de L'Aveyron*. Trans. H. Lane Paladin, Granada Publishing, London, Sydney, Toronto and New York, 1979.

Jauhar, R. and Weller, M.P.I. (1982). Psychiatric morbidity and time zone changes. A study of patients from Heathrow Airport. *Br. J. Psychiatr.* **140**, 231–235.

Janowsky, D.S., Risch, S.C., Huey, L.Y., Judd, L.L. and Rausch, J.L. (1983). Hypothalamic-pituitary-adrenal regulations, neurotransmitters and affective disorders. *Peptides* **41**, 775–784.

Jenkins, D., Watson, A. and Miller, G.R. (1963). Population studies on red grouse *Lagopus lagopus scoticus* (Lath.) in North East Scotland. *J. Anim. Ecol.* **32**, 317–376.

Keller, S.E., Weiss, J.M., Schleifer, S.J., Miller, N.E. and Stein, M. (1981). Suppression of immunity by stress: effect of a graded series of stressors on lymphocyte stimulation in the rat. *Science (NY)* **213**, 1397–1400.

Kendell, R.E. and Kemp, I.W. (1989). Maternal influenza in the etiology of schizophrenia. *Arch. Gen. Psychiat.* **46**, 878–882.

Kiecolt-Glaser, J.K. and Glaser, W. (1986). Psychological influences on immunity. *Psychosomatics* **27**, 621–624.

Kiecolt-Glaser, J.K. and Glaser, W. (1987). Psychological moderators of immune function. *Ann. Behav. Med.* **9**, 16–20.

Kissen, D.M. (1966). The significance of personality in lung cancer in men. *Ann. NY Acad. Sci.* **125**, 820–826.

Knapp, P. (1967). Airway resistance and emotional state in bronchial asthma. *Psychosom. Med.* **29**, 450–451.

Kolvin, L., Garside, R.S., Nichol, A.R., McMillan, A., Wolstenholm, E.S. and Leitch, I.N. (1981). *Help Starts Here: The Maladjusted Child in the Ordinary School*. London: Tavistock.

Kraepelin, E. (1919). *Dementia Praecox*, M. Barclay (trans.), G.M. Robertson (ed.), p. 270. Edinburgh: E. and S. Livingstone.

Kuhn, T.S. (1961). *The Structure of Scientific Revolutions*. Chicago: University of Chicago Press.

Kune, G.A., Kune, S., Watson, L.F. and Bahnson, C.B. (1991). Personality as a risk factor in large bowel cancer: data from the Melbourne colorectal cancer study. *Psychol. Med.* **21**, 29–41.

Lamb, H.R. and Grant, R.W. (1982). The mentally ill in a county jail. *Arch. Gen. Psychiat.* **39**, 17–22.

Lamb, H.R. (1984) (ed.). *The Homeless Mentally Ill.* Washington, DC: American Psychiatric Press.

Lambert, W.E., Libman, E. and Poser, E.G. (1960). The effect of increased salience of a membership group on pain tolerance. *J. Pers.* **28**, 350–357.

Lancet editorial (1981). Social class and ischaemic heart disease. *Lancet* **ii**, 347.

Lashley, K.S. (1929). *Brain Mechanisms and Intelligence*. Chicago: University of Chicago Press.

Lashley, K.S. (1950). In search of the engram. In: *Physiological Mechanisms in Animal Behaviour* (Society of Experimental Biology Symposium No. 4), pp. 454–483. Cambridge: Cambridge University Press.

Levy, S.M. and Wise, B.D. (1988). Psychosocial risk factors and cancer progression. In: C.L. Cooper (ed.) *Stress and Breast Cancer*, pp. 77–96. Chichester: John Wiley.

Lewin, R. (1981). Is your brain really necessary? *Science (NY)* **210**, 1232–1234.

Liddle, P.F. (1990). Prefrontal and subcortical dysfunction in schizophrenia. In: M.P.I. Weller (ed.) *International Perspectives in Schizophrenia*. London: John Libby.

Lloyd, G.G. and Cawley, R.H. (1978). Psychiatric morbidity in men one week after first acute myocardial infarction. *Br. Med. J.* **ii**, 1453–1454.

Lloyd, G.G. and Cawley, R.H. (1980). Smoking habits after myocardial infarction. *J. R. Coll. Physicians, Lond.* **11**, 221–226.

Lorenz, K. (1963). *On Aggression*. London: Methuen.

Maclean, D. and Reichlin, S. (1981). Neuroendocrinology and the immune process. In: R. Ader (ed.) *Psychoneuroimmunology*, pp. 475–520. New York: Academic Press.

Madison, D.V. and Nicoll, R.A. (1982). Noradrenaline blocks accommodation of pyramidal cell discharge in the hippocampus. *Nature (Lond.)* **299**, 636–638.

Maier, N.R.F. (1932). The effect of cerebral destruction on reasoning and learning in rats. *J. Comp. Neurol.* **54**, 45–75.

Mann, L. and Taylor, K.F. (1969). Queue counting: the effect of motives upon estimates of numbers in waiting lines. *J. Personality Social Psychol.* **13**, 79–82.

McBain, C.J., Traynelis, S.F. and Dingledine, R. (1990). Regional variation of extracellular space in the hippocampus. *Science* **249**, 674–677.

McClelland, D.C., Atkinson, J.W., Clark, R.A. and Lowell, E.L. (1953). *The Achievement Motive*. New York: Appleton-Century-Crofts.

McEwen, B. (1979). (Cited in Kolata, G.B.) Sex hormones and brain development. *Science (NY)* **205**, 985–987.

McFall, M.E., Murburg, M.M., Ko, G.N. and Veith, R.C. (1990). Autonomic responses to stress in Vietnam combat veterans with Posttraumatic Stress Disorder. *Biol. Psychiat.* **27**, 1165–1175.

Mead, G.H. (1938). *The Philosophy of the Act*. Chicago: University of Chicago Press.

Meares, R., Mendelsohn, F.A.O. and Milgrom-Friedman, J. (1981). A sex difference in the seasonal variation of suicide rate: a single cycle for men, two cycles for women. *Br. J. Psychiat.* **138**, 321–325.

Mechanic, D. (1975). Sociocultural and social-psychological factors affecting personal responses to psychological disorder. *J. Health Soc. Behav.* **16**, 393–404.

Mednick, S.A., Machen, R.A. and Huttunen, M.O. (1988). Adult schizophrenia following prenatal exposure to an influenza epidemic. *Arch. Gen. Psychiat.* **45**, 189–192.

Mednick, S.A., Machen, R.A. and Huttunen, M.O. (1990). An update on the Helsinki influenza project. *Arch. Gen. Psychiat.* **47**, 292.

Menninger, K. (1928). The schizophrenic syndrome as a product of acute infectious disease. *Arch. Neurol. Psychiat.* **20**, 464–481.

Metz, A. (1983). Changes in platelet alpha-2-adrenoceptor binding post partum: possible relation to maternity blues. *Lancet* **i**, 495–498.

Napalkov, A.V. (1963). Information processes of the brain. In: N. Weiner and J.C. Schade (eds) *Prog. Brain Res.* Vol. 2, pp. 59–69. Amsterdam: Elsevier.

Nature (Lond.) editorial (1981). Neuronal plasticity, learning and remembering, **293**, 525–526.

Needleman, H.L., Gunnoe, C., Leviton, A. *et al.* (1979). Deficits in psychologic and classroom performance of children with elevated dentine lead levels. *New Engl. J. Med.* **300**, 689–695.

Nichols, R.A., Talvinder, S.S., Czernik, A.J., Nairn, A.C. and Greengard, P. (1990). Calcium/calmodulin-dependent protein kinase II increases glutamate and noradrenaline release from synaptosomes. *Nature* **343**, 647–651.

Numan, M., Rosenblatt, J.S. and Komisaruk, B.R. (1977). Medical preoptic area and onset of maternal behavior in the rat. *J. Comp. Physiol. Psychol.* **91**, 146–164.

Nunes, E.V., Frank, K.A. and Kornfeld, D.S. (1987). Psychological treatment for the type A behaviour pattern and for coronary heart disease: a meta-analysis of the literature. *Psychosom. Med.* **48**, 15–73.

O'Callaghan, E., Gibson, T., Colohan, D. *et al.* (1991). Season of birth in schizophrenia. Evidence for the confinement of an excess of winter births to patients without a family history of mental disorder. *Br. J. Psychiat.* **158**, 764–769.

Olney, J.W. (1990). Excitatory amino acids and schizophrenia. *Biol. Psychiat.* **28**, 553–554.

Parkes, C.M., Benjamin, B. and Fitzgerald, R.G. (1969). Broken heart: a statistical study of increased mortality among widowers. *Br. Med. J.* **i**, 740–743.

Pasamanick, B. and Knobloch, H. (1961). Complications of pregnancy. In: G. Caplan (ed.) *Prevention of Mental Disorders in Children*. New York: Basic Books.

Paulman, R.G., Devous, Sr. M.D., Gregory, R.R. *et al.* (1990). Hypofrontality and cognitive impairment in schizophrenia: dynamic single-photon tomography and neuropsychological assessment of schizophrenic brain function. *Biol. Psychiat.* **27**, 377–399.

Penfield, W. and Rasmussen, T. (1950). *The Cerebral Cortex of Man: A Clinical Study of Localization of Function*. New York: Macmillan.

Penrose, L.S. (1938). Mental disease and crime: outline of a comparative study of European statistics. *Br. J. Psychol. Med.* **18**, 1–15.

Pepper, B., Kirshner, M.C. and Ryglewicz, H. (1981). The young chronic patient: overview of a population. *Hosp. Commun. Psychiat.* **32**, 463–469.

Perl, D.P., Gajdusek, D.C., Garruto, R.M., Yanagihara, R.T. and Gibbs, C.J. Jr (1982). Intraneural aluminium accumulation in amyotrophic lateral sclerosis and Parkinsonism —Dementia of Guam. *Science (NY)* **217**, 1053–1055.

Perry, V.H. and Cowey, A. (1982). A sensitive period for ganglion cell degeneration and the formation of aberrant retino-fugal connections following tectal lesions in rats. *Neuroscience* **7**, 583–594.

Petrich, J. (1976). Rate of psychiatric morbidity in a metropolitan county jail population. *Am. J. Psychiat.* **133**, 1439–1444.

Phillips, A.G. and Fiberger, H.G. (1989). Neuroanatomical bases of intracranial self-stimulation: untangling the Gordian knot. In: J.M. Liebman and S.J. Cooper (eds) *The Neuropharmacological Basis of Reward*, pp. 66–105. Oxford: Oxford Science Publishers.

Polanyi, M. (1962). Life's irreducible Structure. In: M. Grene (ed.) (1969). *Knowing and Being, Essays by Michael Polanyi*. London: Routledge & Kegan Paul.

Post, R.M., Rubinow, D.R. and Ballenger, J.C. (1986). Conditioning and sensitization in the longitudinal course of affective illness. *Br. J. Psychiat.* **149**, 191–201.

Post, R.M., DeLisi, L.E., Holcomb, H.H., Unde, T.W., Cohen, R. and Buchsbaum, M.S. (1987). Glucose utilization in the temporal cortex of affectively ill patients: Positron emission tomography. *Biol. Psychiat.* **22**, 545–553.

Price, J.S. (1969). Personality differences within families: Comparison of adults, brothers and sisters. *J. Biosoc. Sci.* **1**, 177–205.

Raisman, G. and Field, P. (1973). Sexual dimorphism in the neurophil of the pre-optic area of the rat and its dependence on neonatal androgens. *Brain Res.* **54**, 1–29.

Rangel-Guerra, R.A., Perez-Payan, H., Minkoff, L. and Todd, L.E. (1983). Nuclear magnetic resonance in bipolar affective disorders. *Am. J. Neuroradiol.* **4**, 229–231.

Ravenholt, R.T. and Foege, W.H. (1982). 1918 Influenza, encephalitis lethargica. Parkinsonism. *Lancet* **ii**, 860–864.

Reinberg, A., Lagoguey, M., Cessalin, F. *et al.* (1978). Circadian and circannual rhythms in plasma hormones and other variables of five healthy young human males. *Acta Endocr. (Copenh.)* **88**, 417–427.

Report of Working Group on Suicide Prevention (1986). London: HMSO.

Rich, K.M. and Hollowell, J.P. (1990). Flunarazine protects neurons from death after axotomy or NGF deprivation. *Science* **248**, 1419–1421.

Risch, S.C. (1982). Beta-endorphin hypersecretion in depression. Possible cholinergic mechanisms. *Biol. Psychiat.* **17**, 1071–1079.

Roberts, G.W. (1990). Brain development and CCK systems in schizophrenia: a working hypothesis. In: M. Weller (ed.) *International Perspectives in Schizophrenia*. London: John Libbey.

Roberts, G.W. (1991). Schizophrenia: a neuropathological perspective. *Br. J. Psychiat.* **158**, 8–17..

Roos, R.P. and Johnson, R.T. (1977). Viruses and dementia. In: C.E. Wells (ed.) *Dementia*, 2nd edn. pp. 93–112. Philadelphia: Davis.

Rosanoff, A.J., Handy, L.M. and Plesset, I.R. (1941). The aetiology of child behaviour difficulties, juvenile delinquency and adult criminality with special reference to their occurrence in twins. *Psychiatric Monographs*, State Printing Office for the Department of Institutions. Vol. 1. Sacramento: California.

Rosenthal, J., Strauss, A., Minkoff, L. and Winston, A. (1986). Identifying lithium-responsive bipolar depressed patients using nuclear magnetic resonance. *Am. J. Psychiat.* **143**, 779–780.

Rosenzweig, M.R. (1969). Effects of heredity and environment on brain chemistry, brain anatomy and learning ability in the rat. In: M. Manosevitz, G. Lindzey and D.D. Thiessen (eds) *Behavioural Genetics*. New York: Appleton-Century-Crofts.

Royal College of General Practitioners (1981). *Survey of Primary Care in London*. Occasional Paper 16. London: Royal College of General Practitioners.

Rutter, M., Birch, H.G., Thomas, A. and Chess, S. (1964). Temperamental characteristics in infancy and the later development of behavioural disorders. *Br. J. Psychiat.* **110**, 651–661.

Rutter, M., Graham, P. and Yule, W. (1970). *A Neuropsychiatric Study in Childhood*. London: Heinemann.

Sagen, J., Sortwell, C.E. and Pappas, G.D. (1990). Monoaminergic neural transplants prevent learned helplessness in a rat depression model. *Biol. Psychiat.* **28**, 1037–1048.

Sanua, V.D. (1960). Sociocultural factors in responses to stressful life situations: the behaviour of aged amputees as an example. *J. Health Human Behav.* **1**, 17–24.

Sapolsky, R.M. (1990). Adrenocortical function, social rank, and personality among wild baboons. *Biol. Psychiat.* **28**, 862–878.

Scarone, S., Pieri, E., Gambini, O., Massironi, R. and Cazullo, C.L. (1982). The asymmetric lateralisation of tactile extinction in schizophrenia: the possible role of limbic and frontal regions. *Br. J. Psychiat.* **141**, 350–353.

Schleifer, S.J., Keller, S.E., Bond, R.N., Cohen, J. and Stein, M. (1989). Major depressive disorder: role of age, sex, severity and hospitalization. *Arch. Gen. Psychiat.* **46**, 81–87.

Schmale, A.H. Jr (1958). Relation of separation and depression to disease: 1. A report on a hospitalized medical population. *Psychosom. Med.* **20**, 259–277.

Segal, B.E. (1966). Epideminology of emotional disturbance among college under-graduates: a review and analysis. *J. Nerv. Ment. Dis.* **143**, 348–362.

Segal, B.E. and Phillips, D.L. (1967). Work, play and emotional disturbance. An examination of environment and disturbance. *Arch. Gen. Psychiat.* **16**, 173–179.

Selye, H. (1950). *The Physiology and Pathology of Exposure to Stress*. Montreal: Acta.

Servan-Schrieber, D., Printz, H. and Cohen, J.D. (1990). A network model of catechol-amine effects: Gain, signal-to-noise, and behaviour. *Science* **249**, 892–895.

Service, A.L., Koval, J.S. and Pursey-Day, C. (1981). *Final Report: Mental Health Systems Study*. Submitted to the Joint Budget Committee of the Colorado General Assembly, December 1, cited Warner (1985), *ibid*.

Shaikh, A.A., Naqvi, R.H. and Shaikh, S.A. (1978). Concentrations of oestradiol-17 beta and progesterone in the peripheral plasma of the cynomolgus monkey (*Macaca fascicularis*) in relation to the length of the menstrual cycle and its component phases. *J. Endocr.* **79**, 1–7.

Shearer, M. and Finch, S. (1964). Periodic organic psychosis associated with recurrent herpes simplex. *New Engl. J. Med.* **271**, 494–497.

Shekelle, R.B., Raynor, W.J. Jr, Ostfeld, A.M. *et al.* (1981). Psychological depression and 17-year risk of death from cancer. *Psychosom. Med.* **43**, 117–126.

Sherif, M. and Sherif, C.W. (1956). *An Outline of Social Psychology*. New York: Harper.

Sherrington, C. (1906). *The Integrative Action of the Nervous System*. New York: Schrieber's.

Simon, R.H., Lovett, E.J. III, Tomaszek, D. and Lundy, J. (1980). Electrical stimulation of the midbrain mediates metastatic tumour growth. *Science (NY)* **209**, 1132–1133.

Skodak, M. and Skeels, H.M. (1949). A final follow-up study of one-hundred adopted children. *J. Genet. Psychol.* **75**, 85–125.

Slater, E., Beard, A.W. and Glithero, E. (1963). The schizophrenia-like psychosis of epilepsy. *Br. J. Psychiat.* **109**, 95–97.

Sperry, R.W. *et al.* (1969). In: P. Vinken and G.W. Bruyn (eds) *Handbook of Clinical Neurology*, Vol. 4, pp. 273–289. Amsterdam: Elsevier/North-Holland.

Stein, M., Miller, A.H. and Trestman, R.L. (1991). Depression, the immune system, and health and illness. *Arch. Gen. Psychiat.* **48**, 171–177.

Sterman, M.D. (1982). EEG biofeedback in the treatment of epilepsy: an overview circa 1980. In: L. White and B. Tursky (eds) *Clinical Biofeedback: Efficacy and Mechanisms*, pp. 311–330. New York: Guilford Press.

Stevenson-Hinde, J. and Hinde, R.A. (1986). Changes in associations between character-istics. In: R. Plomin and J. Dunn (eds) *The Study of Temperament: Changes, Continuities and Challenges*. Hilldale, NJ: Lawrence Erlbaum.

Strole, L., Langer, T., Michael, S., Opler, M. and Rennie, T.A.C. (1962). *Mental Health in the Metropolis*. New York: McGraw-Hill.

Swank, G.E. and Winer, D. (1976). Occurrence of psychiatric disorder in a county jail population. *Am. J. Psychiat.* **133**, 1331–1333.

Talbot, J.D., Marrett, S., Evans, A.C., Meyer, E., Bushnell, M.C. and Duncan, G.H. (1991). Multiple representations of pain in human cerebral cortex. *Science* **251**, 1355–1358.

Templer, D.I. and Veleber, D.M. (1982). Seasonality of schizophrenic births: harmful effects or genetic morphism? *Br. J. Psychiat.* **140**, 323–324.

Tetrud, J.W. and Langston, J.W. (1989). The effects of Deprenyl (Selegiline) on the natural history of Parkinson's diseases. *Science* **245**, 519–522; and (1990) **249**, 303–304 (letter).

Thomas, C.B. and Greenstreet, R.L. (1973). Psychobiological characteristics in youth as mediators of five disease states: suicide, mental illness, hypertension, coronary heart disease and tumour. *Johns Hopkins Med. J.* **132**, 16–43.

Tindall, J.S. (1978). In: S.L. Jeffcoate and J.S.M. Hutchinson (eds) *The Endocrine Hypothalamus*, pp. 253–292. London: Academic Press.

Tollefson, G.D. (1990). Short-term effects of the calcium channel blocker nimodipine (Bay-e-9736) in the management of primary degenerative dementia. *Biol. Psychiat.* **27**, 1133–1142.

Torrey, E.F., Yolken, R.H. and Winfrey, C.J. (1982). Cytomegalovirus antibody in cere-brospinal fluid of schizophrenic patients detected by enzyme immunoassay. *Science* (*NY*) **216**, 892–894.

Ts'o, D.Y., Frostig, R.D., Lieke, E.E. and Grinvald, A. (1990). Functional organization of primate visual cortex revealed by high resolution optical imaging. *Science* **249**, 417–420.

Tyron, R.C. (1963). Experimental behavioural genetics of maze learning and a sufficient polygenic theory. *Am. Psychol.* **18**, 442.

Valsik, J.A. (1965). The seasonal rhythm of menarch. A review. *Hum. Biol.* **37**, 75–90.

Vickers, R.R. Jr (1988). Effectiveness of defences: a significant predictor of cortisol excretion under stress. *Psychosom. Res.* **32**, 21–29.

Wai, L., Richmond, J., Burton, H. and Lindsay, R.M. (1981). Influence of psychosocial factors on survival of home-dialysis patients. *Lancet* **ii**, 1155–1156.

Warner, R. (1985). *Recovery from Schizophrenia: Psychiatry and Political Economy*. London, Boston and Henley: Routledge and Kegan Paul.

Watson, JM., Greer, S., Rowden, L. *et al.* (1991). Relationships between emotional control, adjustment to cancer and depression and anxiety in breast cancer patients. *Psychol. Med.* **21**, 51–57.

Weinberger, D.R., Berman, K.F. and Zec, R.F. (1986). Physiologic dysfunction of dorso-lateral prefrontal cortex in schizophrenia. 11. Regional cerebral blood flow evidence. *Arch. Gen. Psychiat.* **43**, 114–124.

Weinberger, D.R., Wagner, R. and Wyatt, R.J. (1983). Neuropathological studies of schizophrenia: a selected review. *Schizophrenia Bulletin* **9**, 193–212.

Weiner, H., Thaler, M., Reiser, M.F. and Mirsky, I.A. (1957). Aetiology of duodenal ulcer 1. Relation of specific psychological characteristics to rate of gastric secretion (serum pepsinogen). *Psychosom. Med.* **19**, 1–10.

Weiss, B., William, J.H., Margen, S. *et al.* (1980). Food dyes impair performance of hyperactive children on a laboratory learning test. *Science* (*NY*) **207**, 1485–1489.

Weiss, J.M. (1972). Psychological factors in stress and disease. *Scient. Am.* **226**, 104–113.

Weller, M.P.I. (1989). Mental illness—who cares? *Nature* **399**, 249–252.

Weller, M.P.I. and Jauhar, P. (1981). Travel induced disturbances in circadian rhythms as precipitants of affective illness. In: G. Perris, G. Struwe and B. Jansson (eds) *Biological Psychiatry*, pp. 1253–6. Amsterdam: Elsevier/North-Holland.

Weller, M.P.I. and Latimer-Sayer, D.T. (1985). Increasing right hand dominance with advancing age on a motor skill task. *Psychol. Med.* **15**, 867–872.

Weller, M.P.I. and Montagu, J.D. (1979). Electroencephalographic coherence in schizophrenia. In: *Hemisphere Asymmetries of Function and Psychopathology*. J. Gruzelier and P. Flor-Henry (eds), pp. 285–292. Amsterdam, New York and London: Elsevier.

Weller, M.P.I., Peatfield, R.C., Glover, V., Littlewood, J., Clifford-Rose, F. and Sandler, M. (1982). Monoamine oxidase and personality features in migrainous patients. Abstracts Vol. II, Collegium Internationale Neuro-Psychopharmacologicum, 13th C.I.N.P. Congress, Jerusalem, June 20–25; p. 757.

West, D.J. (1977). The chronic offender. *Hosp. Med.* October, 48–50.

Williams, J.M.G., Watts, F.N., MacLeod, C. and Mathews, A. (1988). *Cognitive Psychology and the Emotional Disorders*. Chichester: John Wiley.

Wilson, J., Ping, A.J., Kraus, J.C. *et al.* (1990). Correction of CD18-deficient lymphocytes by retrovirus-mediated gene transfer. *Science* **248**, 1413–1416.

Wolf, S. and Wolff, H.G. (1947). *Human Gastric Function*. London: Oxford Medical.

Wolff, C.T., Friedman, S., Hofer, M. and Mason, J. (1964). Relationship between psychological defences and mean urinary 17-hydroxycorticosteroid excretion rates. *Psychosom. Med.* **26**, 576–588.

Wood and Darling (Cited in Boyd, W. (1961). *A Textbook of Pathology*, p. 952. London: Kimpton.)

Yalom, I.D., Lunde, D.T., Moos, R.H. and Hamburg, D.A. (1968). 'Post partum' blues syndrome. *Arch. Gen. Psychiat.* **18**, 16–27.

Young, A.H., Blackwood, D.H.R., Roxborough, H., McQueen, J.K., Martin, M.J. and Kean, D. (1991). A magnetic resonance imaging study of schizophrenia: brain structure and clinical symptoms. *Br. J. Psychiat.* **158**, 158–164.

— 2

Historical Introduction to Psychiatry

P. Pichot

In my attempt to survey the development of psychological medicine during the entire past century I am confronted by the necessity of selecting certain facts while neglecting others. I am aware of the dangers implicit in such a process. I only can hope that you will forgive me if, in spite of my best efforts, my prejudices seemingly distort historical reality.

First, in accordance with the present fashion amongst historians, let us consider the demographic data. In 1881 France had 120 psychiatrists, one for about 300 000 inhabitants. Today there are 4000 recognized specialists, one for less than 14 000 inhabitants, a 23-fold increase of the ratio. In the United States of America, the trend has been ever stronger: the proportion of psychiatrists to the population has been multiplied 50-fold in one century. Equally striking is the representation of psychiatrists among American physicians. In 1881 there were only two American psychiatrists out of 1000 medical practitioners; today there are 75. Such growth, which has taken place with minor variations everywhere, deserves a careful examination of its background and of its phases.

One tends to explain the traditional division of history into periods of one century by the fact that three generations are considered necessary to complete a cultural mutation. Whatever the truth of this proposition it has the advantage of providing us with a convenient framework. We shall examine three periods during the past century of approximately the same duration whose divisions are marked by great historical events. The first goes from 1881 to 1914, the second spans the time between the two world wars and the third consists of the period from 1945 to the present.

In 1881 French psychiatry could feel proud of its continuous development during the preceding century: the French school, first with Pinel, then with Esquirol, had taken the world leadership. The Salpêtrière and the Bicêtre General Hospitals in Paris, where Pinel had delivered the insane from their chains, were still, in their psychiatric wards, the Mecca where, according to a later historian, 'every French or foreign psychiatrist visiting Paris went as a pilgrim'. Of the former Esquirol pupils, Baillarger, then at the Salpêtrière, was the most famous, and if he was approaching the end of a brilliant scientific career, he had in both hospitals younger colleagues who had been trained in the prestigious French clinical tradition: Falret, Bourneville, Legrand du Saule, to name but a few.

In 1879 the first University Chair of Psychiatry had been opened in the only psychiatric hospital located inside Paris, Sainte Anne Hospital, and the teaching of 'mental medicine', as it was called, had received the seal of academic respectability.

A law of 1838 had legislated the building of an asylum for the insane in each 'Department' of France, that is, about 80 for the whole country, and the patients were there under the care of full-time specialists in psychological medicine, selected and paid by the State. Although many of these 'asylum physicians', as they were called, contented themselves with custodial routine, some achieved scientific eminence. Benedict Morel, who died in 1873, after being superintendent of an asylum, published his epoch-making work 'Treatise of the Degeneracies of the Human Species', in 1857. In this volume he presented a general theory of the causes of mental diseases which was to play a prominent role in psychiatric discussions until the First World War.

In 1881, the most influential living 'asylum physician' was Valentin Magnan. He was head of the admissions wards at Sainte Anne Hospital where he was to remain for more than 50 years. Through his and his school's work he gained a large influence in France and abroad.

One usually forgets today that in the period under consideration the psychiatrists, whether working in psychiatric wards of general hospitals or in asylums, were concerned only with the most severe cases of mental illness, with what we now call psychotic conditions, since all their patients had to be legally committed. The large group of relatively minor disorders, the neuroses, were under the care of the neurologists. In 1881 the leading neurologist in the world, the founder of the new discipline, was Jean Martin Charcot. He was one of the physicians of the Salpêtrière but in charge of non-psychiatric wards. After having described new neurological diseases and thus achieved fame, he became interested in the problem of hysteria, an interest which was to have important consequences.

A superficial observer would have thought, in 1881, that the position occupied by the French psychiatric school was secure and would be maintained during the next decades. In fact, at precisely this moment, it had begun to be challenged by the German school. The German psychiatrists at the beginning of the nineteenth century had been divided into two contending groups: the 'psychologists' and the 'somaticists'. The first, whose main exponent had been Heinroth, influenced by the romantic movement and by the 'Naturphilosophie' of Schelling, considered the mental disorders as disturbances of the soul and as the consequence of sin. Around 1850 the somaticists, under Griesinger, gained the advantage. The formula coined by their leader, 'psychic diseases are diseases of the brain' became the credo of the whole German school. Historians of psychiatry interpret the ascendancy of Germany over France as the result of the victory of Prussia in 1870. The explanation, however brilliant, remains superficial. The basic factor seems to lie in the organization and the development of the German university system. The social prestige of the pompous 'Herr Professor' was a favourite theme of jokes in France and elsewhere.

However, after 1870, and during the so-called 'Years of the Founders', the 'Gründerjahre', the numerous well-endowed German universities were producing scientific and technological achievements that were becoming a source of awe and sometimes of fear for the rest of the world. One may add that there were

German-speaking universities outside of the boundaries of the Reich. These included the German-speaking part of Switzerland and the whole of the Hapsburg Empire. There were German Chairs of Psychiatry in Prague as well as in Vienna and in Zurich, and professorships were given irrespective of nationality. In 1881, while France had only one Chair of Psychiatry, that in Paris (the second was created in 1892 in Toulouse, the third in 1913 in Bordeaux), there were already more than 14 in the German-speaking countries. It is also striking that in 1872, as soon as Alsace was taken over by Germany, a Chair of Psychiatry was founded in Strasbourg. The career of its first professor, Krafft-Ebing, is typical: born in Mannheim in Germany, he studied psychiatry in Zurich under the German Griesinger, became professor in Strasbourg, accepted the same position in the Austro-Hungarian Empire, first in Graz and finally in Vienna. German psychiatry, from 1881 on, was, in contrast to French and also English psychiatry, university related and its power and influence was a result of the German university system.

Victorian England was, in 1881, both economically and politically, the most powerful country in the world. The industrial revolution at the end of the eighteenth century, born out of a series of technical discoveries and the easy availability of coal and iron ore, gave England a large advantage over its continental competitors. This was the basis of its worldwide commercial expansion, which was greatly aided by its supremacy as a maritime power, undisputed since the fall of Napoleon. One would have expected its contribution to psychiatry to have been commensurate with its scientific, technical, economic and political positions. It is a puzzling paradox that the English left psychiatric leadership, first to the French, then to the Germans. I may venture to suggest that one possible explanation lies in the previous century.

If Pinel is credited with the birth of psychiatry in France during the revolution, William Tuke assumed the same status in England. The ideas of the Quakers, or the Society of Friends, were his inspiration. These included the relief of the poor, sound education, prison reform, the battle against alcoholism, the abolition of slavery, and the care of the insane. The opening of the 'Retreat' near York by William Tuke in 1796 parallels Pinel's reforms at Bicêtre and at the Salpêtrière. But whereas Pinel was a physician who considered insanity as basically a medical and scientific problem, William Tuke was a successful tea and coffee merchant, inspired by his religious convictions and by social ideals. Although in 1881 Henry Maudsley had already published his most important works and gained in his country the reputation of being England's Griesinger, the only internationally-known British psychiatrist was John Conolly. His book, 'Treatment of the Insane Without Mechanical Restraint', introduced a policy that rapidly became known and admired in public institutions on the continent and in the United States even though it was not consistently followed. There is a link between Tuke's York Retreat, Conolly's no-restraint, and present day social preoccupations in psychiatry. The English school was respected for the humanity of its methods of care, but it was confined to the mental hospitals and had no real scientific prestige.

However, two contributions made prior to 1881 and not directly related to medicine were later to have a basic influence on psychiatric thought. The first was the publication of 'The Origin of Species', in 1857. The 'Copernican revolution' initiated by Darwin in biology not only brought about a drastic revision of the anthropocentric view of the position of man amongst the living beings, but also proposed a hierarchical and evolutionary model whose impact on psychology and social sciences was immediate. In 1881, Theodule Ribot, the 'father of French psychopathology', published his book 'Diseases of Memory', based on a systematic use of the principles of evolution and dissolution borrowed from Darwin through Spencer. The same year Hughlings Jackson, a neurologist at the National Hospital in London, presented in a paper a hierarchical theory of the functions of the nervous system, of obvious Darwinian origin, and his model was later to become directly or indirectly an inspiration for psychopathological theories.

The second English contribution was even more remotely related to psychiatry. Francis Galton, a cousin of Darwin, had given birth to biometrics, the science of the measurement of biological, including psychological, phenomena. A typical Victorian genius, a man of independent means without any official university position, Galton had devoted his life to many different and apparently unconnected fields of inquiry. Suffice it to say that he was the founder both of meteorology and of eugenics. In 1878 he published two papers, 'Psychometric Facts' in *Nineteenth Century* and 'Psychometric Experiments' in *Brain*. In the latter, one finds a sentence that sums up the philosophy of his efforts: 'Until the phenomena of any branch of knowledge have been submitted to measurement and number, it cannot assume the status and dignity of science.' In adopting these principles his successors created a British tradition whose influence was extended first to psychology and then to psychiatry. It is customary today to relate the importance given to quantitative techniques and to statistical methods in psychiatric research since the end of the last war to American influence. The truth is that the base had been already laid in 1881 in England.

Outside of the French, the German and the British schools, only individual psychiatrists had made themselves known internationally. These included Beard in the United States with his description of 'neurasthenia' in 1880 and Lombroso in Italy with his theory of the 'born criminal', to mention only two.

The period between 1881 and 1914 is a turning point in the history of art, of literature and also of science. The same applies to psychiatry: discoveries were then made, trends were launched, whose influence is still felt today.

At the beginning of the period, brain anatomy was the accepted basis of psychiatry. Since Broca had proposed his theory of cerebral localizations, the neuroanatomists had described with more and more refined methods complex nervous pathways, and had given to the psychiatrists the conviction that it was now possible to realize Griesinger's dream, to explain mental diseases through specific abnormalities in cerebral functioning. In 1884 there appeared a book by Meynert, the Professor of Psychiatry in Vienna, with the significant title, 'Treatise of Psychiatry: Clinical Studies of the Diseases of the Forebrain'. Previously, in 1880 his pupil, Karl Wernicke, then a Professor in Breslau, had published a manual in which he 'explained' pathological behaviour by definite abnormalities of the reflex arc connecting sensory and perceptual centres with motor pathways through cerebral fibres.

The theories of Meynert and Wernicke did not last and are only of historical interest. It was soon realized that they were only brilliant speculations, or to quote Kraepelin, 'brain mythologies'. But the neurophysiological tradition thus created remained and became a lasting characteristic of the Russian psychiatric school. Its founder, Sergei Korsakov, became internationally known in 1887 by describing a neuropsychiatric disease to which his name was later given. Wernicke's ideas of 'cerebral reflexes' had already been developed by Setchenov. This was continued by Bekhterev, appointed Professor in Saint Petersburg in 1893, a precursor of behaviourism and the father of reflexology. Ivan Pavlov, another pupil of Setchenov, received the Nobel Prize in 1905 for his discovery of the conditioned reflexes.

Pavlovism was to become, half a century later, the adversary of psychoanalysis. Both doctrines, however, stem from a common origin: the neurophysiological trends of the late nineteenth century. Sigmund Freud was a neurologist, a neuroanatomist, a pupil of Meynert for whom he always retained a great veneration. He became converted to the study of neuroses during a short stay with Charcot at the Salpêtrière in 1885. That was the great period of Charcot's studies on hysteria which have since become the theme for historical and literary commentaries. The neurological wards of the Salpêtrière thus became the cradle of the modern psychopathology of the neuroses as developed by Freud and by his French contemporary, Pierre Janet.

If one tries to define psychiatry between 1881 and 1914 by a work of paramount importance, one has to invoke the name of Emil Kraepelin, who was to exemplify the rise of the German school of psychiatry. He served as Professor in Heidelberg until 1903, then in Munich. He was known for his 'Handbook of Psychiatry', whose first edition appeared in 1883, and the ninth immediately after his death in 1927. Kraepelin shaped progressively a general classification of mental diseases which was to remain practically unchanged until today. The elements were often taken from his predecessors, mainly French and German psychiatrists, but Kraepelin's genius lay in his ability to systematize a heterogeneous puzzle of independent concepts. In 1896 he reached his final synthesis by using as criteria for classification both the symptoms and the course of the disorder. It was the victory of sound clinical observation over the speculation of Meynert and Wernicke. At the same time Magnan and his pupils made similar efforts on the basis of the French tradition. But if their concepts were accepted in France, where they are still used today, they could not easily fit into the Kraepelinian system because the principles on which they rested were of a different nature. French psychiatrists, reluctant to accept *in toto* Kraepelin's psychiatry—the mounting nationalism of the period played a role in this antagonism—tried to compromise and to keep their original position. The rest of the world progressively accepted the ideas of the German school while French psychiatry became relatively isolated.

If Kraepelin was the principal catalyst of the rise of German-speaking psychiatry he did not stand alone in the world. In Austria Freud, after his visit to Charcot, laid the basis of psychoanalysis and his fundamental works were written for the most part before 1914.

In Switzerland Eugen Bleuler, Professor in Zurich, published in 1911 his classical work 'Dementia Praecox or the Group of Schizophrenias'. He not only coined a new word, 'schizophrenia', to describe Kraepelin's dementia praecox, but also introduced a dynamic element into the more static views of his predecessor by borrowing ideas from freud through his assistant Carl Jung. His brilliant delineation of some of the basic manifestations of the disease, such as autism and ambivalence, his distinction of primary symptoms produced by the disease, and of secondary symptoms as reactions of the patient's personality, were to shape our outlook of this psychotic disorder in the following decades.

At about the same time psychopathology became an autonomous chapter of psychiatry. The philosopher Karl Jaspers, then a young psychiatric assistant in Heidelberg, and a pupil of Dielthey and of Husserl, created what he called in a paper of 1912 'the phenomenological perspective in psychopathology'. The next year saw the publication of the first and still most famous survey of the subject, 'General Psychopathology'.

With Kraepelin, Freud, Bleuler and Jaspers, to mention only its most prestigious figures, the German-speaking school of psychiatry had become the recognized leader. Sir Aubrey Lewis, in describing the work of Henry Maudsley, informed us that the idea of creating a 'University psychiatric hospital in England which should be devoted to early treatment, research and postgraduate training' was due to the suggestion of Sir Frederik Mott after the latter's visit to Kraepelin's clinic in Munich. The offer of £3000 by Maudsley was accepted by the London County Council and the University of London in 1908, and the present Institute of Psychiatry, which was fully opened in 1923, was in some way a tribute to German leadership.

On the other side of the Atlantic one could already discern the birth of trends which, after a period of maturation, were to characterize the American school when it achieved pre-eminence after the Second World War. A young Swiss psychiatrist, Adolf Meyer, emigrated to the United States in 1904. Professor at Cornell University in New York in 1911, he accepted the Henry Phipps Chair of Psychiatry created for him at the Johns Hopkins University. He rapidly became the leading figure of American psychiatry. Under the influence of the philanthropism of his Swiss teacher, August Forel, and of the optimistic pragmatism of his American philosopher friends, John Dewey, George Mead and Charles Cooley, he advocated as early as 1911 the 'Community Psychiatry' system. He rejected Kraepelin's medical model in favour of the concept of 'reaction types', the background of the antinosological movement after the Second World War. He met Freud at Clark University in 1904 and, without adhering to the new doctrine, displayed an understanding and tolerance towards it. His pupils later significantly influenced American psychiatry, from Harry Stack Sullivan to Jules Masserman, from Oscar Diethelm to Franklin Ebaugh, not to mention Sir David Henderson in England.

The period which begins with the First World War and ends with the Second can be viewed in many aspects as transitional. Although defeated in the field, Germany had retained its scientific prestige. In 1917 a Research Institute of Psychiatry opened in Munich. Emil Kraepelin, at the same time Professor at the

University, became its Director. It was the first autonomous psychiatric research organization and it was to become a model. Here psychiatric genetics was born in Rudin's Department, where all the future world specialists were trained: Essen Moller and Sjögren from Sweden, Eric Strömgren from Denmark, Eliot Slater from Great Britain, and the German Franz Kallman who, after his emigration, continued the tradition in the United States.

During the 1920s, the massive 'Handbook of the Mental Disorders' was published under the editorship of Bumke. This work seemed to symbolize the undisputed supremacy of Germany in the field, a position recognized even by the Soviet Union which asked German neuropathologists to study the structure of the brain of its founder, Lenin.

One often says that National Socialism was indirectly responsible for the decline of German psychiatry. It is true that, by compelling many psychiatrists and psychoanalysts to emigrate, the Nazi regime played such a role, but it also indirectly modified the evolution of both British and American psychiatry. It is also true that the expulsion of Freud from Vienna and his death in London were symbolic of this tragedy. But the main consequences of racist persecutions were of a more ethical nature. The programme of extermination of the so-called 'incurable insane' and the misuse of pseudo-scientific genetic concepts have had a lasting influence on the conscience of psychiatrists the world over. The decline of German psychiatry probably antedated the advent of Hitler and was only accelerated after 1933. German psychiatry was still active in the post First World War period. The Heidelberg school under Kurt Schneider and the Tubingen school under Ernst Kretschmer tried to bring new perspectives to Kraepelin's tradition. The 'anthropological school' of von Gebsattel and the 'comprehensive anthropology' of Zutt were born in 1928 under the influence of the philosopher Max Scheeler and Heidegger's book 'Sein und Zeit'. The latter formed the basis of Binswanger's Daseinsanalyse. Those trends would have, after the Second World War, a localized and short-lived success but none could be compared in importance to the works of Kraepelin, Freud, Bleuler and Jaspers.

The same need for new ways is to be found in France. Henri Claude, the Professor of Psychiatry in Paris, and Gaetan de Clerambault continued the French clinical traditions whereas Eugene Minkowski developed a phenomenological psychopathology based on Bergson's philosophy. Henri Ey, a pupil of Henri Claude, began to build his 'organodynamic' psychiatry, based on the Darwinian model, as transmitted by Hughlings Jackson, whose main period of success would come later.

American psychiatry was still relatively unknown, although it had now reached maturity. In 1940 there were more than 2500 psychiatrists in the United States, an impressive number if compared with the situation in Europe. Psychiatry had become respectable with the creation of prestigious university departments at Johns Hopkins and Harvard. From 1934 on, the American Board of Psychiatry and Neurology controlled the quality of postgraduate teaching. Adolf Meyer's department was open to many influences. His laboratory of psychology was directed by John B. Watson, the father of behaviourism, and in 1930 W. Horsley Gantt introduced Pavlov's ideas into the Phipps Clinic. Although Meyer's 'psychobiology' was not so close to psychoanalysis as it is sometimes claimed, its general trends probably facilitated the acceptance of Freud's theories. Although many European psychoanalysts came to the United States after 1933, the growth of the new school had begun much earlier. Otto Rank came in 1924, and Sandor Rado, who organized the New York Psychoanalytic Institute on the Berlin model, in 1931. In 1931 Franz Alexander founded the Institute of Chicago and attracted Karin Horney. In 1939 the American psychoanalytic school felt strong enough to declare its independence from the International Psychoanalytic Association.

The period 1914–1945 marks a transition in general psychiatry, but a turning point in its biological aspects. For the first time somatic treatments with real efficacy in the most severe psychiatric disorders, namely the psychoses, appeared. Around 1900 about one-quarter of all admissions in the psychiatric hospitals were cases of general paralysis, a syphilitic dementia for which no treatment existed and which brought death in a few years. In 1917 Wagner von Jauregg, Professor in Vienna, discovered that by provoking high fever in the patient by the inoculation of malaria, the course of the disease could be stopped and eventually reversed. The impressive character of such results is difficult to realize today. At a time when mental diseases were generally considered as incurable, Wagner von Jauregg's discovery was hailed as a scientific revolution and he was awarded the Nobel prize, the only psychiatrist so honoured until now.

In 1932 the treatment of schizophrenia by insulin coma was proposed by Manfred Sakel in Vienna; in 1936 Metrazol shock was described by von Meduna, and finally just before the outbreak of the war, Cerletti and Bini in Rome introduced electroshock therapy, a method still used today as a treatment of severe depressive states. Around 1940, at a time when descriptive psychiatry was making efforts to propose new concepts but was unable to displace the fundamental ideas laid down by the preceding generation, the discovery of effective somatic therapies had convinced some psychiatrists that biology would open the way to an explanation of psychiatric illnesses. On the other hand, the rise of psychoanalysis testified to the faith of others that the doctrine of Freud would bring about an understanding of the mechanisms of the abnormalities of the mind.

With the end of the Second World War, the world situation changed radically and the new economic and political situation was reflected in the scientific scene. One of the obvious consequences is the place taken by the English language in scientific exchanges. Science, and especially medicine, have used in their history several languages for international communication: Greek in Antiquity continuing through the duration of the Roman Empire, later Arabic and finally Latin. From the eighteenth century on, with the advent of nationalism, no common scientific language was accepted any longer. French was then the language of culture and diplomacy but never recognized internationally as the instrument of scientific literature. After 1945, English, until then used outside its geographical frontiers mainly for business matters, became, through the influence of the United States, the international scientific idiom. I shall not discuss here the problems raised by such a situation but I want to mention it only as an expression of the new American influence which was immediately evident in psychiatry after 1945. I am not referring here to basic discoveries, such as those connected with psychopharmacology where the original contribution of the United States has been minimal, but to general trends starting from America and followed with some delay and local modifications all over the world.

The most obvious fact in post-war psychiatry has been the increase of the number of specialists. In the United States, the growth curve had been more or less constant until 1945. Then it changed abruptly. There are today more than 30 000 American psychiatrists, more than one-third of the world's total number, a factor of influence not to be lightly dismissed. The same trend can be recognized in the industrial countries but with enormous differences linked with economic development: one psychiatrist serves 6500 people in the United States, about 13 000 in Europe, 500 000 in the People's Republic of China and 17 million in Ethiopia.

Behind this development there appeared a change in public attitude, symbolized by the general adoption after 1945 of the concept of 'mental health'. The new interest in psychiatry can be best described by the succession of governmental measures taken in the United States. During the war, the Veterans' Administration had already started an ambitious treatment programme. In 1945 the National Mental Health Act was adopted, and 1949 saw the foundation of the National Institute of Mental Health. It has been said that 'by that time, with typical American enthusiasm and urge for action, the issue of mental illness was becoming national'. In February 1963 the well-known message to Congress was delivered by President Kennedy and a few months later the Community Mental Health Act was adopted. In most industrial countries, with local variations, the same changes took place: in the United Kingdom within the National Health Service; in France after 1950 with the transformation of the public psychiatric care. One can find an international expression of this trend in the elevation by the World Health Organization of its Section of Mental Health to the dignity of an autonomous division.

One of the most original aspects of the change has been the place taken by psychiatric research. The example set by the Munich Research Institute was followed after 1950. In 1973 the American National Institute of Mental Health had a budget of 112 million dollars for financing the Bethesda centres and other laboratories all over the country. The Medical Research Council in Great Britain, the Institut National de la Santé et de la Recherche Médicale, and the Academy Research Institutes in the socialist countries have created a system of psychiatric support, generally independent of the teaching functions of the universities. Although the connections between the care of patients, the pre- and postgraduate training of the psychiatrists and the research itself still raises many problems, the new structures testify to the widespread current faith that scientific progress in psychiatry can best be obtained by full-time specialists.

The most remarkable transformation occurring during the last decades in the general organization of psychiatry is, however, the radical change in the system of care. The role of hospitalizations, especially in the large mental hospitals located away from population centres, has everywhere been reduced, and in some countries drastically. Compulsory treatment has become much less common and the laws about commitment are now subject to discussion and revision. The opening of psychiatric wards in general hospitals, the extension of ambulatory treatment through dispensaries located near the homes of the patients, and the creation of special centres for rehabilitation to social life have become a common goal with the purpose of abolishing the former segregation of the mental patient, thereby giving him the possibility of better integration in the community. These trends, with national variants, have many origins. One is the necessity of answering the increasing requests for psychiatric care: in the United States 5% of the population has at least one psychiatric contact every year.

On the other hand, the ideas that had been advocated in 1911 by Adolf Meyer, the British tradition of social psychiatry, and the French and Italian movements against long-term hospitalization, to name but a few, have also played a role. These trends toward a better availability of psychiatric care irrespective of social class, and towards more tolerance to deviance have been decisively favoured by the therapeutic progress. It has also had a consequence: the increased participation by non-medical personnel in the care of mental patients. To take an example, the clinical psychologists have gradually occupied more and more important positions. In the United States, where there were only about 200 in 1945, there are now 20 000, two-thirds of the number of psychiatrists. They receive 40% of the research grants of the NIMH, against 19% to the psychiatrists. They play an important part in teaching, and many states in the United States give them the legal right of independent diagnostic and therapeutic private practice. The tensions arising from such a situation are not limited to the United States.

From a more general point of view, the end of the war marked the expansion of psychoanalysis. In 1945, symbolically, Sandor Rado became Professor at Columbia University and the Director of the first University Institute of Psycho-analysis. The movement spread first over American psychiatry, then, with of course different modalities, over the other national schools, with the exception of the socialist countries. Space does not permit an adequate description of the history of this evolution, of its institutional and social aspects, and of its impact on the practice of psychiatry. Suffice it to say that in a few years psychoanalysis gained such a prestige that it was often equated by the general public with psychiatry. In the 1960s a large number of the Heads of Departments of Psychiatry in the United States had been psychoanalytically trained. The only systematic opposition came from the USSR.

During the Cold War, psychoanalysis was formally condemned as an idealist and reactionary doctrine, and the work of Pavlov was presented as the only acceptable scientific basis of psychiatry, defined as the pathology of the higher nervous functions. However, both the United States and the USSR were in agree-ment on one point at that time: the absence of hereditary factors in the mental diseases. A causal role was attributed, either in the USSR to the imperfect social structure, or in the United States by many to faulty family relations in early infancy. In the latter country, it had as a consequence the opposition to the medical model. The only accepted perspective for this group was the comprehension of the psychodynamics of the individual case. The study of the symptoms and the classification of patients was of little interest. Such an extreme point of view was not accepted by all even in the United States, but it infiltrated into psychiatric thinking everywhere even if the practical necessities in the treatment of patients compelled the physicians to forget their theoretical attitudes sometimes.

It is a fact that, even during the period of dominance of psychoanalytic thinking, the biological orientation maintained its position thanks to its therapeutic efficacy. Insulin coma in schizophrenia, electric shock in depression were still in common use. The situation was, however, radically transformed by the discovery around 1953 of psychopharmacology. In a few years drugs appeared which were beneficial for the schizophrenic, depressive and anxiety disorders. The empirical discovery of these agents was the result of the joint efforts of pharmacologists and clinical psychiatrists, and it took place mostly in Europe: in France with the introduction of chlorpromazine by Delay and Deniker, in Switzerland with the work of Kuhn on the antidepressants, in Belgium and elsewhere. The initial scepticism was rapidly replaced by widespread use. Psychopharmacology has been largely responsible for changes in the organization of psychiatric practice. However, paradoxically, until the mid 1960s the growth of psychodynamic and environmentalist ideas continued in the United States. With a suddenness not uncommon in the movement of ideas in America, a change took place. Psycho-analysis lost its dominant position. Brain biochemistry, stimulated by psycho-pharmacology, and fortified by the discoveries of molecular biology, took a leading place in research. Genetics, after being discredited by its misuse in Nazi Germany, was also on the ascendancy, and the radical environmentalism of the 1950s was on the wane. The reversal of the trend was not only evident in the award of research grants by governmental organizations in most countries, but became apparent to the lay public. In 1979, the well-known American magazine *Time* published under the title 'Psychiatry on the Couch' an editorial analysing accurately the new situation.

The relative decline of psychodynamics left room in the clinical field for the resurgence of a movement of ancient origin, descriptive psychiatry, now rein-forced by the use of statistical methods. Since Galton had initiated their appli-cation to psychological phenomena, statistics had given birth to the tech-niques of mental testing, first introduced in practical psychiatric use by the French psychologist, Alfred Binet, in 1905. The trend towards an objective and communicable description of pathological symptoms, the availability of mathematical methods for treating the data gathered, and the development of computers were the background of a movement first stimulated by the necessities of therapeutic trials of the new drugs and also to some extent by the birth of psychiatric epidemiology. It is significant that Great Britain, thanks to her strong tradition here, took one of the first places. I need only to mention the English contributions to the dimensional description of personality, to the development of instruments for an objective appraisal of the symptomatology, which have become internationally recognized, and to the socio-epidemiological research combining the two elements of social and statistical tradition. The United States follows in its own way the same trend. The publication in early 1980 of the new official American classification of mental disorders crowns an evolution that began around 1965. It reflects some present basic ideas: a relative scepticism towards the former psychodynamic concepts, the adoption of a medical model and, in many respects, a return to the clinical descriptive perspective in vogue before the First World War.

This survey of the last hundred years of the history of psychiatry at first glance suggests an optimistic view of its future development. The increase of the number of psychiatrists, of their role within medicine, and of their therapeutic efficacy are obvious facts. One must not, however, remain blind to less comforting recent events. The so-called antipsychiatric movement, which a few years ago appeared under various forms in many countries, has been one of several expressions of a loss of prestige of psychiatry amongst physicians and general public alike. The paper published by *Time* Magazine in 1979 was not only a questioning of the value of psychoanalysis but also of psychiatry itself. Since 1967 the percentage of psychiatrists among physicians has ceased to increase in the United States and the proportion of students choosing psychiatry as their specialty has decreased from 12% to 3% today. In that country where its success has been the greatest one speaks today of a crisis and the loss of contact with the medical model during the years following the war is blamed.

'Remedicalization of psychiatry' is the current slogan in national and international meetings. It is of course too early to say if we are witnessing only a small and transient reversal on a continuous growing curve or if we are at the beginning of a downward trend. In the long run I am convinced that psychiatry will continue to progress. Divergent trends in the national schools, conflicting tendencies according to the theoretical orientations inside the same country are always and will always be present. They are a stimulant and their confrontation leads to new discoveries. For that reason it is necessary that each national school maintains its own tradition but, at the same time, integrates the progress made by the others. I have tried to show how with the passage of time different countries have led the way, but I firmly believe that each has and will have something to contribute to our knowledge. In the present world, even more than before, international cooperation is the prerequisite of scientific progress.

Methodology

Rating Scale Methods: Validity and Reliability

B.T. Kugler

Rating scales are used a great deal in psychiatry, yet psychiatrists are rarely psychometricians and may know relatively little about the rationale on which such methods of assessment are based. The present chapter hopes to convey something of that rationale as a background against which specific rating scales (regularly encountered in psychiatric journals!) can be evaluated. The exercise, if not overly exciting, is assuredly useful.

Measurement of Psychological Characteristics

Attempts to measure psychological characteristics stem from a desire to evaluate individuals by accurate description of attributes or qualities that are of relevance to a particular investigation. The evaluations made may be based on the results of tests appraising correct/incorrect performance, or on the results of assessment procedures for which no 'right' or 'wrong' answers exist. In the former case (encountered in testing specific aptitudes and cognitive processes) the definition of right and wrong is quite independent of both rater and ratee, although results may still not be free from bias. Evaluations in the latter case (and rating scales fall into this category) are largely based on observation and judgement.

As a result of this distinction, many of the technical, and much of the theoretical, bases of cognitive and aptitude testing procedures do not apply to this latter group of 'tests'. Nevertheless, there are some issues—notably those of validity, reliability and standardization—which apply to all measurement techniques. The question of *what* a test measures is the concern of validity; *how well* measurements are made is the concern of reliability. Interpretation of test scores is assisted by standardization.

Validity

Validity raises the question of whether a test measures the attribute it is *supposed* to measure. A test is valid to the extent that there is a high correlation (or degree of relationship) between it and the quality it is claimed to measure. The validity of a test must be expressed in relation to suitable external criteria. If the quality in question is neither directly observable nor universally understood (and there are disagreements as to what such terms as 'intelligence' and 'anxiety' mean), there are serious difficulties in test validation. Recourse is sometimes made to correlations with alternative or indirect indices of the quality. Thus, we might compare scores obtained on the Stanford–Binet with those obtained on the Wechsler Scale supposing both to measure intelligence. A high correlation will indicate that the two tests are measuring something similar but whether that something is 'intelligence' will remain an open question.

Distinctions have been made (e.g. Cronbach, 1960) between various types of validity, the most frequently differentiated being content validity, concurrent validity, predictive validity and construct validity. *Content* (or face) validity usually refers to whether the items of a test *look* as if they are relevant indicators of the quality the test is designed to measure and, as might be expected, the appropriateness of this form of validation in the context of psychological testing has been seriously questioned.

Concurrent and *predictive* (or criterion-related) validity both refer to comparisons between test scores and suitable criteria. For concurrent validation, both comparison measures are made at about the same time—a new test, designed to improve on and replace a former one measuring the same quality, might be validated in this way. In predictive validation, the test is used to predict some future outcome relating to scores on the test and actual outcome is compared with the prediction. Criterion measures, whether other tests or predicted outcomes, must be known to be valid if these procedures are to be meaningful. Chosen criteria need to be relevant, reliable and free from bias (Thorndike and Hagen, 1969)—a tall order for many psychological tests!

Construct validity presupposes that a test is derived from some theory which can be used to generate other testable hypotheses. The degree to which these hypotheses are confirmed—in conjunction with measures made by the test—reflects the validity of the test as an adequate index of the attribute with which the theory is concerned. In attempting to elucidate the meaning of a test, this form of validity is very important. If predicted hypotheses are *not* confirmed, the test, the theory, or both are invalidated.

Reliability

Not only should tests be valid, they should also be reliable. As measuring instruments, they should be accurate in the sense of producing consistent results whenever they are used (under the same conditions) to assess the same individuals. Two different aspects of consistency are subsumed under the term reliability. Cronbach (1960) distinguishes between the *stability* and the *internal consistency* of a test.

The stability of a test could be evaluated by repeatedly measuring the same individual and examining the distribution of the scores. Little variation between scores would indicate high reliability. It is more usual, however, to give the same test (or equivalent forms of it) to the same people on two occasions and correlate the scores. Such test–retest reliability procedures assess the extent to which the people tested maintain the same relation to one another on separate occasions. The actual scores each person obtains on the two occasions may well not remain the same but each person should do as well, *relative to the other people tested*, on the second occasion as on the first.

The performance of human beings is not stable as chance elements are introduced by factors such as memory, practice and guesswork and by 'good' and 'bad' days. If equivalent forms of the test (instead of the same test twice) are used to counter memory and practice effects, no matter how carefully items are 'matched' they will not be identical and some people may do better on one test than on the other.

People may, of course, change from one occasion to the next. Indeed, Fransella (1975) points out that high reliability may sometimes be nothing more than 'a measure of failure to reflect change'. While it is reasonable to expect relatively stable characteristics to give high reliability coefficients, a test measuring a change in symptoms could only be reliable, in this sense, if there had been *no* change.

If the items of a test are believed to be different indicators of the same underlying quality, then their summation will give a more reliable measure of that quality than can be given by any one item in itself. Internal consistency can be assessed by 'split-half' reliability. The test, in this case, is only given once but is later subdivided into two or more 'equivalent' parts which are correlated with each other. The subdivision may involve balancing items for content and difficulty or may be random. In this sense, reliability reflects the degree of homogeneity of the test items, the danger being that spuriously high reliabilities may be obtained if the test contains *redundant* items. A more sophisticated development of split-half reliability is the Kuder–Richardson procedure (Thorndike and Hagen, 1969) which, in giving the average coefficient which would be obtained if the items of the test were subdivided in *every* possible way, provides a conservative estimate of internal consistency.

Clearly, it is possible to be highly reliable in a method which has little validity. Nevertheless, reliability does set limits on validity. If a test is unreliable, it cannot be giving precise information about anything, so questions of *what* it is measuring are largely irrelevant.

Standardization

In dealing with *physical* measures, we are dealing with accepted and meaningful measuring instruments and units of measurement. Length, for example, is measured with a tape measure in inches which are equal and additive. Two inches *are* twice the size of one inch. 'Twice as long' is, therefore, a meaningful statement. How meaningful, however, is a statement such as 'twice as intelligent'?

The scores obtained in psychological measurement are *relative* and can be given meaning only by reference to other scores drawn from the general population or designated subgroups of it. Such systems of reference may allocate the person to a particular subgroup of similarly-scoring individuals in a series of subgroups ('mental age' assigns the child to an established level of performance in this way), or may place him along an ordered continuum of scores *within* a group.

Intelligence tests, for example, yield a spread of scores (IQs) in the general population from which we obtain an 'average' score and an index of the variation between scores (the standard deviation, SD) such that approximately two-thirds of the scores in the population fall between $+1$ SD and -1 SD from the average score. As the average IQ is nominally 100 and the SD is about 15, two-thirds of the population obtain IQs between 85 and 115. The results of subsequent intelligence tests can be referred to these 'norms' for interpretation. Clearly, the population on which we choose to standardize a test must be comparable to that on which the test is to be used in the future. The availability of suitable normative data against which further test results can be compared determines the degree of standardization of the test.

Rating Scale Methods

Validity, reliability and standardization, however, are all easier to establish for tests of specific aptitudes and cognitive processes than for rating scales based on judgement or observation. Rating scale methods have been widely used for assessing particular characteristics of people *and* objects and extensive coverage of this area can be found elsewhere (e.g. Cronbach, 1960; Guilford, 1954; Nunnally, 1967). Rating scale methods in psychiatry have been used to facilitate appraisals of self or others by providing the rater with statements or adjectives (which are quantifiable in some way) from which he can select those which most closely describe the ratee. Ratings may represent an individual as he sees himself (self-report), or as others see him (observer scales). In psychiatry, they might be concerned with the patient's behaviour ('signs' of the illness), the patient's complaints ('symptoms' of the illness), or both. Where patients are believed to be lacking in insight or in motivation, questions arise as to the value of self-report ratings. It has been suggested, for example, that 'patients sick enough to require hospitalization cannot be objective enough to do their own ratings' (Cutler and Kurland, 1961). Many ratings, nevertheless, are of *necessity* based on judgements and inferences drawn from what the patient says about himself in interviews with the rater.

In the 1950s, reviews of rating scales in psychiatry discussed around a dozen scales which had appeared in the previous decade (Lorr, 1954). The proliferation of such techniques over the years makes such a review in the 1990s unwieldy and, because there is still need for improvement in terms of the validation, reliability and standardization of available rating scales, impractical. The present discussion provides a context to which specific appraisals may be referred.

Rating scales differ in the ways in which they are constructed. Some rating scale methods involve the simple endorsement or rejection of a statement on an all-or-none basis (checklist methods), while others require the assignment of a number to a statement (numerical scales). Still other methods require the rater to make choices among carefully described alternatives (forced-choice methods). The Delusions–Symptoms–States Inventory (Foulds and Bedford, 1975) or DSSI, for example, is a self-report scale of the checklist variety and asks subjects to endorse statements which have 'recently' applied to them. Sample items are:

Worrying has kept me awake at night.
I have been quite unable to bring myself to go out alone.
I have felt I must tell the whole world of my brilliant ideas.
Someone else has been doing the thinking that goes on in my head.

The Nurses' Observation Scale for Inpatient Evaluation (NOSIE) (Honigfeld and Klett, 1965) illustrates numerical rating scales. The nurse is asked to estimate whether, over a specified period of time, various descriptions of a patient's behaviour were true:

0 Never
1 Sometimes
2 Often
3 Usually
4 Always

Sample items on which ratings are made by circling the correct number before each statement are:

0 1 2 3 4   Resists suggestions and requests.
0 1 2 3 4   Is cheerful and optimistic.
0 1 2 3 4   Sleeps, unless directed into activity.
0 1 2 3 4   Is alert and attentive.

The APQ, or Activity Preference Questionnaire (Lykken *et al.*, 1973), asks subjects to 'pretend' that one of two situations has to happen to them and to decide which alternative would be the 'lesser of evils'. Every item in the test has to be answered and the method is one of 'forced choice'. Sample items are as follows:

(a) Finding out people have been gossiping about you.
(b) Working all day in the hot sun.

(a) Having to stand up on the bus.
(b) Introducing yourself to a total stranger.

Rating scales have often been presented *graphically* and such presentation may serve to increase discrimination by asking for degree to be indicated by a mark anywhere along an unbroken line. Thus, an item from NOSIE, for example, may be represented as follows:

Is alert and attentive
NEVER ——————————— ALWAYS
0   1   2   3   4

There are indications, however, that graphic scales may have little to commend them (other than attractiveness and convenience) over the other methods of rating (Blumberg *et al.*, 1966).

Response categories (as opposed to statements acting as stimuli) usually refer to frequency or to severity/intensity. Items on NOSIE are rated on a five-point *frequency* continuum while items in the Brief Psychiatric Rating Scale or BPRS (Overall and Gorham, 1962) are rated on a *severity* continuum as follows:

MOTOR RETARDATION   Reduction in energy level evidenced in slowed movements. Rate on the basis of observed behaviour of the patient; do not rate on basis of patient's subjective impression of own energy level.

| NOT PRESENT | VERY MILD | MILD | MODERATE | MODERATELY SEVERE | SEVERE | EXTREMELY SEVERE |

The rater is asked to mark the term which best describes the patient's condition. Other scales—the HRS, or Hamilton Rating Scale for depression (Hamilton, 1960, 1967), for example—may not make clear distinctions between intensity and frequency.

Similarities and differences between various rating scale methods are apparent from the above examples. There are known difficulties with such techniques and, for a fuller discussion of these and further details of scale construction, the interested reader is referred to Guilford (1954). Some difficulties apply especially to self-report scales, others to observer scales and some to both.

A major source of difficulty lies in the descriptive statements which form the items of the scales. Bare trait names such as 'anxiety' are somewhat abstracted from observable behaviour and are open to different interpretations by different raters. Attempts should be made to make rated items as 'tangible' as possible with clear, relevant and precise definition or description. Unfortunately, replacing trait names in this way increases both the length and, to some extent, the intricacy of the scale. Some rating scales restrict themselves purely to observable behaviour but such a restriction in psychiatry might well preclude ratings of a large and relevant section of symptomatology. Ratings such as that of 'Motor Retardation' on the BPRS (which despite its construction for use by skilled psychiatrists does attempt to define concepts for standard use) depend on observable behaviour but ratings of other items on the same scale depend very much on the verbal report of the patient. The following item is given as an example of the latter:

ANXIETY   Worry, fear, or over-concern for present or future. Rate solely on the basis of verbal report of patient's own subjective experiences. Do not infer anxiety from physical signs or from neurotic defence mechanisms.

The response categories for the rating are identical to those given for 'Motor Retardation'.

The idea behind the BPRS was that each item should, in itself, represent a relatively discrete symptom area. Where *several* items are combined to tap one area, as in the previously mentioned DSSI, it is possible to phrase individual items in a more specific and limited way.

Not only are descriptive statements open to numerous different interpretations, but the response categories by which ratings are made are also open to variation in rater standards. One rater's idea of 'mild' may well be that of another's 'moderate'. While too few steps (limiting responses to 'always' and 'never', for example) may make ratings impossible, too many may overtax the rater's powers of discrimination. Unless the distinction between 'very mild' and 'mild' is clearly and explicitly made (and the BPRS provides a handbook which attempts exactly this), raters may use the two categories indiscriminately. Not only is response clarification necessary but, in most situations, 'end-categories' should not be defined so extremely as to be rarely used.

Some items may, by their nature, require more steps for appropriate rating than other items. The HRS, for example, rates items on either a five-point scale or a three-point one. Agitation is rated 0—absent; 1—slight/doubtful; or 2—clearly present. Retardation, on the other hand, is rated 0—absent; 1—mild/trivial (slight retardation at interview); 2—moderate (obvious retardation at interview); 3—moderate (interview difficult); or 4—severe (complete stupor).

Attempts to resolve the issue of 'how many steps?' have not been altogether successful although seven steps are reported as optimal for most purposes (Nunnally, 1967; Symonds, 1931). Whether it is preferable to have an odd or an even number of steps has also been a matter for debate. An odd number allows the incorporation of a 'neutral' step which may be used if, for whatever reason, the item does not apply to the ratee and without which the rater may either not rate the item at all or may rate incorrectly in the belief that all items must be rated. It is generally believed that a 'neutral' step introduces rater bias. Some raters prefer to tread a middle road, rating neither high nor low, and may, therefore, over-use a neutral category if it is available. However, other raters tend to make extreme ratings in any circumstances so rater bias exists no matter how many steps are supplied by the scale. This variability in the *raters*, which does appear to reflect rater characteristics (e.g. Klores, 1966) as opposed to chance factors or faulty scaling, makes comparisons between raters difficult.

Clearly, rater idiosyncrasies misrepresent ratings, lower reliability and cast doubts on validity. Various 'errors in ratings' have been identified (see Guilford, 1954), the major ones being (a) the leniency error, where there is a constant tendency to rate too high or too low; (b) the error of central tendency which, due to an unwillingness to make extreme ratings, displaces the ratee towards the mean of the total group; (c) the halo error where the tendency is to rate *all* specific qualities itemized in terms of the overall *general* impression the rater has formed of the ratee; (d) the logical error by which traits that 'go together' in the rater's mind are rated in similar ways; and (e) the contrast error which reflects the rater's tendency to rate on the assumption that 'everyone is different from me' or, conversely, that 'everyone is like me'.

Careful training of raters which explains the aims of the ratings and the sources of error, clarifies the ambiguities and allows for supervised practice (Anastasi, 1968) minimizes errors, as do techniques which allow one trait at a time to be rated for *all* ratees or for each trait to be rated on a separate page. If the raters are highly motivated and have had adequate opportunity to observe the qualities being rated, and if these qualities have been defined in a way that means the same thing to all the raters, it is possible to minimize errors still further.

Once rating scales have been completed, scoring systems range from simple summations of all rated items to more complicated methods of subscaling and weighting. With the BPRS, for example, it is possible to group items into thought disorder core symptoms, thought disorder associated symptoms, anxiety-depression core symptoms and anxiety-depression associated symptoms. It is also possible to weight items differentially according to the diagnostic group that is the subject of the investigation.

The validity of ratings

Most rating scales 'look' relevant and hence have high content or face validity. Self-assessment scales tend to have lower concurrent validity than observer scales possibly because skilled observers are trained in a 'standard' interpretation of item and response categories and because they are less likely to 'fake' ratings in an attempt to give a distorted impression (Hamilton, 1976a).

Scales which measure one dimension of psychiatric illness, such as the HRS, can be submitted to a factor or component analysis to test whether or not some such dimension *is* being measured and emerges as a general or common factor (e.g. Hamilton, 1967). Such techniques involve complicated matrices of correlations by which relationships among a group of variables may be assessed and the interested reader is referred to Cronbach (1960, Chapter 9) for further details.

It has been pointed out that, insofar as ratings are used to illustrate how someone appears to others, such scales are, by their nature, pertinent and 'the validity of ratings is axiomatic' (Thorndike and Hagen, 1969). However, ratings are mostly commonly employed for some kind of prediction and, in such situations, predictive validity can and should be assessed. Generalization is usually not warranted and the validity must be considered separately for each specific situation.

The fact remains that ratings are frequently used because there is simply no other way in which the information they provide can be obtained. In such cases, there is obviously nothing else against which ratings can be validated. As mentioned earlier, reliability in itself limits validity and 'errors in ratings' are not conducive to high reliability.

The reliability of ratings

Reliability, as applied to rating scales, is most commonly taken as a measure of agreement *between raters* rating the same people. Although the inter-rater reliability of certain scales can be favourable (reports for the HRS, for example, range from 0.88 to 0.98: Hamilton, 1976a), for most rating procedures they are not high. Generally, the average correlation between ratings made by pairs of independent raters has been reported to be in the region of 0.55 to 0.60 (Symonds, 1931).

Reliability coefficients can be improved, however, by pooling the *independent* ratings of a number of raters. Procedures such as the Spearman–Brown Prophecy Formula (Thorndike and Hagen, 1969) are used for estimating this type of reliability. If the reliability of one rater is already known, the formula can be used to estimate reliabilities for any number of raters. Taking the correlation coefficient quoted by Symonds as representative (and time has afforded scant reason for revising it), the reliability of five independent raters would be around 0.86. It is important, however, that the ratings *are* independent and that the raters are equally skilled and have equivalent knowledge and experience of the ratee. Reliability is improved in this way because individual rater idiosyncrasies are cancelled out in the process of pooling (Remmers *et al.*, 1927). Unfortunately, however, large numbers of equally skilled raters are not often available when ratings are being made.

Test-retest reliabilities of rating scales in psychiatry are of little use as the scales are most commonly designed to measure *change*. Split-half reliability is also problematical. The items of a scale such as the HRS should indeed correlate among themselves because they are all measuring depression. The items of the BPRS or the DSSI, on the other hand, either represent discrete symptom areas or do so in particular item combinations. For scales such as the BPRS, estimates of inter-rater reliability are given separately for each item and split-half reliability estimates would have little meaning.

Types of Rating Scale in Psychiatry

One reason for the proliferation of rating scales in psychiatry lies in dissatisfaction with the free-ranging interview as *the* method of assessment in psychiatry. Factors such as style-of-interviewing and conceptual differences between psychiatrists have led to low reliability estimates (e.g. Beck, 1962; Kreitman *et al.*, 1961) and predictive validity studies have been rare (Marzillier, 1976). Structured interview techniques and rating scales were developed, therefore, to ensure that the same range of topics would be covered whenever patients were assessed and that the information obtained would be recorded in standard ways (Kendell, 1975). This would then allow comparison between different patients and between the same patients on different occasions, thus facilitating comparison and combination of research results from different studies.

Four main types of rating scale have been used in psychiatry although such use has been in research rather than day-to-day clinical practice (Garside, 1976; Hamilton, 1976b). The four types are: (1) differential or discriminatory scales for diagnosis and classification; (2) intensity or descriptive scales for assessing the severity of illness; (3) prognostic scales predicting the course and outcome of the illness; and (4) selection scales for predicting outcome as a result of a specific treatment.

The DSSI is a differential scale which attempts to discriminate between twelve putative clinical syndromes. As these syndromes do not stand in direct correspondence to diagnostic categories, attempts at validation against clinical ratings rather than diagnosis have been made (Bedford and Foulds, 1977). Results have been only tentative.

Psychiatry lacks technical aids to diagnosis but the development of the Present State Examination (Wing *et al.*, 1974) as a structured method of assessment has shown that the 'symptoms' of mental illness can be reliably recognized by trained psychiatrists and that rules can be formulated with sufficient precision for patients with particular symptom clusters to be reliably classified. Although usually referred to as an interview technique rather than a 'rating scale', the PSE has much in common with certain rating scale methods. The presence and extent of symptomatology is elicited by structured, predetermined questioning at interview (although without a total loss of flexibility) and is rated in a standard way which later translates (via the Catego computer programme) into a diagnosis. The interview setting is akin to that for completion of the BPRS and, in fact, the PSE procedure is considerably more structured than the BPRS. The ensuing improvement in reliability (possibly due to the arduous training of 'raters' both in the interpretation of terms used and in the use of appropriate response categories) over that of free-ranging interviews has been salutary.

Reliability of diagnosis is crucially important in the general validation of rating scales in psychiatry. Because of difficulties in finding suitable criteria against which rating scales may be evaluated, one way of determining validity is to use the scale on groups of people who are *known* to differ in the quality tested and to show that the scale can indeed differentiate between the scores of the different groups (Hamilton, 1976a). Thus, scales that rate depression should clearly discriminate between depressed patients and 'normals' *if* reliable criteria have separated these groups in the first place. Thus far, attempts to validate scales of depression in this way have been made against clinical judgement (Hamilton, 1976a).

Descriptive or intensity scales are the most frequently used in psychiatry, particularly in the assessment of change during clinical trials. The BPRS is a scale specifically designed for this purpose and has been widely used in this way (e.g. Gorham and Pokorny, 1964; Overall *et al.*, 1964; Yorkston *et al.*, 1981). Sensitivity to change such that changes in scores on the rating scale accurately mirror changes in symptomatology is an important consideration here and the validity of such tests is measured by the precision with which different scores reliably represent different levels of severity of illness (Hamilton, 1976a). Diagnoses are invariably made before such scales are used and need to be valid if the ratings made in the course of the trial are to be useful.

Prognostic and selection scales are predictive and, in the light of the increasing variety of possible treatment procedures, are of potential importance in determining the 'best' treatment for a particular patient. Although diagnosis itself has obvious implications for treatment, patients with a shared diagnosis do not always respond similarly to the same treatments. Scales predicting outcome after ECT (Carney *et al.*, 1965) and after treatment with imipramine (Kiloh *et al.*, 1962) in depression are concerned with clarification of this issue. It has been pointed out that, if rating scales are to supplement diagnosis in determining treatment choice, separate rating scales for each available treatment would be needed (Garside, 1976). The practicality of such an undertaking—in development *and* administration—raises the question of whether the potential of such rating scale methods can ever be realized.

Rating scales have proved problematical as reliable and valid methods of assessment but, in the absence of alternative standardized and objective techniques, do provide useful information. The construction of *useful* scales, standardized on appropriate patient populations, is very much dependent on an appropriate body of theory. On the other hand, reliable and sensible *use* of ratings may, despite the slight circularity of the argument, actually help to elucidate theoretical controversies in psychiatry.

References

Anastasi, A. (1968). *Psychological Testing*, 3rd edn. London: Macmillan.

Beck, A.T. (1962). Reliability of psychiatric diagnoses. I. Critique of systematic studies. *Am. J. Psychiat.* **119**, 210–216.

Bedford, A. and Foulds, G.A. (1977). Validation of the Delusions–Symptoms–States Inventory. *Br. J. Med. Psychol.* **50**, 163–171.

Blumberg, H.H., De Soto, C.B. and Kuethe, J.L. (1966). Evaluation of rating scale formats. *Personn. Psychol.* **19**, 243–260.

Carney, M.W.P., Roth, M. and Garside, R.F. (1965). The diagnosis of depressive syndromes and the prediction of ECT response. *Br. J. Psychiat.* **111**, 659–674.

Cronbach, L.J. (1960). *Essentials of Psychological Testing.* New York: Harper & Row.

Cutler, R.P. and Kurland, H.D. (1961). Clinical quantification of depressive reactions. *Arch. Gen. Psychiat.* **5**, 280–285.

Foulds, G.A. and Bedford, A. (1975). Hierarchy of classes of personal illness. *Psychol. Med.* **5**, 181–192.

Fransella, F. (1975). Studying the individual. In: P. Sainsbury and N. Kreitman (eds) *Methods of Psychiatric Research*, 2nd edn. Oxford: University Press.

Garside, R.F. (1976). The comparative value of types of rating scale. *Br. J. Clin. Pharmacol. Suppl.*, 61–67.

Gorham, D.R. and Pokorny, A.D. (1964). Effects of a phenothiazine and/or group psychotherapy with schizophrenics. *Dis. Nerv. Syst.* **25**, 77–86.

Guilford, J.P. (1954). *Psychometric Methods*, 2nd edn. New York: McGraw-Hill.

Hamilton, M. (1960). A rating scale for depression. *J. Neurol. Neurosurg. Psychiat.* **23**, 56–62.

Hamilton, M. (1967). Development of a rating scale for primary depressive illness. *Br. J. Soc. Clin. Psychol.* **6**, 278–296.

Hamilton, M. (1976a). Comparative value of rating scales. *Br. J. Clin. Pharmacol. Suppl.*, 58–60.

Hamilton, M. (1976b). Editorial: The role of rating scales in psychiatry. *Psychol. Med.* **6**, 347–349.

Honigfeld, G. and Klett, C.J. (1965). The Nurses' Observation Scale for Inpatient Evaluation. A new scale for measuring improvement in chronic schizophrenia. *J. Clin. Psychol.* **21**, 65–71.

Kendell, R.E. (1975). Defining diagnostic criteria for research purposes. In: P. Sainsbury and N. Kreitman (eds) *Methods of Psychiatric Research*, 2nd edn. Oxford: University Press.

Kiloh, L.G., Ball, J.R.B. and Garside, R.F. (1962). Diagnostic factors in treatment of depressive states with imipramine. *Br. Med. J.* **i**, 1225–1227.

Klores, M.S. (1966). Rater bias in forced-distribution performance ratings. *Personn. Psychol.* **19**, 411–421.

Kreitman, N., Sainsbury, P., Morissey, J., Towers, J. and Scrivener, J. (1961). The reliability of psychiatric assessment: an analysis. *J. Ment. Sci.* **107**, 887–908.

Lorr, M. (1954). Rating scales and check lists for the evaluation of psychopathology. *Psychol. Bull.* **51**, 119–127.

Lykken, D.T., Tellegen, A. and Katzenmeyer, C. (1973). *Manual for the Activity Preference Questionnaire (APQ)*. Reports from the Research Laboratories of the Department of Psychiatry, University of Minnesota, Report Number PR-73-4.

Marzillier, J.S. (1976). Interviewing. In: H.J. Eysenck and G.D. Wilson (eds) *A Textbook of Human Psychology*. Lancaster: MTP Press.

Nunnally, J.C. (1967). *Psychometric Theory*. New York: McGraw-Hill.

Overall, J.E. and Gorham, D.R. (1962). The Brief Psychiatric Rating Scale. *Psychol. Rep.* **10**, 799–812.

Overall, J.E., Hollister, L.E., Meyer, F., Kimbell, I. and Shelton, J. (1964). Imipramine and thioridazine in depressed and schizophrenic patients. *J. Am. Med. Ass.* **189**, 605–608.

Remmers, H.H., Shock, N.W. and Kelly, E.L. (1927). An empirical study of the validity of the Spearman–Brown formula as applied to the Purdue Rating Scale. *J. Ed. Psychol.* **18**, 187–195.

Symonds, P.M. (1931). *Diagnosing Personality and Conduct*. New York: Century.

Thorndike, R.L. and Hagen, E. (1969). *Measurement and Evaluation in Psychology and Education*, 3rd edn. New York: Wiley.

Wing, J.K., Cooper, J.E. and Sartorius, N. (1974). *The Measurement and Classification of Psychiatric Symptoms*. Cambridge: University Press.

Yorkston, N.J., Zaki, S.A., Weller, M.P., Gruzelier, J.H. and Hirsch, S.R. (1981). DL-Propranolol and chlorpromazine following admission for schizophrenia. *Acta Psychiat. Scand.* **63**, 13–27.

The Rationale of Clinical Trials

S.R. Hirsch

This chapter describes the organization and rationale of clinical trials. It is intended as a guide for those who wish to plan a research study, and for clinicians who should be able to evaluate critically research reports in scientific journals. The chapter will deal with basic concepts and definitions to enable the reader to gain an understanding of the rationale behind such procedures as randomizing, double-blind techniques, independent assessments, etc., and to provide some basic standards by which he or she can judge research reports. The chapter is not intended to be an extensive exposition of research methodology but is rather an introduction to it.

Aims of the Research

The touchstone of any research is a clear definition of its aim. What is to be achieved, and for what purpose? When one is able to say 'the study is being carried out *in order to* . . .', one has gone a long way to clarifying the aim. The selection of subjects, the methods to be used, the way the results are to be analysed, etc., should all be seen as a function of why the research is being carried out. When one is only able to say that the study is being done 'to look at . . .' or 'to see a relationship between a and b', the aim has in all probability not been sufficiently clarified. This should be obvious but the pressure to 'publish or perish' is so strong that this basic point is often lost sight of.

Background

A statement of the background which has led up to the research is a most useful starting point. It should include a survey of the previous literature relevant to the research, with particular emphasis on those studies which bear on the present aims. The previous work which sets the background for the current study and indicates why it is being done is particularly important.

Hypotheses

Having formulated the general purpose of the study, it is helpful to state the specific hypotheses which the research sets out to test, and go on in the analysis section of the protocol to indicate how the methodology will be analysed to test the hypotheses. If the hypotheses can be formulated in advance of the research, particularly if one is able to make a prediction which can be tested, then the importance of one's findings is strengthened. Discoveries made in the course of the research or at the time of the analysis of the results are not true results in the sense that they do not test hypotheses which have been formulated before. They are useful because they generate new questions and possibly new hypotheses but conclusions can only be drawn if a further study is mounted to test and confirm them.

Key Variables—Independent and Dependent

It is sometimes useful to identify the independent variable or variables which are operating in the study. These are factors which act independently to have an effect on other factors, called dependent variables, which are expected to vary or be affected by the action of the independent variables. The most important independent variable is of course the experimental one which is under study. For example, chlorpromazine treatment would be an independent variable if the experimenter wished to alter its presence, absence, or the strength of the dose, in order to see the effects on dependent variables such as the patient's symptoms, or side effects. Other independent variables may or may not be identifiable but are almost certainly present. For example the patient's age, sex, body weight, liver function, or environmental factors are all independent factors which could have an effect on such dependent variables as symptoms and side effects.

The purpose of modern research methodology is to control the effects of all independent variables other than the experimental one under study. The assumption is that if there is only one independent variable which changes under different conditions, then any change which is observed must be due to the change in the independent variable. Thus if the patients can be divided into three truly identical groups and each is given a different treatment, A, B or C, any difference between the groups subsequently noted in their condition must be due to the difference in the treatments A, B or C which were independently varied. In practice, one of the difficulties is in controlling the infinite number of other ways the groups could vary and this is the object of a controlled trial.

Definitions

In setting out the aims of the study and identifying the main variables under consideration, a number of operational concepts will have been mentioned which require definition for the sake of clarity and precision, particularly if the terms do not have a universally accepted use. For example, a study of the prevalence of alcoholism and 'at risk drinking' in the brewery industry requires a clear definition of the terms 'alcoholism' and 'at risk drinking'. Thus, for such a purpose 'alcoholism' might be operationally defined in terms of the signs and symptoms of physical dependence following withdrawal, such as tremor, hallucinations and delusions, and/or a strong physical craving for drink. 'At risk drinking' might be defined as imbibing on average 70 units of alcohol per week in a man or 35 units in a woman, one unit being equivalent to a glass of wine, or a single pub measure of whisky or other spirit.

Similarly, diagnostic concepts such as the diagnosis of schizophrenia or manic depression, should be operationally defined as well. An operational definition is one which indicates the operation one must carry out to establish the presence or absence of something, and in this case establishing the criteria for diagnosis. Various criteria are available to operationally define schizophrenia such as the CATEGO computerized rules used by the MRC Social Psychiatry Unit, the DSM-III United States Diagnostic Manual, the Feighner Criteria, or the Research Diagnostic Criteria of Spitzer, to name a few examples. However, each definition identifies a somewhat different group of individuals, and excludes others. One states the operational rules for defining concepts to be used in the research so others can know exactly what is meant and can, if necessary, repeat the experiment themselves. This is very important if others are going to be able to repeat the results. A trial which shows that drugs are useful to treat depression or that counselling is useful for school phobia is of little use if it does not inform the reader of the necessary information about the drug and its dose, or adequately describe the kind of counselling and which patients are suitable for which treatment. Unfortunately, papers are still being submitted to journals and sometimes published which do not provide such basic information as is necessary for the results to be useful.

Why Establish a Protocol?

This is extremely helpful to the research worker who wishes to work out in advance how he will go about his work and identify many of the snags beforehand which might be difficult to rectify if left till later. For example, having decided to use the Feighner Criteria to diagnose schizophrenia, when setting these down one will realize that first admission schizophrenics will be excluded from the study because the Feighner Criteria require that the symptoms of schizophrenia have been present for at least six months.

Methods

The rest of the chapter deals with the methodology, analysis and interpretation of results. Remember that the prime test of each step along the way is whether the methods which have been chosen help to achieve the aim and test the hypotheses that were established ahead of time. If not, they must be changed accordingly. If one wished to ask whether benzodiazepines as used by general practitioners are effective, one must ask 'effective for what?'. There is a difference between a study of benzodiazepines for anxiety state and presenting for minor emotional upsets. The criteria for entry into this trial would be different and depend on the question to be answered.

Choice of Subjects

It follows from the above that one must first of all choose selection criteria with the overall aim of the project clearly in mind. Clear selection criteria enable the reader to appreciate the applicability of the result to his patients. In order to avoid bias in the selection of the subject, it is often useful to choose an epidemiologically-based population from which to draw a sample. Thus a study of the efficacy of depot neuroleptics as maintenance medication for chronic schizophrenics would yield a better measure of its overall effectiveness if the sample consisted of all the patients from a given geographical population for whom the treatment is relevant. A sample of patients from a teaching hospital practice which has a special interest in schizophrenia would include a bias; a non-representative population. It could test the efficacy of the drug in the patients but it would be difficult to generalize from their experience because the patients could be unusually difficult, or include a disproportionate number of mild cases, depending on the rating of the practice. If the practice specialized in difficult, tertiary referrals, the treatment response could appear to be worse than it would in an epidemiologically-based catchment area sample.

When the number of potential cases is small a total sample chosen consecutively as they arise helps to avoid a selection bias. When the number of potential cases is large, one must take a randomly selected subsample in order to have as representative a subsample as possible and avoid including excessive numbers with either a good or a poor prognosis.

Sometimes it is important to control for other independent variables such as whether the patients are employed or at home during the day, or whether they are old or young. A stratified sample allows for pre-selection of the required numbers of patients for each subgroup according to certain criteria, e.g. whether patients are older or younger than 65. One then attempts to select a representative unbiased group of patients from within each of these subgroups.

How Many Patients Are Required?
Tests of Significance and Power

Enough subjects must be included in any experiment to achieve a definitive result. The number depends on the purpose of the study. If, for example, one wishes to compare the effectiveness of two treatments, one needs to decide ahead of time the magnitude of the difference one wants to detect between the treatments. To detect small differences and show they are statistically significant one needs very large numbers. To detect large differences the numbers can be small. One must choose a sufficient number of subjects to be sure that it is possible to show that if a critical minimal difference between treatments turns up in the result, the statistical evaluation will be able to demonstrate that it could not have occurred merely as a matter of chance.

The calculation to estimate this is called 'power analysis'. For example, if one is comparing a new antidepressant with an old one it may be decided that it is important not to overlook a difference between the two treatments as small as 15%. Tables can be consulted (Paulson and Wallis, 1947) to determine the number of patients required in each of the two groups for a difference between two treatments of 15% to occur by chance less than 5% of the time—'statistically significant at the 5% level'.

The tables show that one would need at least 73 subjects in each group for a difference of 15% to be significant at the 5% level if say 70% of one group showed improvement compared to 85% in another (chi-square test). According to the tables if there were 70 patients in each group instead of 73 and 85% improved on treatment A while 70% improved on treatment B, the difference would *not* be significant; it could occur by chance more than 5 times out of 100. This does not of course mean that the 15% difference between the two treatments would then not be a real one, but only that it could be shown statistically to be a chance result. When there is a real difference between treatments which is missed because the groups are too small, a 'type 2' error has occurred.

Type 2 errors are the most common errors in clinical research literature. This is where the study fails through inadequate design to demonstrate a statistically significant effect which does in reality exist. They arise when an effective treatment is compared to a possibly less effective one using samples that are too small to detect the difference. One is unable to detect the difference because the variation in scores within the groups (within-group variance) is greater than the difference between the groups. Using small numbers of subjects many experimenters fail to find a statistically significant difference between, say, a new antidepressant and a well-established one, and falsely conclude that the two are equal in effectiveness when actually the sample sizes are too small to be able to detect differences between treatments.

Equally, one does not wish to choose samples which are much larger than is necessary, as it is important to minimize the number of subjects involved in any experiment. If one wishes to test whether a new antipsychotic agent is pharmacologically more active for acute schizophrenics than placebo, one may only be interested if the response rate on the neuroleptic is at least 75%, as compared to an expected placebo improvement of say 25% over three weeks. Tables would reveal that if there are twelve subjects in each group, one group showing 75% improvement and the other 25%, this would be statistically significant (unlikely to occur by chance) in less than 5% of cases. If one had only ten subjects in each group, such a difference could occur by chance in more than 5% of trials. Thus, it would be false to conclude that a difference between two groups of 50% is significant if the two groups were smaller than 11. To regard a difference as significant when in fact it is not, is called a 'type 1' error. This is the error usually tested in clinical trials in order to avoid falsely concluding that a result is significant when it is not.

Strictly speaking, to exclude type 1 errors, one is testing the significance of *differences* observed in order to see that they could not have occurred by chance. When one is testing for a type 2 error, one is using the test of 'power' to determine that the equivalence of two treatments is unlikely to be merely a matter of chance at, say, the 95% confidence level.

Power analysis is fairly straightforward and can in most cases be performed on a pocket calculator. It is increasingly recognized as a crucial part of any research design aiming to compare an experimental group with a control group with regard to a particular dependent variable. This variable is usually a measure of outcome or improvement in the case of clinical trials. First, it is necessary to look at one's proposed outcome variable: is it categorical (a yes/no type measure) or is it continuous (a graded measurement such as a depression score)? The methods of calculating power differ slightly for the two sorts of variables because the statistical tests used to deal with categorical data (non-parametric tests such as chi-square) differ from those used with continuous data (parametric tests such as a t-test of means). In each case you will need to enter into the calculation an estimate of the size of the difference you are likely to be producing (with standard deviations, in the case of continuous data). You will also need to enter the level of statistical significance you want to see in your results (usually set at $p = 0.05$), as well as the level of confidence you want to have that your study is big enough. In other words, setting the confidence value at 0.80 means you wish to be at least 80% confident that your planned study will show a statistically significant difference, if a difference does in reality exist. The equations for calculating sample size in a power analysis are easy to follow and the reader is referred to Pocock (1983) or Altman (1980). The latter article gives a simple graphical nomogram to simplify things further.

Thus, in order to determine how many patients in each group are necessary for a clinical trial, one must decide what response rate is expected for each treatment, and how large a difference would be wanted to be detected as significant and not missed. It is wise to consult a statistician for advice before embarking on a clinical trial. When assessing reports in journals, look for the test of significance differences if the results say the outcome of the two treatments is different. Look for the tests of power if the results claim they are not different. The latter is unfortunately rarely reported.

Selection of Subjects

This is perhaps the most important variable. Leff (1973) was the first to illustrate from published clinical trial data that the factors which determine which patients are chosen for a clinical trial can be more important in determining whether a group has a good or poor outcome than the actual treatment itself. In a previous study (Leff and Wing, 1971) of the value of oral phenothiazines used to prevent relapse in schizophrenic patients from the time they left hospital, Leff and Wing demonstrated a significant advantage of active medication over placebo; 35% of patients on medication relapsed compared to 80% on placebo. However when they looked at the outcome for the patients whom the consultants would not allow into the trial, which comprised 70% of admissions, they found an opposite result. There were 40 patients to whom the consultants insisted on giving medication, and 37 patients for whom medication was not prescribed or the patient refused to take it. There were 4 patients lost to follow-up.

Examining the outcome for all patients who had had active medication 69% relapsed, while only 47% of patients who did not have active medication relapsed. This suggests that medication was more strongly associated with the relapse than no treatment! The association, though correct, is spurious. The critical variable is not medication but the fact that those who received medication had not been allowed into the trial because they were a poor prognosis group, and those who did not receive medication had not received it because they were a good prognosis group. Leff concluded that the medication offers protective advantage for the middle group who were not bound to relapse but were still at risk if they did not have medication and went on to illustrate how the same principle applies to other trials including maintenance medication for depression.

Criteria for Selection of Subjects

It is important that these are spelled out so that anyone interpreting the results of the trial is able to know the type of patient selected and therefore to whom the results can be applied clinically. Thus diagnostic criteria, age, sex, and reason for excluding certain groups, such as drug addiction, physical illness, etc., all need to be specified. Patients extraneous to the aims of the trial are of course excluded. To include patients with, for example, psychotic depression in a trial for a new drug, thought to be useful for schizophrenia, would only confuse the interpretation of results.

Procedures for Avoiding Bias

The need to routinely employ procedures to avoid factors which may bias the outcome of the trial is summed up in the phrase 'randomized double-blind placebo controlled trial'. Such trials embody procedures to avoid bias in the selection of patients and the evaluation of the effects of treatment. The individual components of these procedures require definition and explanation:

Matching

Matching is done prospectively when one wishes to exclude the effect of a specific known independent variable which might have an effect on the outcome. In a trial of psychotherapy, for example, one might wish to exclude the effect of the sex of the patient by separately allocating males and females to the randomization procedure in order to ensure that equal numbers of each are separately allocated to experimental and control treatment. Thus matching removes the effect of an anticipated specific variable by seeing that it occurs equally in both treatment groups.

Randomization

Randomization removes the effect of any unspecific and unidentifiable variables on the result. It is assumed that if the patients are randomly assigned to treatments, any unspecified variables will have an equal chance of occurring in each of the treatment groups. In this way all variables not accounted for in other ways, such as diet, weight, exercise, occurrence of life-events, living situation, employment, etc., will be accounted for on the basis that they will occur equally in all groups by random chance. However, it is normal practice to check the analysis of the result to see whether any variables considered to be possibly important did in fact occur equally in all groups. When by chance this is not the case, the effect of the experimental variable on differences which were present at the beginning of the trial can sometimes be accounted for statistically when analysing the results by cross-tabulation or analysis of covariance. Advice on these and other statistical techniques can be sought elsewhere.

Blind procedures

This implies that the patient is kept unaware of which treatment he or she is having so that the patient's prejudice in favour of or against the treatment will not influence either his or her willingness to continue with the treatment or any of the dependent variables being studied, such as his or her symptoms, level of activity, recovery rate, or whatever.

Double-blind procedure

This refers to the fact that everyone treating the patient is also kept ignorant of the true nature of the treatment being given to any particular patient. This is done in order to avoid any difference in handling the patient, or administering the treatments which could occur as a result of bias towards the treatment or assessment of the treatment's effect. In practice it is often difficult to keep patients and/or the doctors completely blind because of the side effects of treatment. An additional safeguard is to use a completely independent observer who has no knowledge of the patient's treatment or side effects to make the ratings.

Placebos

Placebos offer a number of advantages, not all of which are always appreciated. By including a placebo, or inactive dummy treatment, one is able to get a measure of the response of the patient to the psychological aspects of being treated—the so-called 'placebo response'. The difference between the placebo response and the response to active medication gives a measure of the specific treatment effect of the active drug. However, the response to the placebo medication is not just response to the psychological aspects of the treatment, such as the colour of the tablets and the doctor–patient relationship, but also to all the unspecified aspects of the treatment programme, such as the patient's faith in the doctor, nursing care, diet, the season of the year, etc., which might be influencing the result. Thus the difference between the response to the experimental treatment and the placebo is a useful indicator of the specific treatment effect.

The placebo response is strictly speaking a measure of the psychological effects of the effect of being treated, as opposed to a measure of the response of patients who have had no treatment whatsoever. The difference in the response to no treatment and to having placebo gives an indication of the placebo effect; this in turn is a measure of all the specific and unspecific aspects of being treated except the specific pharmacological action of the drug under test.

In psychiatry at least 20% of schizophrenics and manic-depressives respond to hospitalization alone over a period of a month. Given sufficient time it is said that over 60% of patients with affective illness will significantly improve without medication. Another 10–20% show very poor response to any treatment, particularly in the short run. Though difficult in practice, any trial of a new medication for schizophrenia or depression should ideally also include, for comparison, a group of patients taking standard medication to see if the subjects chosen have any potential to respond. In general, it can be said that the problem in clinical trials is to generalize from the results of the small sample under test. A placebo group gives a measure of the response to non-specific factors, and a standard treatment group indicates the extent to which the patients under test are responsive to treatment. The experimental treatment should ideally be compared with both to show that improvement is not just a placebo effect and to compare the treatment to established alternatives.

Treatment regime

It is important to choose a treatment regime which is suited to answer the question posed by the study. A fixed dose study might be desirable if one is studying dose–response relationships but giving a clinician freedom to choose the best dose for the patient would be a better test of a drug used in outpatients, because under these conditions it is best to test what actually takes place in clinical practice.

Rating scales and measuring instruments

Be sure that the rating scale is not just chosen because it is one commonly used but that it is the one that actually serves the purpose of the study. The problems of rating instruments are discussed elsewhere (see Chapter 10).

Assuming that the validity of the instrument or its ability to serve the purpose for which it is employed has already been proven elsewhere, then the experimenter should ensure that the instrument is reliable in the hands of the research workers carrying out the study. Advice on how to establish reliability should be sought elsewhere.

Results

It is not the aim of this chapter to discuss the statistical aspects of research but certain points on type 1 and type 2 errors are discussed in an earlier section. Results should be reported honestly and where possible confined to those tests and analyses which were planned in advance. Serendipitous results should be reported as such because their statistical validity may be in doubt, though they may prove to be important for establishing the basis of future research.

Where possible, the author should try to consider all the alternative explanations which could equally lead to the same result. Where it is possible to dispose of these by argument or further analysis, by all means do so. However, almost no research design can meet every possible criticism. It is far better to be aware of the shortcomings of one's work and set them out so that oneself or future workers can avoid them in the future. This is the way progress is made. There is no excuse for making interpretations on non-statistically valid trends or trying to construct long-winded implications for one's results, particularly if they have not gone in the direction anticipated. Honesty, clarity and self-criticism are the hallmarks of a good research report. There is no room for rationalization but succinct interpretations and recommendations for further work are always appreciated. A sign of a bad paper is one which provides conclusions in the summary for which there is no factual basis in the data reported.

References

Altman, D.G. (1980). Statistics and ethics in medical research: how large a sample? *Br. Med. J.* **281**, 1336–1338.

Leff, J.P. (1973). The influence of selection of patients on results of clinical trials. *Br. Med. J.* **4**, 156–158.

Leff, J.P. and Wing, J.K. (1971). Trial of maintenance therapy in schizophrenia. *Br. Med. J.* **iii**, 599–604.

Paulson, E. and Wallis, W.A. (1947). *Selected Techniques of Statistical Analysis.* New York: McGraw-Hill.

Pocock, S.J. (1983). *Clinical Trials: A Practical Approach.* Chichester: John Wiley.

For further reading on methodology of clinical trials in psychiatry, covering statistical and methodological issues see:

Hirsch, S.R. and MacRae, K.D. (1986). Essential elements in the design of clinical trials. In: *The Psychopharmacology and Treatment of Schizophrenia*, Ch. 8. Oxford: Oxford University Press.

— 5

Statistics in Psychiatric Research

K.D. MacRae

Introduction

Three quite distinct areas of knowledge or expertise can be distinguished when the use of statistics in medical research is considered. First, there is the question of why we use statistics—what questions are addressed by a statistical analysis and what do the answers mean. Second, there is the matter of deciding which type of analysis to apply to the study data—i.e. choosing the 'correct' statistical method. Third, there is the issue of how to perform the calculations involved in carrying out the 'correct' analysis.

Fortunately, the last of these three sorts of expertise no longer requires the user of statistics to work through the various formulae in detail—whether to do so or not is now largely a matter of taste. In practice, the execution of a statistical analysis nowadays is a matter of being able to use a suitable computer statistical 'package'. The practical knowledge needed consists of knowing the instructions needed to make the computer perform the calculations, rather than a knowledge of how the calculations are performed. Widely used statistical 'packages' include the Statistical Package for the Social Sciences (SPSS), the Statistical Analysis System (SAS) and Biomedical Data Processing (BMD). All three of these exist in versions that can be run on a personal computer (PC). A relatively recent development is the publishing of a set of computer programs (on a computer-readable disc) to accompany a statistics textbook—such as the Confidence Interval Analysis (CIA) programs that accompany Gardner and Altman (1989) and the set of programs that can perform the analyses described in Tallirada and Murray (1987). Therefore, computational details will not be given a great deal of prominence in what follows, although important and relatively simple calculations will be demonstrated whenever they help understanding. Instead, the intention is to explain the rationale for the use of statistics, the interpretation of the results of a statistical analysis, and the choice of appropriate methods of analysis.

However, before the discussion of statistics can begin, it is necessary to consider first what sorts of data might be obtained in a study. From a statistical viewpoint, data can be classified as belonging to a particular scale of measurement. It is essential to consider the scale of measurement of the data to be obtained in a study in calculating how large the study needs to be, and also in choosing the methods to be used in analysing the results when the study is complete. The following section will therefore consider measurement.

Measurement

In order to study something, it has to be measured. For statistical purposes, measurements can be thought of as being qualitative, ordinal or quantitative. This classification is based on the formal mathematical properties pertaining to different types of data.

Qualitative data

Qualitative data fulfill the mathematical property of equivalence. Events, outcomes or characteristics of the study subjects belong to categories. Perhaps the commonest example of such a measurement in clinical research is the categorization of individuals as being 'successes' or 'failures' following treatment. All patients who are classified as 'successes' are considered as being equivalent; similarly, all the 'failures' are classed as equivalent to each other. Of course, how the judgement that a patient is a success or a failure is made is a most important matter—more will be said about this in due course.

In oncological and cardiovascular research the qualitative measurement of interest is often whether the patient is 'alive' or 'dead'. Other examples include the categorizations 'pain' versus 'no pain', 'depressed' versus 'not depressed', and 'anxious' versus 'not anxious'.

Qualitative data are also known as 'nominal' or 'classificatory' data. The examples above are all binary (two-valued). Usually, if not invariably, when there are three categories, they form a natural ordering and therefore the data are ordinal—the next type of data to be discussed.

Ordinal data

Ordinal data consist of at least three categories that have the formal property that the relation 'greater than' applies to all possible pairs of categories. This means, of course, that the categories form an ordered sequence. So, for instance, the categories 'not depressed', 'slightly depressed', 'moderately depressed' and 'very depressed' form an ordinal scale—a four-point scale, as there are four categories. Ordinal data are very common in medical and behavioural research, and the statistical methods used for the analysis of such data are often referred to as being 'non-parametric' (for reasons to be discussed later). Such data are often referred to as being 'ranked'.

Quantitative data

The essential property of a quantitative scale is that it has a unit of measurement that is of constant size throughout the range of possible scale values. For obvious reasons, such data are sometimes referred to as being on an 'equal interval scale'.

If, in addition to having a unit of measurement, a particular type of data has a true origin or zero point, the data belong to a ratio scale. This means that ratios between any two points on the scale are meaningful. For example, if an object is twice as long as another object, the ratio of the two lengths will be exactly 2 regardless of whether the lengths have been expressed in centimetres, inches or whatever.

However, despite having a unit of measurement, certain types of data do not have a true zero point that is unambiguously fixed by nature. A well-known example of this is provided by the Celsius and Fahrenheit scales for temperature—zero in the former denotes the temperature at which water freezes, but in the latter zero is 32 Fahrenheit degrees below the freezing point of water. This means that the ratio between two temperatures on one of these scales will not hold true for the other scale. For example, 20 degrees Celsius is twice 10 degrees. However, the Fahrenheit equivalents are 86 and 50 degrees, respectively. Such data are therefore said to belong to an interval scale. It is probably the case that, at best, all psychometric tests give interval scale data. How depressed, anxious, intelligent, introverted or psychotic one has to be to score positively on a particular test depends on what part of the range of possibilities the test constructor has designed his test to assess. Is it, for example, intended to assess individuals who are severely depressed, to an extent that merits medical intervention, or is it a test to look at variations in mood that fall into the 'normal' range for individuals who would not be thought to be ill?

In practice, the interval–ratio distinction is often unimportant, and the statistical methods for quantitative data usually require just that the data have been measured on at least an interval scale.

Why Do We Use Statistics?

A statistical analysis of a data set can be thought of as having three functions, namely description, estimation and hypothesis testing. The starting point for any analysis will, of course, be a complete listing of the data—what is often called the 'raw' data. A simple example might look like this:

Patient	Sex	Age	Severity	Treatment	Outcome
1	M	47	Mild	A	Success
2	F	35	Moderate	B	Success
3	F	58	Moderate	B	Fail
4	F	61	Severe	A	Success
5	M	44	Mild	A	Fail
.	.	.	.	.	.
40	F	52	Moderate	A	Success

There are just 40 patients in the data set, and the full listing could be squeezed onto a single sheet of paper. It would be possible to inspect the raw data in detail and to form some impression of what the data set amounted to. However, even with such a small data set, it would be helpful to produce a summary table such as this:

Outcome	Treatment	
	A	B
Success	16	8
Fail	4	12

Such a table is an example of the statistical task of *description*. The description of the results of such a study would be improved by quoting the percentages of patients who were successful with each treatment, namely 80% with A and 40% with B—a difference of 40% in favour of A. This is just a concise and clear summary of the data. Graphs, tables and summary statistics are the standard methods for producing descriptions of study data. These methods will be elaborated on below.

A good description of the data is essential, but research aims to do more than just document what occurred in a study that has been completed. These further aims are addressed by *estimation* and *hypothesis testing*.

To illustrate what is being attempted in *estimation*, we can use the data given in the table above to produce the following statement:

I have treated 20 patients with treatment A.
80% of those were successes.
Therefore (I estimate that) treatment A produces a success rate of 80%.

A similar statement could be made using the data from treatment B, and the following statement could be made using both A and B:

I have treated 20 patients with A and 20 patients with B.
The difference between the percentages of successes was 40%, A being better.
Therefore (I estimate that) treatment A produces a success rate 40% higher than B.

These are examples of attempting to generalize from the results of a particular study —i.e. inductive reasoning. If, instead of 20 patients with each treatment, the success rates had been based on 200 patients per treatment, we would feel our 'estimates' were in some way more 'accurate' or closer to the 'truth'. As we shall see, expressing the 'accuracy' of the estimate is a salient feature of the use of statistics for estimation.

Hypothesis testing is an attempt to make a decision when faced with a data set. In comparing two treatments, the decision addresses the question of whether it is plausible that the difference (if any) seen in the data of the study might just be due to chance. So, if one had a very small study giving the following:

Outcome	Treatments	
	A	B
Successes	1	0
Failures	0	1

Without performing any sophisticated calculations, it is apparent that such a difference between the treatments might well be purely fortuitous—and that it would be rather foolish to conclude there is a 'real' difference.

However, the following data set might be more persuasive:

Outcome	Treatments	
	A	B
Successes	10	0
Failures	0	10

Finally, in the data that follows, it would be highly implausible that the difference is simply a chance effect:

Outcome	Treatments	
	A	B
Successes	100	0
Failures	0	100

Hypothesis testing in statistics consists of procedures for assessing whether the results of a study could plausibly be simply chance effects or whether (whatever the reason might be) chance is not a credible explanation for what is seen.

Description, estimation and hypothesis testing will now be considered in turn.

Description

In describing a set of data, three methods are used, namely tables, graphs and summary statistics.

Tables

Tables are an ideal method for describing a set of qualitative data, as in the example in the previous section:

Outcome	Treatment	
	A	B
Success	16	8
Fail	4	12
Total	20	20

If the data are ordinal or quantitative the table will be more complicated, and will show the frequency distribution of the data set. For example, each individual value could be shown:

Height (cm)	Frequency	Percentage	Cumulative frequency	Cumulative percentage
150	1	0.4	1	0.4
151	0	0.0	1	0.4
152	1	0.4	2	0.8
153	0	0.0	2	0.8
154	0	0.0	2	0.8
155	2	0.8	4	1.6
:	:	:	:	:
198	1	0.4	249	99.6
199	0	0.0	249	99.6
200	1	0.4	250	100.0
Total	250	100.0		

Of course, this is a very lengthy method of presentation if there are many different values in the data set, so a grouped frequency distribution is often used:

Height (cm)	Frequency	Percentage	Cumulative frequency	Cumulative percentage
140–150	0	0.0	0	0.0
150–160	6	2.4	6	2.4
160–170	56	22.4	62	24.8
170–180	124	49.6	186	74.4
180–190	59	23.6	245	98.0
190–200	4	1.6	249	99.6
200–210	1	0.4	250	100.0
Total	250	100.0		

Grouping data is to some extent a rather arbitrary process—the choice of the starting point and width for each interval will affect the distribution that results.

Graphs

Graphs can make it very easy to look at frequency distributions such as those in the previous section, the most widely used graph being a histogram. The histogram for the grouped data distribution would look like this:

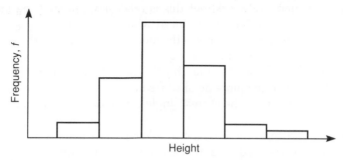

Note that the height of each rectangle is the frequency for a class interval and the width is the width of the class interval.

A very useful method for showing ordinal or quantitative data graphically is the box and whisker plot (Tukey, 1977). The data set consisting of the heights of 250 persons might look like this on such a graph:

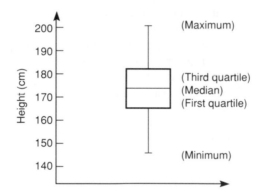

This type of graph introduces certain summary statistics, which will be explained in the next section.

Summary statistics

Although tables and graphs are very useful, it is necessary for many purposes to summarize data sets using numbers called summary statistics. For example, the maximum value and the minimum value shown at the ends of the 'whiskers' in the box and whisker plot give a description of an aspect of the data set in numerical form—variability being the aspect described.

With quantitative data sets, four features of the data can be described numerically, namely, central tendency, variability, symmetry and shape.

Central tendency

In everyday English, this concept is referred to as the 'average'. Three summary statistics are in common use to express this feature of a data set—the mode, the median and the (arithmetic) mean. Occasionally, the geometric and harmonic means appear in statistical work, but this is relatively rare and the mean (type unspecified) will be the arithmetic mean in what follows here.

The simplest of the three averages is the mode—derived from the French word for fashion—which is simply the most frequently occurring value or class interval in the data. In the histogram for the grouped height data, the modal interval is the 170–180 cm one. If the more detailed frequency distribution were presented, the mode could be found to the nearest single centimetre—let us suppose a value of, say, 176 cm.

The average shown in the box and whisker plot as being the line inside the 'box' is the median. The median is the value above and below which half the data lie—i.e. it divides the data into the top 50% and the bottom 50% (hence it can be referred to as the 50% partition value). In the data set above, the median would be close to the mode—it might be, say, 175.5 cm.

The mean is found by adding up all the individual values and dividing by the number of values. In the height data set the mean would be close to the other two averages—suppose it is, say 175.3 cm.

The frequency distribution of heights has a shape that is commonly found with biological data—namely a single peak or mode in the middle of the range of values with a progressive and approximately symmetric tailing off on either side of the mode. The data are thus unimodal (1 peak or mode) and (approximately) symmetrically distributed about the mode. Under these circumstances the mean, median and mode will be close to each other—if there is perfect symmetry, they will have the same value. A summary statistic to describe symmetry/asymmetry will be considered later, but at this point it is worth noting that a comparison of the mean, median and mode is a simple way of detecting asymmetry—or 'skew' in statistical parlance. In the diagrams below, A is the mean, B is the median and C is the mode.

The distribution on the left is said to be positively skewed, there being a long 'tail' to the right indicating that a few relatively high values are present. In this situation, the mean (A) is the highest of the three averages and the mode (C) is the lowest. The distribution on the right is said to be negatively skewed, and now the mean (A) is the lowest of the three averages and the mode (C) is the highest.

Variability

Variability (or spread or dispersion) means simply that all the individuals are not the same on the characteristic being measured. This is self-evident in a description of a data set by a table or a graph.

With ordinal and quantitative data a very simple way of indicating variability is to quote the minimum and maximum values in the data set. The difference between the minimum and maximum is known as the 'range'. This is especially valuable when the data have been entered into a computer, as a simple check that these values make biological sense—i.e. that no error in data entry has been made. It is also a way of showing that the study subjects comply with an eligibility criterion (e.g. whether they are all within the age range specified in the study protocol). However, these two extreme values do not give a representative picture of the variation in the data as a whole.

Useful descriptions of variability with ordinal or quantitative data are the interquartile range and the semi-interquartile range. Both of these are based on the difference (i.e. range) between the first (or lower) quartile (referred to as Q1) and the third (or upper) quartile (referred to as Q3). Quartiles are partition values (as in the median): the lower quartile is the value below which 25% of values lie, and above which 75% lie; the upper quartile is the value below which 75% of values lie and above which 25% lie. The median, it will be recalled, is the 50% partition value—and, although it is rarely referred to as such, is the second (or middle) quartile, Q2. The interquartile range is simply the difference between Q1 and Q3, and the semi-interquartile range is half of the interquartile range. The most detailed partition values in common use are percentiles (or centiles). P25 (or C25) is the 25% partition value i.e. Q1; P75 (or C75) is the 75% partition value, i.e. Q3; P50 (or C50) is the 50% partition value, i.e. the median. To define 'abnormally' low or high values on a particular characteristic, the 5% (P5) or 10% (P10) and 90% (P90) or 95% (P95) partition values are often used. 'Abnormal' is in fact 'unusual', in the sense that the individual is in the bottom (or top) 5% or 10% of the range of values.

With quantitative data, the summary statistic most used to express variability is the 'standard deviation' (SD). The SD is the square root of the 'variance', variance being the average of the squared differences of the values in the data set from their mean. In statistical notation,

$$\text{variance} = \frac{\Sigma(X - \bar{X})^2}{N}$$

where X is the data value, $\bar{X}$ is the mean, and N is the sample size. Thus, the standard deviation is given by

$$\text{SD} = \sqrt{\frac{\Sigma(X - \bar{X})^2}{N}}$$

However, in calculating the SD for a data set, the formula is slightly modified by replacing 'N' in the denominator by '$N - 1$'. This is known as 'Bessel's correction', and the purpose of the correction is to make the SD of a sample an unbiased estimate of the SD of the population the sample 'represents'. More will be said about this matter when estimation is discussed later.

Why do we use the SD? It is because the SD is one of the two parameters of the Normal distribution (the other parameter being the mean). The Normal distribution is the most used and most important distribution in statistics. Its formula is

$$f(x) = \frac{1}{\sigma\sqrt{2\pi}}\, e^{-(x-\mu)^2/2\sigma^2}$$

where e and π are constants and μ and σ are the mean and SD of the distribution, respectively. This distribution is often referred to eponymously as the Gaussian distribution (Gauss lived from 1777 to 1855) but its appearance pre-dates Gauss —Walker (1931) considered that it was discovered in 1721 by Abraham de Moivre (1667–1754) as an approximate formula for the binomial distribution. It was called the 'Normal' distribution by Pearson in 1893.

Why is the Normal distribution so important? There are three reasons. First, many sorts of data are distributed such that the Normal distribution can be used as an adequate or good description of the data—especially in biology. Second, it is often possible to transform data mathematically so that the Normal distribution can be used to describe the data (e.g. positively skewed data can be made to be Normally distributed by taking the square root or the logarithm of the values). Third, and most important of all, sampling distributions are Normal distributions when the sample size is sufficiently large. Explanation of this last reason will be left to the section on estimation.

Suppose that the height data shown earlier has SD = 7.6 cm (the mean being 175.3 cm), and that the heights are Normally distributed (how we would know this will be considered in the following sections on symmetry and shape). Tables of areas under the Normal curve have been produced which enable us to know the proportion of individuals who fall within a given particular range of values. The most commonly used range is the mean ± 1.96 SD, which is the range within which 95% of individual values will fall. So, 175.3 ± 1.96 × 7.6 cm (a range of 160.4 cm to 190.1 cm) is the range within which the heights of 95% of the individuals in the sample would be expected to fall. The 95% range is often approximated to by using the mean ± 2 SD, which would give 160.1 cm to 190.5 cm with the height data. Graphically, the height data (assuming them to be perfectly Normally distributed) would look like this:

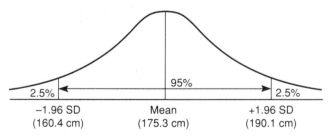

The 5% who lie outside the range 160.4 cm to 190.1 cm are divided equally into those who lie below 160.4 and those who are above 190.1. Thus, the 5% is made up of the 2.5% below 160.4 and the 2.5% above 190.1. The extremes of the distribution are known as the 'tails' of the distribution, and the mean + 1.96 SD defines a two-tailed 95% range.

Of course, interest may be greater in 'abnormality' or unusualness in one direction than in the other direction. If unusually low height was of particular interest, a one-tailed range could be calculated. For example, 95% of individuals lie above the mean − 1.645 SD (here, 175.3 − 1.645 × 7.6 cm, or 162.8 cm), and therefore 5% of individuals would have heights less than 162.8 cm. Graphically:

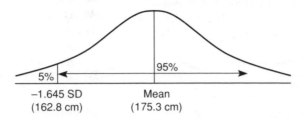

5%   95%

-1.645 SD   Mean
(162.8 cm)   (175.3 cm)

The values 1.96 and 1.645 are known as 'Normal deviates', being the deviation in numbers of SDs. From the mean of a Normal distribution. The usual notation is to use the letter 'z' for a Normal deviate. A small table of useful values of z follows:

z						
	0.84	1.00	1.28	1.645	1.96	2.576
1-tailed area	20%/80%	15.87%/84.13%	10%/90%	5%/95%	2.5%/97.5%	0.5%/99.5%
2-tailed area	40%/60%	31.74%/68.26%	20%/80%	10%/90%	5%/95%	1%/99%

The first percentage is that in the tail or two tails, and the second is the percentage not in the tail or tails.

Symmetry and skew

A Normal distribution is a symmetrical distribution—symmetrical about its mean, median and mode, and, as has been mentioned in the previous section, the fact that the three 'averages' have identical or very similar values indicates that the distribution is symmetrical. A distribution that is not symmetrical is said to be 'skewed', a word which the Collins English Dictionary states originates from the Old Normal French verb 'escuer'—to shun; a Middle Dutch verb 'schuwen'—to avoid—is of similar origin. A symmetrical distribution (such as the Normal distribution) is not skewed or 'unskewed'.

Skew is easy to detect if the data distribution is presented graphically, as was shown earlier. A summary statistic to describe the symmetry or lack of symmetry of a data set is g1.

$$g1 = \frac{m3}{m2\sqrt{m2}}, \quad \text{where } m2 = \frac{\Sigma(X - \bar{X})^2}{N} \quad \text{and} \quad m3 = \frac{\Sigma(X - \bar{X})^3}{N}$$

m2 is, of course, the variance (and is calculated with N rather than $N - 1$ in the denominator in this context); it is known more generally as the second moment about the mean (hence m2). m3 is known as the third moment about the mean (hence m3). As m3 is calculated by raising the $X - \bar{X}$ differences to the power 3, it can have a positive or a negative value, and therefore g1 can be positive or negative. A symmetrical, unskewed, data set will have g1 = 0. As shown below, a positive g1 means that there is a longer 'tail' of relatively high values in the data set (referred to as positive skew) and a negative g1 means that there is a longer 'tail' of relatively low values (referred to as negative skew).

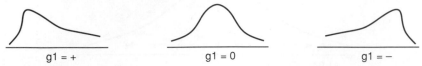

g1 = +   g1 = 0   g1 = −

Obviously, a non-zero value of g1 indicates that the distribution of the data in the sample is perfectly symmetrical about its mean. To consider the interpretation of a calculated value of g1, we must consider the concept of sampling 'error' or variation. The data we have available for analysis are based on one or more samples of individuals—let us confine the discussion to a single sample at this stage. Our intention in the statistical task 'description' is just to summarize the important features of the data relating to that sample. However, we are (almost) always interested in using the sample to tell us something about the 'population' that the sample 'represents', i.e. we would like to use the sample to estimate various characteristics of the population. In the terminology of estimation, we say we would like to use the 'sample statistic' (such as the value of g1 we have calculated from our data) to estimate the 'population parameter' (the 'true' value of the skew coefficient—referred to as $\gamma 1$—in the population). So, if the value of g1 we have calculated from our sample is not exactly zero, does this mean that $\gamma 1$ is also not zero?

Let us assume that the value of $\gamma 1$ for a particular characteristic is, in fact, exactly zero—the distribution is perfectly symmetrical in the population (the 'population' is assumed to be infinitely large, and is therefore hypothetical). If we select a sample of N individuals at random (i.e. a sample of size N), would we expect the value of g1 to be zero? At the level of common sense, we might conclude that zero is the most likely value we would obtain for g1, but by 'chance' the particular sample we have selected might have a value that is not exactly zero. Also, again at the level of common sense, we would expect small differences from the 'true' value of zero to be more likely to occur in our sample than very large differences from zero, i.e. samples will not necessarily reflect exactly the 'truth' about the population, but a sample statistic (such as g1) will be more likely to be close to the population parameter (such as $\gamma 1$) than far away from it. We can represent this graphically:

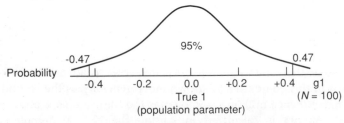

The distribution above represents sampling 'error' or variation—the variation from the 'truth' that we might expect when we take a sample. The sample size assumed here is 100. If we make the sample larger, we would expect the 'error' or variation to be less; if the sample size was 400, the graph of expected sampling error would look like this:

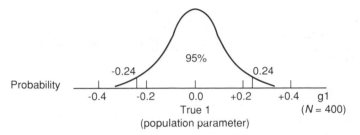

These graphs represent 'sampling distributions'—distributions which describe the variation we expect in the value of a sample statistic around the true value, the population parameter. The distribution for a sample of $N = 400$ shows less variability than that for $N = 100$. At a common sense level, a large sample is more likely to give a value of g1 close to the 'truth' than a smaller sample. Note also that the sampling distributions have been drawn in the shape of a Normal distribution. This is because, with large samples, sampling distributions are indeed Normal distributions. Finally, note also that the 95% range (giving 5% of the two tails) has been marked on each of the graphs.

These sampling distributions can be determined just as if they were data distributions, with, *inter alia*, a mean and a SD. The mean is the true $\gamma 1$, the population parameter (in these cases 0). The SD for the distribution for samples of $N = 100$ is 0.24, while that for the distribution for samples of $N = 400$ is 0.12 (these values have been found from a table of the sampling error of g1, such as Table 34B in Vol. 1 of the *Biometrika Tables for Statisticians* (Pearson and Hartley, 1970). The 95% range for the $N = 100$ distribution is therefore $0 \pm 1.96 \times 0.24$, or -0.47 to $+0.47$; the 95% range for the $N = 400$ distribution is $0 \pm 1.96 \times 0.12$, or -0.24 to $+0.24$. The SD of a sampling distribution is usually called the *standard error* (SE) of the sample statistic. If tables are not available, a good estimate of the SE (the estimate improves as the sample size increases) is given by $\sqrt{6/N}$—the values for $N = 100$ and $N = 400$ being 0.245 and 0.122, respectively.

These sampling distributions can be used in two ways. First a value of g1 outside the 95% range for a parameter $\gamma 1 = 0$ has a probability of occurrence of less than 5% if $\gamma 1 = 0$. By convention, this is taken to be sufficiently improbable for the hypothesis that $\gamma 1$ is indeed zero to be rejected as implausible. This is using the sampling distribution for a hypothesis testing (here, testing the hypothesis that $\gamma 1 = 0$). A value of g1 inside the 95% range is not considered, according to this convention, to be sufficiently improbable for decision to reject the hypothesis that $\gamma 1 = 0$ to be justified. The 95% range for $\gamma 1 = 0$ is -0.47 to $+0.47$ for $N = 100$, so a g1 $= +0.5$ would lead us to conclude that the hypothesis that $\gamma 1 = 0$ should be rejected, but a g1 $= +0.4$ would not permit such a conclusion. Second, just as when $\gamma 1 = 0$ the most likely value of g1 for a sample to have is zero, if $\gamma 1$ is any other value (e.g. $+0.3$) the most likely value of g1 for a sample to have is that value (i.e. if γ1 is $+0.3$, then the most likely single value for a sample g1 is $+0.3$). So, we can use the actual value of g1 as the best estimate of γ1. This can be written thus:

$$g1 \; = \; \hat{\gamma}1 \; = \; 0.3$$

This is called a *point estimate* of γ1. The circumflex over the γ means 'estimate of' and is called 'hat' in statistics.

However, a g1 of 0.3 might occur in a sample if γ1 was not exactly 0.3. That is, other true values of γ1 could give g1 $=$ 0.3 in a sample. Consider the diagram below:

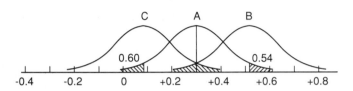

The sampling distribution marked 'A' represents the sampling distribution of g1 for $N = 400$ if $\gamma1 = +0.3$. This shows that values less than $+0.06$ or greater than $+0.54$ fall outside the 95% range. Sampling distribution 'B' represents the possibility that $\gamma1 = +0.54$. The value $+0.3$ is the lower limit of the 95% range for this distribution. So, if $\gamma1 = +0.54$, a value of $+0.3$ for g1 is the most extreme value below $+0.54$ that falls into the 95% range. Distribution 'C' represents the possibility that the true value of γ1 is $+0.06$. The value of $+0.3$ is now the upper limit of the 95% range for this sampling distribution, and therefore a value of $+0.3$ is the most extreme value above $+0.06$ that falls into the 95% range.

From the above it can be concluded that true values of γ1 above $+0.54$ or below $+0.06$ have probabilities of less than 5% of giving a value of g1 in the sample (if $N = 400$, of course). The $+0.54$ and $+0.06$ are given directly by the values of g1 in the sample (namely g1 $= +0.3$). That is, values of γ1 within the 95% range of the sampling distribution of γ1 given by the point estimate have probabilities of greater than 5% of giving g1 in a sample $= +0.3$; values of γ1 outside the 95% range have probabilities of less than 5% of giving a g1 $= +0.3$. Such a 95% range is called a **95%** *confidence interval* for the estimate of γ1. It is a range of possible values of γ1 all of which have probabilities greater than 5% of giving g1 $= +0.3$ in the sample. We take such a range as giving us an estimate of where we think the 'true' value of γ1 'probably' lies—'probably' being taken to be 95% likely as the values of γ1 are within the 95% range of the sampling distribution of the point estimate value of γ1.

In summary then, we can use 0 $\pm$ 1.96 SE to give a range of values of g1 which are consistent with the hypothesis that $\gamma1 = 0$. Or, we can use the value of g1 + 1.96 SE to give us a range of possible true values of γ1 consistent with the value of g1 calculated from the data. The former is hypothesis testing (using a 5% criterion of statistical significance); the latter is estimation (using a 95% confidence interval). The two procedures are consistent with each other, in the sense that when the hypothesis test leads to a rejection of the hypothesis that $\gamma 1 = 0$, the confidence interval will not include the possibility that $\gamma 1$ is zero.

Shape and kurtosis

The term 'kurtosis' comes from the Greek 'kurtos', meaning 'arched'. The term is used to refer to the width of the arch in the middle of a unimodal distribution. The kurtosis of a distribution is described by the statistic g2:

$$g2 = \frac{m4}{m2^2} - 3$$

where m4 is the fourth moment about the mean, given by:

$$m4 = \frac{\Sigma(X - \bar{X})^4}{N}$$

A Normal distribution has a value 0 for g2. Thus, a perfectly Normally distributed data set will have both g1 and g2 = 0. A distribution with g2 = 0 is said to be 'meso-kurtic' (from the Greek 'mesos', meaning middle).

If g2 is greater than 0, the distribution is said to be 'lepto-kurtic' (from the Greek 'leptos', which means literally 'peeled' and hence 'fine or slender'). A lepto-kurtic distribution will have a narrower middle arch than a meso-kurtic distribution, and will also have longer 'tails'. The figure illustrates this:

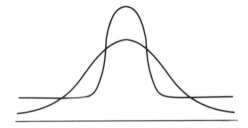

A value of g2 less than 0 shows that the distribution is 'platy-kurtic' (from the Greek 'platus' meaning 'flat, wide or broad'). A platy-kurtic distribution has a flat middle arch, and shorter tails than a meso-kurtic distribution. The meso- and platy-kurtic shapes are compared in the figure:

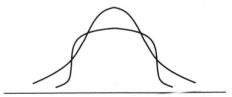

The question of interpreting a value of g2 calculated from the data in a sample arises as it did for a value of g1. If our interest is in whether the distribution is consistent with the hypothesis that the sample comes from a Normally distributed population, a value of g2 = 0 is most consistent with this possibility. The sampling distribution of the statistic must be considered when non-zero values of g2 are found. Unfortunately, the sampling distribution of g2 does not become approximately Normal until N is at least 1000 (when the SE of g2 is given by $\sqrt{24/N}$). For smaller sample sizes a table of g2, such as Table 34C of Vol. 1 of the *Biometrika Tables for Statisticians* (Pearson and Hartley, 1970) should be consulted.

In practice, the interpretation of g1 and g2 is facilitated nowadays by many statistical packages (such as SPSS), which give the probabilities of the calculated g1 and g2 assuming the hypothesis that $\gamma1$ and $\gamma2$ are zero.

Estimation

In estimation, the intention is to use the data available (which are always obtained from a sample, however large) to generalize—to estimate the 'true' or population parameter. When dealing with the interpretation of a value of g1 for the skew of a sample of data we need to know what the g1 of our sample tells us about the g1 of the population. This issue was addressed in the earlier section *Symmetry and Skew.*

With qualitative data, the interest is usually in using the proportion or percentage of individuals having some characteristic or outcome in the sample to estimate the 'true' or population percentage. If we call the sample (the sample statistic) percentage 'p' and the true percentage (the population parameter) 'π', we would be interested in using p to estimate π.

With quantitative data, we would most often wish to use the mean calculated from the sample (the sample statistic) to estimate the true mean (the population parameter). The usual notation is $\bar{X}$ for the sample mean and μ for the true (i.e. population) mean.

Point estimation

The logic here is very straightforward. If the population parameter (whatever it might be—percentage, mean, etc.) has a value θ, what is the most likely value of the sample statistic in a sample drawn randomly from that population? For most parameters in which we are interested, the most likely single value of the sample statistic is the 'true' value—the value of the population parameter. The most important exception to this was encountered earlier in the section *Variability*, in which it was noted that the SD should be calculated with $N - 1$ in the denominator, rather than N, to make the sample SD an unbiased estimate of the population SD. This is because the most likely single value for a sample SD, if the population SD is σ, is

$$\sigma \sqrt{\frac{N}{N - 1}}$$

The $\sqrt{N/N - 1}$, known as Bessel's correction, is usually incorporated into the formula for the SD calculation by replacing the N in the denominator by $N - 1$.

Note the structure of the logic. If the true value (in the population) is σ, the most likely value in a sample is σ. However, the sample value is all that is available in practice; if this has a value of σ, and σ is the most likely single value if the 'truth' is σ, we can conclude that σ is the most likely true value of the parameter. This estimate of the parameter is called a *point estimate* because it is a single-valued estimate. It will be apparent that a deductive argument (if the truth is σ, the most likely sample value is σ) has been converted into an apparently inductive argument (if the sample gives σ, we conclude that the truth is most likely to be σ).

Interval estimation

Consider the following descriptions of three samples:

Sample	A	B	C
Alive	9	90	900
Dead	1	10	100
N	10	100	1000

In all three samples, p, the percentage alive, is 90%. So, the point estimate of π is 90% whether we have the sample with $N = 10$, $N = 100$ or $N = 1000$. At a purely common-sense level, an estimate based on a large sample is preferable to one based on a small sample. The reason for this is that a large sample will be less likely than a small sample to have a value of the sample statistic that is very different from the population parameter, because the variability of a sampling distribution is smaller, the larger the sample. As we have discussed earlier, the SD of the sampling distribution is known as the SE. With large samples, the SE of a sample percentage is:

$$\text{SE } p \;=\; \sqrt{\frac{\pi(100 - \pi)}{N}}$$

Of course, we never know π in practice, so the SE of p is estimated by substituting the point estimate of π, p, for π in the formula, i.e.:

$$\text{estimated SE } p \;=\; \sqrt{\frac{p(100 - p)}{N}}$$

The values for samples A, B and C are 9.5%, 3.0% and 0.95%, respectively.

Again when the sample is large, the sampling distribution is approximately Normal, so it is expected that the sample statistic, p, will lie in the range $\pm 1.96 \times$ SE with 95% probability. Although the logic is based on reasoning from an assumed population parameter to the most likely value (the point estimate) or, now, a range of values in a sample, the logic is reversed so that we conclude that the population parameter has a 95% probability of lying in the range $p \pm 1.96 \times$ SE p. Such a range is referred to as a *confidence interval*, CI. When $\pm 1.96 \times$ SE is used to calculate the interval, it is a 95% confidence interval. In A, B and C, $p \pm 1.96 \times$ SE p are:

A   90% $\pm$ 1.96 $\times$ 9.5%   = 90% $\pm$ 18.6% = 71.4% to 108.6%
B   90% $\pm$ 1.96 $\times$ 3.0%   = 90% $\pm$ 5.9%   = 84.1% to 95.9%
C   90% $\pm$ 1.96 $\times$ 0.95%   = 90% $\pm$ 1.9%   = 88.1% to 91.9%

Two features of these answers are apparent. First, the intervals become narrower as the sample size increases. This is quite straightforward—the larger the sample, the narrower the confidence interval, and therefore the more precise is our estimate of the 'truth'. Second, the answer for A has an impossible upper limit to the interval. This is partly because the sample is very small, $N = 10$, and partly because p is close to 100%. Unfortunately, SE of p depends both on the sample size and on π, which we try to estimate with p. Estimating π with p becomes particularly unsatisfactory when p is close to 0% or 100%—and if p is 0% or 100% the estimated SE of p is 0%. Under these circumstances a more complex procedure is involved —exact binomial estimation—which will not be considered here. However, a general point is worth making here, namely that statistical methods for large samples are relatively straightforward and are based largely on the Normal distribution. With large samples, sampling distributions are Normal distributions even if the population from which the sample has been drawn is not Normally distributed —the theorem relevant to this fact being termed the *central limit theorem* (which states that the distribution of the sum or mean of a number of random variables approaches a Normal distribution as a limit as the number of random variables increases). This theorem is arguably the most important one in statistical inference.

As a further example, let us now consider the following descriptions of three samples (quantitative data):

Sample	A	B	C
Mean	70.0	70.0	70.0
SD	8.0	8.0	8.0
N	10	100	1000

All three samples have the same value, 70.0, for the mean, and thus give the same point estimate for μ, the population mean. The SE of the mean of a sample (SEM) is given by:

$$SEM = \frac{\sigma}{\sqrt{N}}$$

where σ is the population SD. Of course, the population SD is unknown, and has to be estimated by the sample SD (calculated with $N - 1$ in the denominator). The estimated SEM in the samples are therefore 2.5, 0.8 and 0.25, respectively. Using the point estimate $\pm 1.96 \times$ SEM to calculate 95% confidence intervals gives:

A   70.0 $\pm$ 1.96 $\times$ 2.5   = 70.0 $\pm$ 4.9   = 65.1 to 74.9
B   70.0 $\pm$ 1.96 $\times$ 0.8   = 70.0 $\pm$ 1.57 = 68.43 to 71.57
C   70.0 $\pm$ 1.96 $\times$ 0.25 = 70.0 $\pm$ 0.49 = 69.51 to 70.49

Two points should be made here. First, we again find that the larger the sample, the narrower is the confidence interval and therefore the more precise the estimate. Second, although it is not obviously wrong, the interval with the $N = 10$ sample is incorrect; even with a Normally distributed population, the sampling distribution of a sample mean is not Normally distributed if the sample is small (less than 30, say). Instead, another distribution, the 't' distribution, should be used—about which more in due course.

Hypothesis Testing

Statistical significance

In what follows, the situation being considered will be one in which the efficacy of a treatment is being evaluated, i.e. a clinical trial. The essence of treatment evaluation is the concept of control or comparison. The simplest sort of data that can result from a clinical trial might look like this:

Outcome	Treatments	
	1	2
Success	21	15
Failure	10	17
Total	31	32

In the above, $p_1 = 67.7\%$ and $p_2 = 46.9\%$ and the difference, $p_1 - p_2$, is 20.8%. All this is description of the study data. If the data had turned out slightly differently, the following might have been obtained:

Outcome	Treatments	
	1	2
Success	22	14
Failure	9	18
Total	31	32

Now, $p_1 = 71.0\%$, $p_2 = 43.8\%$ and $p_1 - p_2 = 27.2\%$.

So, the first data set presented above shows a 20.8% difference between the two treatments, and the second data set a 27.2% difference. The basic idea in hypothesis testing is the probability that a difference will occur in the data of a study if the true difference is zero. In the jargon of statistics, this idea is stated as the probability of the data assuming the null (i.e. zero difference) hypothesis is true, or, in short the null hypothesis probability. Statistical 'tests' are used to calculate these probabilities. An appropriate statistical test that can be applied to the data sets above is the chi-square test. How this test is calculated will not be considered here, but the results of the calculations are as follows:

First data set (20.8% difference): chi-square = 2.80, df = 1, $P = 0.095$
Second data set (27.2% difference): chi-square = 4.76, df = 1, $P = 0.029$

The results of interest are the values of 'P', the null hypothesis probabilities—the values of chi-square and their degrees of freedom (df) are technical details (important as they are), their reason for existence is the finding of the values of 'P'.

So, the 20.8% difference has a probability of occurrence of 0.095 (or 9.5%: 9.5 in 100 or 95 in 1000 or approximately 1 in 10.5) if indeed the true difference is actually zero. The 27.2% difference has a lower probability of occurrence if the true difference is zero, namely 0.029 (or 2.9%: 2.9 in 100 or 29 in 1000 or approximately 1 in 34.5). Although the calculation of the values of chi-square and finding the values of 'P' therefrom is (unless the reader is already familiar with the process) a technical mystery at this stage, it makes sense that the larger difference was less likely to occur by chance than the smaller difference if indeed the true difference is zero.

How are such probabilities used in practice? The thinking is that if the value of 'P' is very low, this constitutes evidence for disbelieving the truth of the hypothesis that the true difference is really zero—in statistical parlance, a low 'P' will lead us to reject the null hypothesis (and believe the difference is non-zero —of which more later). There is virtually a cultural norm nowadays about a low value being 0.05 (or 5%: 5 in 100 or 1 in 20). This is referred to as the 0.05 (or 5%) *level of statistical significance*. If the calculated value of 'P' is less than 0.05, we conclude that the difference between the two treatments is statistically significant (at the 0.05 level of significance); if 'P' is not less than 0.05, the difference is said to be non-significant.

A significance level is referred to by the Greek letter α (alpha). So, if $P < \alpha$, we reject the null hypothesis. In the two data sets above, the small difference with $P = 0.095$ is not statistically significant at the 0.05 level of significance, but the difference with $P = 0.029$ is.

The idea is a very simple one even if the calculations may sometimes be difficult. If the 'P' from the statistical test is less than α (usually 0.05), we conclude there is a 'real' difference between the treatments. If, however, 'P' is not less than α, we conclude that the true difference may indeed be zero.

Type 1 and 2 errors

The value of 'P' in the data set with the larger difference was less than 0.05, and this permits us to reject the null hypothesis at the 0.05 level of statistical significance. However, the improbable may have occurred, and the difference in the data, unlikely as it is if the null hypothesis is true, could have occurred by chance. If all the null hypotheses we tested using the 0.05 level of significance were true, by chance in the long run we would expect to find values of 'P' less than 0.05 in 5% of these tests, i.e. we would be falsely rejecting the null hypotheses in about 5% of the tests. A false rejection of a true null hypothesis is called a *type 1 error*. In rejecting the null hypothesis in the data set showing a 27.2% difference between the treatments, we might be making a type 1 error —the improbable may have occurred. The level of significance (0.05 usually) is therefore the probability of making a type 1 error when the null hypothesis is true —the probability of falsely rejecting a true null hypothesis.

In the data set with a 20.8% difference between the two treatments, the value of 'P' was greater than 0.05, and we are therefore unable to reject the null hypothesis at the customary 0.05 level of significance. This does not mean that we can be confident that the true difference is exactly zero, however. If the study had been 10 times as large, the following data might have resulted:

Outcome	Treatments	
	1	2
Success	210	150
Failure	100	170
Total	310	320

Chi-square is now 28.0, and $P = 0.00001$ (1 in 100 000). In a study this size, a 20.8% difference between the two treatments is extremely unlikely to be seen in the study data if the true difference is zero. The non-significance of the 20.8% difference in the smaller study may just be because the study is too small. We may be failing to reject a false null hypothesis, an error which is called a *type 2 error*. The diagram below summarizes the foregoing (in the form of a decision matrix):

		The 'Truth'	
		Null hypothesis is true	Null hypothesis is false
Decision based on the data of the study	Accept null hypothesis		Type 2 error
	Reject null hypothesis	Type 1 error	

So, when we reject the null hypothesis, we may be making a type 1 error, and when we fail to reject the null hypothesis we may be making a type 2 error. The probability of making a type 1 error when the null hypothesis is true is, as we have seen, controlled by the level of significance, (i.e. 0.05 usually). The probability that a type 2 error will be made if the null hypothesis is false is denoted by the Greek letter β (beta). Put another way, β is the probability that we will say the difference is not statistically significant when, in truth, there is a 'real' difference between the two treatments. For a given 'real' difference between two treatments, the larger the study, the less likely is a type 2 error.

It is customary to consider the problem of type 2 errors by stating or calculating the probability that such an error will *not* be made, if indeed there is a 'real' difference between the treatments. This probability is referred to as the *power* of the study. The larger the study, the higher its power for a given 'true' treatment difference. Suppose that two treatments are really different, the better one giving a success rate of 80% and the worse one a success rate of 60%, i.e. there is a 'real' difference of 20% between the treatments. The table below shows the value of β, and power expressed as $1 - \beta$, and as a percentage, for various study sizes (N.B. the number shown is the number in each of the two treatment groups, and the power is the probability of obtaining a statistically significant difference between the treatments at the 0.05 level of significance):

Number in each treatment group	β	Power $(1 - \beta)$	Power (as %)
20	0.72	0.28	28
40	0.50	0.50	50
60	0.33	0.67	67
80	0.21	0.79	79
100	0.13	0.87	87
150	0.034	0.964	96.4
200	0.008	0.992	99.2

The larger study sizes are much more likely to reject the null hypothesis when there is a true difference between the treatments. It is therefore very important to consider this matter before the study is begun, so that an appropriate number of patients will be used to give sufficient power. The next section will deal with this matter.

Calculation of study size

Partly because of the importance of the topic, and partly because this subject is not dealt with particularly well in most introductory textbooks, the calculation of the appropriate size of a study will be dealt with in some detail. The basic formula for the number of subjects required in each group in a study comparing two treatments is:

$$N = \frac{2(Z_\alpha - Z_\beta)^2}{T^2} \quad (+1 \text{ if the data are quantitative})$$

where:

N = the number of subjects in each of the (two) groups;

Z_α = the Normal deviate for α, the level of significance to be used in testing if the difference is statistically significant. If $\alpha = 0.05$, $Z_\alpha = 1.96$. The diagram below shows the sampling distribution of the differences between two treatments if the null hypothesis is true:

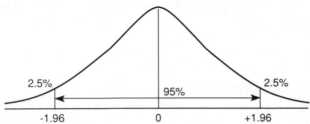

Although the 'true' difference is 0, an individual study may, by chance, show a difference between the two treatments. This difference could be in either direction—chance is impartial. It would be expected that the apparent difference would be small most of the time, but large differences may occur occasionally even when the true difference is zero. For the purposes of statistical significance testing, 0.05 (5%) is considered to be sufficiently unlikely for a difference with a null hypothesis probably less than this to be a basis for rejecting the null hypothesis. If the sampling distribution of differences is Normal (and it is, if the samples are large), $Z_\alpha = 1.96$ defines this level of significance. Note that the Z_α is two-tailed: the 5% probability is made up of 2.5% in each of the two directions from 0.

Z_β = the Normal deviate for β, the probability of a type 2 error. This, of course, determines the power of the study. The diagram below shows the sampling distribution of differences if the null hypothesis is false, and the 'true' difference between the treatments is T:

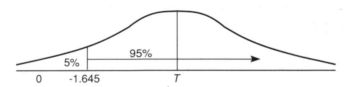

The -1.645 is the Normal deviate that defines the lower tail of the sampling distribution having 5% in it, and the remaining 95% of the sampling distribution lies above this point. A type 2 error occurs when the difference in the study data is too small to be statistically significant, so this error relates to just one tail, the lower tail, of the sampling distribution; if the apparent difference is larger than the true difference, a type 2 error will not be made (if the study is large enough to have a power of more than 50%). So, $Z = -1.645$ is the value for $\beta = 0.05$ (5%), and therefore for a power of 95%. Some values of Z_β for other commonly used powers are as follows:

Power (%)	Z_β
95%	-1.645
90%	-1.28
80%	-0.84
50%	0

T^2 = the standardized treatment difference squared. If the data of interest are qualitative, this is:

$$\frac{(p_1 - p_2)^2}{p(100 - p)}$$

where p_1 is the event rate (e.g. success rate) with one of the treatments (as a percentage) and p_2 is the event rate with the other treatment (also, of course, as a percentage). $p = (p_1 + p_2)/2$. More will be said about this when an example is considered.

If the data are quantitative, T^2 is:

$$\frac{(\bar{X}_1 - \bar{X}_2)^2}{SD^2}$$

where $\bar{X}_1$ is the mean for one treatment, $\bar{X}_2$ is the mean for the second treatment, and SD is the variance within a treatment group. If there is reason to believe the variances of the two treatment groups are likely to be very different, a pooled estimate should be used, pooling thus:

$$SD^2 = \frac{SD_1^2 + SD_2^2}{2}$$

Perhaps some numerical examples will make matters clear. Let us consider the numerator first of all.

The numerator

For the 5% level of significance and 95% power, the numerator will be:

$$2[1.96 - (-1.645)]^2 = 2(1.96 + 1.645)^2 = 25.99205$$

If we choose 90% power instead:

$$2[1.96 - (-1.28)]^2 = 2(1.96 + 1.28)^2 = 20.9952$$

For 80% power:

$$2[1.96 - (-0.84)]^2 = 2(1.96 + 0.84)^2 = 15.68$$

Finally, if the power is to be just 50%:

$$2(1.96 - 0)^2 = 7.6832$$

Putting this in tabular form:

Power	$2(Z_\alpha - Z_\beta)^2$	% of 25.99205
95%	25.99205	100%
90%	20.9952	81%
80%	15.68	60%
50%	7.6832	30%

This table makes the relationship among these commonly used powers and the required sample sizes clear. It can be seen that, for example, we need 81% of the number of patients required for 95% power to give 90% power, 60% of the number for 95% power to give 80% power and 30% of that number for 50% power.

The denominator—qualitative data

Let us deal with qualitative data first of all. The table of powers for various sample sizes was for a comparison in which a 20% difference (between 60% and 80%) was of interest. This could have been chosen if the 'standard' treatment was known to have a success rate of about 60% and a comparison with a new treatment was being planned. The success rate for the new treatment used in the calculation is based on a value judgment—what would the rate need to be in order for the new treatment to be of clinical interest (i.e. the minimum clinically relevant difference is being estimated). In this example, 80% has been chosen. The calculation of T is as follows:

$$p = \frac{60 + 80}{2} = 70$$

$$T^2 = \frac{(60 - 80)^2}{70(100 - 70)} = 0.1905$$

Finally, for 95% power

$$N = \frac{25.99205}{0.1905} = 136.44$$

For 90% power, we would require 81% of 136.44, or 110.52; for 80% power we would need 60% of 136.44, or 81.86; for 50% power the number is 30% of 136.44, or 40.93. These numbers should not be used in an unrealistically precise manner, given the nature of the various quantities used to calculate them. For example, for 95% power, a study with around 135 patients per treatment would be sensible; for 90% power, 110 per group could be used; for 80% power, 80 patients per treatment would be appropriate. The 50% power number is given just for education purposes—one would not choose such a low power in practice.

What is the 'correct' power to use? In practice, 80% is widely used. As only 60% of the number for 95% power is needed to give 80% power, this can be justified on a cost-effectiveness basis. However, it should be borne in mind that the probability of a type 2 error is 0.2 (20%), and also that we are using 5% as the acceptable probability of a type 1 error. The relative importance of type 1 and 2 errors will vary according to the circumstances, but the use of such a high probability of a type 2 error seems hard to justify as a general rule. The author's preference is to use 95% power, making the probabilities of type 1 and 2 errors both 5%. Of course, other error probabilities can be justified according to the precise circumstances relevant to a particular study.

The denominator—quantitative data

As an illustrative example, let us consider a study in which the patients have mild hypercholesterolaemia. The normal range for serum cholesterol is 3.4–6.5 mmol l^{-1}, so the criterion for inclusion into this study would be a serum cholesterol greater than 6.5 mmol l^{-1}—but not to an excessive extent, the maximum permissible being, say, 10 mmol l^{-1}. Suppose the study is intended to see if dietary modification can produce a lower level of serum cholesterol, by randomizing patients to either continue on their present diet or to change to a special diet.

The range of serum cholesterol for the patients at entry to the study, 6.6–10 mmol l^{-1} will be taken as the probable range for those allocated to continue on their present diet. The mid-point of this range will be taken as the group mean, namely 8.3 mmol l^{-1}.

What mean value for the group allocated to the special diet would constitute a clinically worthwhile reduction in serum cholesterol? If the mean was to become 6.5 mmol l^{-1}, the upper limit of normal, about half the patients would now have values within the normal range. So, as an arbitrary value judgment, 6.5 mmol l^{-1} will be taken as the mean for the special diet group that would represent a worthwhile benefit.

To calculate T, SD^2, the variance, is required. An estimate of SD can be made from the Normal range, as this is usually a 95% range and is therefore approximately the mean ± 2 SD, i.e. the normal range is 4 SD wide (assuming that serum cholesterol is approximately Normally distributed). The normal range, 3.4–6.5 mmol l^{-1}, is 3.1 mmol l^{-1} wide, so the SD is approximately $3.1/4 = 0.775$ mmol l^{-1}. SD^2 is $0.775 = 0.6$ mmol l^{-1}. It is worth checking if this SD applies to the patients entered into this study. They lie in the range 6.6–10 mmol l^{-1}, a range of 3.4 mmol l^{-1}. This is a 100% range, as individuals outside this range are excluded from the study. It would appear, therefore, that the estimate of the SD from the normal range is a reasonably appropriate one to use here. Therefore

$$T^2 = \frac{(8.3 - 6.5)^2}{0.6} = \frac{3.24}{0.6} = 5.4$$

For 95% power, $N = 25.99205/5.4 = 4.8$. We must now add 1 to this answer (this correction applies to quantitative data and is of particular importance if N is small, as in this case). The reason for the correction is that the use of Z values in the numerator assumes that the sampling error will be Normally distributed, but with small samples the error will conform to the 't' distribution (see later).

The sensible number of patients to use would therefore be 6 per group (rounding up from 5.8) for 95% power. Five per group (81% of 6, rounded up) would give 90% power, and 4 per group (60% of 6, rounded up) would give 80% power.

These are very small numbers indeed, but T^2 was 5.4, hence T is $\sqrt{5.4}$, or 2.3. That is, the difference we wish to detect between the two means is more than twice the SD. A 1 SD difference could be detected, with 95% power, with

(25.99205/1) + 1, or 27 patients per group. A 1 SD difference is about the difference between the mean heights of men and women, i.e. there is considerable overlap. It obviously depends on the circumstances, but it would often be the case that a difference larger than 1 SD between two means would be clinically interesting, but a difference much smaller than this would often be clinically unimportant.

Estimation of Differences

In the earlier sections *Point estimation* and *Interval estimation*, estimations using a statistic from a single sample (to give an estimate of a single population parameter) were outlined, while in the sections *Statistical significance* and *Type 1 and type 2 errors*, statistical significance testing and power in the context of compairing two treatments were explained. In particular, the two data sets shown again below were discussed.

I

Outcome	Treatments	
	1	2
Success	21	15
Failures	10	17

Chi-square = 2.80;
df = 1; P = 0.095

II

Outcome	Treatments	
	1	2
Success	22	14
Failures	9	18

Chi-square = 4.76;
df = 1; P = 0.025

The data set on the left (I) did not give a value of 'P' sufficiently low for 'chance' to be rejected as a plausible explanation of the difference, i.e. if the true difference were zero, a difference as large as that seen is not sufficiently probable. On the other hand, the data set on the right (II) did give a value of 'P' low enough to reject the 'chance' explanation. It will be recalled that a 'low enough' value of 'P' is one less than 0.05.

So, we have one data set from which we would conclude that the true difference might be zero, and another data set from which we would be prepared to say that the difference is not zero. In the latter case, the question immediately arises 'if the difference is not zero, what is it?' The difference seen in the data is 27.2% (71.0% versus 43.8% successes), and this provides a point estimate of the true difference. However, as with a single sample, we can calculate a confidence interval around the point estimate, using, as before, a standard error. This time the standard error is the standard error of the diffcrence between the two percentages. For estimation, the formula is:

$$\mathrm{SE}_{p_1 - p_2} = \sqrt{\frac{p_1(100 - p_1)}{N_1} + \frac{p_2(100 - p_2)}{N_2}}$$

The calculations for the two data sets are as follows:

I $\qquad$ $SE = \sqrt{\dfrac{67.7 \times 32.3}{31} + \dfrac{46.9 \times 53.1}{32}} = 12.18\%$

II $\qquad$ $SE = \sqrt{\dfrac{71.0 \times 29.0}{31} + \dfrac{43.8 \times 56.2}{32}} = 11.97\%$

As in the section *Interval estimation*, a 95% confidence interval is:

$$\text{Point estimate} \pm 1.96\,SE$$

The calculations are as follows:

I $20.8\% \pm 1.96 \times 12.18\% = 20.8\% \pm 23.87\% = -3.07\%$ to 44.67%
II $27.2\% \pm 1.96 \times 11.97\% = 27.2\% \pm 23.46\% = 3.74\%$ to 50.66%

In II, where zero was rejected as being the true difference, we can be 95% confident that the true difference lies in the range 3.74% to 50.66%. In I, where the zero difference hypothesis was not rejected, the confidence interval is -3.07% to 44.67%. This interval includes zero, which is consistent with the result of the hypothesis test, and suggests that it is conceivable that the apparently inferior treatment could actually be slightly superior (by up to 3.07%). However, it is also conceivable that the true difference is very large indeed in favour of treatment 1.

The foregoing shows all three uses of a statistical analysis. First, there is a description of the data. Then, an hypothesis test to calculate 'P' values for the data is shown. Finally, point and interval estimates of the true difference are given. These three sorts of analysis can be carried out for a wide range of study designs and types of data.

Choosing a Statistical Analysis

A simple table is a good starting point for the topic of choosing an appropriate statistical analysis for a set of data. Here is such a table:

Scale of measurement	Two independent groups	Paired data	Bivariate data
Qualitative Ordinal	Chi-square Wilcoxon/ Mann–Whitney rank-sum test	McNemar's test Wilcoxon matched-pairs signed-ranks test	Chi-square Spearman's rank correlation coefficient
Quantitative	Unpaired *t* test	Paired *t* test	Pearson's product– moment correlation coefficient

Two independent groups

Studies comparing two treatments, in which two groups of patients are used, one group for each of the two treatments, are very common. Data from such studies should be analysed by methods suitable for comparing two independent groups.

Qualitative data

We have already considered such data, in the sections *Hypothesis Testing* and *Estimation of Differences*. The data are presented in a 2 × 2 table, and the hypothesis test most often used is the chi-square test (χ^2). So, here again is such a data set:

Outcome	Treatments	
	1	2
Success	22	14
Failure	9	18

Chi-square = 4.76; df = 1; P = 0.025
p_1 = 71.0%; p_2 = 43.8%; $p_1 - p_2$ = 27.2%.
95% confidence interval for $\pi_1 - \pi_2$ = 3.74% to 50.66%.

Unfortunately, there is a controversy about the way the value of chi-square should be calculated for such a 2 × 2 table, in that there is a correction, known as the Yates or continuity correction, that can be incorporated into the calculation. The effect of the Yates correction is to reduce the value of chi-square; for the data set above, the Yates-corrected chi-square is 3.72, giving P = 0.054. The 95% CI for the estimate of the true difference, corrected for continuity, is 0.52% to 53.9%.

We now have both a general and a particular problem. The general problem is whether or not the Yates correction should be used. The particular problem is that in the data above the Yates-corrected chi-square gives P = 0.054, which is not quite low enough to reject the zero-difference hypothesis at the customary 0.05 level of statistical significance. However, the 95% confidence interval, corrected for continuity, does not include zero.

Taking the general problem first, it has to be said that unchallengeable advice cannot be given here. The controversy still rages (see Colton, 1974; Everitt, 1977; Upton, 1982). Some statisticians consider that the continuity correction should always be used. Others think that if the data are from a randomized trial, the correction is inappropriate, but if the data are from an association study, the correction should be applied. The reason for the latter view is that in a randomized trial the sizes of the groups are fixed before the study begins, but the numbers of successes and failures are subject to random variation, i.e. we would know the column totals in advance, but not the row totals (or vice versa, depending on how we arrange the data). In an association study (e.g. if we ask a number of people (a) whether they smoke cigarettes, and (b) whether they drink gin and tonic), both the row totals and the column totals are unknown in advance.

The two situations have different underlying sampling distribution. The randomized trial is a binomial comparison, whilst the association study is a hypergeometric situation. The writer inclines to the view that the correction should not be used in the analysis of randomized studies, but again it must be said that firm advice cannot be given. It could be argued that as long as there is a controversy, it might be better to 'play safe' and always use the correction.

Let us now look at the particular problem raised by the Yates-corrected analysis of the data shown above. First of all, the Yates chi-square has given $P = 0.054$, while the uncorrected chi-square has given $P = 0.025$. In simple hypothesis testing terms, we now have a non-significant difference instead of a statistically significant one. Second, despite the non-significance of the Yates-corrected chi-square, the Yates-corrected 95% confidence interval for the difference did not include zero. The technical reason for the apparent inconsistency between the hypothesis test and the confidence interval is because there are two different ways of calculating the SE of the difference between the two percentages—one for hypothesis testing (which gives equivalent answers to chi-square) and one for estimation. Let us consider the data set once more:

Outcome	Treatments		Totals
	1	2	
Success	22	14	36 (=57.14% of 63)
Failure	9	18	27 (=42.86% of 63)
Totals	31	32	63

In testing the null hypothesis, it is assumed that the true difference is zero, and any difference seen in the data has arisen by chance alone. Therefore, the best estimate of the 'true' success rate is that provided by all the data, i.e. by pooling the two treatment groups. This is 57.14% in these data. The SE of the difference for hypothesis testing uses this percentage in the calculation, i.e.

$$SE_{p_1 - p_2} = \sqrt{\frac{p(100 - p)}{N_1} + \frac{p(100 - p)}{N_2}}$$

$$= \sqrt{\frac{57.14 \times 42.86}{31} + \frac{57.14 \times 42.86}{32}} = 12.47\%$$

We can use this SE to test the null hypothesis instead of calculating chi-square. Without the continuity correction, the hypothesis test is:

$$z = \frac{p_1 - p_2}{SE_{p_1 - p_2}} = \frac{70.97\% - 43.75\%}{12.47\%} = \frac{27.22\%}{12.47\%} = 2.1828$$

where z is a Normal deviate, defined as the difference divided by its SE. The percentages have been taken to two places of decimals to make the calculation more accurate. The value of 2.1828 can be looked up in a table of areas under the standard Normal curve, from which it would be found that

$P = 0.029$. Note that the square of 2.1828 is 4.76, the value of the uncorrected chi-square, or, put the other way, the square root of the 1 df chi-square is a Normal deviate.

To apply the Yates correction, the quantity $50(1/N_1 + 1/N_2)$ is first calculated. Here, it is:

$$50(\tfrac{1}{31} + \tfrac{1}{32}) = 50(0.03226 + 0.03125)\% = 3.1755\%$$

This correction factor is used to reduce the $p_1 - p_2$ difference in magnitude before it is divided by the SE. Hence:

$$z(\text{corrected}) = \frac{27.22\% - 3.1755\%}{12.47\%}$$

$$= \frac{24.0445\%}{12.47\%}$$

$$= 1.928$$

This gives $P = 0.054$ from a table of the standard Normal curve. Squared, 1.928 becomes 3.72, the value of the Yates-corrected chi-square.

However, in estimation, it is assumed that the best estimate of the true difference is the difference actually seen in the data, the point estimate of the difference. Therefore, the percentages of successes in the two treatments are used to calculate the SE, and, as we saw earlier in *Estimation of Differences*, this gave a value of 11.97%. The 95% confidence interval is therefore being calculated with a slightly smaller SE than that used for hypothesis testing. To correct the confidence interval for continuity, the correction calculated above is applied to the uncorrected interval, to make it wider. Hence:

$$\text{Corrected lower limit} = 3.7\% - 3.1755\% = 0.52\%$$
$$\text{Corrected lower limit} = 50.7\% + 3.1755\% = 53.88\%$$

The correction is subtracted from the lower limit and added to the upper limit in order to widen the confidence interval. The apparent inconsistency between the hypothesis test and the confidence interval here is, in numerical terms, very small, and has arisen because a Normal distribution approximation to the Binomial has been used. After all, the 0.05 border distinguishing statistical significance from non-significance is somewhat artificial, and the conclusions from the hypothesis test and the confidence interval are not markedly in conflict—both suggest that the true difference may not be very different from zero.

Ordinal data

The table at the beginning of *Choosing a Statistical Analysis* indicates that the Wilcoxon/Mann–Whitney rank-sum test can be used to compare two independent groups in which the data are on an ordinal scale. This test is referred to as either the Wilcoxon rank-sum test or the Mann–Whitney test (or by both eponyms) in various textbooks, reflecting the fact that Wilcoxon and Mann and Whitney independently developed this test—it is the same test whichever eponym is used.

This test (which I shall refer to as the W/M–W test here) is often referred to as a 'non-parametric' test. This is because such tests do not estimate a parameter of a sampling distribution, namely a standard error, in calculating P values and confidence intervals. Instead, they are based on a permutation argument. There are two indications for the use of such a test. First, as has been implied above, ordinal data should be analysed using the appropriate non-parametric test. Second, if there is doubt about the validity of using a parametric test (e.g. the unpaired t test) because the data may be markedly non-Normal or the sample SDs are very different, it is advisable to use such a test, especially if the samples are small. If the data are indeed suitable for the application of a parametric test, little power is lost by using a non-parametric test (the power efficiency of such tests is greater than 90% in comparison with the t test under these circumstances). It is often worth carrying out both a parametric and a non-parametric analysis in order to check if the conclusions are similar. If they give very different results, this is usually because the assumptions justifying the use of a parametric test have been violated by that data set.

The use of the W/M–W test will now be illustrated using a small data test:

Groups		
1		2
26		22
27		25
26		21
24		20
26		18
		21
Mean	25.80	21.17
SD	1.10	2.32
N	5	6
g1	−0.87	0.42
g2	−0.27	−0.34

The difference between the two means is 4.63, negative skew is present in the data from group 1 and positive skew in the data from group 2, though the degree of skew is not large in either group. Both groups have slightly platy-kurtic data. The calculation now proceeds by ranking the data (from the smallest to the largest value), treating the data from the two groups as a single series. Hence:

Ranks:	Group	
	1	2
	9	5
	11	7
	9	3.5
	6	2
	9	1
		3.5

Sum of ranks for Group 1 = 44.
Sum of ranks for Group 1 = 22.
Total = 66.

				(3.5)					(9)		
Rank	1	2	3	4	5	6	7	8	9	10	11
Value	18	20	21	21	22	24	25	26	26	26	27

Notice how the ranking was performed. The total study size was 11, so the data will be ranked from 1 to 11. Equal values (often called tied values) are given the average of the ranks they occupy; so the two values 21 are given 3.5 each (mean of 3 and 4) and the three 26's are given 9 each (mean of 8, 9 and 10). The ranks for each group are then summed. As a check, the total of the ranks for the two groups combined is found. If there are N values in all, the total of their ranks is:

$$\frac{N(N + 1)}{2}$$

Here the total should be $11(11 + 1)/2 = 66$, which it is. This little check is said to have been invented by Gauss whilst a schoolboy (aged 8) in Freiburg. The teacher set the class the task of adding the numbers 1, 2, 3, . . . up to 100. Gauss first wrote the series as follows:

$$1 + \quad 2 + \quad 3 + . + 98 + 99 + 100$$

Then he wrote the series in reverse:

$$100 + 99 + 98 + \ldots + 3 + \quad 2 + \quad 1$$

He then noticed that adding the top number to the lower number always gave a total of 101, and therefore the series added up twice consisted of 100 terms each equal to 101. So the series added up once was half of 100×101 (i.e. 5050), hence the formula given above.

The procedure is now to look up the rank sum for the smaller group (here group 1) in a suitable table. Using Table C12 in Brown and Hollander (1977) gives $P = 0.008$ (two-tailed, of course). For $P < 0.05$, the rank sum (in the smaller group) when the group sizes are 5 and 6, respectively, must either be 42 or greater, or be 18 or less. Here the value 44 is greater than 42, and the 'exact' P is 0.008.

The procedure for obtaining a confidence interval for the difference between the two means is a little tedious. It is made somewhat easier if the data are put in rank order within each group first, and then a table is created thus:

Group 1	Group 2					
	18	20	21	21	22	25
24	6	4	3	3	2	−1
26	8	6	5	5	4	1
26	8	6	5	5	4	1
26	8	6	5	5	4	1
27	9	7	6	6	5	2

The entries in the table are the differences between each group 1 value and each group 2 value. The quantity 'L' is now found by:

$$L = \frac{N_1(2N_2 + N_1 + 1)}{2} + 1 - \text{(upper rank sum for } p < 0.05)$$

It is essential that N_1 is the smaller sample size if the sample sizes differ. Here, the calculation is:

$$L = \frac{5(12 + 5 + 1)}{2} + 1 - 42 = 45 + 1 - 42 = 4$$

The value 42 is the rank sum required for $P < 0.05$ in the smaller of the two groups (18 in the lower rank sum for $P < 0.05$, but the upper value is used). This tells us that the confidence interval is given by the 4th lowest and 4th highest differences in the table of differences above. The 4th lowest difference is 1, and the 4th highest is 8. This is not, however, a precise 95% confidence interval, in that the 42 is for $p < 0.05$, not $P = 0.05$. The 'exact' P for the rank sum of 42 is 0.03, so the confidence interval is a 97% interval. A rank sum of 41 gives $P = 0.052$, so the 5th lowest and highest differences would give the 94.8% confidence interval, namely 2–7.

This calculation is readily performed using the Confidence Interval Analysis (CIA) program that can be purchased from the British Medical Association as a companion to Gardner and Altman (1989).

Quantitative data

The same data set as used in the previous section will now be analysed using the unpaired t test, which assumes that the data are quantitative, that the data consist of samples taken at random from Normally distributed populations, and that the SDs of the populations are identical. Of course the assumptions about Normality and equality of SDs will not hold exactly in the actual samples of data, but the samples should not be so non-Normal or unequal in SD that it is inconceivable that the assumptions could be true. Testing for Normality and inequality of SDs is not really possible with very small samples, and is less necessary with large samples because of the robustness of the t test to violations of its assumptions.

As mentioned in the previous section, a practical solution is often to do both a parametric and a non-parametric analysis to see if they give similar conclusions.

Groups	
1	2
26	22
27	25
26	21
24	20
26	18
	21

Mean	25.80	21.17
SD	1.10	2.32
N	5	6
g1	−0.87	0.42
g2	−0.27	−0.34

In order to calculate the SE of the difference between the two means, an estimate of the population SD must be obtained. As has been noted above, it is assumed that the two samples have been taken from populations with equal SDs, so the 'best' estimate of the population SD is an 'average' of the two SDs. The 'average' (or pooled SD) is found as follows:

$$\text{Pooled SD}^2 = \frac{(N_1 - 1)SD_1^2 + (N_2 - 1)SD_2^2}{N_1 + N_2 - 2} = \frac{4 \times 1.10 + 5 \times 2.32}{9}$$

$$= \frac{4.83 + 26.912}{9}$$

$$= 3.527$$

This pooled SD^2 is then used to calculate the SE of the difference between the two means:

$$SE_{\bar{X}_1 - \bar{X}_2} = \sqrt{\frac{SD^2}{N_1} + \frac{SD^2}{N_2}} = \sqrt{\frac{3.527}{5} + \frac{3.527}{6}}$$

$$= 0.7054 + 0.5878 = 1.137$$

The hypothesis test is as follows

$$t = \frac{\bar{X}_1 - \bar{X}_2}{SE_{\bar{X}_1 - \bar{X}_2}} = \frac{4.63}{1.137} = 4.07$$

The degrees of freedom for an unpaired t test are df $= N_1 + N_2 - 2 = 9$. From a table of t, with df $= 9$, the t must be greater than 2.262 for $P < 0.05$. In fact, it can be calculated that $P = 0.003$.

To obtain a 95% confidence interval for an estimate of the 'true' difference between the two means, the expression is:

$$95\% \ \text{CI} \ = \ \text{point estimate} + t.05 \times \text{SE}_{x_1 - x_2}$$

$$= \ 4.63 \pm (2.262 \times 1.137) \ = \ 4.63 \pm 2.57 \ = \ 2.06\text{--}7.20$$

This is almost the same as the 94.8% interval of 2 to 7 given by the non-parametric calculation in the previous section. Note that the appropriate t value for the df for the study for $P = 0.05$ is the multiplier, rather than 1.96.

The history of the t distribution is interesting. W.S. Gossett, who was employed as a statistician by the firm of Arthur Guinness and Company (famous for its Irish stout), published the paper including the t distribution in *Biometrika* in 1908 under the pseudonym of 'Student'. Rumour has it that he used the pseudonym to conceal his identity from his employers, and that the letter 't' came from tea (the drink)—it is possible that under different circumstances this distribution might have been the G (for Guinness and for Gossett) distribution!

This chapter is intended merely to be a brief introduction to general principles. In addition to those books mentioned already as references for specific points, I particularly commend to your attention the book written by Drs Norman and Streiner, who are respectively a statistician and a psychiatrist at McMaster University. This book explains with a minimum of mathematical detail the concepts underlying most of the more advanced statistical techniques used in psychiatry, such as analysis of variance and covariance, regression analysis, and factor analysis (Norman and Streiner, 1986).

References

Brown, B.W. and Hollander, M. (1977). *Statistics: A Biomedical Introduction*. New York: Wiley.

Colton, T. (1974). *Statistics in Medicine*. Boston: Little Brown.

Everitt, B.S. (1977). *The Analysis of Contingency Tables*. London: Chapman and Hall.

Gardner, M.J. and Altman, D.G. (1989). *Statistics with Confidence*. London: British Medical Journal.

Norman, G.R. and Streiner, D.L. (1986). *PDQ Statistics*. Toronto: Decker.

Pearson, E.S. and Hartley, H.O. (1970). *Biometrika Tables for Statisticians*, Vol. 1. Cambridge: Cambridge University Press.

Pearson, E.S. and Hartley, H.O. (1972). *Biometrika Tables for Statisticians*, Vol. 2. Cambridge: Cambridge University Press.

Tallirada, R.J. and Murray, R.B. (1987). *Manual of Pharmacologic Calculations with Computer Programs*, 2nd edn. New York: Springer-Verlag.

Tukey, J. (1977). *Exploratory Data Analysis*. Massachusetts: Addison-Wesley.

Upton, G.J.G. (1982). *Journal of the Royal Statistical Society A*. **145**, 86–105.

Walker, H.M. (1931). *Studies in the History of Statistical Method*. Baltimore: Williams and Wilkins.

— 6

Epidemiology

G. Lewis and A. Mann

Epidemiology is the population-based, quantitative study of the distribution, determinants and control of disease. It is the basic science of public health medicine and provides the methodological principles for the majority of quantitative clinical research. A knowledge of epidemiological methods is therefore essential before embarking upon most medical research.

There are three main ways in which epidemiology is used. Firstly, in describing the amount and distribution of disease in the population. This is the use of epidemiology which is most familiar and is an essential part of understanding any medical condition. In more recent years epidemiologists have become more interested in a second use of epidemiology, that of explanation. Analytical epidemiology, or the investigation of specific etiological hypotheses, is one of the main areas of interest and intervention studies and clinical trials increasingly require the resources of the epidemiologist. The third use of epidemiology is in determining public health policy and the distribution of health care resources. Screening for disease, evaluating public health interventions, and creating balance sheets for decision-making all require epidemiological expertise.

In this chapter, the principles behind epidemiological research will be outlined, study design and interpretation of findings will be discussed and methods of case definition will be described. Finally, there is an account of published health statistics, relevant to mental health.

Fundamentals of the Epidemiological Method

Population at risk

Epidemiology is the population-based study of disease and so epidemiological research is concerned with rates. A rate can be defined as the number of events, perhaps diseased people, occurring in a population at risk. It is important to relate disease to the population at risk to help interpretation.

For instance, a study might report that there were 140 violent incidents with nurses and 10 violent incidents on doctors in a hospital. If one concluded that nurses are 14 times more likely to be victims of violence this would ignore the fact that there are more nurses than doctors in a hospital. This error is often described as that of the 'floating numerator'. To draw conclusions about the risk of violence on nurses or doctors requires the calculation of a rate—so many violent incidents per 100 nurses and doctors.

Standardizing case definitions

Quantitative medical research is concerned with measuring differences between groups. It is therefore important to measure disease and factors of interest accurately. The diagnostic process in epidemiology, case definition, requires standardization. Standardized case definition is characterized by strict and clearly defined criteria which enable patients to be classified in a reliable way. For instance, most scientific papers now use such standardized criteria to define cases of schizophrenia or depression rather than relying upon the clinical diagnoses of the individual physicians. Clinical diagnoses are notoriously unreliable in all areas of medicine, including psychiatry. The benefits of standardization are that it is possible to compare different studies, it is possible to repeat studies on a different population with the same case definition, and it reduces the possibility of biased assessment which would lead to spurious results.

Incidence and prevalence

There are two main measures of disease frequency. Incidence is a true rate in which the number of new cases of a disease are given for the population at risk. In contrast, the prevalence of a condition is the proportion of cases found in a population on a cross-sectional survey. Prevalent cases will therefore include some relatively new cases and some who have had the condition for some time. A sample selected from cases determined by a cross-sectional survey will therefore have individuals with a chronic course over-represented. Characteristics associated with prevalent cases of disease will include factors related to incidence *and* factors leading to a longer duration of the disease. For instance, in a population survey it may be found that twice the number of women than men have a depressive illness. One cannot therefore say that the incidence of depression is twice as common in women. An alternative explanation would be that women have longer duration depressive illnesses.

Relative and attributable risk

In analytical epidemiology one is interested in the association between a factor of interest, usually called an exposure, and the disease. This association is usually measured in terms of the relative risk. For instance, there is an association between adverse life-events (the exposure) and depressive illness (the disease). The risk of depression in those with adverse life-events is about four times that of people without such an exposure and the relative risk is therefore about four. Relative risk gives an estimate of the etiological force of an exposure in that population.

If we want to assess individual risks of disease or treatment effects then we are interested in the attributable risk—in other words the absolute increase in risk associated with the exposure. The same relative risk will have a much larger attributable risk in a commoner condition.

Study Design in Analytical Epidemiology

In attempting to study causes of disease in the community epidemiologists look for associations between possible causative factors (the exposure) and the disease. There are five types of study design which can be relevant.

1. *Clinical description.* It is often valuable to describe a series of cases and if there is a very strong association between the disease and their possible exposure this may be apparent. However, in the vast majority of cases if one wished to discover an association between the disease and an exposure it would require a comparison group.

2. *Case-control studies.* These can therefore be seen as an extension of the classical case series. The proportion of cases giving a history of exposure is compared with that in the controls. The control group therefore gives an estimate of the proportion of exposed people in the population from which the cases were drawn.

3. *Cross-sectional surveys.* A population is screened for both the disease and the exposure, allowing the association to be studied.

4. *Cohort or longitudinal studies.* The researcher selects two groups without the disease but who differ in terms of their exposure to the possible etiological factor. Subjects are followed up and the incidence of disease in the two groups compared. Cross-sectional surveys and cohort studies can only be done for relatively common conditions.

5. *Clinical trials and other experimental designs.* It is rarely ethical to study etiology with an experimental design, although response to treatment can sometimes provide clues to the cause of disorder. The investigator randomly allocates subjects to two or more groups which are treated in different ways. This design therefore randomly allocates all confounding variables, including those of which the researcher is unaware, and though confounding can still occur it does so according to chance and the probability of this can be statistically estimated.

It is extremely expensive to study uncommon conditions with cross-sectional surveys or cohort studies. For instance, the incidence of schizophrenia is less than 20 in 100 000 per year. Case-control studies are therefore more suitable for studying uncommon conditions such as schizophrenia, severe depressive illness, anorexia nervosa, etc.

Explaining associations

It is well known that there are many problems in attempting to interpret associations between a disease and a possible etiological factor (exposure). There are four main explanations to be considered when an association is observed.

1. *Chance.* An association can arise by chance and this is estimated by the '*p*' value, which is the probability that random variation led to the result. A type 1 error occurs when there was no true association but the *p* value was sufficiently small to reject the null hypothesis. This will be more common if repeated tests are performed. When a real association is missed because the variation is too

large and the study sample is too small it is known as a type 2 error. It should always be considered when there are negative results and the increasing use of confidence intervals is designed to avoid such interpretive errors.

2. *Reverse causality.* An association between a disease and an exposure may occur because the disease causes the exposure. For instance, the well-documented association between schizophrenia and low social class may result from the occupational disability produced by schizophrenia. Cohort studies tend to avoid this problem because they start with people without disease.

3. *Confounding and bias.* These are the most important possible explanations for an association and preoccupy most medical researchers. A confounder is associated with both the disease and the exposure and can therefore lead to a spurious association or can eliminate a real association. Bias in measurement has similar results and selection bias in case-control studies is a particular difficulty.

4. *A true causal association.*

Confounding

Confounders can distort the association between disease and exposures in any observational research. A simple illustration is provided by the observation that more women have Alzheimer's dementia than men. This results firstly from an association between age and Alzheimer's disease (that it becomes commoner with age), and secondly from the fact that women's longevity results in there being more old women than old men. Therefore age is said to confound the relationship between gender (exposure) and Alzheimer's disease.

If confounding variables can be measured, then the possible effects of the confounder on the association between the disease and exposure can be estimated and so an adjusted estimate of relative risk can be calculated. It is therefore important at the design stage of the study to consider all potential confounders and to ensure that these are measured in the course of the study or incorporated in the design. There are four main methods of adjusting for confounding:

1. *Restriction.* When designing a study subjects are only selected if they have the same value of the confounding variable. For instance if sex is a confounder, one might only study women.

2. *Matching.* Each case can be matched with a control on the basis of any number of potential confounders, but commonly age and sex. Matching is done to increase the power of a study and is not an essential way of adjusting for confounders. Furthermore matching can introduce bias into a study unless a matched analysis is performed. There are some disadvantages of matching which are beyond the scope of this chapter, but it is most advantageous in small studies where it is important to increase statistical power.

3. *Stratification.* As long as confounders are measured, adjustment for their effects can occur in the analysis. The simplest approach is a stratified analysis in which the association between disease and exposure is estimated within each category of the confounder. For instance, in the case of Alzheimer's disease one would measure the ratio between men and women within each age category. An adjusted estimate is then calculated as a weighted average over the different

categories. It can be seen that this will eliminate the effect of the confounding variable.

4. *Multivariate techniques.* Multivariate analysis is conceptually similar to stratification but uses mathematical models with simplifying assumptions. It is impossible to examine the effects of more than one or two confounders by stratification unless you have enormous numbers in the sample, but this can be done with multivariate methods. There are a variety of different multivariate methods which are all suitable for different study designs; logistic regression is often used in epidemiology.

Selection bias

Selection bias occurs when the controls in a case-control study give a biased estimate of the prevalence of exposure in the study population. A useful rule-of-thumb to guide the design of a case-control study in order to minimize selection bias is that the controls, if they were to become diseased, would be in the sampling frame for the cases under study.

For instance, it is well known that many of those with affective disorder never contact the psychiatric services. Therefore if one chose hospital cases of depression the use of general population controls could lead to very misleading results in a case-control study (Lewis and Pelosi, 1990). Recognition of this fact has led to the widespread use of population-based surveys in studying the common affective disorders in the community. Cross-sectional surveys will eliminate the possibility of selection bias because it is then clear that the cases and controls (in this case those who are not cases in the survey) were drawn from the same population.

Information bias

Information bias occurs when there is a difference between those with a disease and those without in the gathering of data on exposure. Information bias can be divided into that resulting from the subject and that from the observer. One of the most important subject-derived information biases is often called 'recall bias' and is a problem in case-control studies where the subjects' recall of exposure may be influenced by their disease status. One of the best known examples is Stott's (1958) finding that mothers of children with Down's syndrome more frequently reported an emotional stressor during pregnancy than women who delivered a healthy baby. Subsequent work indicated this was a result of the mother's attempt to explain giving birth to a handicapped child. There are many measures in psychiatry including social network measures, personality measures and measures of marital disharmony that are all probably influenced by current mental state. Recall bias would therefore be a problem in any study designed where such data were collected retrospectively.

Observer bias results when knowledge that a subject is a case or has been exposed to a certain factor leads to a biased assessment of either disease or exposure. The main method for overcoming this is the use of 'blind' assessments, a technique widely used in clinical trials. Observer bias is eliminated by self-administered questionnaires but there is often concern that subjects may not fully understand the questions and that those who read poorly or are illiterate may be unable to respond.

Classification and Case Definition in Psychiatry

Principles

Classification is an important and necessary act but can be stultifying unless its results are seen as provisional and open to revision as medical knowledge increases. Feinstein (1972) has summarized the function of classification in medicine as follows: (a) denomination, the giving of a name to phenomena; (b) qualification, the associating of qualifying or descriptive features to that name; and (c) prediction, the making of statements about outcome. Feinstein also points out how medical classificatory systems are constantly under pressure; from the findings of community surveys where subclinical indistinct cases are discovered and from modern methods of statistical analyses which can show how existing data can be recorded.

Jablensky (1988) has given a classification of classificatory systems. Those systems that depend upon observable facts, for example histological appearance, are called empirical; those that depend on commonly shared hypotheses, such as reactive and endogenous forms of depression, are called inferential. Those classificatory systems that arrange units into classes according to variations along one dimension are called monothetic, whereas those that group units because of their sharing of a large proportion of a number of agreed properties are called polythetic. Classification according to level of intelligence would be an example of the former, the classification of the psychoses of the latter. Much of medical classification is polythetic in nature, depending upon symptom clusters and signs, unless the etiology of a disease is precisely known when the polythetic basis is usually superseded by a monothetic system based upon etiological determinants. However, even in a polythetic system, the cluster of attributes against which an object is to be matched for classification must remain consistent between classes. In medicine, there is usually a similar mixture of symptoms, behaviour and background history.

In one sense there are no principles to medical classification. The purpose of classification is to help doctors carry out their work. Any system of classification that proves useful to practising doctors will become widely used.

Classification in psychiatry

Ever since Pinel in the early nineteenth century, there have been attempts at classification of mental disorders. The Kraepelinian system, separating dementia praecox from manic depressive disorders, has been most enduring, even though this system was the result of successive modifications during Kraepelin's professional life. Classification in psychiatry has been made more feasible by means of the science of phenomenology, as promoted by Jaspers (1963), which has enabled the abnormal components of mental life to be defined. Psychiatric systems are evidently polythetic, abnormal subjective mental experiences and deviant social behaviours being brought together to form the various classes. Psychiatry has been slower than the rest of medicine to discover etiological determinants of the illnesses in its domain so that a monothetic system based upon etiology is not yet possible. Psychiatric classification has been criticised from a number of quarters. For instance, the dynamic psychopathologist would regard the person rather than the disease as the unit for classification, while the philosopher might object to the richness of mental life being dissected and reduced to units, objects, for classification. Some sociologists have drawn attention to the disadvantageous nature of the diagnostic label (Scheff, 1963) by arguing that the label itself encourages deviance and introduces stigma (Goffman, 1976).

Despite these criticisms, which cannot and should not be dismissed, psychiatric classification stemming from Kraepelin has proved useful and endured for nearly a century. Furthermore, it seems that the brain, assumed to be the mediator for all mental phenomena or behaviours, can only become dysfunctional in a limited number of ways.

Jablensky (1988), addressing the desirability of classifications in the future, has pointed out there are some quite practical requirements for a successful system apart from a valid theoretical basis. The system should be useful and accessible for a clinician in his daily practice who will be making decisions based upon it and will be recording diagnoses in case notes, which in turn, become the data for statistical returns. If doctors are to communicate with each other it is important that they can agree on the terms they are using and reliable classifications are of fundamental importance.

Current systems of psychiatric classification

The two systems of classifying psychiatric disorders in wide use are the *International Classification of Diseases, Ninth Revision*, Chapter 5 (ICD-9; World Health Organization, 1978) and the *Diagnostic Statistical Manual of Mental Disorders, Third Edition* (DSM-III; American Psychiatric Association, 1980). DSM-III was revised in 1987, the end result DSM-III-R (American Psychiatric Association, 1987) being similar in concept to DSM-III. ICD-9 is a section of the World Health Organization's general classificatory system for all medical conditions and therefore needs to be acceptable to as many member states of the World Health Organization (WHO) as possible. DSM-III, in comparison, represents the national view of the United States, though its influence now extends far beyond that country (Cooper, 1988). Both ICD and DSM-III are polythetic in type, although certain diagnoses have an etiological dimension.

An approach to classification that contrasts these two is hierarchy of personal illness (Foulds, 1967). Foulds regarded mental illness along a dimension of disturbance in interpersonal relationships from mild to severe, the common disorders arranging themselves into a hierarchy with four levels. Symptoms that occur in the lower level may be present in the higher level disorders, but not the reverse. Thus symptoms of delusion (level 3 disorder) may be accompanied by affective changes (level 1), but those disorders at level 1, such as depression or anxiety, may not possess level 3 symptoms. This system most sparingly fits the rules of classification and yet has found little acceptance.

ICD-9 and ICD-10

ICD-9 maintained the classical subdivision between psychoses and neuroses and, for the first time, introduced a section on disorders of childhood and adolescence. Each section is further subdivided into ten units. There is a short glossary of the major terms for the user.

The *Ninth Revision* has functioned well but has become increasingly criticised. A major inconsistency is that the classification is sometimes empirical and sometimes inferential. Some disorders are subdivided according to etiology while others refer to further definitions based upon symptoms, behaviours or outcome. This arrangement is recognized in the introduction as a compromise, reflecting the special problems of psychiatry at the time. Although the basis of classification is not consistent, the system does require the user to behave as though it was unidimensional, to choose between categories and therefore give one diagnosis. This leads to unreliability, as does the vagueness of some of the criteria in the glossary. The ICD-9 system has difficulties in dealing with transient disorders associated with stress and with physical symptoms that probably have no organic basis.

Sartorius (1988) has described some of the pressures that led to ICD-10 that should come into use in 1992. There was the need to describe the patient in terms of symptom state, etiology and disability. There was dissatisfaction of psychiatrists from the Third World countries with the way that psychoses were classified. There was continuing criticism of the concept of neurosis and the general inadequacy of all the categories for use in primary care settings.

One major change in ICD-10 has been the abandoning of the classical divide between psychoses and neuroses as existed in ICD-9. A new broad grouping of somatoform disorders has been created that contains many of the former neurotic disorders and allows psychogenic physical symptoms to be included. Disorders with an affective theme, whether they were previously regarded as a psychoses, neuroses, or even a personality disorder, are grouped together under affective disorders.

This clinical review has been accompanied by a much more sophisticated introduction entitled 'Clinical Description and Diagnostic Guidelines'. These provide details of each clinical concept with diagnostic guidelines for each category into possible differential diagnoses for the user to consider. There will soon be a second set of more stringent guidelines for use when the ICD-10 classification is being used for research. Furthermore, standardized interviews are being developed to collect data, so that the research criteria can be applied internationally. Finally, there is to be a dictionary, to give accurate definitions of the individual phenomena of the diagnostic syndromes.

This is a much more sophisticated system, designed to last and to be the servant rather than the master of its users (Sartorius, 1988). To this end, development has been a bottom-up approach, data coming from global consultation with field trials to inform the final system.

DSM-III and DSM-IV

DSM-III was designed to be empirical rather than inferential, so that some traditional diagnoses, still present in ICD-9, were abandoned. In order to aid reliability, detailed diagnostic criteria were provided, reflecting the 'collective wisdom of the numerous experts in psychopathology' working on advisory committees (Skodol and Spitzer, 1982). To allow for multiaxial classifications, the system consisted of five axes (see below).

The major conceptual changes in DSM-III included the abandonment of the neuroses as a group, each former member being reclassified according to its major clinical feature. The diagnosis of schizophrenia was narrowed, introducing the requirement for active psychotic features to be present and a duration of six months. Other changes were to the categories of affective disorders which are subdivided to major and minor, rather than psychotic and neurotic.

DSM-III-R was published in 1987. Modification of DSM-III is relatively minor, and the principles underlying DSM-III were unchanged. However, DSM-III-R eliminated many of the diagnostic hierarchies stipulated in DSM-III, therefore allowing the existence of 'comorbidity'. Furthermore, the codes given in DSM-III-R are more comparable to those in ICD-9.

DSM-III has an impact beyond its national boundary, its tightly written standardized diagnostic guidelines facilitating intra- and international research. However, for general clinical use, the precision of some of its criteria make DSM-III cumbersome and impracticable. However, it can be seen that ICD-10 has been influenced by DSM-III.

DSM-IV is now in discussion, but is not planned to be radically different from DSM-III. Modifications will be based upon experience with use of DSM-III. DSM-IV and ICD-10 are likely to be closer to each other than DSM-III and ICD-9.

Multiaxial systems

There are many elements of the clinical picture that determine response to treatment and outcome including previous personality, course of illness, social impairment and social support. A multiaxial system can recognize this complexity. Such a multiaxial system has been in use in child psychiatry for nearly 20 years and five axes are included in DSM-III. Axis I refers to the main diagnosis, axis II is used to rate personality disorder, axis III is for physical disorders, axis IV gives the severity of etiologically important stressors and axis V rates the 'highest level of adaptive functioning in the past year'.

There has also been discussion of a multiaxial system for ICD-10, though a consensus has not yet been reached. Symptoms and etiology make two obvious axes; personality, social impairment, severity and certainty of diagnosis have been suggested as others.

Case definition in psychiatry

There has been considerable research into improving the reliability of psychiatric diagnoses. There are two main ways in which people have attempted to define cases of psychiatric disorder: firstly, standardized interviews such as the present State Examination (PSE; Wing *et al.*, 1974); and secondly, using self-administered questionnaires such as the General Health Questionnaire (GHQ; Goldberg and Williams, 1988). Self-administered computerized assessments of psychiatric disorder have also been devised and can perform quite well in assessing neurotic symptoms (Lewis *et al.*, 1988; Greist *et al.*, 1987).

One of the most influential developments in psychiatric measurement was that of the PSE. This is in effect a standardized assessment of the mental state enquiring about both neurotic and psychotic symptoms over the four weeks preceding the interview. The questions, called 'probes', are specified and there is an extensive glossary of terms to assist the interviewer in deciding upon the presence or absence of psychopathology. It was designed for use by psychiatrists, although non-medical interviewers have also been trained in its use. Unlike some of the American interviews such as the Schedule for Affective Disorders and Schizophrenia (SADS; Spitzer and Endicott, 1978), the PSE has a 'bottom-up' design in that symptoms are defined by the interview. In contrast the SADS starts with the research diagnostic criteria (Spitzer *et al.*, 1975) and is in that sense 'top-down'. These two interviews have been designed by hospital psychiatrists and therefore concentrate on severe, mostly psychotic, psychopathology, although they also include questions about the commoner neurotic symptoms. In contrast, the Clinical Interview Schedule (Goldberg *et al.*, 1970) was designed for use in community studies and in general practice and so almost exclusively enquires about neurotic symptoms.

The General Health Questionnaire (GHQ) has been used in a large number of studies in a variety of cultures and has proved a useful measure of neurotic symptomatology in the community and general practice. Similar questionnaires exist, although none have been studied to such an extent as the GHQ. Despite its value, there is some evidence that the physically ill score more highly on the GHQ irrespective of their psychiatric symptoms.

When designing a study the researcher must decide whether to measure psychiatric disorder using an interview or questionnaire measure. Interviews have the disadvantage that they may be contaminated by observer bias and the majority of existing interviews allow on occasions considerable latitude in making ratings about the presence or absence of psychopathology. In contrast, the researcher may be concerned that subjects will not understand the questions of a self-administered questionnaire and some subjects are partially sighted or have poor language. However, there are many circumstances where more random errors resulting from using a self-administered questionnaire are more acceptable to the experimenter than the observer bias which may contaminate interview measures. It is often wise to use both a self-administered and interview measure in a study.

Screening for psychiatric disorder

Questionnaires such as the GHQ are often referred to as screening questionnaires. This arises from the belief that such questionnaires are inferior measures of psychiatric disorder to the lengthy and thorough standardized interviews such as the PSE. Studies are much quicker and cheaper to conduct with questionnaires and so there are occasions when a researcher may wish to screen a large population with a GHQ and then follow up the high scoring individuals with a more detailed assessment. In addition, some psychiatrists have suggested that physicians and general practitioners use the GHQ in their clinical work to detect cases of psychiatric disorder. In practice this has rarely been done except on an experimental basis.

When describing the properties of a screening test the sensitivity (proportion of non-cases accurately classified) and the specificity (the proportion of cases correctly classified) are usually calculated. Often of more importance in a practical screening programme is the positive predictive value of the test. This is the proportion of subjects who score positively on the test and are in fact cases of the disorder. The positive predictive value depends crucially upon the prevalence of the condition, for if the condition is rare the number of false positives increases dramatically. In other words for rare conditions screening for disorder is useless unless one has an *extremely* accurate screening test.

This phenomenon has been illustrated by Williams *et al.* (1982) with the Eating Attitudes Test (EAT; Garner and Garfinkel, 1980). This test appeared to have relatively good sensitivities and specificities in a population in which there was a high prevalence of anorexia and bulimia nervosa. However, when applied to samples from general practice, anorexia and bulimia are so uncommon that the EAT becomes almost worthless screening for cases of disorder.

Mental Health Statistics

National data

The management and evaluation of mental health services requires information on current activities. This is now done using the Hospital In-Patient Enquiry (HIPE), which produces standard data for 10% of all discharges from hospital. In the past, psychiatric hospital statistics were collected separately in the Mental Health Enquiry. The major limitation of HIPE is that it counts admissions, not people; people who are admitted twice will therefore be counted twice in HIPE. The Hospital Activity Analysis (HAA) is a local way of collecting similar data to HIPE on 100% of the discharges.

The General Household Survey and Social Trends can also provide information relevant to psychiatric research. Consultations with general practitioners and alcohol intake are routinely assessed. The National Morbidity Statistics give details of consultations in general practice, where the bulk of mental health activity in the United Kingdom takes place. These data are often ignored by mental health service planners. At the moment, returns from districts provided by public health doctors on their morbidity and service use in their locality rarely mention mental illness.

Brooke (1980) has criticised health service statistics as a means of monitoring mental health service activity on the following grounds. First, they are not complete—data are only gathered from institutions run by the health authorities, as social services and voluntary and private agencies are not included. Second, in-patient activity is emphasized, and the greater amount of day and out-patient activities are not included. Third, it is hard to validate the information, for example, on diagnosis. Fourth, these data are often produced too late for useful decisions on policy to be made. From the point of view of use of these statistics for research, there are two further difficulties. They tend to be group returns by region, their figures probably ironing out many important between-service variations, and the data are often too broad for information about specific patient groups to be obtained.

For these reasons, case registers have been set up (see below) to provide details of service use in restricted geographical areas. However, the broadly based national statistics have had their use in furthering research. The US/UK studies evolved from the observation that admission rates were much higher in the United States than in the United Kingdom for schizophrenia (Cooper et al., 1972) and for organic disorders in old age (Gurland et al., 1983). These studies examined whether these apparent differences reflected prevalence rate differences in the two countries, or differences in diagnostic habit.

Case registers

Case registers are local systems that record the contacts with designated medical and social services for a geographical area (Wing, 1989). The advantages of a register have been summarized by Wing and Hailey (1972). Selection bias and duplicated counts are avoided as case registers collect their data from all residents of a defined district and individual patients are identified to avoid counting the same patient several times. In contrast, HIPE is based upon hospitals rather than geographical areas and may be biased by a hospital's particular local policy. The case register, based upon a defined area, makes it possible to calculate rates of diagnosis per unit of population in a way that allows comparisons with other districts and other countries.

There are, as always, some problems in interpreting the results derived from case registers. First, a register usually covers a relatively small and arbitrarily defined part of a larger conurbation and is therefore unlikely to produce generalizable data. Second, the morbidity recorded is only likely to be an accurate reflection of the community incidence of a disease with high visibility, such as schizophrenia.

The data on, for example, anxiety or depression, will be unrepresentative of the community at large. Third, there are still no data on recovery or outcome. A patient could leave the register for several reasons—because the patient had left the district, the patient was still with symptoms but had stopped attending, *or* the patient had recovered. Fourth, the diagnoses in case registers are poorly standardized.

Despite these disadvantages, case registers have made a considerable contribution to knowledge of the interaction of patients and services and have provided a fertile soil for identifying patient groups for more detailed research. In the United Kingdom there have been successful registers in Camberwell, Salford, Aberdeen and Southampton, and in Oxford there has been a unique linkage system in which all patient contacts with all the arms of the health services can be traced. Case registers have also been set up overseas, in particular in Denmark, Norway and Germany. However, in recent years many registers have closed down because central funding has been withdrawn as each health district is now required to produce its own patient contact or Körner statistics, thereby obviating the administrative need for specific detailed registers to provide data from certain areas. In Europe, on the other hand, registers have been under political attack from pressure groups who see such storing of data about patients with mental illness as an infringement of individual liberty.

References

American Psychiatric Association (1980). *Diagnostic and Statistical Manual*, 3rd edn. Washington, DC: American Psychiatric Association.

American Psychiatric Association (1987). *Diagnostic and Statistical Manual of Mental Disorders*, 3rd edn, revised. Washington, DC: American Psychiatric Association.

Brooke, E.M. (1980). Information in mental health services: a tripartite system. In: E. Strömgren, A. Dupont and J. Achton Nielsen (eds) *Epidemiological Research as Basis for the Organization of Extramural Psychiatry. Acta Psychiat. Scand.* **62** (Suppl. 285).

Cooper, J.E. (1988). The structure and presentation of contemporary psychiatric classification with special reference to ICD-9 and 10. *Br. J. Psychiat.* **152** (Suppl. 1), 21–28.

Cooper, J.E., Kendell, R.E., Gurland, B.J., Sharpe, L., Copeland, J.R.M. and Simon, R. (1972). *Psychiatric Diagnosis in New York and London: A Comparative Study of Mental Hospital Admissions*, Institute of Psychiatry Maudsley Monographs No. 20. London: Oxford University Press.

Feinstein, A.R. (1972). Clinical biostatistics. XIII: On homogeneity, taxonomy and nosography. *Clin. Pharmacol. Ther.* **13**, 114–129.

Foulds, G.A. (1967). *The Hierarchical Nature of Personal Illness*. London: Academic Press.

Garner, D.M. and Garfinkel, P.E. (1980). Socio-cultural factors in the development of anorexia nervosa. *Psychol. Med.* **10**, 647–656.

Goffman, E. (1976). *Stigma: Notes on the Management of Spoiled Identity*. Penguin: Harmondsworth.

Goldberg, D. and Williams, P. (1988). *The User's Guide to the General Health Questionnaire*. Windsor: NFER-Nelson.

Goldberg, D.P., Cooper, B., Eastwood, M.R., Kedward, H.B. and Shepherd, M. (1970). A standardised psychiatric interview for use in community surveys. *Br. J. Prevent. Soc. Med.* **24**, 18–23.

Greist, J.H., Klein, M.H., Erdman, H.P., Bires, J.K., Bass, S.M., Machtinger, P.E. and Kresge, D.G. (1987). Comparison of computer- and interviewer-administered versions of the Diagnostic Interview Schedule. *Hosp. Commun. Psychiat.* **38**, 1304–1311.

Gurland, B., Copeland, J., Kuriansky, J., Kelleher, M., Sharpe, L. and Dean, L.L. (1983). *The Mind and Mood of Aging. Mental Health Problems of the Community Elderly in New York and London.* New York: The Haworth Press.

Jablensky, A. (1988). Methodological issues in psychiatric classification. *Br. J. Psychiat.* **152** (Suppl. 1), 15–20.

Jaspers, K. (1963). *General Psychopathology*, J. Hoenig and M.W. Hamilton (trans.). Manchester: Manchester University Press.

Lewis, G. and Pelosi, A.J. (1990). The case-control study in psychiatry. *Br. J. Psychiat.* **157**, 197–207.

Lewis, G., Pelosi, A.J., Glover, E., Wilkinson, G., Stansfeld, S.A., Williams, P. and Shepherd, M. (1988). The development of a computerized assessment for minor psychiatric disorder. *Psychol. Med.* **18**, 737–745.

Sartorius, N. (1988). International perspectives of psychiatric classification. *Br. J. Psychiat.* **152** (Suppl. 1), 9–14.

Scheff, T.J. (1963). The role of the mentally ill and the dynamics of mental disorder. *Sociometry* **26**, 436–453.

Skodol, A.E. and Spitzer, R.L. (1982). DSM-III: rationale, basic concepts, and some differences. *Acta Psychiat. Scand.* **66**, 271–281.

Spitzer, R.L. and Endicott, J. (1978). *Schedule for Affective Disorders and Schizophrenia.* New York: New York State Psychiatric Institute.

Spitzer, R.L., Endicott, J. and Robins, E. (1975). *Research Diagnostic Criteria.* New York: Biometrics Research, New York State Psychiatric Institute.

Stott, D.H. (1958). Some psychosomatic aspects of causality in reproduction. *J. Psychosom. Res.* **3**, 42–55.

Williams, P., Hand, D. and Tarnopolsky, A. (1982). The problem of screening for uncommon disorders—a comment on the Eating Attitudes Test. *Psychol. Med.* **12**, 431–434.

Wing, J.K. (ed.) (1989). *Health Services Planning and Research: Contributions from Psychiatric Case Registers.* London: Gaskell.

Wing, J.K. and Hailey, A.M. (1972). *Evaluating a Community Psychiatric Service.* Oxford: Oxford University Press.

Wing, J.K., Cooper, J.E. and Sartorius, N. (1974). *The Measurement and Classification of Psychiatric Symptoms.* Cambridge: Cambridge University Press.

World Health Organization (1978). *Mental Disorders: Glossary and Guide to their Classification in Accordance with the Ninth Revision of the International Classification of Diseases.* Geneva: World Health Organization.

Further Reading

Barker, D.J.P. and Rose, G. (1984). *Epidemiology in Medical Practice*, 3rd edn. Churchill Livingstone: Edinburgh.

Hennekens, C.H. and Buring, J.E. (1987). *Epidemiology in Medicine.* Boston: Little Brown.

Lewis, G. and Pelosi, A.J. (1990). The case-control study in psychiatry. *Br. J. Psychiat.* **157**, 197–207.

Rothman, K. (1986). *Modern Epidemiology.* Boston: Little Brown.

Neurological Sciences

Neurophysiological Aspects of Psychiatry

M.D. Craggs and A.C. Carr

Introduction

Half of our hospital beds are occupied by psychiatric patients. At least 20% of these patients are known to have brain damage visible under the microscope; the illnesses of many more probably result from biochemical disturbances. Yet our psychiatric knowledge and treatment remains almost entirely empirical, owing little or nothing to the efforts of a century of neurophysiologists. Why should this be so? The greatest obstacle is undoubtedly the sheer complexity of the brain, immeasurably greater than that of modern computers, perhaps inevitably so—'if the brain were simple enough for us to understand, we would be so simple that we couldn't' (Lyall Watson). Added to this is the brain's astonishing degree of miniaturization and relative inaccessibility. However, modern techniques (notably single-cell recordings with microelectrodes, neurochemical assay and molecular biology) are allowing great progress, and a scientific basis for psychiatry is now taking shape.

Relating psychiatric systems to the underlying physiological disturbance is remarkably difficult. We know, for example, that acute brain damage produces a constant clinical picture of delirium (acute organic reaction), whether caused by trauma, poisoning, metabolic disorders, anoxia or otherwise. The incomplete arousal may arise from impairment of the reticular activating system (RAS), producing clouded consciousness, stupor and coma successively; defective perception leads to disorientation; impaired thinking ability results in confusion; and overactivity and restlessness may result in part from an inability to monitor the success of purposive efforts. Chronic generalized brain damage again produces a constant picture (dementia) regardless of origin. The two main features are diminished intelligence and impaired memory; presumably these are diffusely localized functions.

Localized brain damage may give rise to symptoms characteristic of the area involved, thereby adding to our understanding of brain function. Lesions of the motor or sensory cortex produce neurological defects (paresis and anaesthesia, respectively). More anterior, frontal lobe damage may result in 'frontal' personality changes, notably social disinhibition, impaired judgement and euphoria, for unknown reasons. Moving posteriorly, parietal lobe lesions interfere with the integration of both motor and sensory activity into conscious thought, and

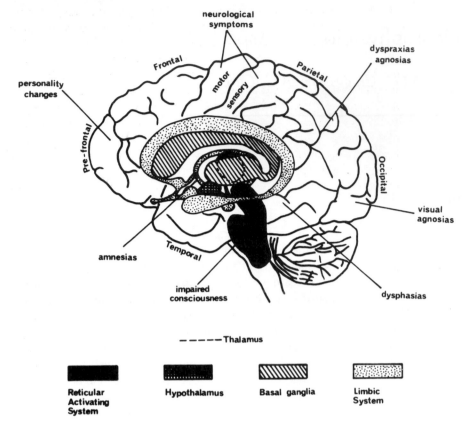

FIG. 7.1   Brain structure and function.

produce a fascinating variety of symptoms. Damage to the dominant (usually the left) parietal lobe may interfere with speech, reading and writing; damage to either side may impair visuospatial appreciation and recognition (agnosia and dyspraxias). Occipital lobe damage can interfere with visual perception at various stages of integration, from blindness to more subtle agnosias—such as an inability to recognize colours. Temporal lobe damage may lead to dysphasias and damage to the underlying limbic system may produce the amnesic syndrome. Basal ganglia damage produces the stiffness, tremor and akinesia of Parkinsonism (Fig. 7.1).

Disappointingly, localized brain damage produces syndromes which are not those of everyday psychiatry. The commonest severe mental illness, schizophrenia, is normally associated with no visible damage whatever (although it is claimed that in some patients the corpus callosum shows enlargement, in others there is cerebral atrophy accompanied by enlarged ventricles and in a small number of patients, disorientation of hippocampal pyramidal cells and their processes can be observed: Scheibel and Kovelman, 1981), yet a schizophrenic syndrome is more likely to occur after localized damage to any part of the brain —a baffling finding. Many schizophrenic patients improve when given any one of numerous drugs which have a dopamine (DA)-receptor blocking action, suggesting that the underlying dysfunction is physiological and perhaps quite specific. This specificity is such that only in acute schizophrenia (type I) are DA-2 receptor populations seen to be elevated (Crow *et al.*, 1984). Depression, too, may be alleviated by any of a large group of drugs with a common action, for example, potentiation of noradrenergic or 5-hydroxytryptamine transmission by re-uptake blockade, and a fairly straightforward physiological disturbance again seems likely. Such disturbances could be influenced by both developmental and environmental factors. Mania may perhaps result from similar neurotransmitter abnormalities. In the dementias, for example of the Alzheimer's type, there could be disturbances to cholinergic function at the receptor. Thus, many psychiatric disorders are probably associated with selective impairment of neurotransmission at receptor sites. An explanation for this impairment is very likely to emerge from new research in the rapidly expanding fields of molecular biology and electrophysiology.

Of the remaining mental disorders very little is yet known of the underlying mechanisms. It is of course true that 'physiological factors' (past and present personal experience of life-events) play a large part in precipitating and maintaining psychiatric disorders: this is true to some extent even in such 'organic' illnesses as epilepsy and dementia. However, an underlying genetic susceptibility has been demonstrated—the children of alcoholics, for example, show an increased tendency to become alcoholics even after adoption at birth—and such a predisposition must reside either in the properties of individual brain cells or their interconnections, or both.

Nerves and Synapses

Studies of recordings of the electrical activity of a single nerve cell, using a microelectrode positioned in or near it, have greatly advanced our understanding of neurophysiology. It has been shown, for example, that a voluntary movement is preceded by discharges in specific cells in many other areas besides the motor cortex, notably the nuclei of the basal ganglia and the cerebellum. Indeed, activity signalling an intended movement can be detected in certain cells of the frontal lobe several hundred milliseconds (ms) beforehand. This is an astonishingly long time for a cerebral event. For comparison, motor impulses traverse the simple two-neurone (myelinated) motor pathway from cortex to leg in 10 ms. Nerve impulses traverse even the slowest cortical neurones within 50 ms or so, and synaptic transmission is rapid (a few milliseconds). Clearly the complexity of the pathway carrying the movement intention from the prefrontal areas to the motor cortex is enormous, involving very many neurones. However, it has been suggested that some very slow potentials such as the contingent negative variation (CNV), which is detectable in the EEG several seconds before an intended movement, might not in fact reflect such activity directly but could result from accompanying biochemical activity in the neuroglial cells (Somjen, 1978).

A cortical neurone may have very intensive and numerous dendrites, which may be longer than the cell axon and may synapse with thousands of other neurones. An incoming impulse is not usually adequate to cause an immediate discharge in the cell, but produces a small excitatory or inhibitory postsynaptic potential. These potentials summate throughout the dendritic tree and discharge occurs when the cell threshold is exceeded, reflecting information integrated from all the contributing neurones. The axon may also divide into collaterals, perhaps of differing diameters, so that the impulses may arrive at several destinations with different conduction velocities. Recent work suggests that the impulses may even be directed down one axonal branch in preference to another, according to the code of impulses being transmitted (Swadlow *et al.*, 1980). An excitatory impulse may be transmitted rapidly across synapses between cortical cells by secretion of acetylcholine, noradrenaline, dopamine or serotonin (Fig. 7.2). Other neurotransmitters (notably GABA—γ-aminobutyric acid) have an inhibiting effect. A variety of other amino acids and polypeptides act as neurotransmitters, and it is also believed that some neurones communicate by direct electrical connection (Bennett, 1972).

A single cell may well receive impulses carried by all of the different transmitters (some exciting and some inhibiting it). Nevertheless, the main physiological pathways appear to depend principally on a single neurotransmitter, and this allows their course to be mapped. For example, there is a noradrenergic pathway ascending from the reticular activating system which maintains the excitability of the cortex (on which consciousness depends). Cells of this particular system may have many axon branches ramifying throughout the central nervous system (CNS), each branch making thousands of synaptic connections with other cells.

Synapses also occur directly between axons. An axo-axonal synapse can inhibit a cell by preventing the release of its transmitter. This 'presynaptic inhibition' plays an important part in modifying sensory inputs. Pain impulses, for example, can be inhibited by the activity in other sensory pathways, providing a possible mechanism for the pain-reducing action of counter-irritants, transcutaneous electrical stimulation and acupuncture (Melzack and Wall, 1989).

Synaptic transmission is not always a simple, short-lived event. When a cell receives an excitatory impulse via a synapse some depolarization can persist for hundreds of milliseconds. The discharge of the cell then depends on information integrated over time as well as over the spatial ramification of its dendrites. Equally long-lasting inhibitory influences have also been demonstrated, e.g. by brain stem cells acting upon the hippocampus and cerebellum. A further influence on the cell's activity is the rapidity with which neurotransmitters are removed from its synaptic clefts by degrading enzymes and other mechanisms. Most antidepressant drugs appear to act by slowing these processes, increasing the effective stimulation of the neurone.

Indeed, it now appears that the concept of a single transmitter conveying impulses along a pathway is an oversimplification. Many workers are identifying various 'coexisting transmitters', which appear to be liberated in parallel with a classical one (probably by different neurones in the same pathway). In some cholinergic systems, for example, a polypeptide (VIP) appears to assist

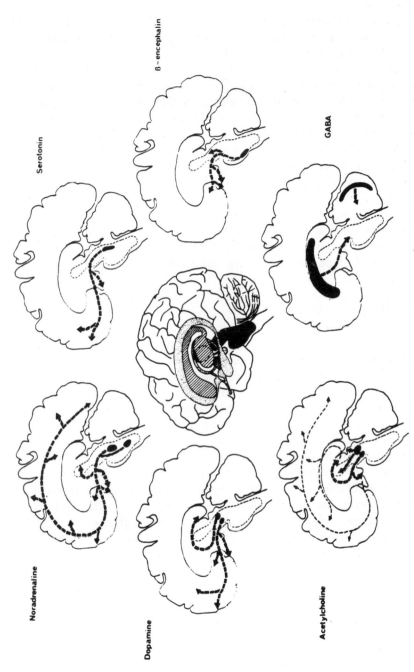

Serotonin

β – encephalin

GABA

Noradrenaline

Dopamine

Acetylcholine

FIG. 7.2   Principal neurotransmitter pathways.

acetylcholine in activating a receptor neurone, perhaps by 'priming' its receptor surface. Serotonin may be released along with another polypeptide (substance P), dopamine with cholecystokinin, and so on.

Recently, our knowledge of receptor sites has been advanced by molecular biology and a new electrophysiological technique called 'patch-clamping'. Patch-clamping permits investigation of single ion channels in nerve membranes. With this technique it is possible to observe the precise nature by which molecules of neurotransmitter cause potential changes at receptors by modifying ionic permeability. However, we now know from cloning studies that there is a baffling array of subtypes of receptors in the central nervous system including GABA and nicotinic ones. For example cloning of the glutamate receptor has revealed at least three different types, of which the ubiquitous NMDA (N-methyl D-aspartate) produces the greatest, but slowest, ionic conductance changes (Howe et al., 1988). The NMDA receptor is of particular interest because it is thought to be involved, among other things, in plasticity of the nervous system during development, considered to be important in learning and memory.

Neuronal Integration

Traditional concepts of neurological function are based on the reflex arc: a sensory stimulus, intermediate cells (interneurones) conducting the impulses, and a motor response. The information can be 'gated' or modulated by the inter-neurones to obtain the appropriate response. The simplest example is the familiar spinal reflex with its Renshaw cell which limits the resulting motor impulses. However, this immediate 'knee-jerk' response is followed by another slower contraction which has clearly traversed several interneurones. Cells in such 'integrated reflex' pathways make up the grey matter in the spinal cord, arranged in layers. As sensory impulses traverse the layer of cells from posterior root ganglia to anterior horn cell they are modified by cortical factors such as anxiety or voluntary movement, modulating the size of the response. The cortex controls sensory impulse conduction in the spinal cord through various descending pathways, such as pyramidal fibres descending from the sensory cortex (these make up about 25% of the pyramidal tract). Recordings of sensory impulses from electrodes over the sensory cortex have shown that motor activity on one hand, for example, reduces the volume of sensory information received from that hand (but not from the other), apparently via inhibitory interneurones at all levels in the neural axis, and also by presynaptic inhibition of the sensory neurones (Rushton et al., 1981).

The mechanisms of such modulation have been studied in cells of the visual cortex. After each discharge these neurones have an appreciable refractory period, during which no impulse can pass. In periods of high arousal (e.g. in states of excitement or fear) these cells receive noradrenergic stimulation from the reticular activating system (RAS) which reduces their refractory period, allowing impulse transmission more frequently but sometimes more selectively (Livingstone and Hubel, 1981). The arousal thus produces disinhibition of the cortex, which becomes more active. States of arousal similarly modify activity in cells of the limbic system (hippocampus, amygdala and related structures), which may explain why aggression occurs more easily during arousal. Normally the brain disregards the vast majority of sensory impulses which bombard it, selectively attending to relevant sensations by suitably adjusting 'gating' interneurones. Without such selective attention the brain would be inundated with information, enough to impede thought. Some failure of this mechanism has been postulated in schizophrenia. Different patterns of sensory impulses can set up specific 'gating' arrangements, allowing cells to specialize in responding only to a certain pattern of information. Successive layers of cells may respond to increasingly complex stimuli ('serial processing'). Thus microelectrode studies suggest there is a hierarchy of cells in primary sensory areas such as the visual cortex. Lowest-level cells respond directly to light stimulation of a corresponding area of the retina; cells at the next level respond only to certain combinations of stimuli (e.g. a line or light–dark edge in the visual field); higher cells respond to more precise stimuli such as an oblique line at a certain inclination or the speed at which it is moving (Hubel and Wiesel, 1965). Such specialization has also been demonstrated in the somatosensory area (Fig. 7.3).

So far we have considered the brain simply as a processor of sensory impulses, a massive sequential reflex pathway. However, this is clearly an inadequate model. Cortical cells display spontaneous activity, and indeed may become even more active when the organism is at rest. Again, rhythmic activity such as breathing or walking can scarcely be imagined to result solely from sensory input. Much activity arises spontaneously in the brain, such as, for example, α rhythm.

The main non-invasive technique for observing brain activity has been the electroencephalogram (EEG), which is often very difficult to interpret. Despite this, most information on normal human brains has been derived from the EEG. The signals are thought to reflect changes in the activity and synchronization of cortical cells. Synchronous rhythmic discharges produce high amplitude 'slow' signals (α waves during quiet thought, spikes in epilepsy), while the scattered asynchronous activity which accompanies perception and movement is recorded as small 'fast' signals (Fig. 7.4). A power spectrum can be derived by computer analysis and the fast and slow activity can be measured quantitatively. (Suggestions that much EEG activity is artificial, due to eye movements, have not been substantiated. It is, however, partly produced by the polarization and depolarization of dendrites as they receive inhibitory and excitatory impulses.) EEG waves due to a specific event are usually obscured by noise, but repeated traces can be computer-averaged to reveal the 'sensory evoked potential' (SEP). When a subject observes a sudden flash of light or other stimulus, the resulting evoked potential consists of several successive waves or components. First, an immediate set of impulses arrive at the appropriate sensory cortex (in the case of a flash, the contralateral visual cortex) within 20 ms. These impulses have evidently traversed very few neurones and appear to be unmodified by mood or activity. A moment later, further activity reaches the same area of cortex, but via interneurones which can modulate it—it is this element which is inhibited by simultaneous movement of the same part of the body, as described above

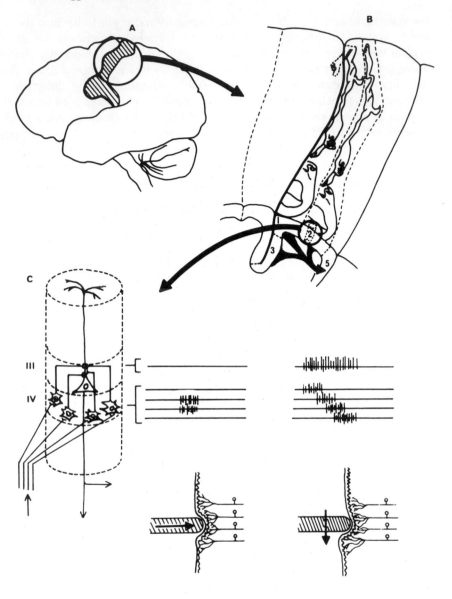

FIG. 7.3   Somatosensory processing. Sensory information arriving at the post-central cortex (A) is distributed topographically along body images in areas 1–3 (B) and then converges on area 5. In each area columns of cells integrate impulses from several neurones to detect a specific pattern such as direction of movement. (C) In this example a cutaneous stimulus (lower left) excites only cells in layer IV; the layer III cells respond only to a temporal sequence of activity in layer IV cells, corresponding to downward movement of the stimulus (lower right). Processed information from skin and joint receptors is then combined in area 5.

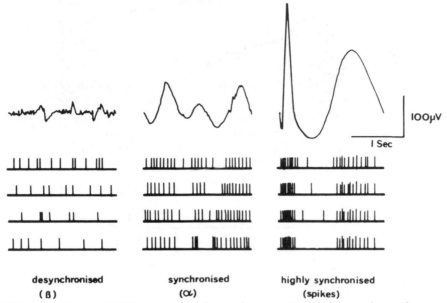

FIG. 7.4 Origin of EEG waves. The figure shows an EEG trace together with micro-electrode records from four underlying cortical cells. In an alert subject cortical neurones appear to fire almost at random, generating an irregular waveform (fast or β-activity) in the EEG. At rest, rhythmic bursts of cortical activity generate larger, slower EEG α waves. In epilepsy, waves of activity spread directly from cell to cell across the cortex, the simultaneous discharge of many cells producing high-voltage EEG 'spikes'.

(Fig. 7.5). Finally, after 150 ms or more, further impulses arrive, which can be detected bilaterally over a more diffuse area of cortex. These vary in amplitude according to the degree of wakefulness and preoccupation of the subject, perhaps showing the effects of selective attention.

Where the stimulus is a signal to prepare to act, the subject's intention to move is associated with further electrical activity, the contingent negative variation (CNV), which outlasts the SEP. The CNV also varies with the subject's attention, and possibly his intelligence.

States of Consciousness

The way the brain carries out its functions is sometimes neatly demonstrated by the effects of localized damage. An animal may show a specific behavioural impairment, and on histological examination after a week or two the course of the damaged pathway may be traced out by staining the degenerating nerve fibres. For example, a lesion in the locus ceruleus (a nucleus in the pons, part of the RAS) will result in degeneration of tracts of fibres projecting to all parts of the cerebral cortex. These fibres are noradrenergic, and their function appears to be one of exciting (disinhibiting) the cortical cells to maintain consciousness. Damage can sometimes result in irreversible stupor or coma. These cells discharge

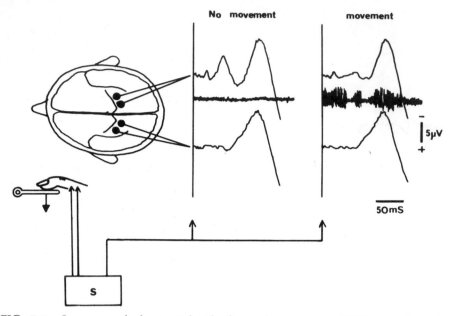

FIG. 7.5   Sensory evoked potentials. The figure shows averaged EEG traces from the right (upper trace) and left (lower trace) somatosensory areas, together with an EMG from the left pollicus longus (middle trace). Sensory stimulation of the left thumb at rest produces evoked potentials over the right cortex with prominent negative peaks at 20, 55 and 140 ms, but only the last of these is seen over the left cortex. If the thumb is stimulated whilst at work flexing a spring-loaded lever, the second negative peak is suppressed.

most frequently in states of high arousal and least during sleep, offering a convenient concept of sleep as a low-arousal state. However, a well-known paradox appears here. When the locus ceruleus cells are least active and the subject is firmly asleep (hardest to arouse, with antigravity muscles fully relaxed but with rapid eye movements—REM) his cortex becomes more active again, according to the EEG.

The traditional explanation was that another activating pathway is responsible for inducing sleep, via serotoninergic cells of the neighbouring raphe nucleus. During its influence, periods of arousal by the noradrenergic fibres would produce this 'paradoxical sleep' (active dreaming, REM sleep), alternating with periods of quiet, slow-wave sleep. In fact microelectrode studies have now shown the converse to be true; raphe cells are less active during sleep than wakefulness, and less active still during REM sleep. It seems that sleep, in particular REM sleep, may depend on yet another pathway, such as cholinergic giant cells of the brain-stem tegmentum. These neurones fire most frequently during REM sleep (Fig. 7.6). Hence, for two populations of cells, the putatively cholinergic (REM-on) and putatively aminergic (REM-off), there appears to be reciprocal interaction. Interestingly, recent histological evidence shows that these two populations of cells may not be segregated but neurochemically mixed. Indeed, it is suggested

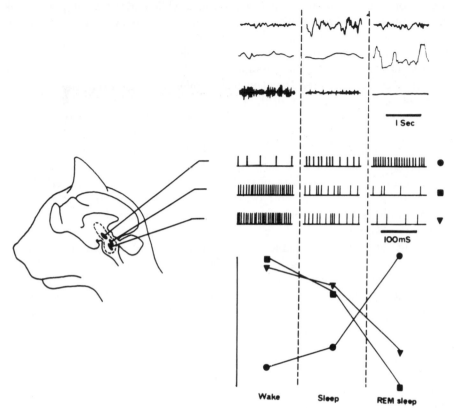

FIG. 7.6 Brain stem activity during sleep. Microelectrode recordings were obtained from nuclei in the RAS (dotted area) of the brain stem of a cat during wakefulness, sleep and REM sleep (columns 1–3). The top three traces show the EEG (with slow activity during sleep), eye movements, and the EMG from an antigravity muscle, respectively. The upper microelectrode trace (●) shows the activity of cholinergic cells in the brainstem tegmentum, which fire most rapidly during REM ('dreaming') sleep and may be partly responsible for its occurrence. Serotoninergic cells in the raphe nucleus (■) and noradrenergic cells in the locus ceruleus (▼) are active during consciousness, quiet during sleep and least active during REM sleep, perhaps explaining why subjects are hardest to arouse from this phase. The cell activities are compared below in graphical form.

that some cholinergic activity may be concerned with the blocking of REM sleep. Such findings make a simple reciprocal-interaction model of sleep unlikely (Hobson *et al.*, 1986). An additional complication is the finding that REM sleep is probably divided into two stages with one stage involving movement. Slow-wave (non-REM) sleep can be separated into at least four stages.

Conscious awareness is closely linked with memory recording, a subject being able to account for his movements unless suffering from a memory disorder due to brain damage. There are, however, states of 'altered consciousness' in which the subject appears awake, yet is left afterwards with no memory of events (despite an intact brain). Hypnosis presents one example. About half the population can be hypnotized quite simply and while entranced can read, speak and act rationally, with a normal EEG yet are afterwards unaware of their actions. The EEG does tend to exhibit more α rhythm (10 Hz waves) during hypnosis, as it does during meditation. Another example is the *fugue*, an hysterical phenomenon in which a patient disappears after some crisis and is found hours or days later. He has often travelled many miles, buying tickets, meals and so forth, yet has no recollection of the trip.

It is interesting that subjects aroused from non-REM sleep (when they are not dreaming) report that they were just lying thinking, and can relate the topic of their thoughts (Cohen, 1979). During non-REM sleep subjects can be woken by quite minor stimuli. We may perhaps speculate that during these periods of sleep the subject is in fact consciously aware but retains no memory of the period next day, in the same way that most dream events fade quickly from memory on waking. If this is the case, 'falling asleep' is simply the point at which permanent memory recording ceases.

During consciousness, a subject is not equally aware of all the multitude of sensory perceptions reaching his brain. How does the brain concentrate? One useful measure of concentration may be the CNV (Fig. 7.7), since it arises when a subject is anticipating a signal to act (having been warned by a preliminary stimulus), and is presumably concentrating closely upon the task. The CNV reflects increased activity mainly in the pre-frontal cortex, a likely site for such concentration since processed sensory information converges upon it from all areas of the brain. This activity also appears when the subject is alerted by an unexpected stimulus, and again might reflect the concentration of his attention upon it.

Concentration presumably involves selectively restricting incoming information, and a possible mechanism could be the control exerted by the reticular nucleus of the thalamus. Much sensory information converging upon the pre-frontal cortex is relayed by the dorsomedial nucleus (DMN) of the thalamus, and this function is inhibited by certain brain-stem reticular cells which activate its reticular nucleus. Incoming sensory information could be picked up by the RAS cells (via brain-stem collaterals) and lead to selective inhibition of the thalamic relay station, preventing extraneous information from reaching the prefrontal cortex. Stimulating these RAS cells electrically causes a CNV to appear over the pre-frontal cortex, in accord with this hypothesis. As expected, this effect can be abolished by prior ablation of the DMN of the thalamus or its connections to the pre-frontal cortex (Fuster, 1989).

Sensory Perception

Sensory perception involves more than simply relaying incoming impulses to the appropriate brain structures. Most incoming information never reaches consciousness but is rejected by a mechanism of 'gating', or selective attention. Only a small fraction is relayed to specialized receiving structures, and reaches several of them rather than a single area of cortex—hence ablations in the classical

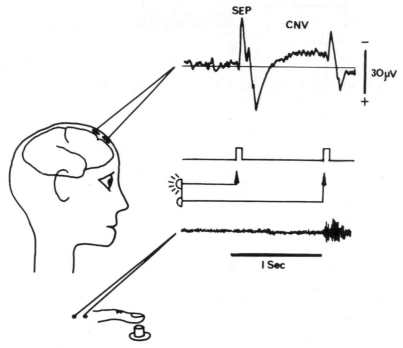

FIG. 7.7 Contingent negative variation (CNV). In an experiment to achieve concentration, a subject has to press a button in response to an action signal which will illuminate shortly after a warning signal. Upper trace: the subject's pre-frontal EEG shows a biphasic sensory potential (SEP) evoked by the warning light, a prolonged negative variation (CNV), and then a second potential evoked by the action signal and motor response. Lower trace: muscle activity immediately follows the action signal.

'sensory cortex' cause only a transient sensory loss. Incoming sensations are integrated to compensate for movement of the stimulus, compared with memory and combined with information from other sensory modalities. How this is done is largely unknown, but clearly involves subcortical as well as neo-cortical processing (Rolls, 1989). Parts of the necessary decoding is done by columns of cells arranged to respond to increasingly complex aspects of the stimulus, as described earlier for the visual cortex; it has also been studied in the somato-sensory cortex (see Fig. 7.3). This process develops during early life through the growth of synaptic connections between the receiving cells; such growth is stimulated by incoming sensory information in infancy, essential for the achievement of normal perception (Blakemore, 1975).

Perception of peripheral stimuli can be detected objectively by observing the SEP, electrical activity evoked in the appropriate area of the cortex. Sensations perceived by an awake subject produce an initial biphasic potential as early as 15–20 ms after the stimulus. Interestingly, this early response can also be detected after a subliminal stimulus too slight to be noticed by the subject, although in this case the wave is not biphasic but lacks an upward (negative) deflection. The

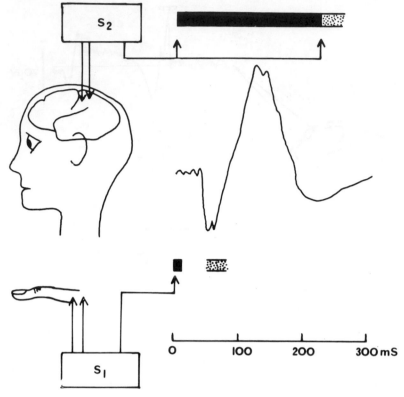

FIG. 7.8   Speed of sensory perception. When a subject's thumb is stimulated electrically (S1) a sensory evoked potential rapidly appears in his EEG (middle trace), and he perceives the stimulus within 50–100 ms (stipple). The evoked potential appears first over his contralateral sensory cortex. If the stimulus is applied directly to the cortex instead (S2) the subject still refers the sensation to his thumb, but perceives it only after a much longer period of stimulation.

negative component might be considered as representing conscious perception of the stimulus, but this is not so. SEPs obtained in sleep and during anaesthesia still have negative components, very large ones in fact.

Sensations may also be induced artificially by direct electrical stimulation of the sensory cortex at operation, and a paradox is then revealed. After peripheral stimulation of a thumb, say, the subject does not perceive the stimulus until well after the signal reaches the cortex, about 50 ms after the SEP begins. If the sensory cortex is stimulated directly instead, contrary to expectation the subject perceives a sensation in his thumb after a much longer delay of 200 ms or more (Fig. 7.8). This suggests that perception is not simply the arrival of signals at the sensory cortex: their passage through the brain stem must also be of importance (Libet et al., 1975).

Selective attention to specific stimuli at the expense of others can also be demonstrated experimentally. In a classical experiment, SEPs were observed in a

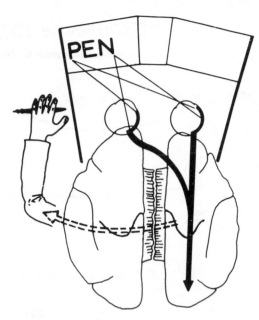

FIG. 7.9 Perception by the non-dominant hemisphere. If connections between the cerebral hemispheres are severed, a word presented in the left visual field cannot be read aloud, the subject being conscious only of a flash of light. Nevertheless, his left hand, controlled by the same hemisphere, can pick out the corresponding object from a hidden tray.

cat's EEG in response to loud clicks—when a mouse appeared the SEPs were abolished! The two cerebral hemispheres appear to direct their attention somewhat differently. Thus, a subject can discriminate between a voice and background noise rather better using his right ear than his left (which radiates primarily to the right, non-dominant hemisphere). Conversely, in the musically unsophisticated the non-dominant hemisphere excels at music discrimination and a tone can be more easily recognized amidst background noise if presented to the left ear. These facts again can be shown objectively by observing evoked potentials; speech sounds generate large SEPs over the left cortex, and vice versa (Friedman, 1978).

Evidence for the importance of brain-stem connections is also provided by experiments on split-brain animals. Independent perception by each hemisphere has been well demonstrated in studies of humans with hemispheres disconnected by section of the corpus callosum and commissures (Sperry, 1974). Such subjects may observe pictures presented to the left visual field and be unable to describe them consciously (i.e. with the dominant left hemisphere), yet can pick out with the left hand corresponding objects from a tray (Fig. 7.9), showing that the right hemisphere has perceived and recognized the picture ('subconsciously' perhaps?). Studies with split-brain cats (Wright et al., 1979) have shown that destruction of the brain-stem–cortex pathway produces a striking contralateral sensory neglect, the animal ignoring cues which previously excited a response despite 'seeing'

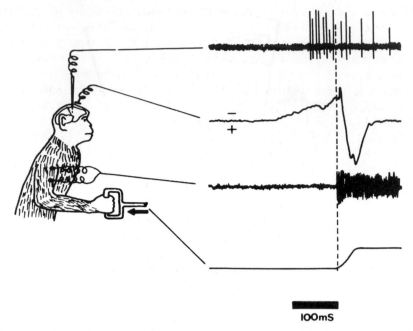

100mS

FIG. 7.10   Cortical activity and movement. When an animal is about to move a lever certain pyramidal cells of the motor cortex begin to discharge (upper trace) appreciably before muscle activity begins (lower trace) and movement occurs. This early activity contributes to the build-up of the motor potential in the EEG (middle trace) associated with the movement.

them normally (as shown by the evoked potentials). The tract destroyed was the medial forebrain bundle, which carries the main outflow of impulses ascending from the RAS. It seems possible that when new sensory information passes through the brain stem it is sensed by the RAS, which then focuses the brain's attention selectively upon the new stimulus. Section of the bundle would then prevent the animal from concentrating on stimuli on the affected side. However, at least one other explanation is possible. The destroyed pathway also carries information to the basal ganglia, and its absence may hinder movements on that side: the basal ganglia are closely involved with voluntary movements.

Motor Performance

In the traditional model, movements are initiated by the precentral 'motor cortex'. It is true that cortical signals can be observed over this area just before muscle activity begins (Fig. 7.10). These motor signals can now be computer analysed to reveal the particular movement intended. Such motor potentials are present even when the intended movement does not occur (in a paralysed subject with, say, spinal cord compression) and could be used to trigger prosthetic devices to perform the appropriate movement (Craggs, 1975).

However, it seems unlikely that purposive movements do in fact originate in the motor cortex. Destruction of this area or of its main outflow (the pyramidal tract) produces only a transient disability in adults, so movement evidently involves other structures. When a subject is waiting for a cue the earliest activity to appear is the CNV, the negative potential detected over the pre-frontal cortex. Movement is perhaps initiated by the effect of this pre-frontal activity on the motor cortex, cerebellum and basal ganglia (in each of which the body is represented topographically) and other structures.

The function of the basal ganglia in controlling voluntary movements appears to be largely an inhibitory one: direct electrical stimulation of part of the caudate nucleus abolishes a movement being executed by the corresponding body part (Hassler, 1978). The basal ganglia appear to refine motor performance. They may abolish unwanted components of a movement simply by interrupting some of the information being fed back to the motor cortex (e.g. sensory impulses passing up the brain stem to the thalamus). Recent studies of the 'no-go' response (inhibiting an intended movement when a negative cue is perceived) suggest that the basal ganglia hold intended movements in check, despite pre-frontal activity, until the subject finally decides to move. The basal ganglia in turn are subject to the inhibitory influence of the RAS principally through dopaminergic pathways (Fig. 7.11). In states of high arousal dopaminergic impulses from the RAS would inhibit the basal ganglia (via the substantia nigra), perhaps explaining poorly controlled impetuous movements during excitement and in hyperactive children.

Conversely, the removal of the inhibitory influence of the RAS would allow the basal ganglia to become overactive and inhibit all voluntary movements. This occurs in Parkinson's disease, where the substantia nigra atrophies, and also during initial blockade by dopamine antagonists such as the phenothiazines (drug-induced Parkinsonism). However, chronic dopamine blockade eventually results in the development of receptor supersensitivity. The basal ganglia then become excessively inhibited, more so if the dopamine-blocking drug is discontinued, presumably explaining the development of abnormal movements (tardive dyskinesia) after long-term phenothiazine administration in schizophrenic patients (Marsden and Jenner, 1980).

Certain individuals have cortical cells which at times become excitable enough to be stimulated by neighbouring neurones. Synchronous waves of activity ('spikes', see Fig. 7.4) can then spread throughout the cortex from a focus such as damaged or scarred brain tissue, producing the symptoms of epilepsy. In epilepsy the normal inhibitory mechanisms involving GABAergic pathways may be impaired and give rise to an unfettered spread of seizure activity (Meldrum, 1988). The excitability of cortical neurones is increased by fever, hypoglycaemia, infection, head injuries, certain drugs and various other factors, increasing the likelihood of a fit occurring. Indeed some combinations of drugs such as imipramine and chlorpromazine together may induce epilepsy in otherwise normal subjects. In some other patients a fit may be induced by lights flashing at about 20 Hz, for example on a cinema or television screen at close quarters. Lights flashing at a slower frequency, around 10 Hz, can 'drive' the brain's normal α rhythm into discharging synchronously with it in many normal individuals.

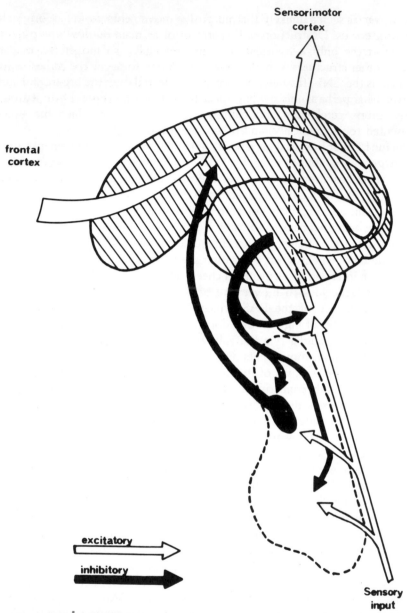

FIG. 7.11   Basal ganglia—postulated control of movement. The caudate nucleus and globus pallidus (shaded) inhibit the thalamus (clear outline), impeding the relay of incoming sensory impulses to the cortex. Voluntary movements appear to depend on sensory feedback, and are thus controlled by these basal ganglia. They in turn are under the inhibitory influence of the substantia nigra of the reticular activating system (RAS, dotted outline) in the brain stem. In states of arousal the substantia nigra inhibits the basal ganglia, relaxing its hold upon the thalamus and allowing some disinhibition of movement. In Parkinsonism the substantia nigra is suppressed, the basal ganglia are fully active and extreme poverty of movement results. After protracted phenothiazine administration, the substantia nigra again becomes overactive and excessive movements occur (tardive dyskinesia).

In a grand-mal epileptic fit, rapid synchronous discharges (about 10 per second) spread directly across the cortex. Involvement of the pre-central (motor) area sends rapid trains of impulses via the pyramidal tracts, producing maximal sustained contraction of all muscle groups, the 'tonic' phase. After several seconds the muscles begin to contract intermittently ('clonic' phase), possibly as the seizure discharges reach deeper brain structures. Consciousness is lost at an early stage as the rhythmic discharges obliterate normal cortical activity. Occasionally an epileptic seizure occurs at a focus in or close to the motor cortex itself; twitching of the corresponding muscles may then occur before consciousness is lost, and as the discharges spread across the motor area successive muscles become involved in a visible progression ('Jacksonian' epilepsy). Even in so-called 'absence seizures' where movement is supposed to be minimal during a brief loss of consciousness, there can be significant overt movement, albeit automatic (Penry *et al.*, 1975).

Autonomic Adjustments

Body organs are often innervated by both divisions of the autonomic nervous system, which act in opposition on glands and involuntary muscles. This balance may be disturbed by psychotropic drugs such as neuroleptics and antidepressants. Many of them block the cholinergic receptors of the parasympathetic system, producing the well-known side effects of dry mouth, blurred vision, constipation and urine retention. A less well-known effect is on sexual function, which depends on both sympathetic and parasympathetic nerves—many drugs can induce impotence and anorgasmia. However, some drugs such as phenoxybenzamine, an α-adrenergic blocking agent, injected directly into the corpus cavernosa of the penis, can be used to promote erections in erectile impotence (Brindley, 1986).

The parasympathetic system can operate quite selectively on different organs, and a topographical representation of the vagus has been identified in the pre-frontal cortex (Fuster, 1989). Electrical stimulation of one site in the posterior orbital region, for example, will dilate splanchnic vessels and lower blood pressure (Fig. 7.12). The autonomic and endocrine effects of such stimulation are probably mediated via the hypothalamus, amygdala and other limbic structures. In contrast, the sympathetic system appears to function mainly as a single unit, preparing all systems for immediate action (raised pulse, blood pressure, blood sugar, diversion of blood flow from gut and skin to muscles, etc.), the 'fight or flight' response. The organism's subsequent action would normally remove the arousing stimulus, allowing autonomic balance to be re-established. In man, however, social inhibitions often interfere with this self-limiting process and allow autonomic arousal to continue for long periods, rendering the subject susceptible to various stress-related diseases (such as hypertension, heart disease and stomach ulcers). These effects can be produced experimentally in animals. For example, a monkey can be placed in an 'executive' situation, where he has to remember to move a lever at intervals, and if he forgets he receives electric shocks. Such a monkey will soon develop peptic ulcers. In one ingenious study (Brady, 1958) a

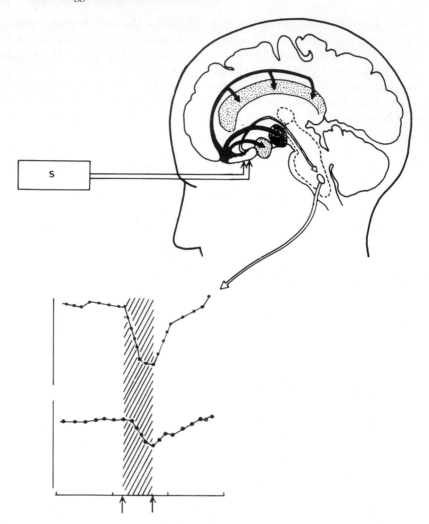

FIG. 7.12 Cortical 'representation' of the vagus. Electrical stimulation of the supra-orbital cortex excites the vagal nucleus in the RAS (dotted line), which dilates splanchnic vessels, slows the heart (upper trace) and lowers blood pressure (lower trace). Interestingly, this area also has inhibitory connections to the amygdala and cingulate gyrus (stippled) and the hypothalamus (cross-hatched).

second 'slave' monkey who simply shared in the electric shocks but had no control over them remained healthy, suggesting perhaps that punishment alone does not cause the same autonomic consequences—preparation for action is also a factor.

Although not directly perceived, autonomic changes may reach awareness through their peripheral effects such as sweating, trembling, blushing, and so on. It has indeed been argued that emotions are actually the result, not the cause, of such perceptions. It is certainly true that intense emotions of fear or anger can be induced by adrenaline injections. From this theory it would appear logical to treat pathological states of arousal, such as anxiety, with agents like propranolol (β-adrenergic antagonist) which would counteract the autonomic imbalance and abolish the peripheral sensations. In practice such treatment has had equivocable success. The observation that acute schizophrenics often exhibit high sympathetic tone has led to trials of adrenaline antagonists in schizophrenia too: their efficacy is disputed although some studies with large groups of patients have shown beneficial effects.

Autonomic differences may account for some aspects of personality, an area which has long interested psychologists. Studies of stress-induced diseases have suggested a fundamental difference between reactive (type A reactors) and unreactive subjects, as measured by the degree to which their autonomic systems respond to stress (Steptoe, 1981). The former subjects have labile autonomic systems and may exhibit, for example, higher rises in blood pressure under stress: they are certainly more susceptible to heart disease and other conditions than the unreactive subjects. The two types also tend to show different temperamental responses to various social situations, and it is interesting to speculate that perception of dramatic autonomic changes (bladder tension, blushing, etc.) leads reactive subjects to adopt more active ways of meeting or avoiding stressful situations, leading to the development of personality characteristics which differ from those of their less labile peers.

Drives and Reinforcements

The mechanisms by which emotions are generated in the brain are difficult to investigate. However, pleasure sensations have been studied in recent years using the self-stimulation electrode. If a small metal electrode is buried in one of certain areas of the brain and electrically stimulated a sensation of 'pleasure' can be induced in the animal, as shown by its willingness to repeat any behaviour which triggers further electrical stimulation (Campbell, 1973). The electrode thus functions as the 'reward' in an operant conditioning procedure. Its efficacy depends on the site of placement. Some sites evidently produce exquisite pleasure, the animal instantly pursuing further gratification after only one or two stimuli, sometimes continuing to do so with great rapidity until completely exhausted, oblivious of food and drink and eventually dying of inanition. These 'pleasure areas' are situated deep in the brain in the hypothalamus and neighbouring limbic structures (Fig. 7.13), and lie in catecholamine pathways (dopaminergic and noradrenergic neurones). Significantly they coincide with areas previously described as the feeding centre, drinking centre, sex centre and others. Such centres were identified by determining where an ablation would reduce the corresponding drive. It now appears that, rather than destroying a 'centre' of brain cells, early ablation experiments interrupted the main drive-reward pathways which pass through these areas. Indeed, careful observation has shown that these nerve fibres rapidly regenerate and reverse the deficit, showing that it was not caused by destruction of whole cell bodies. Thus, lesions in the 'feeding

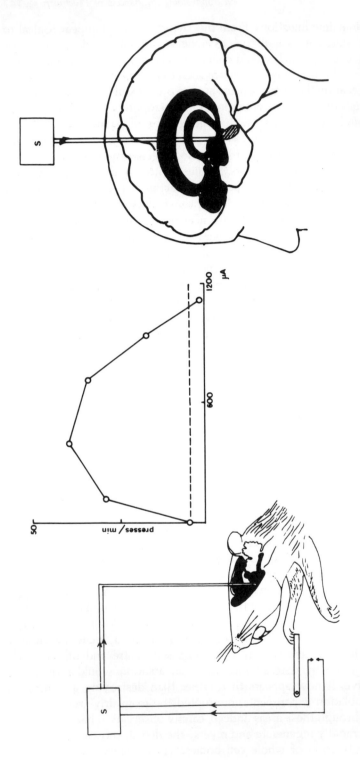

FIG. 7.13 'Pleasure areas' and self-stimulation. If an animal is allowed to press a lever which stimulates electrodes in the lateral hypothalamus, its responses depend on the strength of stimulation. At low currents the animal responds very rapidly, apparently finding the stimulations intensely rewarding. At high currents the response rate falls below even the initial, random rate, indicating that the stimulation has now become aversive. Limited human data suggest that these areas are concentrated in the limbic system and hypothalamus: some areas are principally rewarding (solid shading) while others are mainly aversive (hatched).

centre' in the lateral hypothalamus cause anorexia, by interrupting dopaminergic fibres ascending to the limbic system and basal ganglia (Fig. 7.14). More medial lesions in the 'satiety centre' cause obesity by damaging mainly noradrenergic fibres: again one is probably damaging fibres rather than cell bodies. These two appetite control systems are thought to act in opposition—strangely, *both* act as reward areas for self-stimulation. Crow (1973) has suggested a possible explanation. The dopaminergic fibres may carry impulses generating drive (e.g. appetizing odours arriving through olfactory afferent pathways), which have in themselves become secondary reinforcers by association with eating. The noradrenergic fibres carry satiating information (e.g. taste, stomach fullness) which is also rewarding. Stimulation of the dopaminergic fibres is much more strongly rewarding, contrary perhaps to what one would expect from this hypothesis. The precise mechanisms by which brain stimulation reward and the control of autonomic function are related have yet to be revealed (Halperin & Pfaff, 1982).

Some eating disorders may be produced by abnormal drive and control mechanisms in the hypothalamus: for example in anorexia nervosa, a condition predominantly of young post-pubescent women, there is a severe decrease in eating and loss of weight despite the maintenance of appetite. It is suggested that one possible cause of the symptoms of anorexia nervosa may be the underactivity of noradrenergic neurones in the hypothalamus reducing the drive for eating (Leibowitz, 1983). Abnormal drive-satisfaction mechanisms may also explain the occurrence of habit disorders such as nail-biting, and perhaps even the performance of compulsive rituals. Evidence that dopamine receptors are more numerous in the basal ganglia of schizophrenics (Owen *et al.*, 1978) may suggest that defective drive mechanisms play a part in this illness also.

It is an interesting fact that the 'pleasure' areas of the brain are closely associated with aversive (negative-reward) areas, where electrical stimulation generates unpleasant sensations which the animal will work to avoid. Some of these aversive areas lie medially in the hypothalamus, and contain a mixture of noradrenergic, cholinergic and serotoninergic fibres. However, the predominant noradrenergic fibres do not appear to mediate the aversive effect, since stimulation of the nuclei from which they originate is usually rewarding. This proximity between pleasure and aversive areas make experimentation difficult. The electrodes used are often large enough (0.1 mm across) to contact many neurones, and must be very accurately placed in the pleasure area. Even then, too large a current will involve neighbouring aversive neurones. On many occasions a mixture of sensations is indeed evoked, the animal performing the action compulsively yet with obvious reluctance. The actual mechanisms by which drives are mediated remains obscure. Four pathways ascend through the hypothalamus. Noradrenergic fibres from the RAS pass upwards to the entire cortex and have an arousing effect, compatible with ideas of drive-induced alerting but difficult to reconcile with Crow's suggested satiety role. Dopaminergic neurones of the substantia nigra and ventral tegmentum ascending to the basal ganglia, 'limbic system' and forebrain could perhaps be acting together to prepare for drive-prompted behaviour. Serotonin-secreting fibres from the raphe nucleus of the

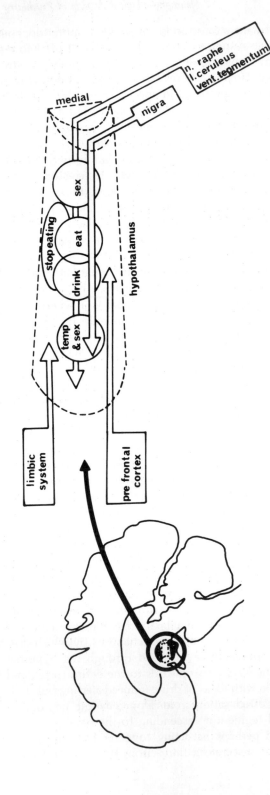

FIG. 7.14 Control of drives in the hypothalamus. Ablations in certain areas of the lateral hypothalamus reduce basic reward-seeking behaviour in animals (eating, drinking, sex). More medial ablations cause obesity by abolishing the aversive effects of satiation. These effects are probably due to interruption of ascending fibres from the reticular activating system, and of descending fibres from the limbic system and pre-frontal cortex. Electrical stimulation in the lateral region is intensely rewarding; more medial stimulation is both rewarding and aversive.

RAS cross the hypothalamus to reach mainly the limbic system and associated areas: it is claimed that stimulation of these fibres produces strong aversion. Finally, cholinergic neurones from the RAS ascend to the thalamus and other areas. These are the cells which appear to arouse the cortex during dreams; they may also play some aversive role or at least moderate the effects of the rewarding adrenergic fibres.

There may be a link between some of these effects produced by electrical stimulation and the behavioural inhibition system hypothesized by Gray (1982). Gray postulates that in a behavioural context the ascending noradrenergic projection to the septo-hippocampal system selects whether certain incoming stimuli are important; the serotoninergic (5HT) pathway then adds information as to whether this stimulus is associated with punishment. The ascending cholinergic pathway would facilitate stimulus analysis; the noradrenergic pathway to the hypothalamus would prime both the somatic and autonomic motor systems for rapid action if appropriate. The relevance of such an hypothesis is in connection with the mechanisms causing anxiety states, and their relief by the use of anxiolytics (Lader, 1983). Gray attributes the therapeutic action of anxiolytics to a reduction in the activity of most of the monoaminergic pathways mentioned above.

Recently interest has centred upon certain 'path neurones' in the medial forebrain bundle (part of the lateral hypothalamus). These wheel-like cells radiate dendrites in all directions and appear to derive information from almost all the fibres in the bundle, both ascending and descending. They radiate to many areas of the cortex and seem intimately connected with drive behaviour (Olds, 1976). Microelectrode studies in the lateral hypothalamus of cats have detected intense activity in some of these cells when the animal is striving for a reward such as food (Fig. 7.15). This activity is usually abolished when eating commences, but continues if the animal is obliged to struggle for more food while eating. Path neurones can also be activated by artificially induced drives such as drug addiction, discharging rapidly during the withdrawal phase produced when naloxone is administered to a morphine-addicted animal. The activity in these cells appears to reflect desire, and is quenched by morphine. Some of the brain cells in this use natural opioids as transmitters (the endorphins or enkephalins); they appear to affect sensitivity to pain, but their precise function is uncertain.

A few self-stimulation experiments have been performed on human subjects (Bishop *et al.*, 1964), but are little more informative than those in animals. A human subject will press a button repeatedly to activate an electrode in his lateral hypothalmus, but if asked why he is doing this cannot usually give a clear explanation. Stimulating this intensely rewarding area does not appear to evoke fully formed sensations of pleasure.

Cognition, Emotional Expression and Language

Cognition appears to occur in three distinct stages, each in adjacent areas of cortex. First, information from a special sense organ arrives at a 'primary sensory

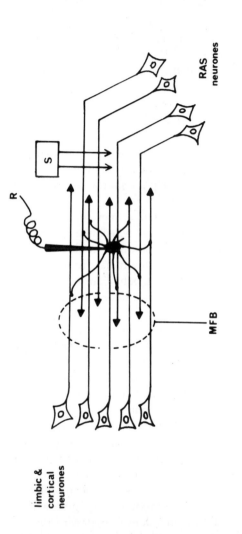
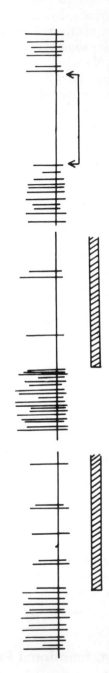

FIG. 7.15 Path neurones and drive. Path or 'wheel' neurones straddle the ascending and descending fibres in the lateral hypothalamus (the medial forebrain bundle), and their activity appears to reflect the presence of desire. Thus activity is diminished when a hungry monkey is given food (left trace) and when an addicted monkey is given morphine (middle trace). These effects are due partly to the arrival of ascending impulses from the reticular activating system, and can be reproduced by stimulating the ascending neurones electrically (right trace).

limbic &
cortical
neurones

R

S

MFB

RAS
neurones

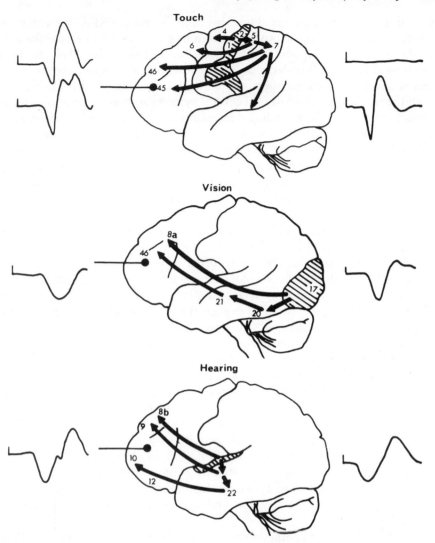

FIG. 7.16 Processing and convergence of sensory information in the cortex. A sensory stimulus perceived by touch, vision or hearing generates a sensory evoked potential (right traces) over the corresponding primary receiving area of cortex (hatched areas). The information is processed in successive association areas of cortex (arrowed) and converges upon the pre-frontal cortex, where the evoked potential may again be detected after a further delay (left traces). If the stimulus is unilateral (upper diagram), evoked potentials can be recorded only from the contralateral primary area (the lower of the paired traces); by the time the sensation reaches the pre-frontal cortex it appears bilaterally.

area' of the neocortex. There are three of these, the visual, auditory and somatosensory areas (smell is relayed to the rhinencephalon, much older in evolutionary terms). Next, the sensation is recognized and interpreted: this occurs in 'association areas' adjacent to each primary sensory cortex (Fig. 7.16). Finally the information from each of the senses must be integrated with memory as it converges on some central processing area in preparation to execute the appropriate behavioural response. This processing system seems likely to be the pre-frontal cortex. Microelectrode and neurochemical studies have shown that this receives many connections from all association areas and is closely linked with the modulatory effects of subcortical systems such as those of the so-called 'limbic system' and the ascending dopaminergic pathways. Interestingly, evoked potentials recorded over these frontal areas are strongly dependent on the subject's degree of attention and can be affected by motivational factors. The main 'outflow' from the pre-frontal area is to the basal ganglia (striatal part) as one would expect, since cognition leads frequently to action and the basal ganglia are the principal controllers of motor performance. However, the pre-frontal cortex does not transmit impulses directly to the motor cortex despite its anatomical proximity. It was indeed from this fact that the term 'silent areas' arose, since electrical stimulation produced no visible effect.

It seems very likely that the frontal cortex with its subcortical connections and dopaminergic modulation is one of the important substrates of psychopathology. Recently, an exciting but controversial unified hypothesis of cortical–subcortical function has been put forward to explain the possible defects underlying major psychiatric illnesses (Swerdlow and Koob, 1987). This simplified hypothesis of the neural circuitry involved (Fig. 7.17), based on clinical and experimental findings, focuses on the central role played by dopaminergic pathways from the ventral tegmentum controlling that part of the striatum called the nucleus accumbens. Overactivity in these pathways, resulting in disruption of thalamo-cortical positive feedback and insufficient filtering of cortical information processing, is proposed to account for the psychotic symptoms of schizophrenia. Conversely, it is suggested that underactivity may give rise to an enhancement of thalamocortical activity, perseveration of a fixed set of cortical processes and the symptoms clinically manifested by depression. Clearly, such an hypothesis cannot account for all types of depression and in particular it is difficult to reconcile with the common finding that depression often accompanies schizophrenia.

Interestingly, this hypothesis parallels a similar model (Penney and Young, 1983) proposed for basal ganglia-dopaminergic dysfunctions associated with several extrapyramidal motor syndromes (dyskinesias). Taken together, these proposals for the integration of cortical and subcortical processes could give us the means to explain how perception, cognition and emotional experiences are translated into the appropriate motor responses of normal behaviour. However, we still have little idea of the mechanisms by which appropriate autonomic responses, both humoral and nervous, are controlled in normal and abnormal behaviour.

How we correlate cognition with neurophysiological measures of cortical and subcortical processing has been achieved by recording averaged evoked responses in subjects performing cognitive tasks involving the detection of novel stimuli (Sutton *et al.*, 1965). These responses, known as the P300 or P3 (occurring about 300 ms after the stimulus), are unlike many other event-related signals in that they

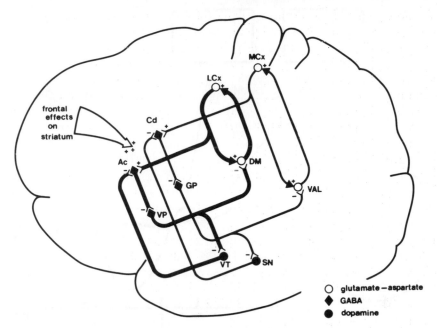

FIG. 7.17 Parallel processing for movement and emotional responses. Dopaminergic pathways from the ventral tegmentum and substantia nigra exert considerable modulatory influence over striatal regions of the basal ganglia to produce the refinement of cortical activation necessary for appropriate behavioural responses. Cognitive and emotional responses involve circuitry (thick lines) that provide a means of sharpening the patterns of 'limbic' cortical and brain-stem activity at the level of the nucleus accumbens in the ventral striatum. Movement on the other hand is refined by parallel circuitry (thin lines) that utilizes the caudate nucleus of the dorsal striatum. This model can be used to explain and show the similarity of various pathological states where dopaminergic dysfunction is implicated. For example, Swerdlow and Koob (1987) have hypothesized that the psychoses and dyskinesias are related to overactivation in the dopaminergic pathways whereas depression and Parkinson's disease result from underactivation.

The plus and minus signs indicate excitatory and inhibitory pathways, respectively. The various neurotransmitter pathways are represented by the different cell body symbols given above. MCx, motor cortex; LCx, limbic cortex; Cd, caudate nucleus; Ac, nucleus accumbens, GP, globus pallidum; VP, ventral pallidum; DM, thalamic dorsomedial nucleus; VAL, thalamic ventral/anterior/lateral nucleus; SN, substantia nigra; VT, ventral tegmentum.

do not require a physical stimulus or motor action to elicit them. In fact the P300 can be elicited by cognitive tasks employing any sensory modality (Fig. 7.18). Because of these findings the P300 is known as an 'endogenous' (internally generated) potential reflecting information processing concerned with stimulus evaluation and task relevance. Indeed, the latency and amplitude measures of the P300 reflect each of these processes, respectively (Donchin *et al.*, 1986).

As cognition depends on the integration of cortical and subcortical processes, in particular those mentioned in the hypotheses above, then it may not be

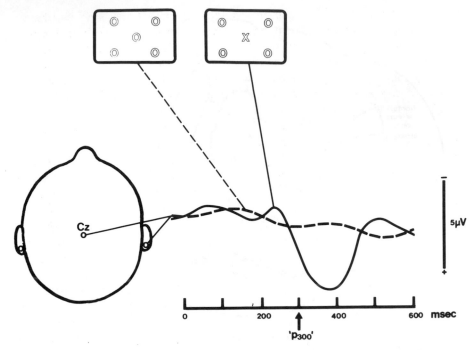

FIG. 7.18 The P300 'cognition' potential. These averaged evoked potentials occur approximately 300 ms after a novel stimulus is presented—an infrequent target stimulus (X) randomly interspersed among frequent non-target stimuli. A cognitive task involving stimuli presented in any sensory modality will elicit the P300 potential. The P300 is also known as an 'endogenous' potential and is said to reflect information processing concerned with stimulus evaluation and task relevance. The latency and amplitude measures of this evoked response reflect each of these processes, respectively. Optimal recordings can be made with a centrally (Cz) placed electrode on the scalp.

surprising to find that neurophysiological signals associated with cognitive tasks can be recorded from depth electrodes placed in various 'limbic' structures. Such signals can be optimally obtained in the hippocampus during simple cognitive tasks (Stapleton and Halgren, 1987). Furthermore, if there are disturbances to cognitive processes, as seen in some psychiatric illnesses, then there is an expectation that P300 measures may give evidence for such disturbances. Confirmation of a possible 'limbic system' dysfunction in schizophrenic patients has been claimed in a study showing that the scalp-recorded P300 in these unmedicated patients was significantly diminished during a cognitive task involving high-incentive stimuli (Brecher and Begleiter, 1983). However, other researchers have found larger P300s to high-incentive stimuli in schizophrenic patients. One such finding has recently been reported (H.B. Andrews, pers. commun.)—curiously, in this study the potentials remained bigger after the patients were told to ignore the stimuli! Perhaps this could be an indication of a defect in the mechanism for switching attention? Medication is certain to be a complicating factor in evoked potential studies on schizophrenic patients but it remains to be seen whether medication can account for any of the disparity in reported results. Schizophrenia, being an illness with a broad range of symptoms, may present different signals in the same task depending on whether the patients are acutely or chronically affected. Results of P300 studies in other psychiatric illnesses are even less clear. So, for example, we are no nearer to understanding the abnormal neurophysiological processes that give rise to the cognitive dysfunctions identified during psychometric testing in children with hyperactivity (Craggs and Taylor, 1987).

Cognition may be impaired or counterfeited at any of the three stages (reception, interpretation and convergence), each with very different effects. Irritation of the primary sensory cortex (e.g. by tumours) may cause primitive 'elemental' hallucinations (flashes of light or colour, noises, etc.), and electrical stimulation has similar effects. These hallucinations are simple and unformed, in sharp contrast with those produced from association areas. In temporal lobe epilepsy, for example, recognizable voices or visions may occur. Penfield and Jasper (1954) stimulated the temporal cortex by applying an electrode directly at operation, and were able to evoke vivid hallucinations of music in some patients who were convinced that they were hearing a concealed gramophone!

Damage to a primary sensory area produces frank loss of function. Extensive occipital damage produces 'cortical blindness', for example, in which pupillary reflexes are preserved. In contrast, damage to an association area causes complex impairments. After visual association area damage a patient may see but be unable to recognize objects (object agnosia), or faces (prosopagnosia), or be unable to make sense of the scene that he sees (simultanagnosia). Damage to the supposed convergence processing area, the frontal lobes, produces little impairment of perception itself but prevents its sensible utilization—a 'frontal lobe' patient may hear or see perfectly yet make a facile or perseverative, purposeless response.

Language may be considered a specialized example of cognition, developed in part of each association area of the dominant hemisphere: the superior temporal cortex is in fact appreciably thicker on the left side in most human brains, even in the fetus. There is thus an auditory area (Wernicke), a visual area and a motor area (Broca), each devoted to language function, with well-developed interconnections (Fig. 7.19). Damage can often be localized to one part of this system by careful clinical observation. A lesion of Wernicke's area, for example, impairs only the comprehension of spoken words. Such a patient can speak spontaneously and fluently, name objects, read aloud and write normally, yet he is grossly impaired at comprehending words spoken to him: he would have great difficulty in repeating what he hears, or in writing it down. Damage to an interconnection, such as the arcuate fasciculus joining Wernicke's and Broca's areas, produces a different syndrome—the patient can speak fluently and comprehend what he hears, but cannot repeat it properly. The sense of his speech is also impaired, since he is unable to 'monitor' what he is saying. However, deficits are rarely so confined and easy to delineate in practice. EEG potentials evoked by specific words or phrases have now been identified over Broca's area in normal volunteers (Brown *et al.*, 1976), but have not so far proved useful in the analysis of speech impairments.

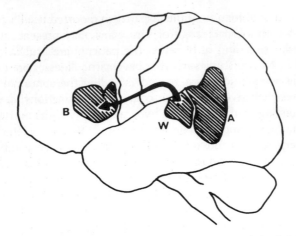

FIG. 7.19   Language processing in the cortex. Three areas of the left hemisphere are dedicated to the recognition and expression of language. The angular gyrus (A) receives information from the visual cortex and translates written words into their auditory form. Adjacent is Wernicke's area (W), which adjoins the auditory cortex and is essential for the recognition and interpretation of spoken words. This communicates via the arcuate fasciculus (arrow) with Broca's area (B), which lies next to the facial portion of the motor cortex and generates movements of speech (and possibly writing). In most human brains language function is almost entirely confined to the left hemisphere, and corresponding areas of the right hemisphere even appear to differ histologically. (The same is true of certain monkeys.)

Conclusion

From a thorough understanding of brain function we might expect several benefits. Knowledge of the interdependence of the brain's functions should allow us to design psychometric tests to isolate and quantify specific abilities, and to detect patterns of impairment peculiar to a particular disease. Topographical knowledge would permit us to interpret the findings from various electrical and radiographic investigations, so as to predict the type of impairment likely to accompany any observed damage. Finally, understanding the neurochemical mechanisms involved might enable us to devise rational treatment for at least some mental illnesses.

Our present grasp of brain function has yielded only a small number of these advantages; of particular note has been the progress made in studying the epilepsies. Despite tantalizing glimpses we have almost no knowledge of practical value. We are still, for example, unable to say exactly how memories are preserved. However, a number of new techniques offer hope for advances in the near future.

The first opportunity to observe the brain in action in close detail is offered by ambulatory and long-term monitoring with telemetry and video, so that EEG changes can be linked to behaviour—a particularly useful technique for studying epilepsy (Binnie, 1987). Microelectrodes can be implanted into the subject's brain and connected to a miniature transmitter, perhaps implanted under the skin. Electrical activity from each site in the brain is broadcast as a multiplexed signal to a nearby receiving system, which decodes it for immediate analysis while the subject carries out any desired actions. The surgical techniques involved have become progressively less injurious, and it should soon become possible to investigate normal human subjects in this way. Durable stimulating electrodes are also being developed which can be triggered remotely, and are capable of exciting or inhibiting groups of cells as a further aid to elucidating their function, and perhaps as a therapeutic tool. Can depression, for example, be relieved or intensified by stimulating certain noradrenergic centres? Perhaps the new, non-invasive, method of stimulating brain structures with magnetic pulses (Barker *et al.*, 1985) could become a way of stimulating these deep brain centres without even implanting electrodes!

Another recent technical advance has been the development of computer methods for analysing and mapping the brain's electrical activity (Pfurtscheller and Lopes da Silva, 1988). EEG surface or depth electrode recordings synchronized with the subject's actions or perceptions can be averaged in order to study the various frequency components present, and their relation to his experience (Fenton, 1980).

Most significantly, but most costly, has been the rapid expansion of several non-invasive brain imaging techniques which now allow us to study the size and metabolic activity of separate areas of the brain in some detail. Of particular interest is positron-emission tomography (PET) and nuclear magnetic resonance imaging (NMR), by which the localized turnover of specific neurotransmitters can be observed. These techniques have become very relevant to studies in psychiatric disorders (Andreasen, 1989) and when linked to the EEG may even help to elucidate the neural substrates and neurophysiological mechanisms underlying the psychoses of temporal lobe epilepsy. Most of the original experimental work has had to be done on animals using both invasive and non-invasive methods, often under anaesthetic. Although such work must continue if we are to advance our scientific knowledge and develop treatments for many as yet intractable diseases, some of the new techniques mentioned above are enabling us to study conscious humans, both sick and healthy. These techniques should help to open the door to major advances in our understanding of brain function and the treatment of psychiatric illnesses.

References

Andreasen, N.C. (1989). *Brain Imaging—Applications in Psychiatry.* New York: American Psychiatric Press Inc.

Barker, A.T., Jalinous, R. and Freeston, I.L. (1985). Non-invasive magnetic stimulation of human motor cortex. *Lancet* **ii**, 1106–1107.

Bennett, M.V.L. (1972). Electrical versus chemical neurotransmissions. In: I.J. Kopin (ed.) *Association for Research in Nervous and Mental Disease*, pp. 58–90. Baltimore: Williams & Wilkins.

Binnie, C.D. (1987). Ambulatory diagnostic monitoring of seizures in adults. In: R.J. Gumnit (ed.) *Advances in Neurology*, Vol. 46, *Intensive Neurodiagnostic Monitoring*. New York: Raven Press.

Bishop, M.P., Elder, S.T. and Heath, R.G. (1964). Attempted control of operant behaviour in man with intracranial self-stimulation. In: R.G. Hall (ed.) *Role of Pleasure in Behaviour*, pp. 58–81. New York: Hoeber Medical, Harper & Row.

Blakemore, C. (1975). Central visual processing. In: M.S. Gazzaniga and C. Blakemore (eds) *Handbook of Psychobiology*, pp. 241–268. New York: Academic Press.

Brady, J.V. (1958). Ulcers in 'executive' monkeys. *Scient. Am.* **199** (4), 95–100.

Brecher, M. and Begleiter, H. (1983). Event-related brain potentials to high-incentive stimuli in unmedicated schizophrenic patients. *Biol. Psychiat.* **18**, 661–674.

Brindley, G.S. (1986). Pilot experiments on the action of drugs injected into the human corpus cavernosum penis. *Br. J. Pharmacol.* **87**, 495–500.

Brown, W.S., Marsh, J.T. and Smith, J.C. (1976). Evoked potential waveform differences produced by the perception of different meanings of an ambiguous phrase. *Electroenceph. Clin. Neurophysiol.* **41**, 113–123.

Campbell, H.J. (1973). *The Pleasure Areas*. London: Eyre Methuen.

Cohen, D.B. (1979). *Sleep and Dreaming: Origins, Nature and Functions*. Oxford: Pergamon.

Craggs, M.D. (1975). Cortical control of motor prostheses: using the cord-transected baboon as the primate model for human paraplegia. In: B.S. Meldrum and C.D. Marsden (eds) *Advances in Neurology*, Vol. 10. New York: Raven Press.

Craggs, M.D. and Taylor, E. (1987). Neurophysiological measures in hyperactive children. In: *Proceedings of the European Brain and Behaviour Society*, Workshop on Attention Deficit Disorder and Hyperactive Syndrome. Oslo, Norway.

Crow, T.J. (1973). Catecholamine-containing neurones and electrical self-stimulation. 2. A theoretical interpretation and some psychiatric implications. *Psychol. Med.* **3**, 66–73.

Crow, T.J., Cross, A.J., Johnson, J.A., Johnstone, E.C., Joseph, M.H., Owen, F., Owens, D.G.C. and Poulter, M. (1984). Catecholamines and schizophrenia: an assessment of the evidence. In: *Catecholamines: Neuropharmacology and Central Nervous-therapeutic Aspects*. London: Alan R. Liss.

Donchin, E., Karis, D., Bashore, T., Coles, M.G.H. and Gratton, G. (1986). Cognitive psychophysiology and human information processing. In: M.G.H. Coles, E. Donchin and S.W. Porges (eds) *Psychophysiology: Systems, Processes, and Applications*, pp. 244–267. New York: Guilford Press.

Fenton, G. (1980). Priorities in research related to neuropsychiatry. In: M. Lader (ed.) *Priorities in Psychiatric Research*, pp. 163–196. Chichester: Wiley.

Friedman, D. (1978). Lateral asymmetry of evoked potentials and linguistic processing. In: D.A. Otto (ed.) *Multidisciplinary Perspectives in Event-Related Brain Potential Research*, pp. 258–260. Washington, DC: US Environment Protection Agency.

Fuster, J.M. (1989). *The Pre-frontal Cortex: Anatomy, Physiology and Neuropsychology of the Frontal Lobe*, 2nd edn. New York: Raven Press.

Gray, J.A. (1982). *The Neuropsychology of Anxiety*. Oxford: Clarendon Press.

Halperin, R. and Pfaff, D.W. (1982). Brain-stimulation reward and control of autonomic function: are they related? In: D.W. Pfaff (ed.) *The Physiological Mechanisms of Motivation*, pp. 337–376. New York: Springer-Verlag.

Hassler, R. (1978). Striatal control of locomotion, intentional actions and of integrating and perceptive activity. *J. Neurol. Sci.* **36**, 187–224.

Hobson, J.A., Lydic, R. and Baghdoyan, H.A. (1986). Evolving concepts of sleep cycle generation: from brain centers to neuronal populations. *Behav. Brain Sci.* **9**, 371–448.

Howe, J.R., Colquhoun, D. and Cull-Candy, S.G. (1988). On the kinetics of large conductance glutamate receptor ion channels in rat cerebellar granule cells. *Proc. R. Soc. Lond. B.* **233**, 407–422.

Hubel, D.H. and Wiesel, T.N. (1965). Receptive fields and functional architecture in two non-striate visual areas (18 and 19) of the cat. *J. Neurophysiol.* **28**, 229–289.

Lader, M. (1983). Behaviour and anxiety: physiologic mechanisms. *J. Clin. Psychiat.* **44**, 5–10.

Leibowitz, S.F. (1983). Hypothalamic catecholamine systems controlling eating behavior: a potential model for anorexia nervosa. In: P.L. Darby, P.E. Garfinkel, D.M. Garner and D.V. Coscina (eds) *Anorexia Nervosa: Recent Developments in Research*. New York: A.R. Liss.

Libet, B., Alberts, W.W., Wright, E.W., Lewis, M. and Feinstein, B. (1975). Cortical representation of evoked potentials relative to conscious sensory responses, and of somatosensory qualities in man. In: H.H. Kornhuber (ed.) *The Somatosensory System*, pp. 289–308. Stuttgart: Thieme.

Livingstone, M.S. and Hubel, D.H. (1981). Effects of sleep and arousal on the processing of visual information in the cat. *Nature* **291**, 554–561.

Marsden, C.D. and Jenner, P. (1980). The pathophysiology of extrapyramidal side-effects of neuroleptic drugs. *Psychol. Med.* **10**, 55–72.

Meldrum, B.S. (1988). Initiation and neuroanatomical spread of seizure activity. In: T.A. Pedley and B.S. Meldrum (eds) *Recent Advances in Epilepsy*, No. 4, pp. 1–19. Edinburgh: Churchill Livingstone.

Melzack, R. & Wall, P.D. (eds) (1989). *The Textbook of Pain*, 2nd edn. London: Churchill Livingstone.

Olds, J. (1976). Reward and drive neurons. In: A. Wauquier and E.T. Rolls (eds) *Brain-Stimulation Reward*, pp. 1–27. Amsterdam: North-Holland.

Owen, F., Crow, T.J., Poulter, M., Cross, A.J., Longden, A. and Riley, G.J. (1978). Increased dopamine-receptor sensitivity in schizophrenia. *Lancet* **ii**, 223–226.

Penfield, W. and Jasper, H. (1954). *Epilepsy and the Functional Anatomy of the Human Brain*. Boston: Little Brown.

Penney, J.B. and Young, A.B. (1983). Speculations on the functional anatomy of basal ganglia disorders. *Ann. Rev. Neurosci.* **6**, 73–94.

Penry, J.K., Porter, R.J. and Dreifuss, F.E. (1975). Simultaneous recording of absence seizures with video tape and electroencephalography: a study of 374 seizures in 48 patients. *Brain* **98**, 427–440.

Pfurtscheller, G. and Lopes da Silva, F.H. (eds) (1988). *Functional Brain Imaging*. Toronto: Hans Huber.

Rolls, E. (1989). Functions of neuronal networks in the hippocampal and cerebral cortex in memory. In: R. Durbin, C. Miall and G. Mitchison (eds) *The Computing Neuron*, pp. 125–159. Wokingham, England: Addison-Wesley.

Rushton, D.N., Rothwell, J.C. and Craggs, M.D. (1981). Gating of somatosensory evoked potentials during different kinds of movement in man. *Brain* **104**, 465–491.

Scheibel, A. and Kovelman, J. (1981). Disorientation of the hippocampal pyramidal cell and its processes in the schizophrenic patient. *Biol. Psychiat.* **16**, 101–102.

Somjen, G.G. (1978). Contributions of neuroglia to extracellular sustained potential shifts. In: D. Otto (ed.) *Multidisciplinary Perspectives in Event-related Brain Potential Research*, pp. 19–24. Washington, DC: US Environmental Protection Agency.

Sperry, R.W. (1974). Lateral specialization in the surgically separated hemispheres. In: F.O. Schmitt and F.G. Worden (eds) *The Neurosciences Third Study Program*, pp. 5–19. Cambridge, MA: MIT Press.

Stapleton, J.M. and Halgren, E. (1987). Endogenous potentials evoked in simple cognitive tasks: depth components and task correlates. *EEG & Clin. Neurophysiol.* **67**, 44–52.

Steptoe, A. (1981). *Psychological Factors in Cardiovascular Disorders.* London: Academic Press.

Sutton, S., Braren, M., Zubin, J. and John, E.R. (1965). Evoked-potential correlates of stimulus uncertainty. *Science* **150**, 1187–1188.

Swadlow, H.A., Kocsis, J.D. and Waxman, S.G. (1980). Modulation of impulse conduction along the axonal tree. *Ann. Rev. Biophys. Biomed. Eng.* **9**, 143–179.

Swerdlow, N.R. and Koob, G.F. (1987). Dopamine, schizophrenia, mania, and depression: toward a unified hypothesis of cortico-striato-pallido-thalamic function. *Behav. Brain Sci.* **10**, 197–245.

Wright, J.J., Craggs, M.D. and Sergejew, A.A. (1979). Visual evoked response in lateral hypothalamic neglect. *Exp. Neurol.* **65**, 178–185.

General Reading

Agranoff, B.W., Albers, R.W. and Molinoff, P.B. (eds) (1989). *Basic Neurochemistry: Molecular, Cellular and Medical Aspects.* London: Raven Press.

Bannister, Sir R. (ed.) (1988). *Autonomic Failure,* 2nd edn. Oxford: Oxford University Press.

Bindman, L. and Lippold, O. (1981). *The Neurophysiology of the Cerebral Cortex.* London: Edward Arnold.

Brodal, A. (1981). *Neurological Anatomy,* 3rd edn. Oxford: Oxford University Press.

Carlson, N.R. (1986). *Physiology of Behavior,* 3rd edn. Boston: Allyn and Bacon, Inc.

Carpenter, R.H.S. (1990). *Neurophysiology,* Physiological Principles in Medicine Series, 2nd edn. London: Edward Arnold.

CIBA (1979). *Brain and Mind,* CIBA Foundation Symposium 69. New York: Excerpta Medica.

Cooper, R., Osselton, J.W. and Shaw, J.C. (1980). *EEG Technology,* 3rd edn. London: Butterworth.

Doane, B.K. and Livingstone, K.F. (eds) (1986). *The Limbic System: Functional Organization and Clinical Disorders.* New York: Raven Press.

Eccles, J.C. (1973). *The Understanding of the Brain.* New York: McGraw-Hill.

Halliday, A.M., Butler, S.R. and Paul, R. (eds) (1987). *A Textbook of Clinical Neurophysiology.* Chichester: John Wiley & Sons.

Hobson, J.A. and Brazier, M.A.B. (eds) (1980). *The Reticular Formation Revisited.* New York: Raven Press.

Kiloh, L.G., McComas, A.G., Osselton, J.W. and Upton, A.R.M. (1981). *Clinical Electroencephalography.* London: Butterworth.

Kruk, Z.L. and Pycock, C.J. (1979). *Neurotransmitters and Drugs.* London: Croom Helm.

Lader, M. (1975). *The Psychophysiology of Mental Illness.* London: Routledge & Kegan Paul.

Lishman, W.A. (1987). *Organic Psychiatry: The Psychological Consequences of Cerebral Disorder,* 2nd edn. Oxford: Blackwell.

Papakostopoulos, D., Butler, S. and Martin, I. (eds) (1985). *Clinical and Experimental Neuropsychophysiology.* London: Croom Helm.

Quinn, N.P. and Jenner, P.G. (eds) (1989). *Disorders of Movement: Clinical, Pharmacological and Physiological Aspects.* London: Academic Press.

Richter, D. (ed.) (1984). *Research in Mental Illness.* London: William Heinemann Medical Books Ltd.

Stalberg, E. and Young, R.R. (eds) (1981). *Neurology I: Clinical Neurophysiology.* London: Butterworth.

Trimble, M.R. and Zarifian, E. (eds) (1984). *Psychopharmacology of the Limbic System,* British Association for Psychopharmacology No. 5. Oxford: Oxford University Press.

— 8

Neuropsychology and the Localization of Cognitive Function

I.C. McManus

The brain being brain must try to establish laws.

Iain Crichton Smith

That the brain, and especially the cerebral cortex, is not anatomically homogeneous is immediately obvious on inspection; the primary concern of this chapter will be whether the brain, and particularly the cortex is *functionally* homogeneous, and if not, how we may ascribe particular functions to particular areas, and how such knowledge may be of use in psychology and psychiatry. A more extensive introduction to the problems of neuropsychology in general will be found in Kolb and Whishaw (1989).

Methodological Problems

Clearly the first priority if we are to have an adequate theory of cerebral *localization* is that we must be able to localize damage in the brain substance. In the absence of lesions of brain tissue (or alternatively of abnormal brain stimulation) we can conclude nothing about localization (and this was probably one of the principal errors of the phrenologists). Until recently, knowledge was based almost entirely on the traditional methods of observing the brain at post-mortem or at operation. The limitations of both are obvious. In the first case one may have to wait a number of years, there may be subsequent or progressive pathology, and there is no question of going back to make further observations in the light of unusual or surprising findings, while the only positive advantage is the ability to make a complete and, if necessary, microscopic analysis of the entire brain. In the case of operative lesions we cannot be assured of the completeness of a lesion, or of its extent, or of the non-existence of other pathology in unexplored areas, and of course we do not have the freedom to make lesions as would interest us or inform us; we are completely dominated by the therapeutic needs of the patient. Recent advances, which are already revolutionizing neuropsychology, allow non-invasive visualization of the living brain. The first major advance was the development of computerized tomography (CT scanning) which allowed one to observe areas of damage, down to a resolution of a millimetre or so. The procedure could be repeated to assess change, although the problem of radiation dosage limited its usage. More importantly from a diagnostic point of view, the technique suffers from being unable to distinguish white and grey matter. Nuclear magnetic resonance imaging (MRI; see Pykett, 1982) circumvents both problems: no radiation is involved, and because of their differing proportions of water, white and grey matter are readily distinguishable. However both CT and MRI only allow the demonstration of structure (that is, of anatomy); more recent techniques such as PET (positron emission tomography; see Ter-Pogossian et al., 1980; Phelps and Mazziotta, 1985) and SPECT (single proton emission computed tomography) not only show structure but also show function (i.e. physiology), by observing changes in local metabolism (generally or of specific substrates) or local cortical blood flow (Lassen, 1982). In each case, by observing changes from a resting baseline whilst carrying out particular psychological tasks, such as speaking aloud or carrying out mental arithmetic, one can obtain detailed information about localization (see e.g. Petersen et al., 1988).

Electrical recordings from the brain are less helpful than might be expected in localizing function due to their being dominated both by the gross electrical activity of the brain (the α rhythm, etc.) and because of confusion with other, simultaneous but unrelated activity. These problems can be circumvented by the method of evoked potentials in which repeated presentation of a carefully timed stimulus (perhaps 256, 1024 or even 4096 times) allows one to average out background and extraneous noise and thereby extract a specific signal (see Chiappa and Ropper, 1982). The method is useful for observing the early stages of sensation and perception (up to 200 or 300 ms) but is otherwise limited, in part by the fact that many psychological events cannot be repeated precisely many times. In recent years the advent of powerful computer imaging methods to EEG activity has resulted in the methods of neurometrics which produces sophisticated maps of cortical activity, albeit at fairly low resolution (e.g. John et al., 1988); at present it is still unclear whether such techniques will contribute substantially to neuropsychology.

Localization as such is not the end but is only the beginning in the cerebral localization of function. To go from the existence of a lesion in a particular place to the function of the lesioned tissue is a giant step. An adequate theory of neuropsychology can only be found in a sound psychological theory of the normal processes, and no reasonable theory is likely to emerge solely as a result of making clinical observations of lesioned individuals.

A further problem of interpretation concerns the necessary and sufficient lesion to produce an effect. In neuropsychology this is a peculiarly difficult problem. A large brain lesion will destroy various abilities, but many of these deficits may be secondary to some other function which has been damaged. To avoid these problems, Teuber introduced the principle of double dissociation: if lesion A damages function P and not function Q and lesion B damages function Q and not function P, then we are entitled to conclude either that the area of lesion A is involved in function P, or that area B is involved in function Q. Clearly, the lesions must be relatively small and not overlapping for such logic to work, and as a general principle small lesions tell us more about the function of the underlying tissue than do large lesions. Despite being the keystone of most neuropsychology, the theoretical implications of the method are still not fully clear (for discussion and developments of the method, see Weiskrantz, 1968; Dunn and Kirsner, 1988).

An important assumption underlies the principle of double dissociation. In general it is highly unlikely that a single individual will have lesion A and then lesion B and it is almost impossible that lesion A will be 'cured' after the subsequent occurrence of lesion B. Hence the principle necessarily deals with lesions in different individuals, and thus assumes that the organization of different brains is similar. Whether this assumption is reasonable is unclear. Obvious counter-examples may be found in the case of language lateralization where, for one reason or another, the majority of the population have their language function in the left hemisphere but a minority (perhaps 8–10%) have right-sided language. More worrying still, there is evidence that left-handers perhaps have a more 'diffuse', and hence qualitatively different, brain organization from right-handers; similar suggestions have been made for differences between the sexes. Such factors complicate the application of the double dissociation principle.

A further complication concerns the assumption that the anatomical site of a lesion corresponds to the extent of its functional effect. However, to remove any portion of a complex system is to affect many other subsystems. Such neural effects have been termed *diaschisis* (a term introduced by von Monakow in 1914) and involve both a functional interrelation, and perhaps also a more physiological interaction, akin to the phenomenon of spinal shock. In either case the functional extent of a lesion may shrink with time, even though the anatomical lesion may not vary, and thus apparent recovery of function may occur. The anatomical extent of lesions can also vary, due either to secondary processes such as oedema, or to further extension of the lesion. In general, therefore, neuropsychology is the study of chronic patients in whom lesions have largely stabilized, both pathologically and functionally. The theoretical problems of interpreting recovery of function have been well described by Buffery and Burton (1982) (for a general overview, see Finger and Stein, 1982).

The final problem with the principle of double dissociation is that whilst the lesion may indeed be specific to a particular functional defect, it need not necessarily be responsible for that function. Geschwind (1965) published two important papers in which he suggested that many of the characteristic syndromes of neuropsychology were actually *disconnection syndromes*, which arise from disrupted fibres of passage between centres rather than damage to the centres themselves.

Disorders of Language

In 1861 Broca described a patient with the aphasia that now bears his name; the synonyms for the syndrome (motor aphasia, non-fluent aphasia and expressive aphasia) contain the essence of the defect, although they all make theoretical assumptions as well. The patients' problem is that they apparently cannot *produce* spoken language adequately, although *comprehension* of spoken language is normal. Spoken language is not entirely absent; the remaining speech is slow and deliberate, and is much abbreviated, sometimes having a 'telegraphic' quality, using only the shortest, commonest words. There is however no defect in actually making vocal sounds, since often the patient can exclaim, or even sing (sometimes producing words which they could not speak). In 1875 Wernicke described his eponymous aphasia, which also has a range of synonyms (sensory aphasia, fluent aphasia, receptive aphasia and jargon aphasia), each of which contrasts with the synonyms for Broca's aphasia. The main problem is in the *comprehension* of speech; the *production* of speech apparently being broadly intact. The contrast between the two types of aphasia is heightened by the fact that in the original observations they were described as being due to small, well-circumscribed lesions of the pre-frontal cortex and of the temporoparietal cortex respectively, and these areas have since become known as Broca's area and Wernicke's area. Clinical descriptions of both syndromes will be found in Hecaen and Albert (1978) and Heilman and Valenstein (1979); a more popular and very readable account is given in Gardner (1976). Modern work has shown that whilst there are differences in localization they are not as clear-cut as was originally thought, although undoubtedly patients with Broca's aphasia tend to have more anterior lesions than do patients with Wernicke's aphasia.

It is tempting, on the basis of the preceding descriptions, and many 'diagram-makers' in the late nineteenth century were so tempted, to conclude that the function of Wernicke's area is to comprehend spoken language and that the function of Broca's area is to produce spoken language. That such theorizing is misguided was shown by work in neurolinguistics, which began with the eminent linguists Jakobson and Halle. Jakobson felt that the deficits of these patients were far more widespread than was immediately apparent, and he suggested that the defects corresponded to what linguists know as the syntagmatic and paradigmatic systems, and which we can approximately refer to as syntax and semantics. Careful study of a patient with Broca's aphasia shows that the problem is often not only in the production of speech, but is far broader, in terms of the overall comprehension of syntax. That the patient does understand sentences is in large part due to the redundancy of much of language, so that syntax is essential for comprehension. Thus one may understand sentences such as 'Put your hand in the air' without using syntax since 'Put the air in your hand' does not make sense. However, if syntax is made critically important to comprehension, then a Broca's patient will fail at the task; for example, in distinguishing 'Put the book on your hand' from 'Put your hand on the book'. Since the comprehension of spoken syntax is also very much dependent upon perception of order and timing, it has been asked whether the primary defect is of sequencing, and hence also of pro-duction of the closely synchronized vocal tract movements involved in speech.

Closer linguistic analysis also suggests that the defect in Wernicke's aphasia is not just of the reception of the spoken language, but might be more extensive. The speech of Wernicke's aphasics shows several abnormalities; the words which are pro-duced show phonemic confusions (paraphonias: /b/ is confused with /p/ and /l/ with /r/) and there are also confusions of meaning (paraphasias: 'chair' may be said instead of 'table'). Note that in neither case is the error completely random, but rather a close approximation to the correct version is produced. Thus in both Wernicke's and Broca's aphasia there is evidence of defects of language as a whole, rather than just of the reception and production of speech, although a comprehensive theoretical account of these defects is still in its infancy. The development of systematic assessments of linguistic ability (such as the Porch Index of Communicative Ability (PICA), the Boston diagnostic aphasia test, and the Minnesota test for differential degrees of aphasia) will help both in research and diagnosis.

Of course most patients with aphasia are neither Broca's nor Wernicke's in type; they instead have a 'global' aphasia, which is due to large lesions and contains features of both of the syndromes. A few other, far rarer, syndromes also occur, and are of particular interest to neuropsychologists. *Conduction aphasia* can often fail to be detected unless specifically searched for. Production and reception are apparently normal, but the defect is in the ability to repeat sentences exactly; instead of exact repetition there is a paraphrasing of the sentence so that meaning is retained but exact form is not. The sentence is thus literally reconstructed from its meaning (which will only retain some of the surface structure of the particular words originally used in it), rather than being remembered verbatim. The classical account of this disorder is in terms of the Wernicke–Geschwind model of speech and language (although see Shallice, 1988, for a more modern view). The lesion is supposed to occur in the arcuate fasciculus, the large bundle of fibres connecting Wernicke's and Broca's areas. These two areas have become disconnected, and information cannot therefore pass directly from one to the other, but instead has to travel via other, more indirect routes, during which presumably the message loses its exact form, although retaining meaning, perhaps having been translated into and back from what Chomsky has called 'deep structure'. Certainly, the lesions of conduction aphasia are compatible with such a theory, but direct proof, in the form of sectioning of the arcuate fasciculus, is lacking, and in recent years there have been some cases reported which at first sight do not seem compatible with the theory (see Mendez and Benson, 1985).

Almost the exact opposite, or complement, of conduction aphasia, is *transcortical aphasia*, in which there is no evidence of spontaneous speech, or of comprehension, but the patient can (and does) repeat sentences (echolalia). Most intriguingly of all, the patient can modify grammatical constructions ('How are you today?' becomes 'How am I today?') and can complete conventional phrases ('roses are . . .'). The explanation of the syndrome in terms of the Wernicke–Geschwind model is that Broca's and Wernicke's areas, and the arcuate fasciculus connecting them, have become disconnected from the rest of the brain due to a diffuse lesion (typically carbon monoxide poisoning, or a multifocal dementia); in consequence the only possible route by which received speech can become spoken speech is by going directly from Wernicke's area to Broca's area, via the arcuate fasciculus, without any possibility of the intervention of thought or cognition *en route*.

The final major type of aphasia is anomic or amnesic aphasia. Comprehension, production and repetition of speech are entirely normal, and the patient is fluent in conversation. The problem is that they are unable to remember names of objects and things. The defect is not one of intelligence or thinking, since the patient is well able to provide circumlocutions, and to process ideas associated with the thing in question, but they cannot retrieve the name of the object from memory. The syndrome can occur in a pure form, but is often found in association with other forms of aphasia, and also with agraphia and alexia (see below).

The account so far given of the classical aphasic syndromes (Broca's, Wernicke's, etc.) has come under attack in the past two decades from the emerging discipline of *cognitive neuropsychology*, whose main concern is with the dissection (or *fractionation*) of psychological functions into discrete processes (or *modules*—see Fodor, 1983),. using the natural lesions produced by brain damage as its scalpel (see Shallice, 1988). It stresses the search for dissociation between different cognitive tasks and emphasizes that it is necessary to examine individual patients in great detail, looking for those key individuals who show dissociation of abilities (see Caramazza, 1986). The corollary is that the study of groups of patients is often not useful and indeed may be positively confusing or misleading, not allowing subtle differences within syndromes to emerge. Indeed when individual patients with conditions such as 'Broca's aphasia' are studied in depth, it becomes apparent that what in classical terms is a unitary syndrome can better be seen as comprised of many subsyndromes which are often dissociated (see Chapter 9 in Ellis and Young, 1988). Nevertheless, such theoretical strictures and problems apply principally to psychologists attempting to dissect function; to busy clinicians there is still little doubt that the classical syndromes provide an heuristically useful way of categorizing function in brain-damaged patients.

The model of language given above has also been attacked during the past decade for its emphasis upon the role of the *cortex* in controlling language. A growing number of aphasic patients have been shown in recent years to have subcortical, particularly thalamic, lesions, and it is thought that these are directly responsible for the aphasia (see Metter *et al.*, 1988).

Language of course does not refer only to spoken speech (as is shown clearly in aphasic deaf patients who lose their ability to produce sign language), but it also includes written language. To a certain extent difficulties in reading (alexia or acquired dyslexia) or in writing (agraphia or dysgraphia) tend to coexist with aphasia. Nevertheless, the correspondence is sufficiently incomplete to produce interesting syndromes which throw light on brain organization. Déjérine, in 1891 and 1892, described the two major forms of alexia; alexia without agraphia often occurs in isolation, the only defect being an inability to read the written word. In particular the patient can write, and hence is in the apparently paradoxical position of not being able to read what they have just written. This syndrome is probably the best example of a disconnection syndrome (although this was not recognized by Déjérine). The lesion is usually in the left primary visual cortex (and hence there is a right homonymous hemianopia), and in the splenium of the cortex callosum. There is therefore no route by which the visual input can reach the dominant hemisphere, since information from the right visual field gets no further than the lateral geniculate nucleus, whilst information from the left visual field passes to the right visual cortex but is then prevented from passing to the dominant hemisphere by the lesion in the splenium.

The syndrome of alexia with agraphia involves defects in both reading and writing, and can be, but need not be, associated with a Wernicke's type of aphasia. The critical lesion seems to be in the angular gyrus of the dominant hemisphere, at a position ideally placed to disrupt the integration of information from visual cortex and Wernicke's area. Pure agraphia (i.e. agraphia in the absence of aphasia or alexia), is rare and controversial. Exner, in 1881, suggested that it was due to lesions in what has since been called Exner's area, at the foot of the second left frontal gyrus (i.e. close to but separate from Broca's area), but this is by no means well accepted.

Finally a very rare syndrome, deep dyslexia, must be mentioned, not because it is clinically very important, but because these patients have been the subject of intense psychological research (Coltheart *et al.*, 1980). The symptoms are bizarre, and of the greatest importance in analysing the underlying mechanisms. The patients have problems in reading, and in particular are unable to read non-words (e.g. 'wux' or 'tud'), find difficulty in reading other words, in particular those which are of low imagability or are simply 'function words' (e.g. 'the' or 'is'), and make semantic errors while reading (e.g. 'play' for 'act', 'food' for 'dinner'). The final surprising thing about the patients, given the limit of their deficits, is the relatively large size of their lesions, which are always left-sided; indeed Coltheart has suggested that in the deep dyslexic we are observing the pure reading ability of the isolated right hemisphere.

Cerebral Dominance

In the mid-nineteenth century Broca and Dax showed convincingly, on the basis of the association between aphasia and right-sided hemiplegia, that language was preferentially associated with the left side of the brain (for an excellent historical account, see Harrington, 1987, who makes it clear that even at that time it was being argued that hemispheric asymmetry may explain psychiatric conditions —a recurrent modern theme: see Gruzelier and Flor-Henry, 1979). Since the time of Broca it has become clear that whilst a majority of the population have left-sided language dominance, a minority have right-sided language dominance; there is also the controversial possibility that some individuals have bilateral speech processes. It is probable that both handedness and cerebral dominance for language are under the genetic control of the same gene (see Annett, 1985; McManus, 1985).

The prediction of which individuals in a population have right-sided dominance is of theoretical and practical importance. Neurosurgeons wish to be able to operate through the non-dominant hemisphere in order to avoid producing post-operative aphasia, and psychiatrists wish to be able to give unilateral ECT to the non-dominant hemisphere in order to be able to minimize verbal memory disturbance. There are four basic methods for assessing dominance:

(1) *The Wada technique.* This involves the unilateral injection of sodium amytal into the one carotid artery and then the other, observing whether speech loss occurs after right or left injection. The method is indubitably effective, but has a sufficiently high morbidity to mean that it is only of use for pre-operative assessment where the risks are justified.

(2) *Unilateral ECT.* The administration of unilateral ECT to the two hemi-spheres, and the observation of verbal difficulties in the minutes after recovery of consciousness, may itself be used as an accurate means of assessment of dominance but is clearly difficult to justify in non-depressed patients.

(3) *Dichotic listening and visual half-field studies.* If information is presented just to one ear, or to one visual field (by means of an exposure short enough to prevent saccadic eye movements, in a tachistoscope), then because of the corpus callosum the information will be transferred to both cerebral hemispheres. If, however, different messages are presented simultaneously either to the two ears or the two visual fields, then there is sufficient competition between the stimuli to mean that the message contralateral to the dominant hemisphere is perceived better (i.e. left language dominance is associated with a right-ear advantage or a right-visual field advantage). The method is easy to use and harmless, and hence has been much used for research purposes (see Hugdahl, 1988). However, it is insufficiently reliable or accurate to be of use for pre-operative assessment of language dominance.

(4) *EEG studies.* If the α rhythm is recorded from both hemispheres during verbal thought then there is a greater suppression on the side which is more active, which is the dominant side. Again, this is primarily a research tool, rather than a routine procedure.

A major advance in the study of cerebral dominance has been work on 'split-brain' patients. These individuals have had a cerebral commissurotomy, involving section of the corpus callosum, for the treatment of severe epilepsy. As a result it is possible, by mean of carefully controlled stimulus presentations, to study just one hemisphere at a time in isolation (thereby fulfilling the criteria for double dissociation within a single patient). From these patients it seems clear that the non-dominant hemisphere does indeed have *some* language but that it is far more restricted than that in the left hemisphere, being limited to concrete rather than abstract words, having a smaller vocabulary, and having poor command or syntax. By contrast, however, the right hemisphere seems to be better at tasks involving visuospatial problems, such as those requiring mental imagery or patterns. This insight is well supported by the clinical effects of right-hemisphere lesions.

Disorders of Perception and Action

The contrast between the cognitive modes of the left and right hemispheres is reflected in the difference between lesions affecting symbolic action (such as the aphasias, alexias, agraphias and some of the apraxias) and the lesions affecting spatial and perceptual processes, such as the agnosias and constructional apraxia. Relatively less is known about these latter syndromes and they appear to be somewhat less common, perhaps in part because they are less looked for.

At the lowest level, disorders of perception result in apparent absence of sensory function. It must, however, be remembered that in, say, the visual system, the primary visual cortex is not the only retinal projection. The projection to the superior colliculus is of great importance in the unconscious detection of movement (whereas the visual cortex is of importance in the conscious recognition of form). Hence individuals with lesions of primary visual cortex cannot see in the conscious sense, but it can be demonstrated that they can use collicular information, albeit unconsciously, and in a way that they feel is random guessing; a phenomenon that Weiskrantz has called 'blind-sight' (see Weiskrantz, 1986).

At a slightly higher level in the visual system, we find a miscellaneous collection of conditions known as the agnosias, often involving lesions of the right occipitoparietal area. They were described originally in experimental dogs by Munck, in 1881, and he called them 'mind blindness', which emphasizes that there is no blindness in the strict sense of seeing lines, edges, etc., but rather there is a general failure to integrate the information. Some of the agnosias are general, whereas others, such as colour agnosia, and prosopagnosia (the inability to recognize faces), are highly specific, and are of great importance in suggesting that the brain has specific systems for dealing with certain types of stimuli. A common denominator of the agnosias, as recognized by Luria, is the inability to carry out the operation of separating figure from ground (or foreground from background), and this means that agnosics are peculiarly poor at disambiguating figures which are embedded in other figures. Agnosias can also occur in the auditory system (agnosia for sounds, in which non-verbal auditory stimuli are incorrectly recognized, and the amusias, which specifically involve defects of musical perception) and in the somatosensory system (such as astereognosia, in which objects can be recognized by touch alone, and asomatognosia, in which the patient fails to 'know' the position and state of their own body, and may even deny the existence of half of it—hemineglect—or apparently be unaware and indifferent to pain in a particular area—pain asymbolia). At the highest intellectual level agnosia can also manifest as a lack of understanding of the spatial environment (see de Renzi, 1982).

There is a sense in which the apraxias are the converse of the agnosias, being defects of motor rather than sensory function. Liepmann, in 1900, described patients who could perform simple actions, but could not integrate the actions into a well-organized sequence (ideomotor apraxia); there were also patients who could perform actual actions, but were unable to imitate them without the actual objects, as for instance in striking an imaginary match (ideational apraxia). There are also specific apraxias, such as buccofacial apraxia in which motor sequences with mouth and face are impaired, once more suggesting the possible existence of specific cerebral subsystems. The apraxias are controversial in that they are usually associated with left-hemisphere damage, and frequently coexist with aphasia; the question therefore arises of whether aphasia and apraxia are independent syndromes, or are perhaps indicative of a more widespread defect of symbolism and gesture (which is of course closely associated with language).

In contrast to the left-sided apraxias described above, there is constructional apraxia, in which the patient is unable to construct objects from building blocks, or is unable to draw, or even to copy simple line drawings. Here the defect is primarily one of the mental reconstruction of the object, rather than in the motor control *per se*, and it is almost always associated with right-sided parietal damage.

By now it must seem that there is an infinity of different syndromes involving specific defects. As a cautionary note on the overmultiplication of syndromes, it is worth considering Gerstmann's syndrome, which was described in 1924, on the basis of a single patient, and consists of the tetrad of finger agnosia (the inability to name or recognize the fingers), acalculia (inability to carry out arithmetic), agraphia and right–left confusion. It is now controversial as to whether there is any fundamental psychological similarity between these heterogeneous defects (see Benton, 1961), and current opinion probably favours the suggestion that these defects had come together by chance, perhaps due to the lesion affecting several different adjacent cortical areas, particularly since patients may be found with just one, two or three of the tetrad of symptoms.

Disorders of Memory

Two very different types of lesion cause permanent amnesia (see Whitty and Zangwill, 1977): bilateral hippocampal removal (as shown in the much studied patient HM), and Korsakoff's syndrome, in which the major anatomic lesions seem to be in the mammillary bodies and the anterior thalamus. In both conditions, despite the lack of coincidence of the lesions, the symptoms are strikingly similar: a loss of the ability to form new memories (anterograde amnesia) and an inability to access old memories (retrograde amnesia). In neither condition is there any deficit of short-term memory. The major psychological interest in these cases has concerned whether the defect is one of the creation of new memories, the storage of memory, or the retrieval of memories from store. Warrington and Weiskrantz have shown that with suitable assistance during recall (using 'fragmented stimuli') such patients can 'learn' (although they are not consciously aware of it), suggesting that the major defect may be in the *retrieval* of memory. For more recent ideas on the defects in amnesia, see Mayes (1987) and Hintzman (1990).

Disorders of Personality and Emotion

Thus far the majority of deficits described have been intellectual or cognitive deficits. In this section we must consider the non-cognitive, or affective and personality effects of lesions. Unlike previous work, much of this area is dominated by particular lobes of the brain (temporal and frontal), partly because it is easy to remove the lobes, in both animals and man, and partly because localized diseases, such as tumours, can readily simulate such experimental and surgical lesions. It has also become apparent in recent years that the two sides of the brain are not equally involved in emotional responses (see Heilman and Satz, 1983).

Temporal lobes

In 1937 Kluver and Bucy bilaterally ablated the temporal lobes of a rhesus monkey. The previously aggressive monkey became tame, and also demonstrated hypersexuality, as well as evidence of visual agnosia. The crucial question of course is whether similar symptoms occur in man, and the answer is, yes. However, the symptoms are also associated with defects in language, and in memory, and these factors necessarily modify the picture. Animal studies now make it clear that the decreased aggression of the Kluver–Bucy syndrome is due to lesioning the amygdala; that the hypersexuality may be due to lesioning of the septal system; and that the visual agnosia is due to lesioning the inferior temporal gyrus. In man the defects of language and memory are probably due to involvement of Wernicke's area and the hippocampus, respectively. The 'syndrome' is thus an artificial collection of symptoms which bear no obvious psychological relationship to one another; nevertheless, gross lesions of the area, due to tumour or trauma, or gross stimulation of the area (due to temporal lobe epilepsy), will necessarily affect them all in parallel.

Frontal lobes

Jacobsen, in 1936, showed that frontally lesioned monkeys showed impairment on delayed response tasks, in which an animal is shown where to find a reward, but is prevented from taking the reward for a few seconds. Similarly, the animals are poor at tasks involving alternation of responses (e.g. the reward is under the left cup and then the right cup on alternate trials). The problem seems not to be one of memory but of the inhibition of responses, a conclusion which is supported by the failure of animals with frontal lesions to habituate as rapidly as normal, and hence they continue to produce responses long after a normal animal has ceased —giving the appearance of stereotypy. Frontal lobe damage in humans is far more dramatic, but may be regarded in part as a continuation of the effects found in animals. Frontal patients show a tendency to produce bizarre antisocial behaviours, involving a lack of awareness of social niceties, and with a child-like interest in repeated stimuli and responses—behaviour which has been termed 'pseudopsychopathic', and may be explained in terms of a lack of response inhibition. An alternative personality change in frontal lesions is 'pseudodepression', in which there is a lack of spontaneous activity or drive, a general loss of emotional expression, and reduced speech. Except for the last feature these symptoms may also be found in animals, where spontaneous behaviours may be reduced, facial expressions absent, and social drive diminished (as shown by the animals tending to fall to the bottom of the hierarchy, or 'pecking order').

The deficits of response inhibition and spontaneous behaviour are not the only problems found in frontal lesions. There are also motor difficulties (shown in the inability to imitate movements), difficulties in control of eye movements (due to lesions of the frontal eye fields), and deficits of memory and spatial orientation. It is this heterogeneity of deficits which makes it difficult to know whether there is a simple unitary psychological defect, or perhaps, as in the temporal lobes, there is a series of independent deficits which are associated merely due to neuro-anatomical contiguity. It is somewhat difficult to see how complete removal of the frontal lobes could be therapeutically useful, and it is worth stressing that

Moniz introduced the operation of frontal lobotomy on the basis of a single 'neurotic' chimpanzee which appeared to be more 'relaxed' after its operation.

Conclusions

In a survey such as this, in which coverage is necessarily superficial, some omissions are inevitable. However some omissions are intentional, and perhaps need stressing. One such is the absence of reference to developmental aspects; the organization of the normal adult brain is far from understood, and that of the individual damaged in childhood is still less well understood, and may indeed be qualitatively different from that of the normal adult. Similarly, all references to alexia and dyslexia are to acquired adult dyslexia; the syndrome of childhood dyslexia is controversial, and almost certainly unrelated to the adult condition. And in a similar vein, there is no detailed discussion of the development of recovery from lesions; again too little is known and the questions are perhaps too complex to answer at present.

Perhaps a surprising omission in a work on cognitive function is any reference to 'intelligence'. Thus there is little evidence that intelligence is reduced in aphasia or after brain lesions of small or even moderate size, including, for instance, bilateral frontal lobotomies. Similarly there is little evidence that certain areas are of particular importance in determining intelligence; intelligence as a whole is robust in the face of damage, although specific abilities are not, perhaps thereby justifying in part Lashley's concept of mass action (or equipotentiality). Certainly there is no need as yet for us to postulate a centre which the mediaeval neuroanatomists would have labelled *ratio*.

An exception to the above rule is in the differentiation of right- and left-sided lesions. In general left-sided lesions produce a relatively greater impairment on the verbal subtests of IQ batteries, and right-sided lesions produce a relatively greater impairment on 'performance' (or visuospatial) subtests, and a difference of 10 or more IQ points on the two scales is probably of importance.

Finally, in a book of this sort, which hopes to provide the relevant scientific background for a student of psychiatry (and there seems little doubt that in the future brain imaging and localization will be of growing importance in psychiatry: see Andreasen, 1988), there has been little direct attempt to provide immediate and practical applications of the information given. Rather it has been assumed that any knowledge of the brain and its actions must be of relevance to the concerned psychiatrist, particularly when dealing with bizarre effects of lesions which can simulate psychiatric problems (see e.g. Benson and Blumer, 1975), and that psychiatrists in training will rapidly make such associations for themselves. There is, however, also a more serious problem; while in principle there should be much relevance, that is not always the case. I will conclude therefore with a quotation from Geschwind, who until his death in 1985 was probably one of the most eminent and influential neurologists to address psychological questions:

> While it has become fashionable to acknowledge the existence of an area of overlap between neurology and psychiatry, this common ground unfortunately bears more resemblance to

a no-man's land than to an open border . . . Unfortunately, few members of either group have in fact really interested themselves in the borderland area, and too frequently interactions between them are educationally disappointing . . . Hopefully, this situation will be corrected in the next few years, but until then, both psychiatrists and neurologists [and one would add, psychologists] will often have to acquire the necessary knowledge themselves.

References

Andreasen, N.C. (1988). Brain imaging: applications in psychiatry. *Science* **239**, 1381–1388.

Annett, M. (1985). *Left, Right, Hand and Brain: The Right Shift Theory*. London: Lawrence Erlbaum.

Benson, D.F. and Blumer, D. (eds) (1975). *Psychiatric Aspects of Neurological Disease*. New York: Grune & Stratton.

Benton, A.L. (1961). The fiction of the Gerstmann syndrome. *J. Neurol. Neurosurg. Psychiat.* **24**, 176–181.

Buffery, A.W.H. and Burton, A. (1982). Information processing and redevelopment: towards a science of neuropsychological rehabilitation. In: A. Burton (ed.) *The Pathology and Psychology of Cognition*. London: Methuen.

Caramazza, A. (1986). On drawing inferences about the structure of normal cognitive systems from the analysis of patterns of impaired performance: the case for single-patient studies. *Brain & Cognition* **5**, 41–66.

Chiappa, K.H. and Ropper, A.H. (1982). Evoked potentials in clinical medicine. *New Engl. J. Med.* **306**, 1140–1150; 1205–1211.

Coltheart, M., Patterson, K. and Marshall, J.C. (1980). *Deep Dyslexia*. London: Routledge & Kegan Paul.

de Renzi, E. (1982). *Disorders of Space Exploration and Cognition*. New York: John Wiley.

Dunn, J.C. and Kirsner, K. (1988). Discovering functionally independent mental processes: the principle of reversed association. *Psychol. Rev.* **95**, 91–101.

Ellis, A.W. and Young, A.W. (1988). *Human Cognitive Neuropsychology*. London: Lawrence Erlbaum.

Finger, S. and Stein, D.G. (1982). *Brain Damage and Recovery*. New York: Academic Press.

Fodor, J.A. (1983). *The Modularity of Mind*. Cambridge, MA: MIT Press.

Gardner, H. (1976). *The Shattered Mind: The Person After Brain Damage*. New York: Vintage Books.

Geschwind, B. (1965). Disconnexion syndromes in animals and man. *Brain* **88**, 237–294; 585–644.

Gruzelier, J. and Flor-Henry, P. (eds) (1979). *Hemisphere Asymmetries of Function in Psychopathology*. Amsterdam: Elsevier.

Harrington, A. (1987). *Medicine, Mind and the Double Brain*. Princeton, NJ: Princeton University Press.

Hecaen, H. and Albert, M.L. (1978). *Human Neuropsychology*. New York: Wiley.

Heilman, K.M. and Satz, P. (1983). *Neuropsychology of Human Emotion*. New York: Guilford Press.

Heilman, K.M. and Valenstein, E. (eds) (1979). *Clinical Neuropsychology*. Oxford: Oxford University Press.

Hintzman, D.L. (1990). Human learning and memory: connections and dissociations. *Ann. Rev. Psychol.* **41**, 109–139.

Hugdahl, K. (ed.) (1988). *Handbook of Dichotic Listening: Theory, Methods and Research.* New York: Wiley.

John, E.R., Prichep, L.S., Fredman, J. and Easton, P. (1988). Neurometrics: computer-assisted differential diagnosis of brain dysfunctions. *Science* **239**, 162–169.

Kolb, B. and Whishaw, I.Q. (1989). *Fundamentals of Human Neuropsychology*, 3rd edn. San Francisco: Freeman.

Lassen, N.A. (1982). Measurement of cerebral blood flow and metabolism in man. *Clin. Sci.* **62**, 567–572.

Mayes, A. (1987). Human organic memory disorders. In: H. Beloff and A.M. Colman (eds) *Psychology Survey 6*, pp. 170–191. Leicester: British Psychological Society.

McManus, I.C. (1985). *Handedness, Language Dominance and Aphasia: A Genetic Model. Psychol. Med.:* Monograph Supplements, No. 8.

Mendez, M.F. and Benson, D.F. (1985). Atypical conduction aphasia: a disconnection syndrome. *Arch. Neurol.* **42**, 886–891.

Metter, E.J., Riege, W.H., Hanson, W.R., Jackson, C.A., Kempler, D. and von Lanckner, D. (1988). Subcortical structures in aphasia: an analysis based on [^{18}F] fluorodeoxyglucose positron emission tomography and computed tomography. *Arch. Neurol.* **45**, 1229–1234.

Petersen, S.E., Fox, P.T., Posner, M.I., Mintun, M. and Raichle, M.E. (1988). Positron emission tomographic studies of the cortical anatomy of single-word processing. *Nature* **331**, 585–589.

Phelps, M.E. and Mazziotta, J.C. (1985). Positron emission tomography: human brain function and biochemistry. *Science* **228**, 799–809.

Pykett, I.L. (1982). NMR imaging in medicine. *Scient. Am.* **246** (5), 54–64.

Shallice, T. (1988). *From Neuropsychology to Mental Structure.* Cambridge: Cambridge University Press.

Ter-Pogossian, M.M., Raichle, M.E. and Sobel, B.E. (1980). Positron emission tomography. *Scient. Am.* **243** (4), 141–155.

Weiskrantz, L. (1968). Treatments, inferences and brain function. In: L. Weiskrantz (ed.) *Analysis of Behavioural Change.* New York: Harper and Row.

Weiskrantz, L. (1986). *Blindsight.* Oxford: Clarendon Press.

Whitty, C.W.M. and Zangwill, O.L. (1977). *Amnesia: Clinical, Psychological and Medico-legal Aspects.* London: Butterworth.

The Synapse, Receptors and Alzheimer's Disease

A.N. Davison

The encoding and storage of behavioural information as well as other complex aspects of mental function is dependent on the neuronal network within the brain. In some neurological and psychiatric disorders perturbation due to loss of nerve cells or their connections may occur with selective changes in particular neurotransmitter systems. An example is loss of dopaminergic nerve cells from the basal ganglia in Parkinson's disease, or more controversially altered brain morphology in schizophrenia or autism. In the brain of the elderly and in dementia anatomical changes result in biochemical modifications, which to some extent reflect alterations in cognitive function. One aspect of research in neuro-degenerative disease is focused on the mechanism of selective neuronal loss and the molecular biology of the associated cytoskeletal changes. The resultant alterations in neurotransmitters, found in the brain, can sometimes be detected in the cerebrospinal fluid. However positron emission tomography is much more useful, especially in providing a non-invasive alternative to brain biopsy. At post-mortem, measurement of potential synthesizing enzyme ability and receptor binding capacity is valuable since catabolism of neurotransmitters occurs after death. This chapter includes a review of current concepts of the mechanism of synaptic transmission and receptor activity with reference to neuropathological and neurochemical observations in Alzheimer's disease (AD).

The Synapse

Nerve cells communicate with one another through axon terminals which form a network of synapses on the surface of recipient neurones. Synaptic interaction may be with the cell body, axons and dendrites, or even with other nerve endings. As many as 50 000 synapses may emanate from one neurone. In the extreme case of the human striatum, there may be some five million terminals per dopaminergic neurone. Clearly, synaptic architecture is of great complexity, with excitatory and inhibitory signalling mechanisms in which one nerve cell may exert considerable control over many others. D.O. Hebb (1949) proposed that synaptic modification in learning and memory occurs as a consequence of coincidence between pre- and postsynaptic activity.

TABLE 9.1   Some possible neurotransmitters.

Monoamines and amino acids	Peptides
Acetylcholine	Enkephalin, β-endorphin
Dopamine	Substance P
Noradrenaline	Neurotensin
Serotonin	Adrenocorticotrophic hormone (ACTH)
Histamine	Angiotensin
γ-Aminobutyric acid (GABA)	Oxytocin, vasopressin
Glutamic acid	Somatostatin
Glycine	Vasoactive peptide (VIP)
Taurine	Luteinizing hormone-releasing hormone (LHRH)
	Thyrotrophic-releasing hormone (TRH)
	Cholecystokinin
	Galinin

Ultrastructure of the synapse

Electron microscopic examination shows that the synapse is an expansion of the terminal axon branch. The terminal has a continuous outer plasma membrane with a specialized contact zone facing the synaptic gap. A postsynaptic thickening is present on the surface of the receiving neurone. Within the cytoplasm of the terminal there are mitochondria and numerous microvesicles, usually spherical, with a diameter of 40–50 nm. These are surrounded by a membrane containing synaptophysin, an integral glycoprotein which acts as a suitable marker for the synapse. The synaptic vesicles contain bound neurotransmitter and other molecules. In some inhibitory terminals, the vesicles appear to be flattened rather than spherical. In neurosecretory chromaffin cells and in peripheral noradrenergic varicosities, vesicles of different sizes with dense cores are present.

Neurotransmitters

Transmitters are low-molecular-weight substances (Table 9.1) released across the synaptic cleft in response to an action potential passing down the nerve axon. Before the next cell fires or is inhibited, a minimum number (quanta) of transmitter molecules have to be released. Certain criteria are necessary to identify a substance as a neurotransmitter. It must be shown to be released on stimulation under physiological conditions and the isolated transmitter must act in a similar way to normal nervous transmission. The neurotransmitter should be synthesized or accumulated in nerve cells or their synapses. There should be specific antagonists or analogues which interfere with or mimic the action of the proposed transmitter. In addition, mechanisms need to be available to inactivate excess released transmitter either by enzymic activity or by high-affinity re-uptake systems localized in neurones, or possibly in glia enveloping the nerve terminal. Although there are many neurotransmitters, it has been thought that only one is secreted or released by an individual neurone. Now there is evidence that at certain terminals neuroactive peptides may also be present with the neurotransmitter. However, the peptides are thought to function as synaptic modulators by modifying the action of biogenic amines and amino acids with which they coexist. Thus, enkephalins may act in this way in some cholinergic neurones and substance P in nerve cells containing serotonin. Classical neuro-transmitter synthesis principally occurs within the synaptic terminal by enzymes which are generated within the perikaryon and transported down the axon, whereas the peptide cotransmitters are synthesized in the cell body from larger precursors and are transported in vesicles to the terminals (Boarder, 1989).

Transmitter release

It is believed that stored neurotransmitter is released into the synaptic cleft to interact with specific receptor sites on the postsynaptic region of the receiving neurone. Thus, following nerve stimulation, there is a reduction in the proportion of charged vesicles, and an appearance of omega-shaped profiles on the pre-synaptic membrane. The emptied vesicles seem to be coated in a protein network, and these complex vesicles appear in the synaptosomal cytoplasm. There seems to be an active zone involved in transmitter release in which large intramembrane particles (calcium channels) are involved in the initiation of calcium-mediated transmitter release.

Acetylcholine

Acetylcholine is the one substance which satisfies all the various experimental criteria for an established neurotransmitter. The classic example of a cholinergic neurone is the Renshaw cell, which responds to acetylcholine and has muscarinic receptors as well as nicotinic synapses.

Acetylcholine has been shown to be released from brain tissue on stimulation and acts at neuromuscular junctions, in autonomic ganglia and at postganglionic parasympathetic nerve endings. The transmitter is synthesized in the cytoplasm of the nerve terminal by the enzyme choline acetyltransferase which catalyses the acetylation of choline by acetyl-CoA. In the synapse, acetylcholine is stored in vesicles and some is free in the cytoplasm. There is a sodium-dependent high-affinity uptake system for choline. Convincing evidence has not yet been obtained to show unequivocally that the released quanta of transmitter in the cholinergic synapse (estimated at about 6000 molecules of acetylcholine) are derived directly from the vesicles in the central nervous system. It has been shown that on stimulation recently labelled high-specific activity cytoplasmic acetylcholine is released. After release into the synaptic cleft acetylcholine is hydrolysed by the enzyme acetylcholinesterase localized on the postsynaptic surface. Different molecular forms of the enzyme have been characterized—the homologous class of identical globular subunits and in the central nervous system (CNS) the less abdundant heterologous association of up to 12 catalytic subunits with collagen-like filamentous units or a tetramer with lipid-linked tails.

Our knowledge of the biochemistry of the cholinergic system has been helped by extensive investigation of the electric eel, with its massed array of cholinergic electromotor terminals. The vesicles from *Torpedo* contain six main protein components which include ATPase, calmodulin (the calcium receptor protein) and actin. Acetylcholine (in this case about 200 000 molecules) and ATP are present in the lumen of the vesicle. In addition, a glycosaminoglycan is found which may serve to provide negative charges to neutralize the positive charges on the stored acetylcholine ions.

Acetylcholine may induce persistent changes in certain learned behavioural changes in cortical neurones. However, long-term potentiation in the hippocampus is thought to be an important basis for learning, possibly mediated through the transmitter glutamate (Gustaffson and Wigstrom, 1988). Many studies have implicated acetylcholine in memory processes, for example cholinergic antagonists impair memory tasks and lesioning of the basal forebrain disrupts memory in animals.

Neuroanatomy

There are five major cholinergic systems in the vertebrate brain: those of the medial basal forebrain, the extrapyramidal, parabrachial, cranial motor and reticular cell groups. Damage to cholinergic hippocampal circuits originating in the septum and basal areas results in profound memory deficits. The basal forebrain contains nuclei of large cholinergic neurones in the medial septum, the diagonal band of Broca and the nucleus basalis of Meynert. The medial septum and diagonal band have cholinergic projections to the hippocampus although there are also large numbers of non-cholinergic cells. The nucleus basalis provides cholinergic innervation widely to the cerebral cortex and amygdala. There are also projections from cortex to the nucleus basalis. A small number (1–2% of the total neurones) of giant cells in the striatum and nucleus accumbens are cholinergic. Thus choline-acetyltransferase and acetylcholinesterase activities are very high in the caudate, putamen and accumbens.

Other neurotransmitters

Other small molecular substances, such as various amino acids, peptides and amines, are thought to act as neurotransmitters. In the CNS glutamate and the inhibitory transmitter γ-aminobutyric acid (GABA) are quantitatively of particular importance. Glutamic acid is widely distributed within cells, but it has been shown to be excitatory when applied to isolated neurones. Excitatory amino acids such as glutamate and aspartate are major transmitters of the cerebral cortex and hippocampus and appear to be involved in learning and memory. It seems probable that the pyramidal neurones, which constitute the major cell type in the cortex, are glutamatergic cells. Since glutamate is a product of intermediary metabolism within the cell, it is difficult to delineate the amino acid's role as a neurotransmitter, but some information can be obtained by measurement of N-methyl-D-aspartate (NMDA) receptors. NMDA receptors are concentrated in the hippocampus. There is evidence that glutamatergic pathways include cortical association fibres, corticofugal and hippocampal pathways. The catecholamines (dopamine, noradrenaline and adrenaline) and indoleamines (serotonin) are now well recognized as transmitter substances. Noradrenaline has been shown to be synthesized and stored in sympathetic neurones. Well-defined chromaffin granules have been isolated from the adrenals and analysed to show the complex make-up of the vesicles which, besides the transmitter, contain various components including dopamine-β-hydroxylase, the enzyme that catalyses the conversion of dopamine to noradrenaline. Histochemical methods have been successfully used to trace the distribution of the catecholaminergic tracts in the CNS. In contrast to the extracellular action of acetylcholinesterase, inactivation of released biogenic amine is mainly by the action of monoamine oxidase within the cell. Metabolism is also affected by methylation mediated by catechol-O-methyltransferase, which acts within the cytoplasm and possibly extraneurally (e.g. within the synaptic cleft). Re-uptake mechanisms are also of importance in removing excess transmitter. Certain neuropeptides act as neuromodulators and some have been implicated in learning and memory (e.g. vasopressin, adrenocorticotropin hormone and possibly somatostatin).

Receptors

It has been found that some hormones, drugs and transmitter molecules interact as selective binding sites (Fig. 9.1). Some drugs mimic the effect (agonists), while antagonists block the activity. Transmitters act with high affinity at the specific recognition sites, which are coupled to an effector system leading to a signal. For example, released acetylcholine combines with a specific cholinergic receptor protein, mainly nicotinic receptors in the peripheral nervous system and predominantly muscarinic receptors in the CNS. It seems likely that acetylcholine induces conformational changes in the receptor protein resulting in the opening and shutting of pores, or 'gating', of the membrane, with participation of phosphatidic acid and calcium-sensitive Na^+, K^+-activated ATPase. As a result of ATPase action, there are changes in intracellular concentrations of sodium, potassium and calcium ions, with alterations in the resting potential. Guanine nucleotide binding proteins (G proteins) are ubiquitous features of signal transduction mechanisms (Ross, 1989) controlling intracellular calcium concentration and second messenger function (Fig. 9.2). The cholinergic postsynaptic receptor system may involve ionic pores with movement of ions following transmitter stimulus. Other types of receptor interaction result in metabolic changes through the action of a second messenger. An example of this is the postsynaptic system where receptor protein is linked to the enzyme adenylate cyclase. Cyclic adenosine monophosphate is released through the action of the first messenger (which may be one of a number of transmitters or hormones). The cyclic AMP is capable of altering enzyme activities, protein synthesis and membrane permeability. At certain synapses, it is proposed that the cyclic AMP stimulates a membrane protein kinase, leading to depolarization of the postsynaptic neurone. An example is the dopamine

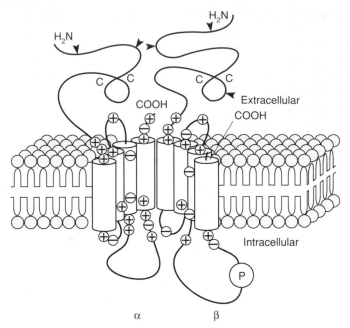

FIG. 9.1   Schematic model of the GABA$_A$ receptor in the cell membrane. In this model four membrane-spanning helices in each subunit are shown as cylinders. The possible conformation of the extracellular domain and potential extracellular sites for N-glycosylation (indicated by triangles) are shown. It is proposed that two copies of each of the subunit structures are complexed in the receptor molecule to align the membrane spanning domains, only some of which will form the inner wall of a central ion channel (Schofield *et al.*, 1987). (Reprinted by kind permission of Dr. E.A. Barnard).

(DA-1) receptor which is adenylate cyclase linked and regulated by guanine nucleotides. Dopamine also may combine with DA-2 receptors which are not linked to adenylate cyclase. A wide range of multiple neurotransmitter receptors have been identified.

Dementia

The diagnostic and statistical manual of mental disorders (DSM-III-R; American Psychiatric Association, 1987) defines dementia as a loss of intellectual ability with resulting occupational and social handicaps. Defective memory is accompanied by one or more of the following: impaired thinking or judgement; aphasia; apraxia; agnosia; constructional difficulties; changes in personality but unclouded consciousness. Other causes of organic mental illness must be excluded. AD is the commonest cause of dementia although exact diagnosis is difficult and ultimately depends on neuropathological examination (Table 9.2). Vascular or multi-infarct dementia accounts for about a quarter of patients with dementia. In addition some individuals have mixed vascular and AD. Regional cerebral blood flow methods using the xenon-133 inhalation method are valuable in predicting vascular

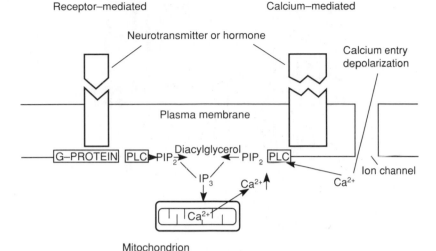

FIG. 9.2 Communication can be effected by direct receptor-mediated mechanism or by calcium influx activating the phospholipase C (PLC) cascade. This may be via the GTP-binding protein (G). PIP$_2$, phosphatidylinositol 4,5-bisphosphate; IP$_3$, inositol triphosphate.

dementia. Reduction in cerebral blood flow occurs in AD but such measurements have been superseded by advances in three-dimensional imaging techniques capable of determining cerebral blood flow and metabolic rate in different brain regions. Positron emission tomography has been used for estimating energy metabolism. Hypometabolism of glucose has been seen, particularly in the parietal and posterior temporal regions in early Alzheimer patients; later the frontal association areas are equally affected. The levels of glucose and oxygen utilization correlate with the degree of dementia. However, some of these effects may be due to atrophy of brain tissue and lack of activation in the association area (see Fig. 9.3).

Neuropathology

Commonly, brain atrophy with enlarged ventricles is a feature of AD, the brain weight dropping from between 1200 and 1350 g to 1000 g or less. There is usually symmetrical cortical atrophy, especially of the frontal lobes and temporal lobe. It has been suggested that a decrease in the length of the cortical ribbon in a columnar fashion contributes to the overall atrophy (Duyckaerts *et al.*, 1985). Using 'biochemical indices', Bowen and his colleagues (1977) have analysed whole temporal lobes from normal elderly and matched demented subjects and found that about one-third of nerve cell components are lost from the temporal lobe at the endpoint in the pathological process. Such losses are in agreement with the histological studies showing loss of predominantly large pyramidal cells from the temporal cortex as well as from the hippocampus and amygdala. In the subcortex there is a significant loss or shrinkage of large cholinergic neurones in

TABLE 9.2 Diagnosis of dementia, showing diagnostic levels I–VI (by courtesy of Professor C.G. Gottfries).

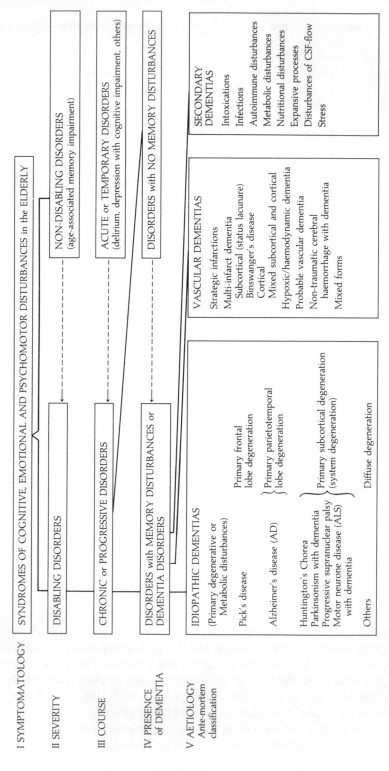

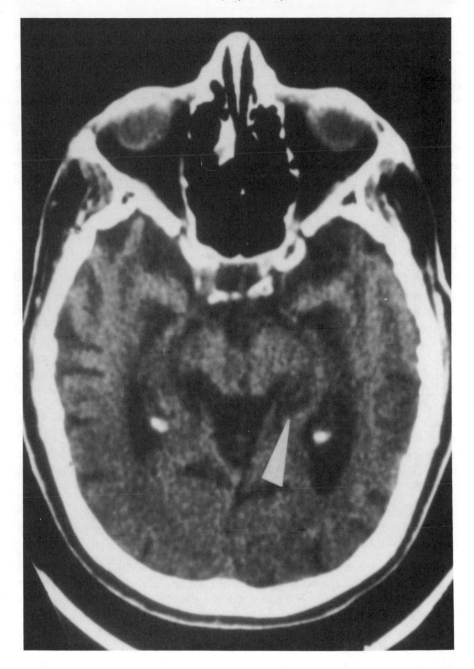

FIG. 9.3 Computerized tomographic scan of patient with Alzheimer's disease. Dilation of the hippocampal (arrow) and choroidal fissures are shown by negative angulation imaging (de Leon *et al.*, 1989). Atrophy of the hippocampus serves as an early indication of memory impairment and is predictive of progressive dementia in AD. (Reprinted by kind permission of Dr M.J. de Leon.)

the nucleus basalis of Meynert. The population of neurones in the locus ceruleus and the raphe nuclei is reduced (for review see Mann, 1988) in comparison to age-matched controls. Microscopic examination shows that as nerve cells degenerate there are reductions in nucleolar volume and cytoplasmic RNA content. Accompanying neural loss (detectable by staining for neurofilament protein) there is reduction in the neuropil and a marked decrease in synaptic innervation—as measured by the concentration of synapsin 1 and synaptophysin.

Alzheimer first described the characteristic inclusion bodies visualized by silver staining in dementia. Neuritic plaques and tangles are found, especially in the association areas of the cortex, hippocampus, amygdala and within certain subcortical nuclei. In the hippocampus granulovacuolar degeneration is a special feature.

Tangles

Neurofibrillar tangles accumulate within the neuronal perikaryon, their twisted paired helical filaments extending into the axon and dendritic processes. In the cortex tangles are found in clusters in the pyramidal neurones of layers III and V. There are also tangle ghosts suggesting that the paired helical filaments interfere with intracellular transport and metabolism leading to cell death. The main components of the tangle are microtubule-associated phosphoproteins (tau). On the basis of amino acid sequences it has been claimed (Beyreuther et al., 1988) that the paired helical filament protein is derived from the amyloid precursor (APP). There are two distinct pathways involved. Intracellular proteolysis of APP give rise to aggregates of A4 (42 amino acid peptide with a trans-membrane domain) which form tangles. The extracellular processing of APP results in formation of amyloid plaques or congophilic angiopathy. Intraneuronal accumulations of aluminium have been found close to the nucleus in tangle-bearing neurones.

Neuritic plaques

Senile plaques are extracellular aggregates of diameter up to 200 μm. They are localized in the cortical association areas but are rare in regions such as primary visual, auditory, somatosensory and motor cortices. There is evidence that plaque formation occurs before tangles appear. Immature plaques containing preamyloid deposits may be detected by using a monoclonal antibody (Glenner and Wong, 1984) directed against an amyloid epitope and there is some evidence to show that plaques form round microglia (Wisniewski et al., 1989). The classical plaque contains a dense core of amyloid, probably with a central 'star' of aluminium silicate and a halo of degenerating swollen neurites and astrocyte processes. Many plaques are acetylcholine and butyrylcholinesterase positive. There is evidence that the amyloid A protein component of the plaque is derived by proteolysis of a larger precursor protein.

Genetics of Alzheimer's Disease

Familial AD is an autosomal dominant inherited condition affecting 15–20% of Alzheimer patients, especially those with an early age of onset (St George-Hyslop *et al.*, 1989). Since most patients with Down's syndrome (trisomy 21) eventually develop the pathological features of AD, this pointed to chromosome 21 as a likely locus. This was confirmed in studies revealing a restriction fragment length polymorphism at the proximal region of chromosome 21. There is no doubt that the same locus does not apply to sporadic forms of the disease. The gene encoding for the 695 amino acid precursor amyloid protein has been localized some 10 million base pairs distant on the long arm of chromosome 21, suggesting that an understanding of regulation of expression at this site may prove informative since the larger amyloid precursor form (APP) contains a domain with homology to the serine proteinase inhibitors. This implies that abnormal peptide formation may occur in AD, for the inhibitor is found in neuritic plaques.

Neurotransmitter Activity

The cholinergic hypothesis

Following screening of post-mortem AD brain for a number of biochemical constituents, Bowen and his colleagues found a reduction in choline acetyltransferase activity which correlated with the degree of pathological damage to the temporal lobe. Shortly after, Davies and Maloney (1976) and Perry and her group (1977, 1978) confirmed and extended these observations. They showed that loss was greatest in the temporal and parietal cortex, the hippocampus and amygdaloid nucleus. Perry and her colleagues demonstrated reduction in choline acetyltransferase and acetylcholinesterase activities in parallel with an increase in neuritic plaque density and pre-mortem intellectual impairment. Muscarinic cholinergic receptor binding was unaffected in the cerebral cortex although butyrylcholinesterase activity actually increased. These observations were extended to fresh cortical biopsy samples (Sims *et al.*, 1983) where it was found that choline acetyltransferase activity, choline uptake and acetylcholine synthesis (stimulated and resting) were significantly reduced within a year of the onset of cognitive symptoms. More recently the M2 (but not M1) subtype muscarinic receptor concentration has been found to be reduced as well as the concentration of the presynaptically located nicotinic receptor (Table 9.3). These and related findings have been interpreted as indicating widespread loss of presynaptic cholinergic terminals in AD, in contrast to multi-infarct dementia where neurotransmitter changes relate to areas of ischaemic damage.

The basal forebrain

The discovery (Whitehouse *et al.*, 1982) that there was in AD an apparent loss of the large cholinergic cells from the nucleus basalis of Meynert explains the loss

TABLE 9.3 Neurotransmitter and receptor concentrations in Alzheimer's disease.

Parameter	Brain area	% Control	Parameter	Brain area	% Control
Cholinergic system			**Serotoninergic system**		
Choline acetyltransferase	Parietal cortex	18[a]	Serotonin	Frontal cortex	78
Acetylcholine synthesis	Temporal cortex (biopsy samples)	36[a]	Serotonin	(Familial AD)	<50
			Serotonin uptake	Temporal cortex	28[a]
Nicotine receptor	Parietal cortex	60[a]	Serotonin	Parietal cortex	74[a]
	Frontal cortex	74	Receptor S1	Entorhinal cortex	42[a]
Muscarinic receptor M1	Hippocampus	79[a]	S2		
M2		81			
Glutamate transmission			**Catecholaminergic system**		
D-Aspartate binding	Parietal cortex	63[a]	Dopamine	Frontal cortex	78
			Noradrenaline	Frontal cortex	60

[a]Significantly different from normal.
Data from various sources.

of presynaptic terminal cholinergic markers. Neuronal loss correlates with neuritic plaque density in the cortical terminal fields, although loss or shrinkage of magnocellular basal neurones appears to be a relatively late phenomenon. The viability of the basalis cells may be dependent on retrograde transport of a trophic factor from target organs in the cortex and hippocampus. Thus shrinkage in the nucleus basalis follows lesioning of the neocortex, leading to the possibility that retrograde degeneration is due to loss of target cells within the cortex. Lesioning experiments have been interpreted to show that reduced innervation by dicarboxylic amino acid-releasing fibres from the amygdala could be a factor in reduction in the activity of nucleus basalis neurones in AD.

Nerve growth factor

Seiler and Schwab (1984) showed specific retrograde transport of nerve growth factor (NGF) from the neocortex to nucleus basalis and NGF has been shown to stimulate neurite formation as well as to prevent the lesion-induced degeneration of cholinergic cells. The protective effect of NGF is exerted in the medial septal nucleus after partial transection of the fimbria. Fischer and his colleagues (1987) continuously infused NGF into the brain of aged rats with spatial memory impairment. This resulted in some prevention of cholinergic cell body atrophy in the nucleus basalis and striatum with recovery of spatial memory as measured in a water maze test. In addition, in animals with unilateral lesions to the nucleus basalis or fimbria physostigmine facilitated memory improvement can be shown with NGF infusion or after transplantation of fetal cholinergic tissue. This recovery is associated with acetylcholinesterase positive innervation of the hippocampus. Cholinergic neurones of the forebrain have a high density of NGF receptors and may thus be dependent on this factor for survival. Of considerable interest is the demonstration that cholinergic neurones of the pontomesencephalotegmental system (brain stem) neither degenerate in AD nor do these neurones have receptors for nerve growth factor. In the rat the highest concentrations of NGF and NGF (mRNA) are found in the hippocampus and cerebral cortex. So far in post-mortem AD brain no difference has been found in available cholinergic stimulation factor or in NGF (mRNA) but there may be atrophy and localized changes (for review, see Hefti *et al.*, 1989).

The cortex

A feature of AD is the loss of large pyramidal cells (up to 60%) in the cortex, especially in the parietal and occipital regions. Pearson and his colleagues (1985) have suggested that AD spreads along projection neurones from the olfactory cortex to the association areas, sparing the occipital and motor cortex. This hypothesis has been strengthened by the observed pathological changes in olfactory neurones in AD patients (Talamo *et al.*, 1989). Thus changes in the cortex may precede those in the subcortex and indeed loss of cortical choline acetyltransferase activity can exceed loss of neurones in the nucleus basalis. The serotoninergic system is dramatically altered in familial cases of AD, levels of

5-hydroxytryptamine sometimes being undetectable in post-mortem brain, correlating with a major loss of neurones from the raphe dorsalis (Herregodts et al., 1989). In sporadic AD the loss is less. The catecholaminergic system is less affected but changes (e.g. in the limbic system) may be related to behavioural abnormalities.

Conclusion

Although the cholinergic system is markedly affected in Alzheimer's disease, dysfunction of subcortical cholinergic projections may be secondary to changes in the cortex. Possible mechanisms of tangle and neuritic plaque formation have been proposed but the etiology of Alzheimer's disease remains obscure. Since trophic factors have been shown to be essential for nerve cell viability, reduction in the concentration of such factors may contribute to the loss of neurones in specific loci.

References

American Psychiatric Association (1987). *Diagnostic and Statistical Manual of Mental Disorders*, 3rd edn, revised. Washington, DC: American Psychiatric Association.

Beyreuther, K., Beer, J., Hilbich, C. et al. (1988). Molecular pathology of amyloid deposition in Alzheimer's disease. In A.S. Henderson and J.H. Henderson (eds) *Etiology of Dementia of Alzheimer's Type*, pp. 125–134. Chichester: John Wiley & Sons.

Boarder, M.R. (1989). Presynaptic aspects of cotransmission: relationship between vesicles and neurotransmitters. *J. Neurochem.* **53**, 1–11.

Bowen, D.M., Smith, C.B., White, P., Flack, R.H.A., Carrasco, L., Gedye, J.L. and Davison, A.N. (1977). Chemical pathology of the organic dementias. II. Quantitative estimation of cellular changes in post-mortem brains. *Brain* **100**, 427–453.

Davies, P. and Maloney, A.J.F. (1976). Selective loss of central cholinergic neurons in Alzheimer's disease. *Lancet* **ii**, 1403.

de Leon, J.J., George, A.E., Stylopoulos, L.A., Smith, G. and Miller, D.C. (1989) Early marker for Alzheimer's disease: the atrophic hippocampus. *Lancet* Sept 16, 672–673 (letter).

Duyckaerts, C., Hauw, J.-J., Piette, F., Poulain, V., Rainsgard, C., Berthaux, P., and Escourolle, R. (1985). Cortical atrophy in senile dementia of the Alzheimer type is mainly due to a decrease in cortical length. *Acta Neuropathol.* **66**, 72–74.

Fischer, W., Wictorin, K., Bjorklund, A., Williams, L.R., Varon, S. and Gaye, F.H. (1987). Amelioration of cholinergic neuron atrophy and spatial memory impairment in aged rats by nerve growth factor. *Nature* **329**, 65–68.

Glenner, G.G. and Wong, C.W. (1984). Alzheimer's disease: initial report of the purification and characterization of a novel cerebrovascular amyloid protein. *Biochem. Biophys. Res. Commun.* **120**, 885–890.

Gustaffson, B. and Wigstrom, H. (1988). Physiological mechanisms underlying long term potentiation. *Trends Neurosci.* **11**, 156–162.

Hebb, D.O. (1949). *The Organization of Behaviour*. New York: John Wiley & Sons.

Hefti, F.J., Hartikka, J., and Knusel, B. (1989). Function of neurotrophic factors in the adult and aging brain and their possible use in the treatment of neurodegenerative disease. *Neurobiol. Aging* **10**, 515–533.

Herregodts, P., Bruyland, M., DeKeyser, J., Solheid, C., Michotte, Y. and Ebinger, G. (1989). Monaminergic neurotransmitters in Alzheimer's disease. An HPLC study comparing presenile familial and sporadic senile cases. *J. Neurol. Sci.* **92**, 101–116.

Mann, D.M.A. (1988). Neuropathological and neurochemical aspects of Alzheimer's disease. In: L.L. Iversen, S.D. Iversen and S.H. Snyder (eds) *Psychopharmacology of the Ageing Nervous System*, pp. 1–67. New York: Plenum Press.

Pearson, R.C.A., Esiri, M.M., Hiorns, R.W., Wilcock, G.K. and Powell, T.P.S. (1985). Anatomical correlates of the distribution of the pathological changes in the neocortex in Alzheimer disease. *Proc. Natl. Acad. Sci. USA* **82**, 1–4.

Perry, E.K., Perry, R.H., Blessed, G. and Tomlinson, B.E. (1977). Neurotransmitter enzyme abnormalities in senile dementia—choline acetyltransferase and glutamic acid decarboxylase in necropsy brain tissue. *J. Neurol. Sci.* **34**, 247–265.

Perry, E.K., Tomlinson, B.E., Blessed, G., Bergmann, K., Gibson, P.H. and Perry, R.H. (1978). Correlation of cholinergic abnormalities with senile plaques and mental test scores in senile dementia. *Br. Med. J.* **2**, 1457–1459.

Ross, E.M. (1989). Signal sorting and amplification through G protein-coupled receptors. *Neuron* **3**, 141–152.

Schofield, P.R., Darlison, M.G., Fujita, N., Burt, D.R., Stephenson, F.A., Rodriguez, H., Rhee, L.M., Ramachandran, J., Reale, V., Glencorse, T.A., Seeburg, P.H. and Barnard, E.A. (1987). Sequence and functional expression of the $GABA_A$ receptor shows a ligand-gated receptor super-family. *Nature* **328**, 221–227.

Seiler, M. and Schwab, M.E. (1984). Specific retrograde transport of nerve growth factor (NGF) from neocortex to nucleus basalis in the rat. *Brain Res.* **300**, 33–39.

Sims, N.R., Bowen, D.M., Allen, S.J., Smith, C.C.T., Neary, D., Thomas, D.J. and Davison, A.N. (1983). Presynaptic cholinergic dysfunction in patients with dementia. *J. Neurochem.* **40**, 503–509.

St George-Hyslop, P.H., Myers, R.H., Haines, J.L., Farrer, L.A., Tanzi, R.E., Abe, K., James, M.F., Conneally, P.M., Polinsky, R.J. and Gusella, J.F. (1989). Familial Alzheimer's disease: progress and problems. *Neurobiol. Aging* **10**, 417–426.

Talamo, B.R., Rudel, R., Kosik, K.S., Lee, V., Neff, S., Adelman, L. and Kauer, J.S. (1989). Pathological changes in olfactory neurons in patients with Alzheimer's disease. *Nature* **337**, 736–739.

Whitehouse, P.J., Price, D.L., Strubie, R.G., Clark, A.W., Coyle, J.T. and Delong, M.R. (1982) Alzheimer's disease and senile dementia: loss of neurons in the basal forebrain. *Science* **215**, 1237–1239.

Wisniewski, H.M., Wegiel, J., Wang, M., Kujawa, M. and Lach, B. (1989). Ultrastructural studies of the cells forming amyloid fibres in classical plaques. *Can. J. Neurol. Sci.* **16**, (4 Suppl.) 535–542.

General Reading

Bartus, R.T. (ed.) (1989). Alzheimer's disease: current and emerging topics on age-related neurodegeneration. In: *Neurobiology of Aging*, Vol. 10, pp. 381–659.

Iversen, L.L., Iversen, S.D. and Snyder, S.H. (eds) (1988). Psychopharmacology of the aging nervous system. In: *Handbook of Psychopharmacology*, Vol. 20. New York: Plenum Press.

Siegel, G., Agranoff, B., Albers, R.W. and Molinoff, P. (1989). *Basic Neurochemistry*, 4th edn. New York: Raven Press.

— 10

Some Aspects of the Use of the EEG in Psychiatry

P.B.C. Fenwick

The EEG and Psychiatry

One of the most significant discoveries of the twentieth century is that neural activity is accompanied by changes in the electrical fields surrounding the neurone. These electrical fields can also be measured on the surface of the scalp. Hans Berger, a German psychiatrist, was the first person to make a detailed study of these fields in man and in 1929 he published the first paper on the electro-encephalogram (EEG). Since that time, monitoring of the scalp EEG has become routine. Changes in technology now allow the recording of the electrical rhythms of the brain throughout the 24 hours, during both waking and sleeping. Of more significance, modern telemetry and lightweight tape recorders allow the EEG to be recorded during the day, away from the hospital, at home or at work.

In the late 1940s Dawson showed that stimulating a peripheral nerve can result in a change in activity on the surface of the scalp. These changes are usually of such low amplitude that it is difficult to distinguish them from the ongoing background activity of the brain. Dawson's contribution was that he provided the first method of detecting these potentials by the principle of averaging, which has opened up the field of evoked-potential study. The advent of modern digital computers has extended this field.

Advances in neurosurgery brought about the possibility of recording the electrical activity at the surface of the cortex, the electrocorticogram (ECoG). Depth-electrode recording from leashes of chronically implanted electrodes has revealed the presence of electrical activity deep within the brain, which at times is seen to correlate with different subjective experiences. Behavioural correlates of these discharges have led to some understanding of the role played by these deeper structures in personal experience.

Advances in videotape recording and split-screen viewing, in which the EEG and patient can be viewed side by side, have led to a precise correlation between the behavioural changes seen during a seizure and abnormal electrical discharges. It is to be hoped that these techniques, when extended to patients with psychiatric illness, will also improve our understanding of the disease.

Finally, the expansion in computing facilities and the application of mathematical methods to signal analysis have allowed features of the EEG to be extracted and quantified. This has led to a better understanding of the cognitive changes that occur during the presence of abnormal cerebral activity. For the future it will be important to study the way that abnormal cerebral activities can be modified by the progression of mental illness and the relationship between mental illness, changes in neurotransmitters and changes in cognition.

Genesis

The electrocorticogram measured on the surface of the cerebral cortex is the spatial average of the underlying dendritic fields of the cells in the superficial layer of the cortex. These dendritic fields are generated by the inhibitory and excitatory postsynaptic potentials (IPSP or EPSP).

Microelectrode recordings from the cell bodies of cortical neurones show that the hyper- and hypo-polarization of the cells that are related to the IPSPs and EPSPs can be detected outside the cells so long as the recording electrode remains within the vicinity of those cells. As soon as the electrode is withdrawn beyond the dendrites, the potential fields of neighbouring cells interfere and the original correlation is lost (Creutzfeldt et al., 1966). Creutzfeldt showed that the waveform of these potential fields depends on the cells that generated them. Thus at a cellular level there is information about cell type and neural activity coded within the EEG waveform. The spatial average of these dendritic fields, all of which have random phase to each other, could be expected to sum to zero, as predicted by the central limit theorem. However, this does not occur because groups of cells become synchronized, and it is this activity which forms the electrocorticogram. If spindles of coherent activity are the potentials which go to make up the electrocorticogram, which systems are responsible for this spindling and synchronization of these cell populations?

Andersen and Andersson (1974) have shown that spindle activity in the non-specific nuclei of the thalamus is transmitted to the thalamic-projection areas of the cortex. Thus the EEG generators can be regarded as thalamocortical in structure; although the actual potential fields are created by the cells in the superficial layers of the cortex, the synchronization of those cells is derived from the thalamus. What then controls thalamic activity?

Thalamic activity is modulated by a tonic bombardment from the reticular activating system of the midbrain and brain stem. Depression of reticular tone leads to synchronization of the thalamic rhythms and so to synchronization and slowing of the cortical rhythms. An increase in reticular tone leads to desynchronization of the EEG, due to a breaking up of thalamic spindle activity (Andersen and Andersson, 1974).

The relationship between the electrocorticogram and the scalp EEG has been studied by several groups of workers (see a most important paper by Cooper et al., 1965). In summary, they have shown that the ECoG shows a difference in electrical activity from point to point on the surface of the cortex, even when these points are only 1–2 mm apart. This indicates a lack of spread of activity within the cortex, similar activity of two or more electrodes being due either to an underlying synchronization of the cortical generators or to a physiological connection between them. The scalp EEG is a spatial average of the activity of these small cortical areas, the larger the cortical area involved in synchronized activity, the higher the amplitude of the EEG. An estimate given by Cooper *et al.* (1965) is that it requires $6\,cm^2$ of coherent activity on the surface of the cortex to be 'seen' in the scalp EEG.

Although the above description relates specifically to the ongoing background activity or to the spontaneous EEG, it also holds true for evoked activity. In evoked activity a sensory stimulus—visual, auditory or somatosensory—is given. The stimulus enters the central nervous system by specific sensory pathways, relays in the thalamic nuclei and is then transmitted to the cortex. Wide pools of cortical neurones are synchronized by the stimulus and it is the activity of these pools that is seen as the evoked response.

A further group is that of slow cortical potentials. In a forewarned reaction-time task, a negative shift in cortical potential develops between the warning stimulus and the second imperative stimulus to which a motor response is mandatory. These negative shifts in potential are called contingent negative variations (CNV), and are thought to be related to cortical excitability (Tecce, 1972).

Thus the scalp EEG shows, par excellence, patterns of synchronization of cortical activity and is therefore well suited for the investigation of epilepsy. Its sensitivity to changes in level of consciousness and mild cerebral dysfunction make it an ideal tool in psychiatric practice to help distinguish between organic pathology and a functional illness.

Recording and Terminology

The EEG is recorded from electrodes placed on the scalp. It is not necessary to be totally familiar with the details of the system, although some knowledge is helpful. The electrodes are usually silver discs coated with silver chloride, which are stuck to the cleaned scalp with collodion. Platinum intradermal needles are used by some laboratories, usually if the patient is unconscious, while there is a fashion in the United States to use gold-plated silver discs. The electrodes are placed on the scalp in certain positions, which are defined by the distance from a fixed landmark, such as the nasion or inion. This system placement is called the International 10–20 system, since the distance between the landmarks is divided into intervals of 10% and 20% of the major distances (Sannit, 1963).

One electrode is connected to each of the two inputs to every EEG amplifier channel. It is conventional to label one of the inputs as black and the other as white. The names define the direction (up or down) in which the pens will move when a voltage is applied across the input. The convention states that the black input lead is the lead that causes an upward deflection of the pen when it is negative compared to the other input lead (BUN—black up negative). The electrodes are connected together in standard runs called a montage and a diagram detailing the montage in use during the recording is placed in the EEG record before every section.

EEG activity can be broken down into a number of bands, depending on its frequency. The first rhythm to be discovered was a rhythm measured between

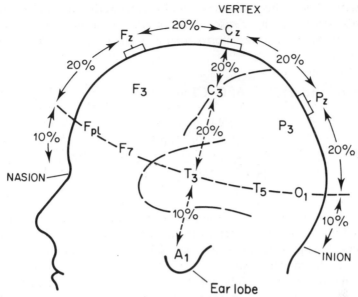

FIG. 10.1 Standard electrode positions labelled according to the International 10–20 system. Right-side electrodes are even-numbered (e.g. C_4 instead of C_3). (From Callaway, 1975.)

the forehead and the occiput by Hans Berger—no mean feat as he only had a sensitive Einthoven string galvanometer. The rhythm he found was at 10 Hz and came to be known as the Berger rhythm. Later this rhythm was called the α rhythm, as it was the first to be named. Subsequently, other Greek letters were applied to the difference bands in the EEG spectrum. It is agreed internationally that the EEG bands should be designated as follows:

β	Band	> 13 Hz
α	Band	8–13 Hz
θ	Band	4–7.9 Hz
δ	Band	0.1–3.9 Hz

(For more information, see Hill and Parr, 1963.)

A knowledge of certain concepts helps in the understanding of EEG reports. If the activity on the scalp is arising from a localized area of the cortex, it will produce changes in potential in only a few electrodes. The channels connected to these electrodes produce a distinctive pattern of activity, which is mirror-imaged in two or three other channels, e.g. down in one channel and up in the adjacent channel. This pattern is called a focal change and indicates a localized change in potential on the scalp.

Sometimes bursts of cerebral activity are seen for a few seconds only: this activity is called paroxysmal, either localized, if seen in one area, or generalized, if occurring over the whole scalp.

Higher-voltage, spike-like waves standing out from the background activity are called spikes. Officially, a spike must not last longer than 70 ms; if it does last longer, but has the same waveform, then it is called a sharp wave.

Principal Underlying EEG Changes

The normal rhythmic pattern of activity is altered in very specific ways by disease, insult, and changes in metabolism. If it is understood that the actual generators of the EEG are the cells in the superficial layers of the cortex and that large numbers of these cells need to be synchronized by subcortical mechanisms before changes are seen in the scalp EEG, then what follows may be more easily understood:

1. Cortical lesions are more likely to be picked up from the EEG than lesions deep within the cortex. The larger the lesion, the more easily it is 'visualized'.
2. Discharging cortical lesions are more obvious than those which cause effects through pressure.
3. Tumours are electrically silent, but large cortical tumours may show themselves by a flattening of the EEG over them. The appearance of abnormal activity occurs at their edges, due to pressure, anoxia or irritation of surrounding neural tissue.
4. The speed of development of the lesion is crucial for its effect on the EEG. Rapidly expanding lesions, whether they are an abscess, tumour or bleeds, always cause marked focal EEG changes. A chronic slow growing glioma or meningioma, although huge in size, may produce only slight EEG changes. The changes seen will be either at the edges of the lesion or due to pressure (probably brain stem distortion) and occur generally. This is called false localization.
5. Small lesions deep to the cortex may cause little or no EEG change. A small internal capsule bleed, which may lead to a devastating hemiplegia, is likely to produce only minimal EEG changes.
6. Any lesion, either structural (tumour) or biochemical (depressant drug), which depresses the function of the reticular formation will produce widespread EEG changes by altering recruitment in the cortico-thalamic projection systems.
7. Any alteration in the level of consciousness will be reflected by widespread EEG changes, again due to alteration of reticular activating system activity on thalamic recruitment.
8. As a general rule, damage to the cortex leads to rhythms in the area of damage. These show a reduction in frequency compared to those present in the alert subject. The greater the degree and rapidity of onset of the damage, the slower the cerebral rhythms. Thus localized slow activity is usually found over areas of damage.
9. Generalized slowing is found in the EEG when there is either a metabolic abnormality affecting the brain generally or damage to or depression of the reticular formation.

10. Epileptic activity may be transmitted over long distances within the brain, so the presence of an epileptic focus in the scalp EEG does not necessarily indicate the presence of an underlying cortical lesion. A spike's localizing value should be treated with caution.

11. Spikes do not always indicate an epileptogenic lesion, as they can frequently occur in patients without epilepsy. Thus the presence of spikes should never be taken to make the diagnosis of epilepsy without a history of clinical seizures.

12. From what has been said, it can be seen that EEG changes cannot, except in rare circumstances, provide a definite diagnosis. The brain responds electrically to different insults in much the same way, e.g. an abscess, tumour or thrombosis produces focal δ rhythms. The likely diagnosis in the presence of an abnormal EEG is suggested by the clinical situation. Thus the EEG's strength is that it can suggest to the clinician that an organic syndrome is present even with normal brain structure (e.g. normal CAT scan). It can also suggest some possibilities as to what this is likely to be, if interpreted in conjunction with the clinical problem.

Development

Electrical activity has been measured from the brain of the human fetus as early as the 20th week after conception (Eeg-Olofsson, 1970). Little rhythmic activity is present until 36 weeks. At birth, the EEG is dominated by slow rhythmic activity at about 3–4 Hz when the infant is awake, although the pattern is different if he is drowsy or asleep. By 6 months, the EEG increases in frequency posteriorly and has reached about 5 Hz; this rises to nearly 7 Hz by the end of the first year. The increase in frequency continues until the age of seven to eight, although the final frequency may not be attained until the early teens.

The rather simple description above does not reveal the complexity of the human EEG at birth and the large differences in frequency that are found between different areas, which are enhanced as the child matures. It does, however, show that increasing maturity in the child is accompanied by an increase in frequency of the EEG. Studies using frequency analysis show how δ rhythms are dominant in the young infant up to the age of one year. From the age of 2 until 5, θ rhythms are dominant, although δ activity does still appear, albeit with a reducing amplitude. From the age of 6 onwards, θ activity decreases and α activity increases, although θ activity is still present until the early twenties.

These observations about the changing frequencies of the EEG with age have led to the concept of electrical immaturity, meaning that there are slow frequencies present in the EEG that would be more appropriate to a younger age group. Thus an excess of slower rhythms for the age in a child's EEG will lead to it being called immature. This idea has been extended to the EEGs of late adolescents and young adults.

The concept of immaturity has been taken further by Matousek and his colleagues, in Sweden. They analysed the EEGs of a large number of normal

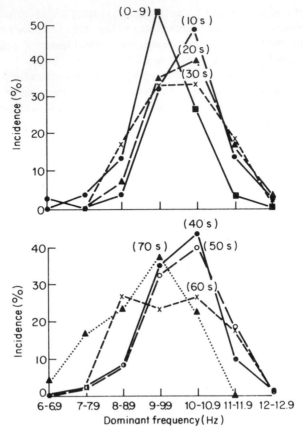

FIG. 10.2   Dominant frequency during wakefulness at different ages (420 normals).

children by the method of frequency analysis, to obtain a spectral (frequency) profile of each age group. From this profile they were able to define statistically the normal frequency composition of an EEG at any age during childhood. They also calculated a weighting function, which could be applied to the analysed spectral profile of any EEG and so allow the electrical age of any child to be calculated. It is thus now possible to give an electrical as well as a chronological age to any child's EEG. However, the concept of immaturity suffers from several drawbacks:

1. Maturation is unlikely to be the same for each child, so one is dealing with a statistical norm.
2. Immaturity is defined as an excess of slower rhythms for the age. Slower rhythms are the non-specific end-result of numerous processes, not only maturation.
3. In a study of normal children, Eeg-Olofsson (1970) showed that 15% of the children and 4.9% of the adolescents had paroxysmal abnormalities. If excess slow was also included, then 32% of the children's and 23% of the adolescents' records were not 'normal'. Thus on the above grounds the limitation of this concept should be clearly understood.

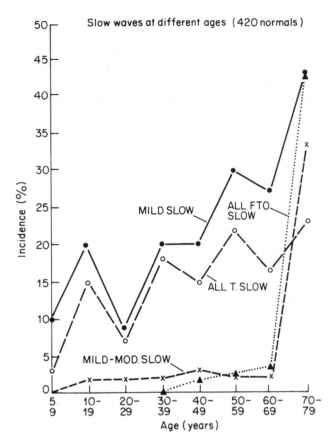

FIG. 10.3   Slow waves at different ages. T, temporal; FTO, frontal temporal and occipital.

The Normal EEG

From the discussion in the preceding section it should be clear that a normal EEG picture, which will fit any particular child, can only be defined with difficulty. The same is true for adults, although here the task is easier. The degree of normality of any population will depend on the group of subjects who are chosen. The abnormality rate is between 5 and 15%. Williams (1941) found a rate of 5–10%, the lower group being the more carefully selected, while Hill and Watterson (1942) found 15% in a group containing mental nurses and psychiatrists! Brazier *et al.* (1945) showed that 5% of RAF flying personnel, 10% of army non-combatants and 15% of civilians had abnormal records. The main abnormalities in abnormal EEGs are an excess of slow activity and/or paroxysmal bursts. This finding suggests that as minor abnormalities in the EEG are common in normal subjects they are best ignored unless they support a definite clinical finding (see Fig. 10.3).

The EEG in Ageing

From the late twenties until the end of the sixth decade, the EEG remains relatively stable. As old age sets in and the sixties approach, a slowing of the α rhythm occurs. In young adults, the mean α frequency is 10.2–10.5 Hz, but this falls to 9.4 Hz in mentally normal men aged 60–74 years and to 8.9 Hz in the 75–94 age group. Women's α rhythms are better preserved, the figures being 9.7 and 9.1 Hz respectively.

The number of people with frequencies over 10 Hz is given as only 16% in one study of 256 people over the age of 60, higher frequencies being much less common. Thus old age slows the dominant rhythm (Obrist and Busse, 1965).

Apart from the slowing, there is also an increase in diffuse slow activity. This is rare under the age of 75 years, but it is reported by Obrist and Busse (1965) to occur in one-in-four of the over-75s.

Finally, the same authors also reported the presence of slow-wave foci in the temporal regions of 30–40% of elderly people. These are rare in the under-forties, but increase in frequency with old age. Commonly these foci are seen in the anterior temporal regions and mainly on the left, or certainly with a left-sided emphasis. Their significance is unknown, but they do not appear to be related to any abnormal clinical picture.

Genetics

Genetic factors are known to play a major part in the determination of EEG patterns. Lennox *et al.* (1942) showed that in a group of 41 monozygotic normal twins, the EEGs were judged identical in 35 pairs. In another group of 53 normal twins, concordance in the EEGs agreed with concordance as judged by physical traits in 87%. A more recent study by Dummermuth (1968), using spectral analysis of the EEGs of identical twins, showed that there was very little difference between the spectral profiles of identical twins compared to the very different profiles of binovular twins. This genetic component determining the EEG is important, as many abnormalities seen in the EEG of patients with epilepsy are inherited.

The Organic Brain Syndromes

Providing the limitations of the EEG as described earlier are clearly understood, then it will be appreciated that the EEG is of great value in helping in the diagnosis of the organic brain syndrome. Any central nervous system lesion may present with confusion, cognitive symptoms, personality change and/or alteration in behaviour, and these are frequently accompanied by EEG changes.

Focal Lesions

Frontal lobe lesions often present with personality change, disinhibition or antisocial and deteriorating behaviour. Some lesions will present with bed-wetting. Basal frontal meningiomas are considered to commonly present with psychiatric symptoms. Occasionally, catatonic features are seen in frontal lesions (Avery, 1971). Lesions of the parietal lobe presenting with object agnosia, disturbance of body image, spatial disorientation and deficits in attention can mimic a hysterical illness (Critchley, 1964). Focal lesions of the temporal lobe can lead to temporal-lobe epilepsy, with disturbances of mood and behaviour, and psychomotor post-ictal confusional states can be mistakenly diagnosed as hysterical fugue states. Tumours of the corpus callosum frequently present with dementia, and disturbances of behaviour, as encountered in some forms of encephalitis, may resemble a functional illness. These organic states can often be differentiated from the purely functional states by the EEG.

Confusional States

Organic mental states usually show some clouding of consciousness. When clouding of consciousness is present, whether the condition is acute or chronic, there is a global change in brain functioning. In the acute onset, clouding of consciousness and mental confusion are commonly seen, and they are always accompanied by EEG changes. Firstly, the α rhythm slows, and then, as the patient becomes more confused, the record is dominated by θ activity. In the early stages the EEG may show a change before an alteration in mental state becomes clinically obvious. A decrease in α frequency may not go outside the normal range and thus even a fall of 2–3 Hz may not be seen as abnormal, unless a control record has already been taken. As confusion increases, the record becomes dominated by diffuse θ activity, which is responsive to eye opening. On the border of unconsciousness, the activity slows still further, and then, with the approach of unconsciousness, δ activity dominates the record, frequently with a bifrontal predominance. In the deeply unconscious patient, the δ activity is no longer affected to any great extent by external stimuli (Romano and Engel, 1944). These EEG changes are non specific and are related to alteration in consciousness. Thus they can be found to different extents in organic mental states due to head injury with cerebral contusion or subdural haematoma, infection, meningitis, abscess, or encephalitis, drugs, and alcohol intoxication, and in post-ictal states. Various metabolic states can cause the same changes, e.g. liver and kidney encephalopathy, porphyria, endocrine disorders, thiamine deficiency, and respiratory disease leading to anoxia or hypercapnia. Acute intercranial pressure can produce marked EEG changes, while surprisingly, gradual increases frequently do not. Should any of the above conditions improve, these will be accompanied by an improvement or increase in the frequency of the EEG.

Dementia

In the pre-senile dementias, EEG changes are common. The abnormalities, as would be expected from the changes seen in old age (see above), are a decrease in α frequency, together with a generalized increase in θ activity. There is

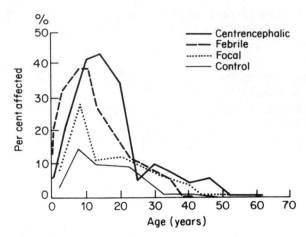

FIG. 10.4   3 Hz spike-and-wave trait. Age distribution of near relatives with the centrencephalic EEG trait for centrencephalic, febrile, focal and control groups. (After Metrakos and Metrakos, 1974, courtesy of Excerpta Medica.)

some correlation between the speed of deterioration and the amount of θ seen in the EEG. In the later stages of the illness, high-voltage δ activity may be seen.

Epilepsy

Inheritance of EEG abnormalities in epilepsy

A comprehensive review is given by Metrakos and Metrakos (1974). Early studies showed that epileptic abnormalities in the EEG could be inherited. The concordance rate for EEG abnormalities in monozygotic twins varied from 40 to 90%, while in dizygotic twins the rate varied between 5 and 20%. In 1961 Metrakos and Metrakos found that of the siblings of epileptic patients, 37% showed abnormal EEGs, compared to 6% for the controls. They suggested the hypothesis that the EEG characterized by 'centrencephalic' EEG abnormalities, i.e. 3 Hz spike and wave, is inherited as an irregular autosomal dominant gene of variable penetrance. They also found that the penetrance of the gene varied with age (see Fig. 10.4).

EEG abnormalities can also be inherited in the focal epilepsies. Rodin and Gonzales (1966) have reported an increased prevalence of EEG abnormalities amongst the near relatives of patients with focal epilepsies.

The frequent occurrence of EEG abnormalities in the seizure-free relatives of patients with epilepsy, up to 45%, emphasizes that the diagnosis of epilepsy must always be a clinical one. Epilepsy should *never* be diagnosed from the EEG alone; *there must always be a clinical history of seizures.*

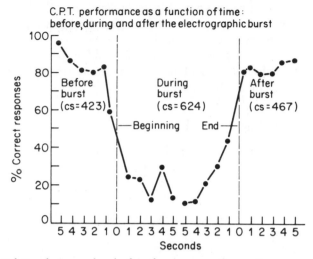

C.P.T. performance as a function of time:
before, during and after the electrographic burst

FIG. 10.5   Relation between level of performance on the continuous performance task (C.P.T.) and onset, development and termination of the electrographic burst. cs refers to the number of correct stimuli. (After Tizzard, B. and Margerison, J.H. (1983). *J. Neurol., Neurosurg. Psychiat.* **26,** 308–313.)

Abnormal epileptic waveforms

Spike-and-wave

The theories explaining the genesis of spike-and-wave activity are at present undergoing considerable modification. A detailed explanation is beyond the scope of this chapter (see Fenwick, 1981, for review), but some knowledge is essential. Recent work on penicillin-induced epilepsy in cats suggests that spike-and-wave activity is generated in the cortex. Spike-and-wave activity is the response of an abnormally excitable cortex to normal thalamic recruiting activity. Thus it would appear that spike-and-wave activity comes from the cortex and is not due to the cortex being passively driven by activity deeper in the brain. If this view is true, then older theories, which suggested a subcortical pacemaker for spike-and-wave activity and from which the theories of 'centrencephalic' epilepsy were derived, should now be viewed with reserve. The names 'primary subcortical epilepsy' and 'centrencephalic epilepsy', which depend heavily on these theories, are best avoided.

Clinical condition. During a spike-and-wave episode, a child may have a petit mal attack. Penry (1973) reviewed the literature relating to the changes in cognition that occur during a spike-and-wave burst. In summary, cognition is usually affected if the burst is longer than 1.0–1.5 s. During the burst, reaction times are lengthened. Complex verbal and mathematical tasks are interfered with more than simple tasks, stimuli that require an immediate response may be missed altogether, and there is a general reduction in the brain's ability to process information. The degree of impairment of cognition will depend on the length of the burst and the degree to which it is generalized over the head. Retrograde amnesia may occur and can persist for 4–15 s. Some studies report a change in cognition 1.0–1.5 s before the burst begins.

Thus the occurrence of spike-and-wave may handicap a child in school by reducing his capacity to learn and attend. Boys are more affected in the classroom by spike-and-wave activity than are girls.

Focal spikes and sharp waves

Focal spikes are not always pathological, as spikes in the EEG can occur normally. Examples are the 14 and 6 positive spikes recorded in adolescents, the spikes found in sleep, and the parietal spikes of childhood. Pathological spikes are generated by pools of damaged epileptic neurones. A damaged epileptic neurone fires in paroxysmal bursts; a group of such neurones, if firing synchronously, leads to the generation of a spike (Lockard and Ward, 1981).

Pathological spikes require careful assessment, as they do not necessarily arise from an area of damaged cortex under the scalp where they appear. Spikes may be conducted across the cortex or projected to the surface from deep structures.

Clinical condition. Little work has been done on the relationship between cognition and the occurrence of cortical spikes and changes in cognition. Some studies report changes, but the picture is not yet clear.

Electroclinical correlation of focal EEG changes and spike-and-wave

This section compares the cognitive changes found in focal and spike-and-wave discharges.

Nuffield (1961) studied 322 children from the Maudsley Epilepsy Unit. Their EEGs were classified according to whether they showed spike-and-wave or focal or mixed EEG activity. The correlation with seizure type was as expected; regular spike-and-wave correlated with petit mal epilepsy, atypical spike-and-wave with grand mal epilepsy, and temporal-lobe foci with psychomotor seizures. The EEG classification was compared with the children's interictal behaviour. It was found that the temporal-lobe group was the most aggressive, but least neurotic, while the true petit mal children were the least aggressive, but most neurotic.

Stores and Hart (1976) looked at a group of epileptic children with general or focal abnormalities and age-matched normal control children. Children with generalized abnormalities did as well at school as their controls. Persistent focal activity was associated with impaired reading accuracy, boys being more affected than girls. A comparison of patients with spike-and-wave or temporal-lobe focal abnormalities on continuous vigilance and memory tasks showed that patients with spike-and-wave activity showed a disorder of attention, whilst the focal group showed a disorder of memory. There is now abundant evidence that dominant temporal-lobe foci are related to a disorder of verbal memory, while non-dominant foci are related to a deficit of visiospatial memory. Taylor (1972) has noted an association between left temporal foci and antisocial behaviour. Lairy (1967) reports the occurrence of parietal sharp-wave foci in epileptic children with psychiatric disorders. Improvement of the children's mental state resulted in the disappearance of the spikes.

Ictal and post-ictal changes

The EEG is helpful in the differential diagnosis of status epilepticus, post-ictal confusional states, automatic behaviour and the epileptic psychoses.

Petit mal status (spike-and-wave status)

This condition presents with a clouding of consciousness and confusion. It lasts from a few minutes to several days and it may wax and wane in intensity, sometimes ceasing abruptly for several minutes. There is a rapid onset and the attack is often terminated by a grand mal seizure. The patient is usually uncoordinated, confused, perseverative and slowed. Not infrequently, the patient appears stuperous and out of contact, remaining motionless and withdrawn.

The EEG record is dominated by spike-and-wave activity, which is very seldom classical. This is an illness of children or young adults only occasionally reported in mature adults (Schwartz and Scott, 1971). In the older age group, it may simulate a retarded depression or a dementing illness.

A similar clinical state is not infrequently seen after one or more grand mal seizures, when the EEG is dominated by diffuse atypical spike-and-wave activity, the continuously abnormal EEG activity indicating status epilepticus.

Automatic states

Automatisms commonly arise during and following the partial phase of temporal-lobe seizures, although Falconer and Taylor (1970) have reported that they may also occur with discharging lesions of the inferior frontal region or the cingulate cortex. A good review of automatisms is given by Fenton (1972).

Automatisms can be divided into three phases: early, middle and late. During the early phase, the subject carries out small stereotyped movements, such as lip smacking or small hand movements. This is accompanied in the EEG by, firstly, a flattening, and then the appearance of low-voltage θ activity at 6–7 Hz, which increases in amplitude and slows in frequency. During the middle phase, the automatisms are more complex, such as handling objects on a table or fumbling with clothes. The EEG shows the abnormal θ discharge, which slows and generalizes to the opposite hemisphere. In the late stage of the automatism, the patient's behaviour becomes more complex and gradually merges into that of everyday life. The EEG shows a post-ictal picture, with bilateral δ waves that frequently have a front-temporal distribution (Gastaut, 1953). However, it is not uncommon for the EEG to show marked differences between patients and not to follow this standard scheme in detail.

Post-ictal states

Following a grand mal seizure, the patient is confused, disoriented and irritable as he regains consciousness. He may lapse into natural sleep or his initially clouded sensorium may slowly clear until full consciousness is regained. The post-ictal state commonly lasts for 5–10 min, with a period of sleep following this. Occasionally, full consciousness may remain impaired for hours, and rarely, for days or weeks. Immediately after the fit, the EEG is dominated by generalized high-voltage activity. Deteriorated cognitive states lasting for several days are frequently seen after grand mal seizures in either elderly patients or patients who have significant associated brain damage. Thus the response to a grand mal seizure will depend on the location of the epileptogenic lesion and on any other associated cerebral pathology.

EEG changes in twilight, psychotic, or post-ictal states

An excellent study by Dongier (1959) analysed 536 psychotic episodes in 516 epileptic patients. Some clouding of consciousness was present in two-thirds of the episodes, delusions in one-third, and hallucinations in 23%. About half the episodes lasted for days and one-third for weeks. The onset was preceded by a seizure in 25% and terminated by a seizure in 10%. There were equal numbers of both cases with generalized epilepsy and psychomotor epilepsy. Confusion was correlated with EEG δ activity or spike-and-wave discharges. Temporal-lobe spikes were mainly associated with delusion, hallucinations and changes of affect.

Bruens (1974) has suggested that all the above-mentioned abnormal states can be divided into the three clinical types: post-ictal twilight states, 'absence' status and psychomotor status. These states frequently have definite EEG correlates.

The post-ictal twilight state is characterized by a disorganized record, dominated by slow-wave activity and very little evidence of epileptic waveforms. 'Absence' status shows 3 Hz spike-and-wave and is readily responsive to intravenous diazepam. Psychomotor status shows a varied picture with or without temporal-lobe spiking, but nearly always an EEG with either excess δ or θ activity. Bruens' classification has yet to be superseded.

Personality Disorders and Psychoneuroses

It was the hope of the early electroencephalographers that the EEG would make a major contribution to our understanding of personality disorders and neuroses. Unfortunately this early expectation has never been fulfilled. No EEG patterns have been found that are diagnostic of psychiatric disorder. Ellingson (1954) (see Ritvo et al., 1970), in a double-blind EEG study of children hospitalized for psychiatric reasons, could find no significant correlation between the EEG findings and the psychiatric diagnosis. The EEG does, however, still have a place in the investigation of psychiatric patients in whom organic cerebral disease is suspected.

Affective Disorders

Patients with affective disorders, like those with other functional illnesses, show a higher prevalence of non-specific abnormalities. When compared with normal control populations, no clear differences are found.

Schizophrenia

Yet again the EEG has shown itself to be disappointing in helping the clinician's understanding of the functional psychoses. The EEG's greatest contribution in this area is the help that it can give, as has already been described, in the separation of the organic mental states from the functional mental states. Some changes in the EEG have been reported in schizophrenia, but these are unlikely to be sufficiently marked to help in the diagnosis of a particular patient. Many of the records tend to be normal, while others show mainly non-specific abnormalities.

Drugs

Most psychotropic drugs cause changes in the EEG. The phenothiazine or tricyclic antidepressants cause an excess of θ and even some δ activity. The tricyclics also reduce α abundance and there is some increase in β activity. Lithium medication can cause an abnormal record, with generalized bursts of δ activity that may even be focal, although the usual picture is similar to that of the tricyclics. Each of these three drugs causes a lowering of the seizure threshold, so that in susceptible individuals paroxysmal bursts of δ activity are seen, while in some individuals frank spike-and-wave or even photo-convulsive potentials may be produced. The opiates, when taken by addicts, produce surprisingly little change in the EEG, the most prominent change being a mild increase in θ activity.

Both the barbiturates and the benzodiazepines produce a low-voltage β rhythm in the fronto-central regions. This is so distinctive that its presence in patients who deny taking the drugs raises the possibility of illicit drug abuse. Diazepam is injected intravenously for status epilepticus and produces a normalization of the EEG record, with a reduction in paroxysmal and epileptic activity. Night sedation by nitrazepam leads to prominent β activity, which is still present the following morning. Alcohol ingestion leads to excess θ in the EEG, and if taken in large quantities, as the level of consciousness starts to fall, so δ activity is seen. Sudden withdrawal in patients who have taken barbiturates, benzodiazepines or alcohol for a few weeks may lead to paroxysmal activity in their EEGs and even to frank fits in susceptible people. Apart from alcohol, all the above drugs may, if given in large doses, produce changes in the EEG that can persist for up to nine weeks after their withdrawal.

ECT

There is a large variation in the change produced in the EEG of patients who are undergoing a course of ECT. Some patients show almost no change after several treatments, while others may show marked changes after only one treatment. In many cases the records will not be entirely back to normal for at least six weeks, while in others it may take three months.

Evoked Potentials

So far this chapter has looked at the ongoing spontaneous EEG rhythms of the cortex. In the 1940s, it was recognized that the brain responds to stimulation of the peripheral sense organs. A flash of light produces a wave over the occipital cortex; a click to the ear over the auditory cortex; and stimulation of the sense organs in the body, an alteration in activity over the sensory motor cortex. These cortical responses are of low amplitude (1–15 μV) and can rarely be seen in the background EEG. Techniques have been evolved to reduce the size of the spontaneous signal so as to improve the resolution of the evoked signals. The most commonly used method is called averaging. As evoked responses are coming to play a more important part in psychiatry, a brief acquaintance with the procedure may be helpful.

Averaging

Averaging is a simple mathematical procedure for allowing any fixed components of the signal to sum, whereas any random components of the signal will tend to diminish to zero. The procedure is very simple. The EEG is recorded, and a signal (flash, click, etc.), is then given to the subject and the EEG is continuously recorded for the next half-second. The procedure is then repeated until a number of stimulus trials have been accumulated. The recordings from each trial are then lined up according to the time the stimulus is given, and the responses summed. The summed responses are then divided by the number of trials, to produce the average. The result is known as the average evoked response or potential. The noise is decreased by the square root of the number of trials. Thus, if the evoked response is 10 μV, and the background EEG is 50 μV, 100 trials will reveal the signal as the background noise will be reduced by a factor of 10 to only 5 μV.

Labelling evoked potentials

The convention usually applied to evoked potentials is to measure the peaks and troughs of the evoked wave and to label them by their polarity and their time from the stimulation of the patient (i.e. the beginning of the evoked response). Conventionally, a negative change is plotted as an upward-going wave, and positive as a downward-going wave. Thus the major downgoing positive peak, 100 ms after the start of the stimulus, is called the P100. Measuring the potential over the scalp, early or short latency potentials, up to 20 ms, reflects activity in the sensory pathways. Late cortical potentials, from 70 to 200 ms, are due to the arrival and elaboration of the sensory volley in the cortex, while late cognitive potentials are those potentials which arise after 200 ms and relate to the stimulus parameters and the behaviour of the subject in the experiment.

Clinical relevance

Early and late potentials are mainly used to help identify pathology in the eyes or ears or conduction deficits in the sensory system. Cognitive potentials have become increasingly used in psychiatry and some familiarity with these is now essential.

P300

The P300 is a positive cognitive potential which occurs around 300 ms after the stimulus. It is usually obtained in an oddball paradigm. The subject listens to a train of high tone beeps which is interleaved with occasional low tone boops. The trials for the beeps and the boops are averaged separately, and the subject is instructed to count the number of boops which occur in the experiment, ignoring the beeps. The ratio is usually 1 : 5. The rare tone evoked response in normal subjects shows a prominent P300 deflection.

Differences in P300 have been found in patients with schizophrenia, behaviour disorders, memory disabilities such as Alzheimer's disease, and attentional disorders. Alteration has also been found as a trait marker in the children of alcoholic parents. In schizophrenia, the amplitude of the P300 is usually decreased and the maximum moves forward from the centre of the head into the frontal region. There are occasionally deficits over the left hemisphere. In the dementias, the P300 shows a significantly delayed latency and reduced amplitude, with, in Alzheimer's disease, again a shift of the main peak and a biparietal reduction in amplitude. There is some early evidence that changes (usually a reduction in amplitude and alteration in the position of the peak) can also be found in patients with affective disorders (for a review, see Maurer, 1989).

Brain mapping or digital EEG

Recent advances in electronics have led to a new generation of EEG machines which convert the EEG into digital information. Because the EEG can now be manipulated by a digital computer, many different forms of presentation are now possible. There is a current vogue for brain mapping. Brain mapping is the plotting out of potential gradients measured from the surface of the scalp onto a map representing the head. These maps are usually coloured, the colours representing bands of equal activity. The maps commonly represent either an instantaneous voltage slice through all EEG channels, or further analysis of the EEG into its frequency bands (usually δ, θ, α and β). Some of these digital EEG machines have large normative data banks. This has resulted in statistical tests being available to test the EEG of individual patients against different diagnostic groups. It is now possible to test each individual patient against a normative data set and also, in some cases, to obtain the probability score that he may belong to some abnormal diagnostic group. These machines are still in their early stages, but they will soon come to dominate all EEG departments, and will have a significant effect on the relevance of EEG to psychiatric practice (John et al., 1977; Duffy et al., 1979, 1981; Maurer, 1989).

Magnetoencephalography

The future of the EEG may lie with the infant science of magnetoencephalography (MEG). MEG is the measurement of the magnetic activity of the brain. When current flows down a conductor, as it does down a nerve fibre, a magnetic field surrounds the conductor. This magnetic field is extremely small, but with modern superconducting technology can be measured at the scalp. Magnetic brain waves unlike the electrical waves of the EEG, have the advantage of passing unattenuated through the brain, CSF, skull and scalp. It is thus possible, by measuring the MEG, to detect deep brain discharges without the necessity of implanting indwelling brain electrodes. MEG technology is still developing, but new multichannel machines bring this goal closer (Sato, 1990).

References

Andersen, P. and Andersson, S.A. (1974). Thalamic origin of cortical rhythmical activity. In: *Handbook of Electroencephalography*, pp. 90–114. Amsterdam: Elsevier.
Avery, T.L. (1971). Seven cases of frontal tumour with psychiatric presentation. *Br. J. Psychiat.* **119**, 19.
Berger, H. (1931). Über das Electroenkephalogramm des Menschen III. *Arch. Psychiatr. Nervenkr.* **94**, 16.
Brazier, H.A.B., Finesinger, J.E., and Cobb, S. (1945). A contrast between the encephalograms of 100 psychoneurotic patients and those of 500 normal adults. *Am. J. Psychiat.* **101**, 443–452.
Bruens, J.H. (1974). Psychosis in epilepsy. In: P. Vinken and G.W. Bruyn (eds) *The Epilepsies*, Handbook of Clinical Neurology, Vol. 15. Amsterdam: North-Holland.
Callaway, E. (1975). *Brain Electrical Potentials and Individual Psychological Differences*. Grune and Stratton.
Cooper, R., Wintter, A.L., Crow, H.J. and Walter, E.G. (1965). Comparison of subcortical and scalp activity using chronically indwelling electrodes in man. *Electroenceph. Clin. Neurophysiol.* **18**, 217–228.
Creutzfeld, O.D., Watanabe, S. and Lasc, H.D. (1966). Relations between EEG phenomena and potentials of single cortical cells. *Electroenceph. Clin. Neurophysiol.* **20**, 19–36.
Critchley, M. (1964). Psychiatric symptoms and parietal disease: differential diagnosis. *Proc. R. Soc. Med.* **57**, 422.
Dawson, G.D. (1947). Cerebral response to electrical stimulation of peripheral nerve in man. *J. Neurol. Neurosurg. Psychiat.* **101**, 134.
Dongier, S. (1959). Statistical study of clinical and electroencephalographic manifestations of 536 psychotic episodes occurring in 516 epileptics between clinical seizures. *Epilepsia* **1**, 117–142.

Duffy, F.H., Birchfiel, J.L. and Lombroso, C.T. (1979). Brain electrical activity mapping (BEAM): a method for extending the clinical utility of EEG and evoked potential data. *Ann. Neurol.* **51**, 455–462.

Duffy, F.H., Bartels, P.H. and Birchfiel, J.L. (1981). Significance probability mapping: an aid in the topographical analysis of brain electrical activity. *Electroenceph. Clin. Neurophysiol.* **51**, 455–462.

Dummermuth, G. (1968). Variance spectra of electroencephalograms in twins—a contribution to the problem of quantification of EEG background activity in childhood. In: P. Kellaway and I. Peterssen (eds) *Clinical Encephalography of Children*, pp. 119–154. New York: Grune & Stratton.

Eeg-Olofsson, O. (1970). The development of the electroencephalogram in normal children and adolescents from the age of 1 through 21 years. *Acta Paediat. Scand. (Suppl.)*, 208.

Falconer, M. and Taylor, D.C. (1970). In: M.H. Price (ed.) *Modern Trends in Psychological Medicine*. London: Butterworth.

Fenton, G.W. (1972). Epilepsy and automatism. *Br. J. Hosp. Med.* **7**, 57–64.

Fenwick, P.B.C. (1981). EEG Studies. In: E.H. Reynolds and M.R. Trimble (eds) *Epilepsy and Psychiatry*, pp. 242–263. Edinburgh: Churchill Livingstone.

Gastaut, H. (1953). So-called 'psychomotor' and 'temporal' epilepsy: a critical study. *Epilepsia* **21**, 59–96.

Hill, D. and Watterson, D. (1942). Electroencephalographic studies of psychopathic personalities. *J. Neurol. Psychiat.* **5**, 47.

Hill, D. and Parr, G. (1963). *Electroencephalography. A Symposium on its Various Aspects*. London: Macdonald.

John, E.R., Carmel, B.Z., Cornigh, W.C. *et al.* (1977). Neurometrics. *Science* **1961**, 1393–1410.

Lairy, G.C. (1967). L'EEG comme moyen d'investigation des modalités individuelles d'adaptation aux situations de stress. In: Recent Advances in Clinical Neurophysiology. *Electroenceph. Clin. Neurophysiol. (Suppl.)* **25**, 282–298.

Lennox, W.G., Gibbs, F.A. and Gibbs, E.L. (1942). Twins, brain waves and epilepsy. *Arch. Neurol. Psychiat. (Chicago)* **47**, 702.

Lockard, J.S. and Ward, A.A. (1981). *Epilepsy: A Window to Brain Mechanism*. New York: Raven Press.

Maurer, K. (1989). *Topographic Brain Mapping of EEG and Evoked Potentials*. Berlin: Springer-Verlag.

Metrakos, K. and Metrakos, J.D. (1974). The genetics of epilepsy. In: P.J. Vinken and G.W. Bruyn (eds) *The Epilepsies*, Handbook of Clinical Neurology, Vol. 15. Amsterdam: Excerpta Medica.

Nuffield, E.J. (1961). Neurophysiology and behaviour disorders in epileptic children. *J. Ment. Sci.* **107**, 438–458.

Obrist, W.D. and Busse, E.W. (1965). In: W.P. Wilson (ed.) *Applications of Encephalography in Psychiatry*. Durham, North Carolina: Duke University Press.

Penry, J.K. (1973). In: M.A.B. Brazier (ed.) *Epilepsy: Its Phenomena in Man*, p. 172. New York: Academic Press.

Ritvo, E.R., Ornitz, E.M., Walter, R.D. and Hanley, J. (1970). Correlation of psychiatric diagnoses and EEG findings—a double-blind study of 184 hospitalized children. *Am. J. Psychiat.* **126**, 988–996.

Rodin, E. and Gonzales, S. (1966). Hereditary components on epileptic patients. Electroencephalogram family studies. *J. Am. Med. Ass.* **198**, 221–225.

Romano, J. and Engel, G.L. (1944). Delirium: I. EEG data. *Arch. Neurol. Psychiat. (Chicago)* **51**, 356.

Sannit, T. (1963). The ten–twenty system: footnotes to measuring technique. *Am. J. Electroenceph. Technol.* **3**, 23.

Sato, S. (ed.) (1990). *Recent Advances in Neurology: Magnetic Measurement.* New York: Raven Press.

Schwartz, M.S. and Scott, D.F. (1971). Isolated petit mal status presenting de novo in middle age. *Lancet* **ii**, 1399–1401.

Stores, G. and Hart, J.A. (1976). Proceedings: reading skills of children with generalized and focal epilepsy attending ordinary school. *Electroenceph. Clin. Neurophysiol.* **39**, 429–430.

Taylor, D.C. (1972). Mental state and temporal lobe epilepsy. A correlative account of 100 patients treated surgically. *Epilepsia* **13**, 727–765.

Tecce, J.J. (1972). Contingent negative variation and psychological processes in man. *Psychol. Bull.* **77**, 73–108.

Williams, D. (1941). The significance of an abnormal electroencephalogram. *J. Neurol. Psychiat.* **4**, 257–268.

Some Issues In Clinical Neurology

M.J. Gawel

A Revision of Basic Neurology

Examination

The neurological examination is well described in the standard textbooks. Most of the problems encountered in neurological diagnosis are based on both faulty history taking and faulty examination. Different observers can easily cause an apparent change in neurological signs and thus create confusion in an essentially straightforward diagnosis. With this in mind, in these introductory paragraphs I will try to help the examiner evoke the appropriate signs with intelligence and avoid being misled. Traditionally, examination of the nervous system is described as a mindless ritual, but in fact it should not be so. If the examiner keeps in mind a general outline of neuroanatomy and neurophysiology, then the neurological examination will follow the clues elicited at various stages. In clinical neurology there are a limited number of combinations of signs and symptoms which should alert the investigator to the correct diagnosis.

Cranial nerves

The first cranial nerve. The first cranial nerve is almost never tested. In a psychiatric context it is of the utmost importance, since one of the treatable causes of dementia is a subfrontal meningioma that can cause anosmia. Testing ought to be carried out bilaterally and with different aspects of smell. If the patient is demented and uncooperative, a strong odour, such as asafoetida, may cause a reaction.

The second nerve. Visual acuity ought always to be tested as a unilateral, uncorrectable loss may suggest optic nerve pathology in the context of other neurological disease. The presence of a field defect is important, but the presence of visual inattention—suggestive of a parietal lesion, most often in the non-dominant hemisphere—is often missed. If compressive pathology in the region of the pituitary is suspected and a bitemporal field defect is not elicited, then it is worth checking colour vision since one of the first signs of this condition is a bitemporal loss of red appreciation. Ophthalmoscopic examination is very important, especially in a situation where raised intracranial pressure is suspected. One of the first

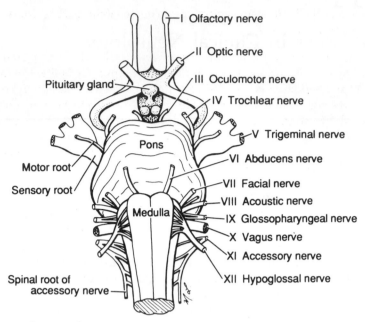

FIG. 11.1   The cranial nerves.

signs of papilloedema is a loss of pulsation of the veins. As the pressure increases there, a visible hyperaemia of the disc or blurring of the margins, primarily evident on the nasal, superior and inferior borders follows. It is important to distinguish papilloedema from pseudo-papilloedema, which is seen in some hypermetropic eyes. Here there is blurring of the disc margins. The surface of the disc is not raised. There is no dilatation of the veins, no hyperaemia and on field testing there is no enlargement of the blind spot as there is in true papilloedema.

The third, fourth and sixth nerves. Eye movements demonstrate the intactness or otherwise of not only the ocular motor nerves and muscles, but also the connections within the brain stem. Bilateral internuclear ophthalmoplegia, when one eye will abduct where the other fails to adduct on conjugate lateral gaze, is suggestive of multiple sclerosis. This is often associated with nystagmus, which is more marked in the abducting eye. Although there are no pathognomonic signs in neurology, such a finding should raise a strong suspicion of multiple sclerosis. Failure of upward conjugate gaze can be due to lesions in the floor of the fourth ventricle or in the posterior part of the third, while the progressive failure of gaze in all directions can be part of the syndrome of progressive supranuclear ophthalmoplegia and is associated with a Parkinsonian syndrome and dementia.

Paralysis of conjugate lateral gaze can be due to a frontal lesion, in which case the gaze cannot be directed away from the lesion and hence is away from the paralysed side. Voluntary components are usually affected in such a case. When the lesion is in the brain stem centre for conjugate lateral gaze, there is a paresis of gaze towards the lesion.

The fifth cranial nerve. Examination of the sensory portion of the fifth cranial nerve can be of help in diagnosing lesion in the cerebellopontine angle. Often in such a case, corneal sensation is lost first and if one encounters facial numbness with sparing of the corneal sensation, it is unlikely that it is due to a compressive lesion intracranially. Headache pain is mediated by the fifth cranial nerve, usually the ophthalmic division. Trigeminal neuralgia, which is a lancinating, stabbing pain along one or more of the divisions of the fifth cranial nerve is not associated with loss of sensation. Trigeminal neuralgia occurring in a young person may be an initial presentation of multiple sclerosis.

The eighth cranial nerve. Probably the commonest cause of minor hearing impairment and dizziness is wax in the ears. It is therefore important to examine the ears with an auroscope before any test of hearing is performed. Impairment of hearing can be found in a number of nervous system disorders, including lesions of the cerebellopontine angle and multiple sclerosis. Nervous system disorders are of course also found in the elderly, where lesions are generally in the end organ. Vertigo is the most characteristic symptom of vestibular disease. It is, however, important to realize that it may be a symptom of general cerebral disease and vertiginous attacks may occur with temporal lobe epilepsy. The most specific involvement of the eighth cranial nerve probably occurs in a cerebellopontine angle neoplasm where it is often associated with other cranial nerve lesions such as seventh and fifth.

The seventh cranial nerve. It is important to distinguish a minimal facial paralysis on one side from a facial contracture on the opposite side and from developmental asymmetry. It is also necessary to remember that muscular weakness can cause facial palsy, as can be found in patients with myopathies. Bilateral lower motor neurone facial palsies, either simultaneous or succeeding each other, can be caused by inflammatory processes, polyneuritis, sarcoidosis or syphilis. The lower motor neurone lesions are distinguished from upper motor neurone lesions by the fact that there is no sparing of the fibres to the forehead.

The ninth cranial nerve. This is rarely involved in an isolated fashion. Severe and lancinating pain originating in the lateral portion of the pharyngeal pouch can occur in glossopharyngeal neuralgias, but palatal reflexes are an important part of the examination of the glossopharyngeal nerve. The pharyngeal or gag reflex is produced by applying a stimulus to the posterior wall, tonsillar region, faucal pillars or even the base of the tongue. The palatal or uvular reflexes can be tested by stimulating the lateral and inferior surface of the uvula or soft palate with a tongue blade or cotton applicator. The motor portion of the reflex arch is carried via the vagus and possibly the glossopharyngeal nerve, whereas the sensory component is via the glossopharyngeal and the vagus nerve. The trigeminal nerve also supplies a part of the soft palate and for this reason the palatal reflex may occasionally be retained in ninth nerve lesions.

The tenth cranial nerve. The vagus nerve is the longest and most widely distributed of the cranial nerves and has parasympathetic components as well as sensory branches. Section of both vagal nerves is incompatible with life. However, unilateral lesions will cause paralysis of the vocal cords and failure of diaphragmatic function on one side. The autonomic functions of the vagus control the heart rate, respiratory rate and these may be tested to some extent by pressure on the eyeball or painful stimulation of the skin on the side of the neck. This will cause the heart to accelerate and is called the oculocardiac reflex.

The eleventh cranial nerve. The spinal accessory, or eleventh cranial nerve, is composed of two parts. The cranial part is smaller and is accessory to the vagus. The major part is the spinal portion which supplies the sternomastoid and trapezius muscles. Generally, the first part cannot be distinguished from the vagus and glossopharyngeal nerves with which it is associated. The spinal part may be involved in such conditions as progressive bulbar palsy. An injury in the posterior cervical triangle will affect only the supply of the trapezius.

The twelfth cranial nerve. The hypoglossal, or twelfth cranial nerve, is the motor supply of the tongue. The real distribution centres are the muscular or lingual branches. They supply the muscles of the tongue and also the genioglossus, myoglossus, hypoglossus and chondroglossus muscles. The cerebral centre for the regulation of tongue movement is the lower portion of the precentral gyrus and within the sylvian fissure. Examination of the tongue will differentiate between upper and lower motor lesions of this type. If the tongue is flaccid and wasted, the lesion is a lower motor neurone type. If the tongue is stiff and paretic, the lesion is an upper motor neurone type. A combination of the two with fasciculations in the tongue is found in amyotrophic lateral sclerosis. The twelfth cranial nerve may be affected in a number of situations: basal skull fractures, subarachnoid or intracranial haemorrhage, meningitis of various types, syphilis, tuberculosis, periostitis, extramedullary neoplasms or abscesses, basilar impression, compression of the medulla into the foramen magnum by increased intracranial pressure and dislocation of the upper cervical vertebrae which may affect the nerve before it leaves the skull.

Trauma of various types can affect it within and at its exit from the hypoglossal canal within the neck. The tongue may also be involved in a variety of dystonic conditions including aphthongia, which is the name given to a form of spasm occurring in speakers and is similar in nature to writer's cramp.

The bulbar musculature

When a patient presents with dysarthria or dysphagia, the following assessments need to be made. Is the lesion a supranuclear or in the lower motor neurone? Is the problem due to incoordination caused by a cerebellar problem? Is it due to muscular weakness? If so, is there fatiguability as in myasthenia gravis? With a supranuclear lesion, the tongue is stiff and the palate arched, being spastic. There is usually a brisk jaw jerk indicating pathology higher up. With a lower motor neurone lesion, the palate is flaccid and the tongue often wasted. Bilateral upper motor neurone lesions involving the bulbar musculature are termed pseudobulbar palsy and may be associated with emotional lability, with the patient altering between laughter and crying for seemingly trivial reasons.

The motor and sensory systems

There is no substitute for formal assessment of strength and sensation in all modalities. There are, however, supplementary procedures which yield a lot of information. One is to have the patient shut his eyes and hold his hands in front of him, fingers together. The palm can be either facing up or facing down. This gives information about pyramidal function, parietal function and cerebellar function, provided the peripheral sensory and motor systems are intact. A minimal pyramidal loss may show itself by spreading of the fingers, especially movement of the little finger away from the rest of the hand. There may be a drift of the whole hand with an abnormal posture, or in more severe cases, drift of the whole arm. Mainly parietal lesions cause the affected arm to drift up and lose position. In cerebellar lesions, the posture of the hand and arm may be abnormal and continually changing. Further information about minimal differences can be gained by asking the patient, with his eyes shut, to bring both arms up to the horizontal as quickly as he can and look for any lag in the movements. Minor differences in motor function in the legs can be brought out by doing dynamic testing causing the patient to walk on his toes or on his heels.

In the absence of any overt abnormalities in the sensory system on formal testing, it is important to test for sensory inattention. This must be done carefully by making sure that the patient is aware of the instructions that are being given. It is sometimes useful to vary the pressure by stimulating fingers to pick up gradations of inattention. There may be inattention occurring in temporal sequence of stimulation as well. Further dynamic testing such as hopping around an object on one foot can bring out abnormalities in cerebellar function not immediately apparent.

Higher mental functions

While it is rare for patients with organic brain disease to be diagnosed as suffering from a mental illness, this occasionally does happen. Since the first edition of this book was written, there have been many changes in our understanding of the nature of mental disorder and an increasing realization that many so-called mental disorders are based on sound neuroanatomical or neurophysiological principles.

This is not the place for an exhaustive description of psychological examination, but the following pointers will aid in diagnosis and treatment.

Dementia

This is defined as a global loss of intellectual function, but the loss may not be even. Thus a demented patient may only present with one aspect of intellectual

TABLE 11.1   Features that distinguish cortical and subcortical dementias. Reproduced from Cummings, J. (1984). *Arch. Neurol.* **41**, 874.

Characteristic	Subcortical	Cortical
Mental status		
Language	No aphasia	Aphasia
Memory	Forgetful (difficulty retrieving learned material)	Amnesia (difficulty learning new material)
Cognition	Impaired (poor problem-solving produced by slowness, forgetfulness, and impaired strategy and planning)	Severely disturbed (based on agnosia, aphasia, acalculia and amnesia)
Slow processing time	Response time relatively normal	
Personality	Apathetic	Unconcerned or euphoric
Mood	Affective disorder common (depression or mania)	Normal
Motor system		
Speech	Dysarthric	Normal[a]
Posture	Abnormal	Normal, upright[a]
Gait	Abnormal	Normal[a]
Motor speed	Slow	Normal[a]
Movement disorder	Common (chorea, tremor, rigidity, ataxia)	Absent
Anatomy		
Cortex	Largely spared	Involved
Basal ganglia, thalamus, mesencephalon	Involved	Largely spared
Metabolism		
Fluorodeoxyglucose scan	Subcortical hypometabolism (cortex largely normal)	Cortical hypometabolism (subcortical metabolism less involved)
Neurotransmitters preferentially involved	Huntington's disease: γ-aminobutyric acid Parkinson's disease: dopamine	Alzheimer's disease: acetylcholine

[a]Motor system involvement occurs late in the course of Alzheimer's disease and Pick's disease.

failure such as memory loss. There is an increasing tendency to divide dementias into two groups, cortical and subcortical. The general characteristics of the two groups are shown in Table 11.1. Generally the ability to perform a complex activity is lost and the one question 'Do you cook your own food?', can help highlight an insidious dementia. There are several standardized questionnaires for the assessment of dementia, such as the mini-mental state.

In elderly people, apart from any neurological lesion, the two commonest causes of dementia are infections and drugs. They may also exacerbate a pre-existing dementia. Treating the first and stopping the second can sometimes cause a dramatic improvement. Drugs commonly implicated as causing dementia in the elderly are those with an anticholinergic action such as antidiarrhoeal preparations and psychoactive drugs in general. However, almost any drug can cause problems.

Three causes of progressive dementia that are potentially reversible are subdural haematoma, a meningioma—either subfrontal or in the sphenoidal ridge—and normal pressure hydrocephalus.

A subdural haematoma may be extremely chronic and not show the classical fluctuations in mental state, nor need there be any neurological signs. There need not be a clear history of head injury either, since in old people even a slight knock can cause subdural bleeding.

Subfrontal or sphenoidal wing meningiomas can also present with dementia with little in the way of focal signs.

Normal pressure hydrocephalus is said to present with a triad of dementia, incontinence and apraxia of gait. The patient is unable to put together the action of walking, although appearing to have normal power, coordination and sensation on formal testing. There appears to be an abnormality in cerebrospinal fluid (CSF) dynamics with increased pressure, especially at night, causing progressive dilatation of the ventricles. This condition can sometimes be idiopathic and occasionally may follow trauma. When the condition is post-traumatic, or follows a bleed, the results of shunting operations are more pronounced. When a CAT scan shows largish ventricles, disproportionately large compared to the size of the sulci, a CSF flow study should be performed to examine the cerebrospinal fluid flow. If it shows little resorption at 24 h from the lateral ventricles, then a shunt ought to be considered. A single photon emission computerized tomography (SPECT) scan may show a diminished perfusion periventricularly. Complications of the shunting operation depend upon the general health of the patient, but also include an increased risk of post-operative subdural haematoma.

There have been great strides in making the diagnosis of other forms of dementia. Alzheimer's disease, characterized by progressive neurofibrillary tangles and senile plaques, described in detail in Chapter 8, is probably the commonest cause of dementia. It can be mimicked clinically by Pick's disease and to some extent the dementia of Parkinson's disease, although the latter is much more of a subcortical dementia, whereas Alzheimer's is cortical. Recently, SPECT scanning has shown that there are characteristic changes in these conditions. In Alzheimer's, the SPECT shows bitemporal perfusion defects, in Pick's disease frontal perfusion defects are seen, while in Parkinson's disease both basal ganglion and frontal perfusion defects are seen. Of course, positron emission tomography (PET) scanning shows particular abnormalities in metabolism of oxygen and cerebral blood flow in these conditions but this form of scanning is still a research tool and not generally available to most clinicians. Some forms of depression mimicking dementia can also show changes on SPECT scanning, reversible by administration of antidepressants. Multi-infarct dementia, which by history should be characterized by progressive step-wise deterioration, will also show a particular pattern on SPECT scan with multiple perfusion defects in various areas.

At present, there is no medical treatment for these dementias, but it is important to differentiate pseudodementia due to depression from true dementia. It is also important to realize that demented patients may be made a lot worse by a variety of extraneous factors such as drugs.

Hemisphere-specific problems

Dominant hemisphere lesions often result in dysphasia. This is well described in Chapter (8). Other problems related to dominant hemisphere lesions are problems with memory, verbal memory, with calculation, left/right orientation and writing.

Non-dominant hemisphere problems

The ability to orientate oneself in space is a property of the non-dominant hemisphere. Other properties are orientation in time and the ability to form a complete body image. For this reason, patients with right hemispheric lesions have much greater problems with rehabilitation following a stroke, even though they are ostensibly less affected, the speech functions being unaffected. They may be totally unaware of the position of their body in space. Irritative foci in the right hemisphere may cause curious syndromes of splitting or feeling that half of one's body is not there. The denial of disability can be another crippling feature of non-dominant hemisphere lesions.

On a higher level, the ability to copy diagrams or to follow a map may be lost. The former can be tested readily with a pencil and paper. The patient can be asked to draw a clock face and put in the numbers and other drawing tasks can be set, e.g. drawing a bicycle. The ability to understand the prosody of speech is also a non-dominant hemisphere property. Thus, patients with lesions in this area will hear the words but be unable to pick up the emotional content which is embedded in the rhythm. This can be extremely disturbing socially, the patient making many interpersonal communication errors, as much of our conversation carries non-verbal information.

Investigations

About 90% of diagnoses in neurological practice can be made on the history alone. The investigations serve to confirm the initial impression.

Skull X-ray

A skull X-ray can be very useful if a fracture is suspected, and indeed many reports just read 'no fracture' with no further comment. However, there is information which can be gained from a skull X-ray which may alert the examiner to further problems.

The vault. Paget's disease can be seen as areas of sclerosis and thickening, or as osteoporosis circumscripta. Lucent secondary deposits, myeloma, etc. can also be seen. Thickening of the skull vault can be due to blood conditions such as thalassaemia. In childhood, expansion of the sutures and the appearance known as copper beating can be due to raised intracranial pressure. Vascular markings may be enlarged due to, for instance, a meningioma and there may be sclerosis over the same area for the same reason. Enlargement of one foramen spinosum on the basal view may also be suggestive of meningioma. Erosion of the sella can be due to pituitary tumour and thinning of the clinoid process can be due to either age or raised intracranial pressure.

The shape of the skull is also important and a shallow posterior fossa with high odontoid process may be found in the condition known as basilar impression or platybasia. This may present with posterior fossa abnormalities·and sometimes hydrocephalus, and be associated with an Arnold Chiari malformation (which results in herniation of the cerebellar tonsils).

Intracranial inclusions. Calcifications within the skull can be due to a calcified tumour such as an oligodendroglioma, a meningioma, a tuberculoma, the wall of an abscess, cysts caused by cysticercosis, *Toxoplasma gondii*, syphilitic gummata, arteriovenous malformations or giant aneurysms.

CAT scan

This rapidly became the investigation in cerebral and spinal cord pathology (in conjunction with myelography). Such problems as may arise are:

1. The posterior fossa is not well visualized.
2. Some lesions may be isodense, e.g. a recent infarct, an isodense subdural or some infiltrating tumours. Contrast enhancement is useful in most cases but not all.
3. The CAT scan gives an anatomical assessment. Patients with gross hemiparesis may have a normal scan. This is because the cells involved have not infarcted but have shut down, being in a state of critical perfusion, as can be demonstrated using other techniques.

The CAT scan is still the most useful and generally available tool in the investigation of a neurological problem. It is, however, necessary to examine the patient first to decide which area needs scanning. Greater detail can be obtained by higher resolution scanning using thinner slices and introduction of contrast around spinal cord or around acoustic lesions. However, the CAT scan has already become obsolete and the investigation of choice for all intracranial and spinal pathology is a magnetic resonance, or MRI. Lack of availability of the latter, however, means the CAT scan will be the most generally used technique for some time to come.

Magnetic resonance imaging

Magnetic resonance imaging has revolutionized neurological investigation. It is able to provide images of anatomical textbook quality of most of the neuraxis.

Stronger magnets have been introduced and the use of orthomagnetic contrast agents such as gadolinium enable even greater detail to be obtained. The combination of CAT scanning, magnetic resonance and surface laser topography promises to give the ultimate in central nervous system imaging. Nevertheless, this is still in the future.

A limitation of magnetic resonance imaging is that the patient must be free of any metal, so that patients who have had previous surgery or, as in one recent case we had, who have shrapnel in them, etc., cannot be imaged. Magnetic resonance imaging is the investigation of choice in multiple sclerosis where bright periventricular lesions are seen on T2 weighted images, and in spinal cord tumours as well as posterior fossa tumours.

PET scan

This involves the tomographic imaging of positron emissions from short half-life isotopes of oxygen-15. These isotopes need to be produced just before the investigation, and thus a cyclotron is necessary. Using the PET scanner, cerebral blood flow and regional metabolism can be assessed. This procedure is still not being used clinically and probably never will be as the development of SPECT scanning progresses.

SPECT scan

The SPECT scan (or ceretic brain scan) is a development of technetium brain scanning. The difference is that once the HMPAO technetium is in the circulation, it fixes in the brain with very little wash-out for significant periods of time. This enables a snapshot of the cerebral perfusion in different areas to be obtained. The resolution of the SPECT scan is down to 3 mm, which is beginning to be comparable to the 1 mm of a PET scan. Thus far, it is too early to describe all the possible clinical applications, since new ones are appearing all the time. Nevertheless, it appears to be very sensitive and relatively specific in the investigation of dementia. Thus, as previously mentioned, Alzheimer's disease shows a bitemporal perfusion defect pattern, Parkinson's disease shows involvement in basal ganglia and frontal lobes, multiple infarct dementia shows multiple areas of diminished perfusion and Pick's disease shows basically frontal abnormalities—while the CAT scan and MRI may be completely normal or show some slight atrophy in all these conditions.

Patients with focal epilepsy may show diminished perfusion in the focus between attacks. Patients with transient cerebral ischaemia with normal CT scans may show perfusion defects in the appropriate clinical areas for some time after the original insult. Recently patients have been described with pseudodementia due to depression, who show specific abnormalities in the basal ganglia.

Doppler ultrasound and transcranial doppler

The evaluation of the extracranial carotid circulation and the larger vessels of the intracranial circulation can be carried out by the use of Doppler ultrasonography.

Two methods are available, continuous wave and pulsed Doppler. The pulsed Doppler is able to give images of the arteries, the vessel walls and show up any evidence of atherosclerotic plaques within the vessel walls, while continuous wave Doppler is very useful in determining Doppler frequency shifts and thus measuring the velocity of the blood corpuscles within the circulation. Integrating the two, it is possible to determine the presence of hemodynamically significant lesions and associate them with stenotic areas caused by sclerotic plaques of different morphology.

A further refinement, using a lower frequency probe, allows the measurement of blood flow velocities within the brain. Further refinements of this technique using provocative techniques such as the inhalation of CO_2 allowed the measure of reactivity of these vessels to be performed. Such studies may be helpful in the elucidation of the haemodynamics in conditions such as migraine, vertebral basilar insufficiency and in alterations in cerebral perfusion in the elderly, where one of the reasons for catastrophic falls may be a drop in cerebral perfusion.

Cerebral angiography

This investigation is very invasive and still carries a significant risk of morbidity. It does, however, provide valuable information. It is now generally used in the assessment of the extra- and intracranial circulation in a patient in whom an aneurysm, arteriovenous malformation or stenotic lesions are suspected.

A development of cerebral angiography called intra-arterial digital subtraction angiography, has superseded standard angiography in the assessment of cerebral vascular disease, as the main area of interest is the extracranial circulation. This enables a much lower volume of contrast to be injected, thus lessening a potential hazard. However, the imaging for lesion such as aneurysms, still requires the use of standard cerebral angiography. Intravenous digital subtraction angiography had a brief vogue but unfortunately the images obtained were not of appropriate quality to allow for assessment for surgical intervention.

It is now possible to obliterate small arteriovenous malformations by the use of intra-arterial embolization during angiography.

Electroencephalogram

Clinically, the value of the EEG is limited to certain fields. It is no longer used for demonstrating space-occupying or vascular lesions. In a diagnosis of epilepsy it can identify specific patterns of discharge, such as spike-and-wave. However, in many cases of clinically proven epilepsy, the inter-ictal EEG may be completely normal and special placements may be necessary to pick up discharges arising from the temporal lobes (sphenoidal leads). Organic brain disease due to toxic and metabolic abnormalities may cause generalized EEG abnormalities, but these are largely non-specific.

Ambulatory monitoring of EEG and ECG and video-controlled telemetry are two methods of assessing the reason for patients' ictal episodes. Hopefully the episode of interest will be experienced while the patient has the monitor on and the search can be made for EEG correlation.

EEG spectral analysis and analysis of visual evoked potentials is a technique which has been developed recently in an effort to quantify the cerebral electrical activity. Many systems for performing this so-called brain electrical activity mapping have been devised, but much work remains to be done in order to determine the usefulness of these techniques despite the claims made for them by their inventors.

Evoked potentials

Stimulation of any sensory modality produces a specific electrical response in the appropriate part of the cortex. Summation of these responses can be achieved using an averager, time-locked to the stimulation that samples pre-set sweeps of the EEG. The resulting trace is called an evoked potential. Visual evoked responses, auditory responses and sensory evoked responses are measured for clinical purposes. The most common use for evoked responses is the diagnosis of multiple sclerosis. If, for instance, there has been demyelination in one optic nerve, even if subclinical, then there will be a delay of the response in that eye. If this result is found in a paraplegic patient, there is evidence for at least two lesions, raising the possibility of multiple sclerosis. Similar principles apply to the other two modalities.

Another important use is the detection of small acoustic neuromas using auditory evoked potentials, the assessment of auditory nerve function during acoustic nerve surgery, and the assessment of spinal cord integrity during spinal cord surgery using somatosensory evoked potentials. The longer latencies of the evoked potentials have been used in a number of psychiatric situations and thus, abnormality in the P300 is said to be abnormal in dementia, both in latency and amplitude.

Recent Advances in Neurological Diseases

Cerebral vascular disease

The term stroke means a focal neurological deficit of vascular cause lasting more than 24 h. This can either mean a cerebral infarction or cerebral haemorrhage. About 80% of strokes are cerebral infarcts. Cerebral haemorrhage may be intracerebral or subarachnoid. A subarachnoid haemorrhage is generally a dramatic event with sudden onset of head pain. Usually, this is followed by signs of meningism and varying degrees of neurological disability. The treatment is usually neurosurgical. However, most strokes are caused by cerebral infarction and are the result of arterial thrombus secondary to embolism from either another artery or from the heart. Cerebral haemorrhage is often associated with hypertension, bleeding tendencies or in the elderly spontaneous on the basis of a small vessel disease called amyloid angiopathy. Clinically it is impossible to distinguish between a haemorrhage or cerebral infarct, and thus a CAT scan at that stage is necessary.

Transient neurological symptoms of the focal sort, e.g. transient monocular blindness or transient weakness in the limb, due to vascular causes and lasting less than 24 h, are called transient ischaemic attacks (TIAs). The onset of these symptoms carries a significant risk, approximately 7% per year, of completed stroke, and also are a risk factor for myocardial infarction. Investigation of patients with TIAs is directed at discerning the source of emboli. Emboli can arise in the left atrium, the mitral valve, the ventricular wall, the arch of the aorta, and the extra- and intracranial carotids. After clinical examination an X-ray, electrocardiography, and 24-h portable cardiac monitoring, and echocardiography are performed. The carotid circulation can be assessed non-invasively by using Doppler imaging techniques and transcranial Doppler. Generally, if the Doppler shows a stenosis of more than 50%, angiography and consideration of surgery may be considered. Currently there is some doubt as to the value of surgery, or at least as to the advantage of having surgery as opposed to medical treatment, and a multi-centre study is under way. This is called NASCET (North American Carotid Endarterectomy Study), where patients are being randomized to either surgical or medical treatment if they are candidates for surgical treatment according to previous criteria. In the United Kingdom endarterectomy is much less common and indeed the galloping rate of increase of carotid endarterectomy in the United States, compared to the United Kingdom, was one of the factors which led to the initiation of this study and its funding by the National Institutes of Health.

Other operative procedures, such as extracranial–intracranial bypass, have also gone by the way since the first edition of this book was published. The EC–IC bypass study demonstrated quite conclusively that patients who had the procedure did worse than those that did not.

Other predisposing factors, such as high platelet activity and hyperlipidaemia, may need to be considered. High viscosity is associated not only with strokes but with impaired mental function in general and venesection can be of value in such patients. Increased lipids are seen to be a risk factor. In some patients, especially young patients who have cerebral infarction, an anticardiolipin antibody, or lupus anticoagulant, may be demonstrated. These patients will have a high activated partial thromboplastin time (APTT). Treatment of these patients is still uncertain, but probably antiplatelet drugs are the treatment of choice. Antiplatelet agents, such as ASA, can certainly abolish transient ischaemic attacks and meta-analysis of their effect demonstrates that they can reduce the incidence of stroke in patients with TIA by about 25%. Women do not appear to benefit as much as men. More recently, a new antiplatelet agent has been shown to be very effective in both women and men, ticlopidine. Its mode of action is uncertain, but it is due to be released in the near future. Anticoagulants such as Coumadin are useful when the emboli come from the heart. Of course, deciding whether the patient has cardiogenic or artery-to-artery emboli can be difficult.

No acute medical treatment has been shown to be effective in reducing the size of the stroke, although calcium blockers such as nimodipine and nicardipine are currently being evaluated. The most valuable procedure is to maintain good cardiorespiratory function in order to optimize cerebral perfusion. Control of hypertension needs to be circumspect, keeping a diastolic of over 110 mm of mercury. Steroids in the acute phase have not been shown to be of any value. As soon as the patient is over the acute phase, early mobilization and physiotherapy produce the best long-term results.

Often the attitudes of the doctors and nurses to the stroke victim need to be retrained. A multi-disciplinary approach is important and the patient's relatives need to be educated as to the effects of the lesion on the patient's personality and abilities. Depression may very frequently accompany a stroke, especially a non-dominant hemispheric stroke, and will respond to standard antidepressant therapy.

Once the patient is mobile and able to go home, follow-up is necessary to prevent further stroke. Risk factors need to be modified.

Multiple sclerosis

Probably the commonest organic disorder with which young patients present in the neurology clinic is multiple sclerosis. The prevalence of multiple sclerosis is 50 to 75 per 100 000 in the Northern Hemisphere. It is most frequently encountered in a temperate climate. It would appear that it is caused by an infectious agent which is picked up before the age of 14. Thus, if somebody is born in the tropics and migrates to a temperate climate after the age of 14, their risk of multiple sclerosis is much less than if they had been born there. Similarly, people born in temperate climates, migrating to the tropics, have an equal risk of developing multiple sclerosis as they would have had in their area of origin.

The pathological lesion is the plaque, an area of focal inflammation leading to total or partial demyelination in the region affected. The initial attack is accompanied by a lot of inflammation which then settles with resolution of symptoms. The symptoms may resolve completely or the patient may be left with some disability. Partially demyelinated neurones are very temperature sensitive and any increase in temperature will cause conduction bloc with consequent alteration in neurological status. Thus, patients with multiple sclerosis may suddenly feel that they are getting much weaker if they develop a cold or fever, or if they are exposed to high external temperatures.

Clinical presentation can include any symptoms of central nervous system involvements. In a large study, weakness of the limb was found to be the presenting feature in 54% of the cases, followed by diplopia in 21%, tremor or ataxia in 19%, paraesthesia in 32% and pain in 10%. Thus, patients presenting with odd feelings of pain, such as trigeminal neuralgia, or curious areas of paraesthesia, need careful evaluation. Occasionally, these areas of involvement do not seem to follow anatomical boundaries and the patient may be diagnosed as being hysterical. Indeed, the pseudo-hysterical presentation of MS is well recognized.

Evoked potential studies may show delay in transmission in one or more modalities. The cerebrospinal fluid may show a specific pattern (oligoclonal banding) on electrophoresis. The MR can show periventricular bright objects and similar objects in other areas on T2 weighted images.

Follow-up studies have shown that 66% of patients are incapacitated by the tenth year and 85% by the fifteenth year of the disease. Seventy-five per cent died within five years of becoming incapacitated.

While there is no definite treatment for multiple sclerosis, there is some advantage in using pulsed megadose steroids in the acute phases. These not only seem to shorten the periods of the acute stage, but diminish the residual deficit. Prolonged treatment with immunosuppressive therapy, such as cyclophosphamide, appears to reduce the number of relapses. This therapy is not without danger, but in rapidly progressing MS, it may well be worth it. It does require continual follow-up and measurement of white cell counts, as well as vigilance in avoidance of infection.

Parkinson's disease

Parkinson's disease is one of the so-called degenerative disorders in the nervous system. The extrapyramidal system including the basal ganglia and striate cortex are involved, with fall-out of dopaminergic neurones. While the etiology is generally unknown, there have been some dramatic advances in our understanding in at least one etiology for Parkinson's disease.

It has been found that a meperidene derivative, MPTP, has the ability to induce Parkinson's, originally in drug addicts and more recently in primates. The Parkinson's disease induced by MPTP will respond to the standard anti-Parkinsonian therapy. As well as this, primate models of the disease develop all the side effects of the therapy, which will be described later. MPTP is specific for dopaminergic neurones, being converted to MPP^+, which is a free radical. It is felt that one of the breakdown products of dopamine at dopaminergic neurones is responsible for the degeneration of the dopaminergic neurones. Because of this, a recent study, Datatop, has demonstrated that inhibition of dopamine break-down by a specific MAO B inhibitor, deprenyl, can slow the rate of progression in Parkinson's by an average one year.

Treatment of Parkinson's disease symptomatically rests still on L-dopa plus a dopa-decarboxylase inhibitor. It is clear now that the lower the dose of L dopa, the fewer side effects there will be, and so there is a general consensus that it is advisable to add a dopamine agonist relatively early on in the disease. The use of anticholinergic therapy is lessening, since it can cause many problems, including memory defects and confusion. L-Deprenyl can be added at any stage, as it does increase the amount of available dopamine, and helps iron out some of the side effects. In the early stages of the disease, patients may respond very well to treatment with L-dopa, although 15% do not appear to respond at all. It is uncertain whether this 15% have true Parkinson's, or whether they have one of the Parkinsonian syndromes.

Adverse effects which occur later on in the disorder include rapid dose–response swings, so-called on–off effects (when the patient alternately freezes and goes hypotonic), end-of-dose akinesia (in which a stiffness towards the end of the dose becomes a problem), and severe orofacial dyskinesia (due to overstimulation of the dopaminergic receptors). All of these problems become more and more severe as the patient gets older, and they are coupled with a decrease in therapeutic efficacy.

Reducing the dose or taking the medication more frequently can help these problems, and shortly, a controlled release form of Sinemet (L-dopa plus carbidopa) will become available. If the patient becomes very confused and develops hallucinations, a drug holiday may be considered. Previously used in patients in whom the symptoms were getting out of control, psychiatric considerations are probably the only indication for a drug holiday at this time. This has to be done in hospital, where the patient's dose of L-dopa is halved for several days and then withdrawn for five to seven days. Following this, the half dosage is restarted.

Thus, the general plan for treating Parkinson's is to introduce L-dopa as late as possible, to keep the dose as low as possible, to introduce a dopamine agonist relatively soon in order to ensure that the dose of L-dopa is as low as possible, and to titrate the medication against the patient's symptoms to avoid overdosing inadvertently.

Depression is an inherent part of Parkinson's disease which in some patients may present before the motor symptoms become evident. This depression is amenable to standard antidepressant therapy and ECT.

Dementia in Parkinson's is commoner than previously suggested. It may be that all Parkinsonian patients eventually become demented. Nevertheless, the dementia is evident in about 40% The dementia of Parkinson's disease is primarily a subcortical dementia, which is different from that of Alzheimer's, although the two may co-exist in the same patient. It seems that the occurrence of hallucinations on anti-Parkinsonian medications may be an indicator of early dementia.

Parkinson's can overlap with other conditions, such as amyotrophic lateral sclerosis (ALS) and Alzheimer's. In Guam, there is a ALS Parkinson's dementia complex in which patients may develop any combination of the three. It appears that the agent responsible for this condition is an excitotoxic amino acid found in a cycad which is used as food in times of famine. This is extremely exciting, since it may be that many of our so-called degenerative diseases are in fact caused by environmental poisoning, coupled with some inherent susceptibility.

Epilepsy

Epilepsy is defined as the tendency to recurrent seizures. It is present in about 0.5% of the population. Most often, epilepsy is idiopathic or familial. However, since intracranial lesions such as tumors can cause epilepsy, epilepsy appearing for the first time is a matter for investigation. It is important to get an idea of what the seizure is like. A description of the actual seizure will enable the physician to classify the seizures into the appropriate classification. The current International Epilepsy Association classification of seizures is given in Table 11.2.

While appearing to ignore the etiology of the seizures, it is a curious fact that the type of seizure, rather than its etiology, is the determinant of the treatment. Certain drugs will produce more favourable results in certain types of seizures, despite the apparent etiology.

TABLE 11.2 Commission on Classification and Terminology of the International League Against Epilepsy. Reproduced from *Epilepsia* (1981), **22**, 489–501

I PARTIAL SEIZURES (seizures beginning locally)
  A Simple partial seizures (consciousness not impaired)
    1. With motor signs
    2. With somatosensory or special sensory symptoms
    3. With autonomic symptoms
    4. With psychic symptoms
  B Complex partial seizures (with impairment of consciousness)
    1. Beginning as simple partial seizures and progressing to impairment of consciousness
    2. With impairment of consciousness at onset
      (a) With impairment of consciousness only
      (b) With automatisms
  C Partial seizures secondarily generalised

II GENERALIZED SEIZURES (bilaterally symmetrical and without local onset)
  A 1. Absence seizures
    2. Atypical absence
  B Myoclonic seizures
  C Clonic seizures
  D Tonic seizures
  E Tonic-clonic seizures
  F Atonic seizures

III UNCLASSIFIED EPILEPTIC SEIZURES (incomplete data)

Investigations of seizures

The investigation of seizures is based on the necessity of characterizing the seizure, by clinical history, EEG pattern and finding the etiology. Structural lesions, such as tumors, can be identified by CAT scan or magnetic resonance imaging. More functional foci may be identified with special electrode placements, SPECT scanning and cortical recording. In some patients, it is very important to identify the focus, since surgical excision of the focus in medically intractable seizures may produce good results.

Treatment of epilepsy

The drugs for the treatment of epilepsy have altered little in the last thirty years. The most commonly used drug for grand mal seizures is Dilantin, with Tegretol and Phenobarbital and Mysoline being also useful in generalized seizures. Sodium valproate is useful in generalized seizures and absence seizures. The current dogma is to use one medication to the full dosage, keeping the blood levels under toxic levels. If this does not succeed, the patient has to be weaned off the medication and tried on the next one in a series. Once all the prime first-line treatments have been tried, then combinations may be attempted. It is generally more sensible to use a combination of a drug which suppresses seizure foci with that which suppresses seizure spread. Thus it does not make sense to combine Tegretol and Dilantin, for instance, since they both do the same thing.

Once the patient is seizure-free on treatment, the medication ought to be continued for at least five years, after which cautious withdrawal may be attempted. This, of course, depends on the reason for the epilepsy.

Status epilepticus is defined as a seizure, or series of seizures, without regaining consciousness, lasting more than half an hour. Status is still a lethal condition, with a mortality of about 8%. When treating status, two areas must be attended to at the same time. The airway must be secured and the patient's breathing unencumbered. This does not mean forcing a tube down the patient's mouth or trying to wrench his teeth apart, but waiting for an appropriate moment when the patient sucks his breath in, at which time the orotracheal airway can be introduced rapidly. An IV must be inserted and blood taken for drug levels and glucose. At the same time, 50 ml of 50% glucose should be injected as well as 10 mg of diazepam. The glucose is necessary to provide for cerebral energy needs, which begin to outstrip metabolic supply at this stage. At the same time that the diazepam is being injected, intravenous Dilantin is administered at a dose of $10-15 \, mg \, kg^{-1}$. This usually works out at about a gram in most people, ranging between 800 and 1200 mg. The diazepam reaches a peak rapidly but then begins to lose its efficacy within half an hour, at which time the effect of the Dilantin becomes apparent. Once control has been achieved, the patient can be dilantinized further if necessary. It does not matter if the patient has been on Dilantin before. The extra Dilantin will not harm them, and the most usual cause for status is failure to take medication, the second commonest cause being withdrawal from alcohol. If the patient does not respond at this stage, intravenous phenobarbitone can be given, or intravenous lignocaine (Lidocaine). If he does not respond then, the patient can be anaesthetized and paralysed, remembering that once the patient is paralysed, seizure activity may not be apparent and damage to the neurones may be continuing.

Most patients with epilepsy are completely normal; however, it has been shown that there is a higher incidence of psychiatric disease in epileptics. Depressive illness appears to be more common in patients with right temporal foci, while psychotic illness is more common in patients with left temporal foci. The cause or relationships between these findings is uncertain and may be circumstantial, indicating two effects of similar destructive processes. Some seizures arising from the temporal lobe may present with a variety of psychic or sensory manifestations, which could be mistaken for psychiatric problems. It is therefore important to take a good history in patients with curious phenomena which are repetitive and relatively short-lived. Attacks of rage may occasionally be caused by seizures, but this is rare.

About 20% of patients with seizures will have pseudo-seizures. Most patients with pseudo-seizures do have occasional genuine seizures. The problem of pseudo-seizures is a difficult one, since they may well be mistaken for genuine seizures. It is important not to make the other mistake of dismissing odd-looking seizures as pseudo-seizures without performing intensive EEG studies. The patient must be in the seizure and have detailed electroencephalographic investigation performed at the same time, including, in some cases, deep electrodes, before one can say for certain that there is no real seizure activity in progress.

Headache

Of all the symptoms which the physician has to manage, headache is probably the most complex and difficult. While the vast majority of headaches are innocent through debilitating manifestations of physiological response, a small percentage are the harbingers of life-threatening diseases.

Mechanisms of head pain

The ophthalmic branch of the fifth cranial nerve innervates most of the intra-cranial contents. Fibres of C2 and C3 innervate the back of the head, and there is some discussion as to whether there is some interchange between fibres of these roots and the intraspinal nucleus of the fifth cranial nerve. The intracranial arteries are innervated by fibres from the locus coeruleus in the brain stem, which are probably vasomotor in function. Fibres from this structure also run into the raphe nuclei in the brain stem, which are involved in pain modulation.

Experiments on this system have raised the possibility that this nucleus may be involved in migraine, since stimulation of this area causes intracranial vaso-construction and extracranial vasodilatation and input into the brain-stem nuclei. Wolff's experiment showed that stimulation of the structures in the posterior part of the cranial cavity caused pain referred to the forehead or eye. This accounts for the observation that lesions in the posterior fossa may present with frontal headache.

Extracranial pain-sensitive structures are the following: extracranial vessels, muscles, skin, articulations of the temporomandibular joint and cervical spin, the nasal sinus, the eye and the periosteum of the skull. Intracranially, the large structures such as the carotid and basilar arteries are still pain-sensitive, but become insensitive as they become smaller and divide into branches. The meninges and venous sinuses are also pain-sensitive. Pain in the head can be caused by traction, displacement, inflammation or erosion of any pain-sensitive structure. Trauma causes headache in the acute stage of contusion and laceration of sensitive structures, and later due to chronic changes which seem to predispose the patient to vascular headache. Mass lesions which raise intracranial pressure cause headache by displacement of meninges and dural sinuses.

The headache of migraine is caused by vascular structures becoming sensitized to pain and involved in presumably a sterile inflammatory process. This is initiated by a variety of predisposing factors and possibly mediated via neural inputs from the locus coereleus.

A plethora of mechanisms can cause diagnostic confusion. In practice, head-aches can be classified most usefully by their mode of onset and temporal pattern. The site of the headache can be useful, but it is not reliable enough to be used in a diagnostic paradigm (Table 11.3).

TABLE 11.3 Common causes of headache.

	Headache	Other symptoms	Diagnosis
Acute	Severe, sudden onset	Focal signs Disturbed consciousness Meningism	Subarachnoid haemorrhage Intracranial haemorrhage Meningitis Encephalitis
		Red eye	Glaucoma (acute)
Subacute	Usually worse in the morning	Nausea Vomiting Dizziness	Raised intracranial pressure
	Worse on stooping or bending Generalized or at back of head	Focal signs Meningeal signs	Meningitis Encephalitis
Chronic	Continuous Generalized Occipital	No other signs or localized trigger points Sleep disturbances	'Tension' Depressive
Paroxysmal	Cranial or hemicranial	Neurological symptoms Neurological signs Nausea and vomiting Psychological disturbances	Migraine
		Worse on standing, better on lying down	Low intracranial pressure
	Retro-orbital continuous	Red eye	Cluster headache
	Variable locations	Older patient Tender arteries	Temporal arteritis

The history is the most important part of the assessment of the headache patient. It is straightforward to diagnose an established typical headache pattern. What is more problematic is the changing pattern or the recent onset of what then turns into a chronic pattern. One such scenario is the young girl who presents to an emergency room with a severe onset of occipital headache with nausea, vomiting, photophobia and some nuchal rigidity. This can cause a degree of panic and the patient is usually fully investigated with a computed tomography (CT) scan and a lumbar puncture. The chronic headache patient who complains that the headache has changed in nature is another diagnostic dilemma.

The approach to these problems should be as follows: patients presenting with new headache patterns, either *de novo* or superimposed on a long-standing problem, whether or not they are associated with any focal neurological signs or changing neurological signs, need a complete assessment or reassessment. The history must be elicited and physical examination performed. The physical examination of the headache patient is not only to exclude or confirm focal neurological features, but to identify painful structures. The skull must be palpated. Are there tender areas over the temporal arteries? Are the carotids tender? Is there tenderness in the muscles or tenderness in the suboccipital areas, and is there tenderness over the trapezii or other muscle groups? Even between attacks, many patients with migraine or tension headache have tender areas over the scalp and in the neck.

Diagnostic tests in headache are designed to exclude or confirm space-occupying lesions in the brain, inflammation or vascular malformations or aneurysms. There is always anxiety (on the part of the patient and physician alike) that the pain is caused by a sinister mechanism. Part of the management of that pain is to allay such fear where appropriate. There is often a conflict between defensive medicine and the desire to perform only the tests which are clinically indicated. Studies suggest that a CT scan is the most cost-effective tool as it will confirm with the greatest sensitivity the one condition that the patient and the physician fear. The electroencephalogram (EEG), skull X-ray and brain scan are second-line tests which may be helpful, but can produce a false sense of security. Recently, there have been developments in diagnostic aids such as thermography which have been claimed to be specific for certain headache syndromes. This has to be confirmed by further studies and specificity and sensitivity determined, but may prove to be useful in the future.

Any patient over the age of 50 who presents with a new headache or a change in headache pattern is a suspect for temporal arteritis. The classic patterns of tenderness in the temporal and occipital arteries are not validated by recent studies. The headaches can take on almost any pattern and be paroxysmal or continuous, hemicranial or occipital. Thus, it is mandatory to perform a sedimentation rate and if appropriate, a temporal artery biopsy. Patients with temporal arteritis who are also on non-steroidal anti-inflammatory drugs (NSAIDs) may have lower erythrocyte sedimentation rates (ESRs) than would be expected. The presence of any muscle stiffness or tenderness is also of help diagnostically, but is not always present. In some patients, the muscle stiffness may develop later on in the course of the disease, while in others it may have presented earlier and been partly treated by NSAIDs, disappeared and then the patient developed headache.

Management of chronic headache

Once the organic headache has been excluded or identified and appropriately managed, the physician is left with a patient who has one of the chronic headache syndromes. Analysis of the symptoms in a large number of headache sufferers concluded that while it was possible to separate cluster headaches as a separate category, and to some extent classic migraine, the vast majority of patients have symptoms which have the characteristics of symptoms previously ascribed to tension and vascular headaches. Recently the International Headache Society has produced a comprehensive classification of headache. This represents a real advance in our ability to differentiate different headache syndromes. I would encourage the reader to obtain a copy (see the reference list at the end of the chapter), since it is beyond the scope of this chapter to delve into these realms. The recognition that muscle tension plays little part in the genesis of so-called tension headache has caused more diagnostic confusion, but has focused attention on the root of the problem—the pathophysiology.

Symptomatic treatment

The infrequent migraine episode is best treated symptomatically. Classically, ergotamine, alone or in combination, is the mainstay of treatment. Unfortunately, 40% of patients find that the side effects preclude its use. Ergotamine should be combined with an antiemetic, such as metoclopramide or domperidone, to be most effective. It has been demonstrated that intravenous metoclopramide helped the absorption of medication, because of the gastric stress during an attack. We use Motilium (domperidone) with analgesics for the acute attack.

Acetylsalicylic acid and acetaminophen, again with an antiemetic, can be very effective. Similarly, combination medications such as Fiorinal, Mersyndol or Flexeril can be extremely useful. Care must be taken when prescribing medications containing sedatives and codeine, because dependence may result. However, judicious use of these compounds with controlled prescription and educated use by the patient should not lead to dependence problems.

Prostaglandin inhibitors such as nonsteroidal anti-inflammatory agents, although useful as prophylactic medication, can also be used symptomatically. Some patients respond well to these, while in others there is no effect.

The aim of symptomatic therapy is to give enough medication early enough, before headache sets in. If oral medication fails and the attack becomes prolonged, parenteral treatment may be necessary. This is often performed in the emergency room of a hospital. Recently, there has been much interest in the non-narcotic treatment of acute attacks.

At Sunnybrook Medical Centre in Toronto, a double-blind trial of intravenous chlorpromazine has been performed. A previous pilot study suggested that 12.5 mg of chlorpromazine intravenously run slowly in saline over 20 min was more effective than the traditional meperidine and dimenhydrinate. The mechanism is possibly related to the dopaminergic block effect of chlorpromazine. One milligram of dihydroergotamine intravenously combined with 10 mg of metoclopramide, repeated at hourly intervals, can abort even chronic vascular headache. This approach has been used in intractable patients, repeating the dose up to 5 times in 24 h with no ill effects. The treatment can be repeated over several days with lower and lower repetitions needed each day. The latter treatment can also be used during withdrawal from chronic analgesic over-use. Currently a new 5HTID agonist, Sumatriptan, is being evaluated worldwide in the treatment of acute migraine.

Prophylaxis

Prophylaxis is based on a pragmatic approach: drugs that work are used, other agents have been postulated on a theoretical basis. For simplicity, the available drugs are classified in the following manner.

Anti-serotonin.
   (a) *Pizotyline.* This drug has probably been the most successful and widely used in migraine prophylaxis. It is a serotonin blocker with some antihistaminic properties. Central blockade of serotonin also has the effect of switching off the satiety centre, and weight gain of 10–20 pounds (4.5–9 kg) may occur in some patients. This can be countered to some extent by taking the medication at night (1–4 mg)
   (b) *Methysergide.* This drug, a serotonin blocker with partial agonist activities, has been available for a long time. Side effects include vasospasms and Raynaud's phenomenon. Retroperitoneal fibrosis was a problem encountered with the drug but can be avoided by leaving the patient drug-free for one month in four.
   (c) *Cyproheptadine.* This drug has weaker antiserotonin properties and is used mainly in the United States where pizotyline is not available. It may be useful in children.

Beta blockers. Worldwide, propranolol is probably the most successful migraine prophylactic medication. The use of beta blockers in migraine came about serendipitously when a cardiologist noticed that a patient put on propranolol for angina was relieved of his migraines. The mechanism by which beta blockers work may be related to their peripheral effect, although a central effect is also possible. Efficacy is related to the slowing of the pulse and hence to beta blockade, although one study showed that the racemic form of propranolol with little beta blocking effects was also useful. Beta blockers with no intrinsic sympathomimetic activity (ISA) are effective; those with ISA are not. Studies have demonstrated the efficacy of nadolol, metoprolol, and atenolol.

Not surprisingly, considering the pharmacological heterogeneity of beta blockers, some people respond better to one beta blocker than to another. In addition, from personal observation, the beneficial effect of the beta blockers can wear off, and at that point, a different beta blocker can work well. Stopping beta blocker treatment abruptly is held by some to be safe, but personal observation has shown that headaches can occur. In one case, rebound hypertension with subsequent cerebral haemorrhage was witnessed in a presumably normotensive patient. In practice, beta blocker dosage should be reduced gradually. Side effects are related to hypotension and fatigue. Remember that the migraine population, i.e. young, active individuals, is more likely to complain of fatiguability, than an elderly population being treated for angina. Recently introduced sustained release beta blockers have been of value to patients for ease of dosage and consistent blood levels of beta blockers.

Tricyclics. Tricyclic antidepressants, such as amitriptyline or nortriptyline, have a definite place in headache treatment. Many patients waken with headache, and in these patients various changes occur during their sleep. They wake from REM sleep, and a release of norepinephrine has been noted three hours before waking. Many of these patients complain of disturbed sleep patterns. A small dose of amitriptyline can be effective. Larger doses are said to be less effective, the serotonin re-uptake blockade being the critical factor. Amitriptyline has also been found to have calcium-blocking properties which may partly explain its efficacy. Combining amitriptyline (up to 100 mg at night) with a daytime beta blocker or calcium blocker can be useful. It is best to start at a small dose, because patients often have side effects early on and may be deterred from continuing therapy. Studies show that amitriptyline is extremely effective in helping patients withdrawing from excessive amounts of analgesic medication.

Monoamine oxidase inhibitors. This class of compound has been maligned in the past and many physicians hesitate to use it because of the possible dangers. These include potential rise in blood pressure and intracerebral bleeding when food containing tyramine is ingested concomitantly. Lance demonstrated the usefulness of phenelzine in patients with chronic vascular headaches, albeit in a non-blind and non-random study. No further studies have been performed. Experience suggests that some patients respond well, although about 25% experience side effects, the most troublesome of which is dizziness. A definite trial is necessary. Deprenyl, a specific MAO inhibitor with no tyramine pressor enhancing effect, may prove valuable in future. Dietary exclusions are not necessarily complex, since the problem foods are often avoided by migraine patients anyway. The most important caveat is the avoidance of injectable narcotics if the patient is taken to emergency.

Non-steroidal anti-inflammatory drugs. Headache is associated with pain. The algesia is probably related to a sterile inflammation mediated by prostaglandins. It would seem reasonable that a prostaglandin antagonist would be effective. Studies have demonstrated no difference between naproxen and propranolol in terms of efficacy in migraine prophylaxis. Mefenamic acid derivatives have been shown to be effective in the acute stage. Curiously, indomethacin does not seem to help migraine, yet is reputed to be the treatment of choice in a variant of cluster headache, called chronic paroxysmal hemicrania. Drugs with action on both prostaglandin synthetase activity and on the peripheral actions of prostaglandins seem to be the most useful. Addition of naproxen to a regime, or its use as interval therapy during menstruation, may be useful to some patients with menstrual migraine; this condition is notoriously difficult to treat.

Calcium channel blockers. The rationale for using calcium blockers is two-fold. First, the cerebral circulation depends on extracellular calcium—hence vasospasms can be prevented with a calcium channel blockade. Why blocking vasospasms should prevent headache is controversial; possibly the whole migraine cycle is blocked, or the vasoconstriction that redistributes the blood during an attack may also be blocked. Another theory is that cerebral ischaemia plays a part in the genesis of migraine and that calcium channel blockers in some way protect against this. Calcium channel blockade may also influence spreading depression, which may play a part in the genesis of classic migraine. Calcium channel blockers may, in future, play a role in the treatment of epilepsy.

In practice, calcium blockers are useful in some patients. Studies of diltiazem and verapamil have demonstrated efficacy. These calcium blockers are not particularly selective. Although nifedipine has been found effective in some studies, in practice it has too many side effects to be well tolerated. Nimodipine is an experimental calcium blocker which has been used in some studies, but no efficacy has been demonstrated. Flunarizine is another calcium blocker recently available in Canada which is also useful.

Calcium blockers seem to have similar effects to beta blockers, in terms of lethargy and loss of athletic performance. However, hypotension rarely results. One curious finding is that calcium blockers take at least a month to start working in migraine patients, in contrast to a rapid onset of action in cardiac indications. This raises some questions about the mode of action. Like other medications, the calcium blockers seem to have a limited period of efficacy. When control is lost, increasing the dose can regain efficacy, but if this does not help, another approach must be tried.

The management of a chronic headache patient, however, follows certain basic principles. One problem which frequently confounds successful treatment is the abuse of symptomatic medication. This has to be identified and faced, since any treatment programme of an addicted patient is doomed to failure. This, of course, implies that the physician and patient develop an ongoing therapeutic relationship. Sleep disturbances occur in about 50% of patients with chronic headache; this may indicate the presence of an underlying depression. Depression may cause headache, may coexist with headache or may be caused by the headache or drugs taken for it. Recognition of depression and treatment play a very vital part in the treatment of chronic pain. Other factors of lifestyle and environment must be identified and discussed. Nevertheless, many patients with chronic vascular headaches have excluded all possible environmental factors and still get headaches.

Non-pharmacological treatment of headache has had a variable degree of success. Biofeedback is the most widely accepted. This modality requires a high degree of motivation on the part of the patient, as well as a fairly high time commitment. Hypnotherapy has some value and this can be carried out by medically qualified practitioners. Other modalities, such as relaxation therapy, all have their uses but there are no clear-cut studies which suggest any definite value. In practice, the combination of pharmacological therapy and some form of non-pharmacological therapy is desirable. However, it must be remembered that some of the medications used in chronic headache, such as amitriptyline, can block the effects of biofeedback.

The problem of chronic headache has two aspects. First, there is the desire on the part of the physician and patient to control the headache without drugs. On the other hand, there is the frequent sheer impossibility of this aim. There exists a fine line between the patient on numerous prophylactic and symptomatic medications and the patient on appropriate prophylactic medication and infrequent symptomatic therapy. What determines the transition into increasing dependence on medication is unknown, but there is evidence that there is a cycle of increasing drug consumption, leading to rebound headache, leading to chronic headache with increased drug abuse. Once the patient is in this situation, withdrawal of the medication can have extremely favourable results. This may have to be done in hospital. The acute attacks may be treated with such non-narcotic medications as dihydro-ergotamine, which has made a bit of a comeback. Postural hypotension is a problem with this, but may not be such a problem when the patient is in a hospital bed. Following this, some form of supportive psychotherapy has to be employed, and then appropriate prophylactic medication possibly reinstituted.

Most patients with headaches can be helped by appropriate medication. However, there does exist a small number who cause an ongoing diagnostic and therapeutic problem to the family doctor and specialist. There is no evidence that this group is any more neurotic or otherwise psychologically abnormal than the other patients. They are probably just at the far end of the spectrum.

In summary, the office management of headache is based on three axioms. Firstly, the exclusion of any organic etiology, such as a space-occupying lesion. Secondly, the identification of the appropriate headache mechanism involved. Thirdly, the appropriate treatment of that mechanism, whether it be a vascular headache such as a migraine, or an inflammatory headache such as temporal arteritis. Finally, in any chronic non-organic headache, the importance of the doctor/patient relationship and the trust which the patient has in the doctor cannot be overemphasized.

Recommended Reading

General

De Jong, R.N. (1970). *The Neurological Examination*. New York: Hoeber Medical, Harper & Row.

Stroke

Hachinksi, V.C. and Norris, J.W. (1975). The acute stroke. In: F. Plum (ed.) *Contemporary Neurology Series*, Vol. 27. Philadelphia: F.A. Davis.

Parkinson's disease

Koller, W. (ed.) (1987). *Handbook of Parkinson's Disease*. New York: Marcel Dekker.

Epilepsy

Wilder, B.J. and Bruni, J. (1981). *Seizure Disorders: A Pharmacological Approach to Treatment*. New York: Raven Press.

Headache

Lance, J. (1982). *Mechanism and Management of Headache*. London: Butterworth.
Hopkins, A. (ed.) (1988). Headache: problems in diagnosis and management. In: *Major Problems in Neurology*. London: W.B. Saunders.
The Headache Classification Committee of the International Headache Society (1988). Classification and diagnostic criteria for headache disorders, cranial neuralgias and facial pain. *Cephalalgia* **8**, (Suppl. 7).

Genetics

— 12

The Principles of Genetics as Applied to Psychiatry

P. Sham, M. Gill and R.M. Murray

Genetics occupies a central position in biology. Genes provide the 'programmes' for assembling the complex molecules necessary for life, and are passed on from generation to generation to enable the reproduction of living organisms. The genetic make-up of a species is determined by past environmental conditions through natural selection. Within a species, genetic differences lead to individual variation, but the passing of genes from parents to offspring produces familial resemblance. In particular, genetic defects are an important cause of familial diseases. This chapter provides an introduction to basic genetic principles and their relevance to psychiatry.

An Overview of Genetic Concepts

Genes and chromosomes

The science of genetics has its origin in Mendel's classic experiments on the garden pea in the 1860s, which enabled him to formulate a theory of inheritance, long before its physical basis was understood (Sturtvant, 1965). Essentially, his theory proposes that certain discrete observable traits (phenotypes) are determined by genes inherited from parents. Each gene can take a number of different forms called alleles, denoted by letters such as A, a. An individual has two genes for each trait, and the alleles of these two genes constitute his genotype for the trait. When the two alleles are identical (AA or aa) the individual is said to be homozygous for the trait, otherwise he is heterozygous. If individuals with genotype Aa are phenotypically indistinguishable from individuals with genotype AA, then allele A is said to be dominant over allele a, or equivalently, allele a is said to be recessive to allele A. If the phenotype of Aa is intermediate between those of AA and aa, then the alleles A and a are said to be co-dominant.

During reproduction, an individual receives with equal probability one of the two genes for every trait from each parent (Mendel's first law, or law of equal segregation). Imagine the genotype of the parent as consisting of two marbles in a box; the law of segregation is equivalent to saying that, in the formation of a gamete, one of the two marbles in the box is picked out at random. Mendel also believed that the segregation of the genes for one trait is not affected by

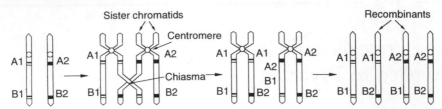

FIG. 12.1   Meiosis. A pair of homologous chromosomes come to lie side by side, each duplicating itself so that four strands are formed (the tetrad). A strand of one chromosome can cross over a strand of the other chromosome. The regions where crossings-over occur are called chiasmata. Genetic material is exchanged in the process, so that genes originally on separate chromosomes (e.g. A1 and B2) can come to lie on the same chromosome.

the segregation of the genes for other traits (Mendel's second law, or law of independent assortment). In the context of our 'box model', this is equivalent to saying that there is a separate box for every trait, each containing two marbles, and that when a gamete is produced, the selection of a marble from one box is independent of the selection of marbles from every other box. Although Mendel's laws were of great importance in the development of genetics, we shall see that they do not always hold.

The significance of Mendel's work was not realized until its 'rediscovery' nearly 40 years later, when the importance of chromosomes in heredity became recognized. Chromosomes are visible in dividing cell nuclei under the light microscope. The usual type of cell division is mitosis, responsible for the increase in the number of cells in the body during growth, and for replacing cells when they are being lost. In a normal mitosis, all the chromosomes are duplicated and distributed equally to two daughter cells, so that each of these contains an identical set of chromosomes to the parent cell.

The second type of cell division is meiosis, and produces sperms and eggs, known as gametes. It is also called reduction division because the number of chromosomes in the cells produced is halved. At an early stage of meiosis (the prophase), each chromosome becomes duplicated to form two sister strands (chromatids) connected to each other at a region called the centromere, as in mitosis. However, the chromosomes also come together in pairs of similar length (homologous pairs). Each resulting complex therefore consists of four strands known as the tetrad (Fig. 12.1). At this stage the non-sister chromatids can cross over each other and exchange material. Two divisions now follow quickly in succession, so that each of the four daughter cells contain one strand of each tetrad. Since these daughter cells have only half the number of chromosomes as normal body cells, they are said to be haploid. Some of these haploid cells develop into gametes. When two gametes, one from each parent, fuse during fertilization, the zygote obtains a complete (diploid) set of chromosome pairs.

Man has 23 pairs of chromosomes. The total display of the 46 chromosomes stained in mitosis is called the human karyotype (Fig. 12.2). Of the 23 pairs, 22 are independent of sex, and are called autosomes. They are numbered in roughly decreasing length from 1 to 22. The remaining pair are the sex chromosomes, and can be of two types: a long type called X, and a short type

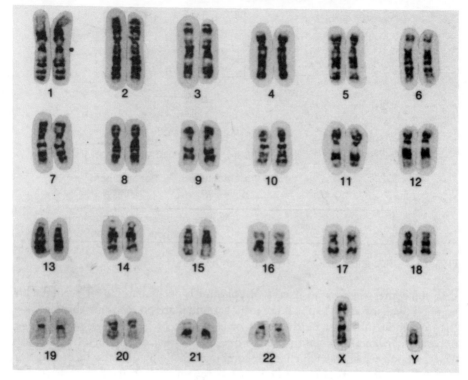

FIG. 12.2 The human male karyotype.

called Y. A normal female has two X chromosomes and a normal male has one X and one Y chromosome. One of the two X chromosomes in each cell of a normal female is inactivated at random early in embryonic development, and appears as a lump in the nucleus called sex chromatin or the Barr body (Lyon, 1968). Females, therefore, are a mosaic of two types of cells depending on which X chromosome is inactivated.

The separation of homologous chromosomes in meiosis closely parallels the equal segregation and independent assortment of the gene pairs in Mendel's theory. This suggests that genes are situated on the chromosomes. However, since the number of genes far exceeds the number of chromosomes, each chromosome must carry many genes, which are then expected to segregate together in meiosis, not independently as Mendel's second law asserts. Suppose that an individual has genotype AB/ab, so that alleles A and B have come from the gamete of one parent and alleles a and b from the gamete of the other; then the possible genotypes of his/her gametes are AB, ab, Ab and aB. Since AB and ab are identical to the parental gametes, they are called parental type gametes. Gametes of genotypes Ab and aB, however, have one gene from each parental gamete, and are called recombinants (Fig. 12.3). Mendel's second law predicts that the four types of gametes occur with equal probabilities, but experiments show

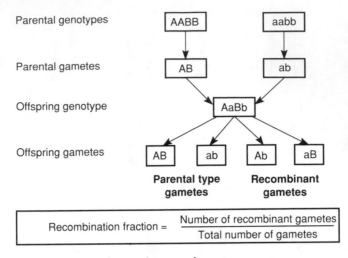

FIG. 12.3   Recombinants and recombination fraction.

that sometimes there is an excess of parental type gametes over recombinant gametes (Bateson *et al.*, 1905). If the loci of A and B are on the same chromosome, then recombinants must be the result of exchange of genetic material between non-sister chromatids when they cross over each other during meiotic prophase. The fraction of gametes which are recombinant is defined as the recombination fraction. The theoretical upper limit of the recombination fraction is $\frac{1}{2}$. At this value the genes at the two loci segregate independently. However, if the recombination fraction is less than $\frac{1}{2}$, then the two loci must be on the same chromosome, and are said to be linked.

Assuming that the probability of a cross-over between two linked loci is proportional to the distance between them, the recombination fraction can be used as a measure of genetic distance. However, because multiple cross-overs do not always result in recombinants, the relationship between recombination fraction and genetic distance is approximately linear only for short distances. The gradient of the curve of recombination fraction versus genetic distance diminishes as genetic distance increases, so that as genetic distance increases indefinitely, the recombination fraction approaches $\frac{1}{2}$. A genetic map unit, or centiMorgan (cM), is defined as the genetic map distance corresponding to a recombination fraction of $\frac{1}{100}$. Map distance does not always correspond to physical distance, because some regions of chromosomes cross over more frequently than others.

Nucleic acids and proteins

Each chromosome contains one very long molecule of DNA. DNA is composed of deoxyribose, phosphate, the purine bases adenine (A) and guanine (G), and the pyrimidine bases cytosine (C) and thymine (T). Watson and Crick (1953) constructed a model in which two chains, each consisting of a sugar-phosphate 'backbone' on which the bases are attached, were joined by hydrogen bonds between T and A, or between C and G. The base pairs, being quite flat, were

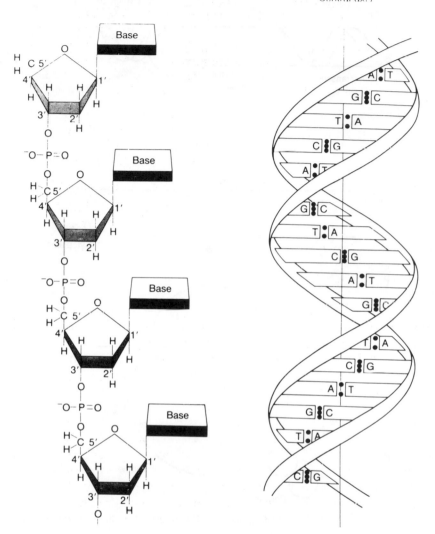

FIG. 12.4 DNA structure. The diagram on the right represents the Watson–Crick double helix model. The diagram on the left represents the molecular structure of part of a DNA chain. Reprinted from Weatherall (1985), with permission.

stacked on each other like the steps of a spiral staircase; and the chains were twisted around each other as a double helix (Fig. 12.4). Since the sequence of either strand is completely determined by the sequence of the other, the two strands are said to be complementary. During cell division, DNA is replicated; the double helix unwinds, splits open, and two new complementary strands are formed against the two old strands.

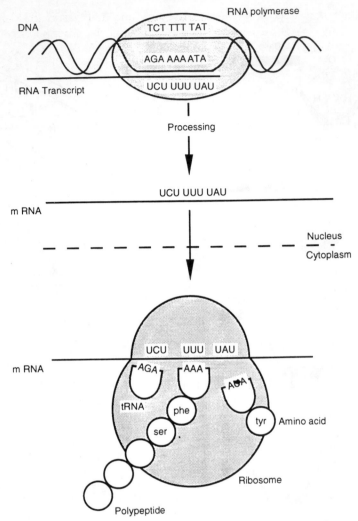

FIG. 12.5   DNA function. Transcription and translation (protein synthesis).

Proteins are chains of amino acids. The inherited sequence of bases in DNA determines the sequence of amino acids in proteins. Thus, the information in a base sequence is decoded into an amino acid sequence (Fig. 12.5). Three bases are decoded into one amino acid, so that there is a sufficient number of unique three-base sequences (called codons) for all amino acids (about 20 in number) to be uniquely determined (Crick, 1962). The code is universal; that is, the same triplet codes for the same amino acid in all living organisms. Decoding begins with the synthesis of a complementary strand of ribonucleic acid (RNA) against a DNA sequence (transcription). RNA differs from DNA in that it is single-stranded, has ribose instead of deoxyribose, and uracil instead of thymine. The newly synthesized RNA is called an RNA transcript. RNA transcripts are processed by the addition of chemicals at their ends ('caps' and 'tails'), and the deletion of certain non-functional sequences ('splicing'). Some of the processed RNA chains are called messenger RNA (mRNA), for they carry the 'messages' of amino acid sequences to ribosomes where proteins are synthesized. The mRNA is transported from the nucleus to the cytoplasm and attaches itself to ribosomes, which are made of ribosomal RNA and proteins. Amino acids are brought to the ribosomes by transfer RNA (tRNA), each of which bears a three-base sequence (called anticodon), and is 'charged' with a corresponding amino acid. The mRNA is 'translated' by lining up a complementary sequence of tRNA, and a corresponding sequence of amino acids, which join up to form a polypeptide chain. The mRNA is then degraded by enzymes.

Since cells require different gene products under different circumstances and at different times in development, the expression of genes requires regulation. In principle, regulation can occur at transcription, processing, transport, translation, or degradation. Many coding genes are normally inactive, and an 'activator' protein is necessary to initiate transcription (Maclean *et al.*, 1983).

Genetic abnormality

The totality of the DNA in a cell is called its genome. The human genome has over 3×10^9 base pairs, corresponding to a total length of about 2 metres. However, most of the genome is non-coding, and the number of protein products coded by genes is probably between 50 000 and 200 000 (Weatherall, 1985).

A change in DNA from a standard type is called a mutation, and the resulting genetic type is called a mutant. When a mutation occurs in a cell destined to differentiate into gametes, it is said to be a germinal mutation and has the potential to be passed on to an offspring; otherwise it is a somatic mutation and cannot be inherited. A mutation involving a single base pair is called a point mutation, and one involving a sequence of base pairs is called a chromosome mutation; the latter may be a rearrangement of a DNA sequence, or a change in the number of chromosomes. Chromosome rearrangements include sequence deletion, duplication, inversion, and translocation (the displacement of a DNA sequence to a non-homologous chromosome).

A set of chromosomes containing one member of each homologous pair is said to be monoploid. The monoploid number in man is therefore 23. A cell is said to be euploid if it contains an exact multiple of the monoploid number of chromosomes. The normal euploid number in man is 46, or diploid. When a cell has a chromosome number which is not euploid then it is said to be aneuploid. Examples of aneuploidy are Turner's syndrome (X0), Klinefelter's syndrome (XXY), and Down's syndrome (trisomy 21). Aneuploidy results from the failure of a pair of chromosomes to separate in meiosis (non-disjunction). Most fetuses with aneuploidy are non-viable and are aborted spontaneously (Creasy *et al.*, 1976). When present, aneuploidy can be detected cytogenetically. For example, Turner's syndrome can be recognized by the absence of the Barr body in the cell nuclei of a female, while Klinefelter's syndrome can be recognized by the presence of a Barr body in the cell nuclei of a male.

The rate of a particular DNA change is called its mutation rate. Agents which increase mutation rate, such as certain types of radiation and chemicals, are called mutagens. High parental age also increases mutation rate. It appears that some regions of the genome have higher mutation rates than others. Indeed, some regions appear to be relatively mobile and frequently change their location. These regions are called transposons (Shapiro, 1983).

The phenotypes which Mendel studied in the garden pea were gross morphological characteristics, and it is remarkable that their pattern of inheritance parallels so closely that of the underlying genes, which act at the molecular level. Of course, phenotypes may also be defined at other levels: molecular, cellular, organ-system, and indeed behavioural. The further a phenotype is away from the molecular level, the more opportunities there are for additional influences, and the less likely that its pattern of inheritance will reflect the segregation of genes at a single locus. For example, severe mental retardation as a whole is genetically complex, but the measurement of underlying morphological and biochemical indices has identified phenotypes caused by single mutations (e.g. phenylketonuria). Diseases in man with clearly identified genetic defects can be classified first by the nature of the mutation: chromosomal or single gene; then by site; autosomal or sex-linked; and then, for single gene defects, by whether the mutation is dominant or recessive (McKusick, 1988). Many diseases do not have an easily identifiable single genetic defect, but a genetic contribution is often implicated when the pattern of occurrence in genetically related individuals is more readily explained by models with a genetic component than ones without.

Biometrical genetics

Many biological traits are continuous, and many of these (e.g. height) follow a normal distribution in the general population. Galton (1889) discovered a linear relationship between the heights of parents and the mean height of their offspring, and invented the concepts of regression and correlation to describe this relationship (Stigler, 1989). Very tall and very short parents had children whose mean heights were closer to the population mean, a phenomenon called regression to the mean. Later, it was found that the inheritance of certain mental traits followed a similar pattern (Pearson, 1904). The normal distribution has long been known to apply when a variable is the sum of a large number of independent variables, and it remained for Fisher (1918) to show that the observed correlations between different classes of relatives were consistent with the hypothesis that continuous traits were determined by many genes, each of small effect (polygenes), together with many environmental factors of small effect. Further developments have led to the disciplines of quantitative genetics (Falconer, 1989) and biometrical genetics (Mather and Jinks, 1982), which are concerned mostly with dividing up the variation of a continuous trait into genetic and environmental components.

It is useful to conceptualize the effect of a gene as consisting of a component that is independent of the other genes present (the additive effect), and a component which depends on the other genes, either at the same locus on the homologous chromosome (dominant interaction), or at other loci (epistatic interaction). The additive effects of genes are more predictable than interactions, so that knowledge of the contribution of additive effects is particularly useful. The proportion of the total variance of a trait in a population explained by the additive genetic component is called its narrow heritability (h^2) in that population. Biometrical analysis has been applied to human intelligence and personality, each showing a substantial additive genetic component, and incidentally causing much controversy (Eysenck and Kamin, 1981; Eaves *et al.*, 1989). The correct interpretation of a high heritability estimate is that existing environmental variation explains little of the current total phenotypic variation; not that additional environmental modification will necessarily have little effect.

The application of polygenic models to discrete psychiatric conditions assumes that the observed trait is a function of an underlying continuous, normally distributed variable (liability), determined by a combination of polygenes and environmental factors (Falconer, 1965). For a dichotomous trait (i.e. one that is either present or absent), a threshold in liability can be postulated such that only individuals with liability above the threshold develop the abnormal condition (Fig. 12.6(a)). With such assumptions, the heritability for the liabilities of disorders like schizophrenia and manic depression can be estimated (Reich *et al.*, 1979).

The assumption of polygenic models that all the relevant genes have only a small effect on the trait is a pessimistic one, for the possibility of understanding the biology of the trait is much increased if a gene with a large effect on the trait can be discovered. Since most common psychiatric disorders cannot be explained by single gene inheritance, much interest has focused on the type of model in which a 'major gene' interacts with other 'minor genes' and environmental factors to produce the condition. Minor genes and environmental factors can be allowed for by postulating 'incomplete penetrance', that is, by postulating that only a proportion of individuals with the vulnerable genotype ever develop the condition (Slater and Cowie, 1971). This 'generalized' single major locus model can be formulated in terms of liability and threshold (Fig. 12.6(b)).

Major genes and minor genes may also act separately to cause a similar phenotype. Thus, in mental retardation a single major cause, genetic or environmental is present in most cases with extremely low IQ, but absent in most moderately retarded individuals, the majority of whom are at the tail end of the 'normal' continuous variation in IQ. Major environmental causes of severe mental retardation include prenatal infection or metabolic problems, and birth complications. Major genetic causes are numerous, and can be classified into chromosomal anomalies and single gene defects (Table 12.1).

Basic Methods of Genetic Research in Psychiatry

Aspects of clinical measurement

An important element in most genetic studies of psychiatric disorders is the clinical assessment of the subjects. It is often from this assessment that the condition for genetic analysis, such as the diagnosis, is derived. To achieve

(a) Liability–threshold polygenic model

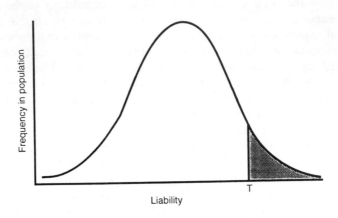

(b) Liability–threshold single major locus model

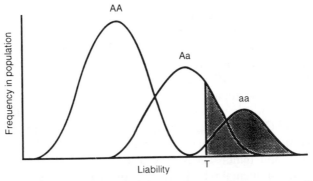

FIG. 12.6   Liability models. (a) The liability in the population is normally distributed. Individuals whose liability is above the threshold, T, are affected. The area under the curve to the right of T represents the proportion of the population affected (i.e. population morbid risk). (b) The population can be divided into three subsets by genotype (AA, Aa, aa). The liability of each of the subsets is normally distributed. Individuals whose liability exceeds the threshold T are affected. Thus the proportion of individuals affected (i.e. penetrance) is largest for those with genotype aa, second largest for those with genotype Aa, and smallest for those with genotype AA.

replicability, standardized psychiatric assessment schedules have been used extensively, most notably the Schedule for Affective Disorders and Schizophrenia or SADS (Endicott and Spitzer, 1978) and the Present State Examination or PSE (Wing *et al.*, 1974). When very accurate information is required, direct interview by a trained interviewer using such schedules is the method of choice. However, sometimes it is necessary, for example, when a subject in a family study is dead,

TABLE 12.1   Some major genetic causes of mental retardation.

Chromosomal defects

Down's syndrome. Trisomy or translocation 21, about 1/600 newborns, IQ 30–50, short stature, hypotonia, upslanting palpebral fissures, speckling of iris (Brushfield spots), fine lens opacities, small nose, protruding tongue, short neck, dermatoglyphic abnormalities (e.g. Simian crease), congenital cardiac defects (in about 40%).

Edward's syndrome. Trisomy 18, about 1/3000 newborns, low birth weight, weak cry, congenital cardiac defect, corneal opacity, only 10% survive 1st year.

Turner's syndrome. XO, about 1/5000 newborns, mean IQ 95, short stature, blue sclerae, cataract, perceptive hearing loss, webbed neck, broad chest with widely spaced nipples, cubitus valgus, ovarian dysgenesis, congenital cardiac defects (in 20%).

Klinefelter's syndrome. XXY, about 1/1000 newborns, mean IQ 85, long limbs, hypogonadism, delayed speech, behaviour problems.

Cri du Chat syndrome. Partial deletion 5p, very rare, IQ 20-30, low birth weight, slow growth, cat-like cry.

X-linked recessive

Fragile X syndrome. Fragile site Xq27, about 1/2000 male newborns, IQ 30–65, large head with prominent forehead and jaws, big ears, macro-orchidism, autistic features common, epilepsy occasionally, many female carriers have mild mental retardation, increased frequency of psychosis.

Lesch–Nyhan syndrome. Disorder of purine metabolism with excessive uric acid production, developmental delay, choreoathetoid movements, self-mutilation sometimes reduced by hydroxytryptophan.

Hunter syndrome (mucopolysaccharidosis type 2). Retardation, deafness, dwafism, grotesque facies, hepatosplenomegaly.

Autosomal dominant

Neuro-fibromatosis. Mental retardation in a minority, neurofibromata, cafe-au-lait spots.

Tuberous sclerosis (epiloia). Variable expression, retardation in about 70%, epilepsy, adenoma sebaceum, retinal phakoma, multiple tumours.

Apert syndrome (acrocephalosyndactyly). Variable degrees of retardation, skull malformation, syndactyly of hands and feet (spoon-shaped hands).

Autosomal recessive

Phenylketonuria. Phenylalanine hydroxylase deficiency, about 1/10 000 newborns, fair hair, blue eyes, retarded growth, epilepsy, eczema, hyperactivity, severe retardation if not treated early by phenylalanine-restricted diet.

Homocystinuria. Cystathionine β-synthase deficiency, retardation in about two-thirds, ectopia lentis, skeletal abnormalities, sometimes treatable by methionine restriction.

Galactosaemia. Galactose 1-phosphate uridyl transferase deficiency, mental retardation, cataracts, hepatomegaly, early treatment by galactose-free diet effective.

Tay Sachs disease. Excess lipid storage, developmental delay, blindness, deafness, spastic paralysis, epilepsy, grey-white area round fovea centralis due to lipid-laden ganglion cells leaves a 'cherry-red' retinal spot, most die aged 2–4 years.

Hurler's syndrome (gargoylism, mucopolysaccharidosis type 1). Retardation, dwarfism, grotesque facies, corneal clouding, hepatosplenomegaly, cardiovascular problems, death before adolescence.

Lawrence–Moon–Biedl syndrome. Moderate mental retardation, pigmentary retinopathy, hypogenitalism, polydactyly.

to rely on second-hand information from another family member. This is often referred to as the family-history method, and a standardized schedule, the Family History–Research Diagnostic Criteria (Andreasen *et al.*, 1986), has been developed especially for this purpose. This method, however, is not as sensitive as direct interviews, particularly when the psychiatric disorder in question is minor (e.g. anxiety neurosis). It may also be less accurate in discriminating between diagnostic categories. In both direct interviews and family history interviews, knowledge of the subject whose relatives are being assessed may lead to bias in their assessment. To avoid this bias, assessment is best performed when the interviewer has no such knowledge. Such an interviewer is often described as 'blind'.

Self-report questionnaires provide a relatively cheap method of clinical assessment, as they can be administered by post. By carefully wording the questions, it is often possible to achieve a high level of reliability. This method is particularly useful when a large number of subjects need to be examined, or as a screening instrument to select subjects for further study (e.g. McKeon and Murray, 1986).

Defining traits for genetic studies

The development of standardized diagnostic criteria such as the RDC (Spitzer *et al.*, 1975) and DSM-III (American Psychiatric Association, 1980), does not imply that the categories so defined constitute disorders most suited for genetic studies. Ideally, syndromes should be classified such that those with considerable genetic overlap are grouped together. If the genetic predisposition to two similar but distinguishable syndromes is caused by the same genes, then the two syndromes should cluster together in families. However, co-aggregation of two syndromes can also be caused by the syndromes sharing environmental factors which are positively correlated between family members (e.g. a family which jointly ran a public house might contain both members with the alcohol dependence syndrome and members with cirrhosis). It is therefore necessary, strictly speaking, to demonstrate co-aggregation between the disorders for family members reared and living apart from each other. An example of co-aggregation, even in family members reared apart, is between schizophrenia and schizotypal personality disorder (Kendler *et al.*, 1984).

Even with one condition, it is often unclear how wide or narrow the definition should be. One possible approach is to define the condition such that familiality is maximized. A recent study, for example, attempted to find the diagnostic criteria for schizophrenia which maximized heritability (McGuffin *et al.*, 1984).

Instead of studying the clinical condition directly, another approach is to study a marker of the condition which is genetically simpler. The marker can be a biochemical abnormality, a physiological dysfunction, a cognitive deficit, or any other stable trait which can be measured reliably. It is hoped that the genetics of the marker will throw light on the genetics of the condition. An example of this approach is the study of smooth pursuit eye movement dysfunction as a marker for schizophrenia (Matthysse *et al.*, 1986).

Confirming a genetic contribution

Family studies

In a family study, sets of related individuals are studied. A set of individuals with the same parents is called a sibship. The inclusion of parents produces a nuclear family. Inclusion of more distant relatives such as grandparents produces what is called an extended pedigree. Within a pedigree, individuals have different degrees of relatedness to each other, measured by the expected proportion of genes in common, called the coefficient of kinship. The parents, siblings, and children of an individual are defined as his first degree relatives, and have a coefficient of kinship of $\frac{1}{2}$. The grandparents, uncles and aunts, nephews and nieces, and grandchildren of an individual are called his second degree relatives, and have a coefficient of kinship of $\frac{1}{4}$.

Having defined a family unit to study, it is possible to obtain a sample of such units from the general population. However, for a rare condition, it is easier to obtain a sample of individuals with the condition and study their relatives. The sampled individuals are called probands, and their affected relatives are called secondary cases.

If a condition has a genetic contribution, the relatives of probands with the condition are expected to have the condition more frequently than (1) individuals in the general population, and (2) relatives of individuals without the condition (control probands). If the relatives of affected and control probands differ in their age, sex or other distributions, it may be necessary to allow for these differences in the statistical analysis. One method of controlling for the effect of age, when a condition has a variable age of onset, is to estimate the proportion of the individuals who would ever develop the condition if they lived through the entire age-range at risk of the disorder. This estimate, often called morbid risk or lifetime expectancy can be obtained most simply by the Weinberg Shorter Method (Slater and Cowie, 1971). In this method, the morbid risk of a set of individuals is estimated by the ratio of the number of individuals observed to have the condition to the sum of the number of individuals above the age-range at risk and half the number of individuals within the age-range at risk. The denominator is often called Bezugsiffer (BZ). A greater morbid risk in the relatives of affected probands than in the relatives of control probands is consistent with a genetic contribution. However, such a result is also consistent with an environmental contribution which is positively correlated between members of a family.

Twin studies

Monozygotic (MZ) twins arise from the division of a fertilized egg, and so have an identical set of genes. Any phenotypic differences must therefore be caused by differences in environment. Dizygotic (DZ) twins, like full sibs, have on average half their genes in common, so that any phenotypic differences may be caused by differences in genes and/or environment. Assuming that environmental differences between MZ twin pairs and DZ twin pairs are equal, then a greater phenotypic difference between DZ twin pairs than MZ twin pairs is evidence that the phenotype has a genetic contribution. For a continuous trait, phenotypic similarity between twin pairs can be measured by a correlation coefficient (r). A genetic contribution is indicated if the correlation coefficient is significantly greater for MZ than for DZ twins.

For a dichotomous trait (e.g. an illness), twin pairs can be classified into those with both members affected (concordant), only one member affected (discordant), or neither member affected. In a sample of twin pairs with at least one affected member, the proportion of concordant pairs is called the pairwise concordance. If the twin pairs are ascertained through affected probands, the proportion of the co-twins affected is called the probandwise concordance. In the calculation of probandwise concordance, concordant twin pairs in which both members are independently ascertained are counted twice, so that the probandwise concordance may be greater than the pairwise concordance. Probandwise concordance is preferred to pairwise concordance, for it is more directly comparable to the risk estimates in other relatives. A genetic contribution is indicated if MZ concordance is significantly greater than DZ concordance. However, an often criticized assumption is that all relevant environmental differences are on average the same for MZ and DZ twin pairs. Common family environment is absent for twins reared apart from birth, but such twins have still shared a common pre-natal and peri-natal environment. As twinning is a special event, many doubt the validity of generalizing from twins to the rest of the population (Elston and Boklage, 1978).

Adoption studies

An adoptee is an individual taken away from his or her biological parents at an early age and reared by genetically unrelated individuals (the adoptive family). It can therefore be argued that any resemblance between the adoptee and his biological relatives is caused by having genes in common, and any resemblance between the adoptee and his adoptive relatives is caused by sharing a similar family environment. Nevertheless, adoptees have spent their pre-natal life in the same uterus as their biological siblings, and this is still a possible source of resemblance.

For rare conditions it is usual to include families for study through affected individuals. One method is to sample affected individuals who have had their offspring adopted away and to study these offspring (the so-called adoptees method). If the morbid risk in these adoptees is greater than that in adoptees born to unaffected biological parents, then a genetic component is often advocated. However, an alternative explanation is that having an affected biological parent is associated with unfavourable adoptive family environment (e.g. the adoption agency may have attempted to find a similar adoptive family). This alternative can be excluded if adoptees with an affected biological parent have a higher morbid risk than adoptees with unaffected biological parents adopted into a family with an affected parent or sibling (the so called cross-fostering method).

Another method is to sample affected adoptees and examine their biological adoptive families (the so-called adoptees' families method). If the morbid risk of the biological relatives of affected adoptees is greater than that of their adoptive relatives, then a genetic component is often advocated. However, alternative explanations are (1) parents with the condition are more likely to adopt their children away than those without the condition, or (2) parents with the condition are less likely to adopt children of other parents than those without the condition. These alternatives can be excluded if the morbid risk in biological relatives of normal adoptees does not exceed that in their adoptive relatives. However, like twinning, adoption has been criticized as being an ill-understood complicated event (Clerget-Darpoux *et al.*, 1986b), so that it may not be possible to generalize the results of adoption studies to the general population.

In theory, family, twin and adoption studies can each infer a genetic component when it is in fact absent. However, when all three types of studies point to a substantial genetic component (as in schizophrenia and affective psychosis), then it is reasonable to conclude that a genetic component does indeed exist.

Finding an appropriate genetic model

The set of hypotheses which Mendel proposed to explain his experimental findings was an abstract model, though most components of his model now have physical meanings. Thus, if after stringent tests, the pattern of occurrence of a condition in families is consistent with a Mendelian model, then a single gene is the likely cause of the condition. This allows one to predict the future pattern of the occurrence of the condition in families, and promises eventual success for molecular genetic studies attempting to locate and identify a defective gene. The most important simple Mendelian models are:

Autosomal dominant. All individuals with the mutant allele are affected. Thus: (a) children of two affected parents have a morbid risk of $\frac{3}{4}$; (b) children of one affected and one normal parent have a morbid risk of $\frac{1}{2}$; (c) children of two normal parents have a morbid risk of 0; (d) the parents and siblings of affected individuals have a morbid risk of $\frac{1}{2}$; and (e) the morbid risks are equal in males and females.

Autosomal recessive. All individuals with two copies of the mutant allele, one from each parent, are affected. Individuals with only one mutant allele do not become affected, but can pass it to their children. Thus: (a) siblings of affected individuals have a morbid risk of $\frac{1}{4}$; (b) parents and children of affected individuals have near 0 morbid risks; (c) children of two affected parents are all affected; (d) there is an excess of consanguineous marriages in the parents of affected individuals; and (e) the morbid risks are equal in males and females.

X-linked recessive. All males with the mutant allele are affected. Females with one mutant and one normal allele are unaffected, but may transmit the mutant allele to their offspring, and are therefore called carriers. Thus: (a) the male siblings of affected males have a morbid risk of $\frac{1}{2}$; (b) the female siblings of affected males have a morbid risk of 0 if the father is unaffected, or $\frac{1}{2}$ is the father is affected; (c) the male children of affected males have a morbid risk of nearly 0; (d) the male

TABLE 12.2 Approximate predictions of simple Mendelian models.

Model of Inheritance	Morbid Risk in			
	Parents	Brothers	Sisters	Children
Autosomal dominant	$\frac{1}{2}$	$\frac{1}{2}$	$\frac{1}{2}$	$\frac{1}{2}$
Autosomal recessive	0	$\frac{1}{4}$	$\frac{1}{4}$	0
X-linked recessive (proband male)	0	$\frac{1}{2}$	0	0

children of daughters of affected males have a morbid risk of $\frac{1}{2}$; and (e) the morbid risk is greater in males than in females.

These predictions, summarized in Table 12.2, can be used to test whether a condition is transmitted as a simple Mendelian character.

Generalized single major locus (SML) model

If the predictions of simple Mendelian models are incompatible with observations, then these models must be rejected and a less specific model proposed. One such model is the generalized single major locus (SML) model. It postulates that the condition is caused by a single locus with two alleles, A and a. The morbid risks of individuals with the three possible genotypes, AA, Aa, and aa, are allowed to take on any values from 0 to 1. These three morbid risks are known as penetrance parameters, and are denoted as p_1, p_2, and p_3, respectively. Clearly, if $p_1 = 1$, $p_2 = 1$, and $p_3 = 0$, the model is autosomal dominant, if $p_1 = 1$, $p_2 = 0$, and $p_3 = 0$, the model is autosomal recessive. For a given set of values of penetrance parameters and gene frequencies, the model predicts the morbid risks of various classes of relatives of affected individuals. The discrepancy between a set of predicted and observed morbid risks can be assessed statistically (for example, by chi-square statistics). The parameter values corresponding to the least discrepancy can be found. This type of analysis, sometimes called morbid risk analysis, gives some indication about whether the model is appropriate for the condition, and provides estimates for the parameters. However, it loses information through grouping the relatives into classes.

Segregation and pedigree analysis

Another type of analysis does not group relatives into classes, but assesses directly the compatibility of the familial data with various models. In general, these methods are based on the statistical theory of likelihood. The rationale is that, if we have two models of similar complexity, we should favour the one under which the observed data is more probable. From a genetic model, an algebraic expression involving the parameters of the model (such as gene frequencies and penetrances), which gives the probability of observing a set of families, can be derived. The values of the parameters which maximize this likelihood function are called the maximum likelihood estimates (MLE) of the parameters. After obtaining the MLE of the parameters of the most general model (usually by iterative procedures using computer programs), simpler models can be tested by fixing certain parameters, obtaining the MLE of the remaining parameters, and then calculating the ratio between the maximum likelihood of the simpler model to the maximum likelihood of the general model. The smaller this likelihood ratio, the less likely is the simpler model compared to the general model. The statistical significance of this ratio can be assessed by a chi-square test. For example, an autosomal dominant model may be accepted if fixing the penetrance parameters to autosomal dominant values does not result in a significant decrease of the maximum likelihood from the generalized SML model.

A problem with the generalized SML model is that the hypothesis of a single locus is the most general model and cannot be tested using the likelihood ratio test. One solution is to construct a more general model, so that the SML model can be tested against it. One model, known as the general transmission model (Elston and Stewart, 1971), allows the probabilities of transmitting an A allele given the genotypes AA, Aa, and aa to be specified by parameters called transmission parameters, denoted as t_1, t_2, and t_3, respectively. If parent to offspring transmission is caused by a single (Mendelian) locus, then $t_1 = 1$, $t_2 = 0.5$, and $t_3 = 0$. Testing this restricted model against the unrestricted general transmission model with the likelihood ratio test provides a test for single major locus inheritance. Another model, known as the mixed model (Morton and McLean, 1974), incorporates a polygenic component to the basic SML model. In this model, to infer that a single major gene is responsible for some parent/child resemblance, it is necessary to show that restricting the model to polygenic (by setting the SML component to 0) significantly decreases the maximum likelihood from the unrestricted mixed model.

Polygenic-multifactorial inheritance

It is conceivable that there is no major gene effect for some psychiatric disorders. A polygenic trait is determined by a 'large' number of genetic loci and environmental factors whose effects are small, independent and additive. Under these assumptions, the trait will have approximately a normal distribution. We can designate the sum of the genetic effects as G, and the sum of the environmental effects as E. An individual's phenotypic value, P, is defined by $P = G + E$. If G and E are independently distributed in a population, then the variance of P is the sum of the variances of G and E. In symbols, $V(P) = V(G) + V(E)$. Thus, ignoring dominant and epistatic effects, we measure the importance of genetic factors by the ratio $V(G)/V(P)$, i.e. heritability (h^2). The environmental effects shared by siblings reared together (common environment) is also a source of familial resemblance. Assuming that common environment is the only source of familial resemblance other than additive gene effects, then h^2 can be estimated from the correlations of MZ and DZ twins by the equations $r(MZ) = h^2 + c^2$, and $r(DZ) = h^2/2 + c^2$, where c^2 is the proportion of phenotypic variance explained by common environment (Falconer, 1989). The polygenic-multi-factorial model can be applied to discrete conditions by postulating that a condition develops when an underlying polygenic-multifactorial liability exceeds a certain threshold (Reich et al., 1979). It can also be combined with the generalized SML model (Morton and McLean, 1974).

Most mental disorders, being common and defined at the level of symptoms and signs, are likely to have complex or even heterogeneous etiology. The relationship between gene and disorder is unlikely to be one-to-one. It is probable that several genes may contribute to one disorder, and that one gene may contribute to several disorders (pleiotropism). Furthermore, the interaction between genes and environment may be complex. For example, a gene may lead to a disorder if and only if a particular environmental event occurs at a particular time in development. It would be unrealistic to expect statistical modelling of familial data on the occurrence of mental illness to completely elucidate such complex etiology. The assumptions of genetic models represent a compromise between the presumed complexity of nature and the effects which one can realistically resolve with the familial data available. The value of genetic modelling lies in (1) resolving major genetic or environmental effects for further research, (2) providing parameter estimates for linkage and association studies, (3) predicting recurrence risks (i.e. the risks for future offspring given information on the pedigree) for genetic counselling.

Identifying environmental factors

The existence of an environmental component in most psychiatric syndromes is indicated simply by the existence of MZ twin pairs discordant for the syndrome. For instance, MZ twin concordance for schizophrenia is less than 50% (see Chapter 31, this volume). The study of the effect of the environment on the distribution of diseases in a population is traditionally the province of epidemiologists. However, for disorders with substantial contributions from both genes and environment, an approach incorporating both genetics and epidemiology is appropriate. Thus, the pattern of occurrence of a disorder in families is studied in conjunction with potential environmental risk factors (Dorman et al., 1988).

Since MZ twins share all their genes, any phenotypic differences must be environmental. Thus, any consistent environmental differences between the well and the ill twins may be related to why they are discordant. Furthermore, traits which are consistently similar in the well and the ill twins must either be unrelated to the disorder, or related to the common predisposition; on the other hand, a trait which is found only in the affected twin must be related to the environmental factor responsible for the discordance, or the disease process itself (Rosenthal, 1970).

Another approach is to study sets of related individuals identified to be of high genetic risk, for example, children of an affected mother (Goldin et al., 1986). Environmental factors can be examined, retrospectively or prospectively, to identify correlates of the later development of the disorder. However, if the 'latent' period between exposure and development of the disorder is long, then a prospective study will take a long time to complete. Despite this, high risk prospective studies for schizophrenia are being conducted, and have produced interesting preliminary results (see Chapter 13, this volume).

Locating genetic defects

Cytogenetics

The standard notation for gene locations specifies firstly the chromosome number (1, 2, . . . , 22, X, Y); secondly, whether the gene lies on the short arm (p) or on the long arm (q); and thirdly the segment number on the arm (1, 2, . . .), numbered from the centromere.

The microscopic examination of the chromosomes can provide clues to the location of defective genes. For example, the first assignment of a gene to an autosome was due to the co-segregation of an unusual looking chromosome 1 with a particular version of the Duffy blood group in a large pedigree (Dohahue *et al.*, 1968).

In psychiatry, cytogenetic abnormalities have already led to some important findings. For example, a fragile site (i.e. a narrowing on a chromosome which appears under special staining, see Sutherland *et al.*, 1985) on Xq27-28 has been found to be closely related to a syndrome with mental retardation (the fragile-X or Martin–Bell syndrome: Nussbaum and Ledbetter, 1986). The location of the fragile site is interesting, as it is near X-chromosomal markers (e.g. red–green colour blindness and G6PD deficiency) claimed to be linked with manic-depressive psychosis (Baron *et al.*, 1987).

Another example arose from the frequent early occurrence of Alzeimer's dementia in individuals with Down's syndrome. This led to speculation of an 'Alzheimer gene' on chromosome 21; and this has now been confirmed by linkage studies (St. George-Hyslop *et al.*, 1987). Similarly, the co-segregation of a partial trisomy of 5q11-q13 and a schizophrenia-like psychosis in a small Chinese pedigree (Basset *et al.*, 1988) led to linkage studies looking for evidence for a 'schizophrenic locus' on chromosome 5 (Kennedy *et al.*, 1988; Sherrington *et al.*, 1988). More recently, co-segregation of balanced translocations involving 11q and major psychiatric disorders have been reported (Holland and Gosden, 1990; St. Clair *et al.*, 1990), suggesting an etiologically important gene on 11q. There is evidence to suggest that chromosomal abnormalities in general are more common in psychiatric patients than in the general population (Wahlstrom *et al.*, 1989).

Molecular genetics

It is now possible to study DNA directly due to the development of recombinant DNA technology (Old and Primrose, 1989). Recombinant DNA is produced by inserting a fragment of foreign DNA into 'vectors' such as circular plasmid or cosmid DNA; the inserted fragment is multiplied as the vector replicates itself in bacteria. Specific DNA fragments can also be amplified enzymatically by DNA polymerase, in a series of reactions known as the polymerase chain reaction (Erlich, 1989).

The discovery in bacteria of restriction enzymes, which cleave DNA at sequence specific sites like chemical scissors, has made it possible to break down a very long DNA molecule into manageable fragments (Smith, 1979). Two single-stranded DNA fragments whose base sequences are complementary will, under certain conditions, hybridize with (i.e. 'stick to') each other to form a double-strand. The presence of a particular DNA fragment can therefore be detected by a complementary strand which has been rendered radioactive, often referred to as a probe.

If the DNA of an individual is broken down by a restriction enzyme and the fragments separated according to size by electrophoresis, a probe can be used to find out whether a particular sequence is present, and the lengths of the fragments which it occupies (Southern, 1975). Chromosomes vary in their base sequence, so that they also vary in the number and locations of restriction enzyme cleaving sites, and the lengths of the fragments containing a DNA sequence. The variations in fragment lengths, called restriction enzyme fragment length poly-morphisms (RFLPs), are inherited along with the chromosomes in a Mendelian fashion, and so can be used as genetic markers for linkage and association studies (Botstein *et al.*, 1980). Thousands of RFLPs have already been discovered in the human genome (Human Gene Mapping 9.5, 1988), thereby giving a vast selection of markers.

Physical gene mapping

A gene of known sequence (Hindley, 1983) can be mapped to its position on the chromosomes by a DNA probe containing its complementary sequence. This method, called *in situ* hybridization, was used in the localization of the dopamine D2 receptor gene to the long arm of chromosome 11 at 11q22-23 (Grandy *et al.*, 1989).

Another method of physical mapping, called somatic cell hybridization (Puck and Kao, 1982), is based on the observation that, when human cells are fused with mouse cells, the hybrid cells tend to lose some of the human chromosomes in subsequent cell divisions. It is possible to influence which chromosomes are conserved by using mouse cells with various genetic defects. The chromosome on which a gene is located can then be deduced from the expression of the gene in a panel of such hybrid cells, or the use of a probe on DNA from these cells.

These methods generally require some knowledge about the products of the gene to be localized. The study of proteins and mRNA in the brain tissue of patients and controls may reveal abnormalities which may lead to the localization of the defective gene. This approach involving the localization of genes from knowledge of their protein products is called 'forward genetics'.

Linkage

When the protein product of a gene is unknown, another approach to gene localization, called 'reverse genetics', is often used. This approach is particularly attractive in those psychiatric conditions where a genetic contribution has been established but its nature is unknown. The first step is to establish linkage of the gene with a genetic marker. As we have seen, a recombination fraction of less than $\frac{1}{2}$ implies that two genes are 'linked' on the same chromosome. Moreover, the smaller the recombination fraction, the more closely the two genes are situated. Thus, if a disorder is linked to a genetic marker of known location, then a locus on the same chromosome must be contributing to the disorder. Obviously, the smaller the recombination fraction, the nearer the disorder locus is to the marker gene. The recombination fraction is usually studied indirectly through the pattern of co-segregation of the disorder and the genetic marker in pedigrees.

Lod-score method. Having assessed members of pedigrees with regard to a disorder and a marker, a statistical method to assess the probability of linkage is necessary. The most widely used method of linkage analysis, as in segregation analysis, is based on the theory of likelihood. However, the parameter to be estimated is now the recombination fraction, while the genetic models and parameters (including gene frequencies and penetrances) of the disorder and the genetic marker are taken as known parameters. Under these assumptions, the likelihood of the observed data is calculated for various values of recombination fraction (θ) in the permissible range of 0 to 1/2. The Lod (*log* of the *od*ds) scores for various values of θ are then defined as:

$$\text{Lod} \ (\theta = \theta_1) \ = \ \log_{10} \frac{L(\theta = \theta_1)}{L(\theta = \frac{1}{2})}$$

where L represents likelihood and θ_1 is a series of values between 0 and $\frac{1}{2}$. The maximum likelihood estimate of θ, denoted as θ^*, is that value of θ with the highest likelihood and hence the highest Lod score. A well established criterion for significant linkage requires the Lod score at $\theta = \theta^*$ to be greater than 3 (Morton, 1955).

A Lod score of 3 means that the observed familial data are 1000 times more likely to have arisen under linkage than under no linkage (since $\log_{10} 1000 = 3$). This seemingly stringent criterion is necessary to keep the probability of falsely inferring linkage at less than the conventional level of $\frac{1}{20}$, since it can be estimated from the number and lengths of human chromosomes that, if two loci are selected at random, the probability of linkage is about $\frac{1}{50}$. In betting terms, we start with the odds of about 50 : 1 against linkage, but after observing data with a Lod score of 3, we change the odds to about 20 : 1 in favour of linkage. A similar argument applies for the rejection of linkage, so that a Lod score of less than -2 is taken as sufficient evidence for excluding linkage. If the Lod score lies between -2 and $+3$, then we do not have sufficient evidence either to conclude or reject linkage, and more familial data are needed.

When data on several loci are available in the same families, the loci can be analysed together so that their relative positions can be estimated to give a 'multipoint map' (Pascoe and Morton, 1987). When such a map is available, a disorder can be tested for linkage to several markers simultaneously, giving extra statistical power (Lathrop *et al.*, 1985).

Since the appropriate genetic models and parameters of most major psychiatric disorders are unclear, they cannot be specified with certainty for linkage analysis. It has been claimed that the effect of model mis-specification is usually to decrease the power for detecting linkage, rather than to increase the chance of a falsely inferring linkage (Clerget-Darpoux *et al.*, 1986a). However, if the Lod score is maximized by employing a variety of different parameter values (e.g. penetrances), then this can give rise to false positive results. Under these circumstances, a Lod score of 3 is not a sufficiently stringent criterion. Furthermore, if linkage analysis is repeated for many different markers, then the chance of falsely inferring linkage is again increased, and it has been advocated that the Lod score for inferring linkage should be increased accordingly (Edwards and Watt, 1989). These methodological issues have been thrown into prominence by the claims of linkage of schizophrenia to chromosome 5 markers (Sherrington *et al.*, 1988), and of manic depression to chromosome 11 markers (Egeland *et al.*, 1987). The former claim has not been replicated (Kennedy *et al.*, 1988; St. Clair *et al.*, 1989; Detera-Wadleigh *et al.*, 1989; Crowe *et al.*, 1990), and the latter has been retracted by the original group, after further study of the pedigrees (Kelsoe *et al.*, 1989).

Sib-pair method. As Kelsoe *et al.* (1989) have shown in their study on manic-depression, the Lod score method is very sensitive to diagnostic errors. Thus, the Lod score may be excessively influenced by a few individuals occupying 'key positions' in the pedigree. If these individuals are incorrectly diagnosed, then false inferences about linkage can be made. A possibly more 'robust' method of linkage analysis is the sib-pair method (Penrose, 1935). The principle of this method is that, if a disorder and a genetic marker are not linked, then whether pairs of siblings are alike with respect to the disorder will be independent of whether they are alike with respect to the marker; on the other hand, if the disorder and the marker are linked, then we expect there to be an excess of sib-pairs alike or unlike for both disorder and marker, and a relative deficit of sib-pairs alike for disorder but unlike for the marker and vice versa.

The original sib-pair method has the advantage that the genetic model or parameters do not have to be specified. Furthermore, no data on parents are necessary. Howrver, this simplicity is achieved at the expense of some loss of power, since information on parents and other family members should clearly be utilized if it is available. Also, if the disorder is not fully penetrant, some sib-pairs alike with respect to the genetic predisposition for the disorder will be erroneously classified as being unlike. A modification of the sib-pair method, called the affected sib-pair method (Suarez *et al.*, 1978), remedies some of these problems. A sib-pair may share 0, 1 or 2 of the genes at any locus. For example, consider a pair of sibs whose genotypes are the same, Aa; and whose parents have genotypes AA and Aa. It is obvious that gene a of the sib-pair must have descended from gene a of the second parent (we say that gene a is identical by descent); whereas gene A need not necessarily have descended from the same A gene of the first parent, since he/she has two A genes. From this example, it is clear that identity by descent cannot always be established with certainty. However, there will be fewer ambiguous cases if the marker locus can have many different alleles (i.e. highly polymorphic), so that the chance of parents carrying more than one copy of an allele is small. For sibs, we expect on average 1 of the 2 genes at any locus to be identical by descent. However, if both members of a sib-pair have the disorder, and if the disorder is linked to a marker locus, then we expect on average more than 1 of the 2 genes at the marker locus to be identical by descent. From a sample of affected sib-pairs, the total number of genes identical by descent at a marker locus can be counted, and tested against the expected number on the null hypothesis of no linkage.

Association

Consider a locus with alleles A,a and a second locus with alleles B,b. We say that allele A is associated with allele B if individuals with allele A have allele B with probability greater than expected from the gene frequency of B. In meiosis, recombinations ensure the 'reshuffling' of genes, so that associations between alleles in one generation tend to diminish in subsequent generations. However, for closely situated loci, recombinations are rare, and associations tend to persist for many generations. This phenomenon is sometimes known as linkage disequilibrium. Thus, if a disorder is associated with an allele at a marker locus, then we should consider the possibility that there is a gene predisposing to the disorder near the marker locus. However, there are other causes of association, which must also be considered. For example, if both the disorder and the allele are more common in a particular large ethnic group than in the rest of the population, then the disorder and the allele will have an apparent association in the entire population, even though no such association exists within the ethnic group or the rest of the population. Of course, another explanation of association is that the allele has a causal role to the disorder.

One problem of using association studies is that, because only close linkage leads to appreciable association, the prior probability that any randomly chosen locus is associated with the disorder is very small. Thus, either we use a very stringent criterion before accepting association, or there will be many false positive results. Association studies are probably more useful for loci for which we have reason to believe may be involved in the disorder (i.e. 'candidate loci').

Identifying, characterizing and elucidating the function of the genetic defect

Having discovered a genetic marker closely linked to a disorder, the next step is to identify the disorder gene itself. This can be a difficult task, since even very closely linked markers are very far apart on the molecular scale. For example, a genetic distance of 1 map unit (i.e. a recombination fraction of 0.01) is roughly equivalent to 10^6 base pairs. In order to search for the disorder gene in the vicinity of its linked marker, a series of overlapping DNA fragments (of about 50 000 base pairs each) can be produced and examined, starting from a fragment containing the marker itself. This method of 'chromosome walking' gives a 'library' of DNA fragments, one of which may contain the defective gene. These fragments can thus be examined for potential gene sequences, for example, by screening the fragments against cDNA libraries (DNA produced by reverse transcription from mRNA) or by sequencing the fragments and looking for a sequence which would start transcription. Any gene sequence identified can be studied further to see if it is the disorder gene. This approach has been successful in identifying the gene for cystic fibrosis (Kerem et al., 1989, Riordan et al., 1989; Rommens et al., 1989).

Once the defective gene is identified, then the structure and function of the protein it codes for can be studied. This may help us to understand the pathogenesis of the disorder.

Clinical Applications

The practical impact of genetics on medicine has so far been largely confined to genetic counselling and prenatal diagnosis. A few genetic disorders can now be treated effectively by environmental manipulation. For example, the severe mental retardation of phenylketonuria can be prevented by restricting dietary phenylalanine from birth. However, for most other genetic disorders, such as the haemoglobinopathies, effective treatment has yet to be developed, despite the fact that the molecular genetics of these disorders is now well understood (Weatherall, 1985). Current research on the direct genetic manipulation of somatic cells or germ cells (gene therapy) may revolutionize the treatment of genetic disorders, although the ethics of such treatment are still controversial (Susuki and Knudtson, 1988). Progress in the genetics of psychiatric disorders has lagged behind that of physical conditions, but we believe that, with further progress, genetic knowledge will eventually contribute to effective prevention and treatment of psychiatric disorders.

References

American Psychiatric Association (1980). *Diagnostic and Statistical Manual of Mental Disorder*, 3rd edn. Washington DC: American Psychiatric Association.

Andreasen, N.C., Rice, J., Endicott, J., Reich, T. and Coryell, W. (1986). The family history approach to diagnosis: How useful is it? *Arch. Gen. Psychiat.* **43**, 421–429.

Baron, M., Risch, N., Hamburger, R. *et al.* (1987). Genetic linkage between X chromosomal markers and bipolar affective illness. *Nature* **326**, 289–292.

Bassett, A.S., McGillivray, B.C., Jones, B.D. and Pantzer, J.T. (1988). Partial trisomy chromosome 5 co-segregating with schizophrenia. *Lancet* **i**, 799–801.

Bateson, W., Saunders, E.R. and Punnet, R.C. (1905). Experimental studies in the physiology of heredity. *Rep. Evol. Comm. R. Soc.* **2**, 1–131.

Botstein, D., White, R.L. and Skolnick, M. (1980). Construction of a genetic linkage map in man using restriction fragment length polymorphisms. *Am. J. Hum. Genet.* **32**, 314–331.

Clerget-Darpoux, F., Bonaiti-Pellie, C. and Hochez, J. (1986a). Effects of misspecifying genetic parameters in lod score analysis. *Biometrics* **42**, 393–399.

Clerget-Darpoux, F., Goldin, L.R. and Gershon, E.S. (1986b). Clinical methods in psychiatric research III: Environmental stratification may simulate a genetic effect in adoption studies. *Acta Psychiatr. Scand.* **74**, 305–311.

Creasy, M.R., Crolla, J.A. and Alberman, E.D. (1976). A cytogenetic study of human spontaneous abortions using banding techniques. *Hum. Genet.* **31**, 177–196.

Crick, F.H.C. (1962). The genetic code. *Scient. Am.*, October.

Crowe, R.R., Black, D.W., Andreasen, N. and Huether, M. (1990). The Iowa Multiplex family study of schizophrenia.: linkage analysis on chromosome 5. *Eur. Arch. Psychiatry Neurol. Sci.* **239**(5), 290–292.

Detera-Wadleigh, S.D., Goldin, L.R. and Sherrington, R. (1989). Exclusion of linkage to 5q11-13 in families with schizophrenia and other psychiatric disorders. *Nature* **340**, 391–393.

Donahue, R.P., Bias, W.B. and Renwick, J.H. (1968). Probable assignment of the Duffy blood-group gene to chromosome 1 in man. *Proc. Natl. Acad. Sci. USA* **61**, 949.

Dorman, J.S., Trucco, M., LaPorte, R. and Kuller, L.H. (1988). Family studies: the key to understanding genetic and environmental etiology of chronic disease? *Genet. Epidemiol.* **5**, 305–310.

Eaves, L.J., Eysenck, H.J. and Martin, N.G. (1989). *Genes, Culture and Personality*. London: Academic Press.

Edwards, J.H. and Watt, D.C. (1989). Caution in locating the gene(s) for affective disorder. *Psychol. Med.* **19**, 273–275.

Egeland, J.A., Gerhard, D.S., Pauls, D.L. *et al.* (1987). Bipolar affective disorder linked to DNA markers on chromosome 11. *Nature* **325**, 783–787.

Elston, R.C. and Boklage, C.E. (1978). An examination of fundamental assumptions of the twin method. In: W.E. Nance (ed.) *Twin Research: Psychology and Methodology*, pp. 189–200. New York: Alan Liss.

Elston, R.C. and Stewart, J. (1971). A general model for the analysis of pedigree data. *Hum. Hered.* **21**, 523–542.

Erlich, H.A. (1989). *PCR Technology: Principles and Applications for DNA Amplification*. New York: Stockton Press.

Endicott, J. and Spitzer, R.L. (1978). A diagnostic interview: the schedule for affective disorders and schizophrenia. *Arch. Gen. Psychiat.* **35**, 837–844.

Eysenck, H.J. and Kamin, L. (1981). *Intelligence: The Babble for the Mind*. London: Pan Paperbacks.

Falconer, D.S. (1965). The inheritance of liability to certain diseases, estimated from the incidence among relatives. *Ann. Hum. Genet.* **29**, 51–76.

Falconer, D.S. (1989). *Introduction to Quantitative Genetics*. New York: Longman Scientific & Technical.

Fisher, R.A. (1918). The correlation between relatives on the supposition of Mendelian inheritance. *Trans. R. Soc. Edinburgh* **52**, 399–433.

Galton, F. (1889). *Natural Inheritance*. London: Macmillan.

Goldin, L.R., Nurnberger, J.I. and Gershon, E.S. (1986). Clinical methods in psychiatric genetics II: The high risk approach. *Acta Psychiatr. Scand.* **74**, 119–128.

Grandy, D.K., Litt, M. and Allen, L. (1989). The human dopamine D2 receptor gene is located on chromosome 11 at q22-q23 and identifies a taq1 RFLP. *Am. J. Hum. Genet.* **45**, 778–785.

Hindley, J. (1983). *DNA Sequencing: Laboratory Techniques in Biochemistry and Molecular Biology*. Amsterdam: Elsevier Science Publishers.

Holland, A. and Gosden, C. (1990). A balanced chromosomal translocation partially cosegregating with psychotic illness in a family. *Psychiat. Res.* **32**, 1–8.

Human Gene Mapping 9.5 (1988). Update to the Ninth International Workshop on Human Gene Mapping. *Cytogenet. Cell Genet.* **49**, 1–260.

Kelsoe, J.R., Ginns, E.I., Egeland, J.A. *et al.* (1989). Re-evaluation of linkage relationship between chromosome 11p loci and the gene for bipolar affective disorder in the Old Order Amish. *Nature* **342**, 238–243.

Kendler, K.S., Gruenberg, A.M. and Strauss, J.S. (1984). An independent analysis of the Danish adoption study of schizophrenia IV. *Arch. Gen. Psychiat.* **38**, 982–984.

Kennedy, J.L., Giuffra, L.A., Moises, H.W. *et al.* (1988). Evidence against linkage of schizophrenia to markers on chromosome 5 in a Swedish pedigree. *Nature* **336**, 167–169.

Kerem, B., Rommens, J.M., Buchanan, J.A. *et al.* (1989). Identification of the cystic fibrosis gene: genetic analysis. *Science* **245**, 1073–1080.

Lathrop, G.M., Lalouel, J.M., Julier, C. and Ott, J. (1985). Multilocus linkage analysis in humans: detection of linkage and estimation of recombination. *Am. J. Hum. Genet.* **37**, 482–498.

Lyon, M. (1968). Chromosomal and subchromosomal inactivation. *Ann. Rev. Genet.* **2**, 31–52.

Maclean, N., Gregory, S.P. and Flavell, R.A. (1983). *Eukaryotic Genes: Their Structure, Activity and Regulation.* London: Butterworths.

McGuffin, P., Farmer, A.E., Gottesman, I.I. *et al.* (1984). Twin concordance for operationally defined schizophrenia: confirmation of familiality and heritability. *Arch. Gen. Psychiat.* **41**, 541–545.

McKeon, P. and Murray, R.M. (1986). Familial aspects of obsessive–compulsive neurosis. *Br. J. Psychiatry* **151**, 528–534.

McKusick, V. (1988). *Medelian Inheritance in Man,* 8th edn. Baltimore, MD: Johns Hopkins University Press.

Mather, K. and Jinks, J.L. (1982). *Biometrical Genetics.* London: Chapman and Hall.

Matthysse, S., Holzman, P.S. and Lange, K. (1986). The genetic transmission of schizophrenia: application of Mendelian latent structure analysis to eye-tracking dysfunctions in schizophrenia and affective disorder. *J. Psychiat. Res.* **20**, 57–76.

Morton, N.E. (1955). Sequence tests for the detection of linkage. *Am. J. Hum. Genet.* **7**, 277–318.

Morton, N.E. (1956). The detection and estimation of linkage between the genes for elliptocytosis and the Rh blood type. *Am. J. Hum. Genet.* **8**, 80–96.

Morton, N.E. and McLean, C. (1974). Analysis of family resemblance III. Complex segregation of quantitative traits. *Am. J. Hum. Genet.* **26**, 489–503.

Nussbaum, R.L. and Ledbetter, D.H. (1986). Fragile X syndrome: a unique mutation in man. *Ann. Rev. Genet.* **20**, 109–145.

Old, R. and Primrose, S.B. (1989). *Principles of Gene Manipulation,* 4th edn. Oxford: Blackwell Scientific.

Ott, J. (1986). *Introduction to Human Linkage Analysis.* Baltimore, MD: Johns Hopkins University Press.

Pascoe, L. and Morton, N.E. (1987). The use of map functions in multipoint mapping. *Am. J. Hum. Genet.* **40**, 174–183.

Pearson, K. (1904). On the laws of inheritance in man II. *Biometrika* **3**, 131–190.

Penrose, L.S. (1935). The detection of autosomal linkage in data which consist of pairs of brothers and sisters of unspecified parentage. *Ann. Eugenics* **6**, 133–138.

Puck, T.T. and Kao, F.T. (1982). Somatic cell genetics and its applications to medicine. *Ann. Rev. Genet.* **16**, 225–272.

Reich, T., Cloninger, C.R., Wette, R. and James, J. (1979). The use of multiple thresholds and segregation analysis in analyzing the phenotypic heterogeneity of multifactorial traits. *Ann. Hum. Genet.* **42,** 371–390.

Rommens, J.M., Iannuzzi, M.C., Kerem, B. *et al.* (1989). Identification of the cystic fibrosis gene: chromosome walking and jumping. *Science* **245,** 1059–1065.

Rosenthal, D. (1970). *Genetic Theory and Abnormal Behaviour.* New York: McGraw Hill.

Riordan, J.R., Rommens, J.M., Kerem, B. *et al.* (1989). Identification of the cystic fibrosis gene: cloning and characterization of complementary DNA. *Science* **245,** 1066–1073.

Shapiro, J.A. (1983). *Mobile Genetic Elements.* New York: Academic Press.

Sherrington, R., Brynjolfsson, F., Petursson, H. *et al.* (1988). Localizations of a susceptibility locus for schizophrenia in chromosome 5. *Nature* **336,** 164–167.

Slater, E. and Cowie, V. (1971). *The Genetics of Mental Disorders.* Oxford: Oxford University Press.

Smith, C.A.B. (1963). Testing for heterogeneity of recombination fraction values in human genetics. *Ann. Hum. Genet.* **27,** 175–182.

Smith, H.O. (1979). Nucleotide sequence specificity of restriction endonucleases. *Science* **205,** 455–462.

Southern, E.M. (1975). Detection of specific sequences among DNA fragments separated by gel electrophoresis. *J. Mol. Biol.* **98,** 503–517.

Spitzer, R.L., Endicott, J. and Robins, E. (1975). *Research Diagnostic Critera.* New York: Biometrics Research, New York State Psychiatric Institute.

St. Clair, D., Blackwood, D., Muir, W. *et al.* (1989). No linkage of chromosome 5q11–13 markers to schizophrenia in Scottish families. *Nature* **339,** 305–309.

St. Clair, D., Blackwood, D., Muir, W., *et al.* (1990). Association within a family of a balanced autosomal translocation with major mental illness. *Lancet* **336,** 13–16.

St. George-Hyslop, P., Tanzi, R. and Polinsky, R. (1987). The genetic defect causing familial Alzheimer's disease maps on chromosome 21. *Science* **235,** 885–889.

Stigler, S.M. (1989). Francis Galton's account of the invention of correlation. *Stat. Sci.* **4,** 73–86.

Stromgren, E. (1950). Statistical and genetical population studies with psychiatry: methods and principal results. Congrès International de Psychiatrie, 6, Paris, pp. 155–188.

Sturtvant, A.H. (1965). *A History of genetics.* New York: Harper and Row.

Suarez, B.K., Rice, J. and Reich, T. (1978). The generalized sib pair IBD distribution: its use in the detection of linkage. *Am. J. Hum. Genet.* **42,** 87–94.

Susuki, D. and Knudtson, P. (1988). *Genethics, The Ethics of Engineering Life.* London: Unwin Hyman.

Sutherland, G.R., Hecht, F., Mulley, J., *et al.* (1985). *Heritable Fragile Sites on Human Chromosomes.* New York: Oxford University Press.

Wahlstrom, J., Axelsson, R. and Johannesson, T. (1989). Chromosome aberrations as tools for gene mapping. In: L. Wetterberg (ed.) *Genetics of Neuropsychiatric Diseases.* London: Macmillan.

Watson, J.D. and Crick, F.H.C. (1953). Molecular structure of nucleic acids. *Nature* **171,** 737–738.

Weatherall, D.J. (1985). *The New Genetics and Clinical Practice.* Oxford: Oxford University Press.

Weisseman, M.M., Merigangas, K.R., John, K. *et al.* (1986). Family-genetic studies of psychiatric disorders. *Arch. Gen. Psychiat.* **43,** 1105–1116.

Wing, J.K., Cooper, J.E. and Sartorius, N. (1974). *Measurement and Classification of Psychiatric Symptoms.* Cambridge: Cambridge University Press.

— 13

The Genetics of Psychiatric Syndromes

C.J.A. Taylor, A.M. Macdonald and R.M. Murray

In the previous chapter, Sham *et al.* reviewed the basic genetic principles of relevance to psychiatry. Here we describe how these principles have been applied to the various psychiatric syndromes, together with the resulting advances in our understanding of their inheritance. The chapter begins with an examination of those neuropsychiatric conditions (such as Huntington's Disease) where the approximate chromosomal location of the responsible gene is known. There follows a discussion of the functional psychoses, where a genetic contribution is proven but the mode of transmission unknown, and of the neurotic conditions where any genetic component is either uncharacterized (as in the anxiety disorders) or absent (as in conversion hysteria).

We wish to emphasize at the beginning that it is not the function of psychiatric geneticists to prove a role for nature over nurture. Rather, they seek to establish whether hereditary factors contribute to the development of the disorder in question, and if so, how these interact with any relevant environmental influences. Indeed, paradoxically, genetic studies have been of great significance in discovering the etiological importance of an adverse environment, sometimes enabling genetic effects to be discounted altogether.

It is also important to recognise that at present psychiatric disorders are largely classified according to their clinical presentation rather than etiology. It is quite possible, for example, that what we currently regard as schizophrenia may have no more permanence than dropsy, and that genetic studies might contribute to the delineation of more discrete disorders. In the meantime, however, geneticists can only work within the constraints of present day knowledge. This chapter is therefore entitled 'The Genetics of Psychiatric Syndromes'. For more detailed discussions of the state of current research, the interested reader is referred to recent specialist publications (e.g. Owen and Murray, 1989; McGuffin and Murray, 1991).

Huntington's Chorea

Huntington's chorea (HC) is a progressive neurodegenerative disease inherited as an autosomal dominant trait. It provides an interesting model for some of the issues that may arise as developments in genetic epidemiology and molecular genetics increase our understanding of the hereditary component of the etiology of other psychiatric disorders. Although penetrance in HC is complete (i.e. all those with the disease gene will develop the illness), the age of onset is delayed until between the third and fifth decade of life. Hence, sons and daughters of individuals affected by HC may reach adulthood (and have their own children) before it is discovered that they themselves have HC, and consequently, that the chance that each of their offspring may have inherited the mutant gene is 50%. So although the prevalence of HC is low, with only about 6000 people in the UK being affected, there are another 50 000 at risk of developing it.

Despite numerous searches for a peripheral biochemical abnormality and studies of post-mortem brain tissue, the biochemical defect in HC remains unknown. Before the advent of the new molecular genetic techniques, the search for the gene mutation had not been fruitful, although classical linkage studies had excluded about 20% of the genome. In the early 1980s, Gusella *et al.* (1983) began a systematic linkage study using polymorphic DNA markers. They were able to study two large multiply affected kindreds, one in Venezuela and another in the USA. Quite by chance, one of the first probes they used identified a polymorphism on the short arm of chromosome 4 which was linked to the disease in these pedigrees. The disease gene for HC is now known to be very close to the tip of chromosome 4. This has made it difficult to localize precisely, as the usual way of pin-pointing a gene is to find new markers close to, but on either side of it. Since Gusella's discovery other, more tightly linked markers have been identified proximal (nearer the centromere) to the locus (Hayden *et al.*, 1988), but the chances of randomly isolating distal probes are small. It is likely that the much slower process of physically mapping the region will be required before the gene can be precisely identified.

The identification of tightly linked markers has, however, enabled pre-symptomatic testing of many of those at risk. Several programmes have been set up in the UK and the USA offering this service. At the present time, there must be sufficient older, living relatives to establish which allele at the marker locus is linked to the disease gene in the particular family. Ideally, DNA should be available either from both parents and one grandparent, or from two close relatives of the affected parent, who are either definitely affected or well past the age at risk. It has been estimated (Craufurd, 1989) that only about 40% of adults at risk have these key relatives living. Additionally, the marker must be informative (i.e. sufficiently polymorphic) in the family. In practice, this is almost always the case, given the current availability of several tightly linked markers. Assuming these two criteria are satisfied, and that all key relatives agree to testing, the margin of error in pre-symptomatic testing is about 2%, allowing for the possibility of recombination (Craufurd, 1989). Obviously, a test which potentially identifies one as the future victim of such a devastating disease is not to be undergone lightly. All families are offered pre-test information and counselling, and regular follow-up and psychological support afterwards (Brandt *et al.*, 1989). By no means all 'at risk' individuals wish to undergo testing.

Pre-natal exclusion testing is an alternative option for 'at risk' couples who plan to have children. In such cases, when pregnancy is established, amniocentesis is used to provide material allowing linked markers to be used to test whether the gene inherited by the fetus from the 'at risk' parent was donated by the unaffected or affected grandparent. The risk to the offspring would be either low (although not zero because of the possibility of recombination) or almost 50% (i.e. the same as the 'at risk' parent), respectively. In the latter case the parents have the option of requesting termination of pregnancy, although of course there is a 50% chance that the fetus is in fact unaffected. However, should the pregnancy remain unterminated and the 'at risk' parent subsequently become ill, the risk to that child would then rise to nearly 100%. The fact that he or she has undergone pre-symptomatic testing without being able to give informed consent presents a difficult ethical dilemma.

Once the disease gene is identified, accurate pre-natal testing will become a possibility, enabling parents to terminate affected pregnancies only, if they so wish. Given the very low rate of spontaneous mutation in HC, this, together with adequate genetic counselling, could lead to a dramatic fall in the prevalence of the illness. Whether this actually proves to be the case depends, of course, on the take-up rates of these services by families carrying the mutant gene (Holloway and Smith, 1975).

Alzheimer's Disease

The cause of Alzheimer's disease remains unknown, but two lines of evidence suggested that genetic factors might be important: first, the results of family and twin studies and second, the observation that all individuals with Down's syndrome who live long enough develop a dementing disorder with neuro-pathological changes identical to those in Alzheimer's disease.

Classical genetic studies

Individuals with a positive family history of Alzheimer's disease are known to be at increased risk of developing the illness themselves (Heyman et al., 1984). Although many cases appear to be sporadic, some large pedigrees have been reported where familial patterns of the disorder seem to be consistent with autosomal dominant inheritance (e.g. Nee et al., 1983). Such pedigrees have been called 'familial Alzheimer's disease' (FAD), or 'early onset' families, because the age at first presentation tends to be between 45 and 65 years. In a study of relatives of probands ascertained on the basis of autopsy data, Heston et al. (1981) estimated that the cumulative incidence of Alzheimer's disease in members of early onset families approaches 50% by 90 years of age. Again, this is consistent with autosomal dominant inheritance.

Such clear evidence of inherited factors is less easy to find in late onset families. Some authors (Breitner et al., 1986) believe that the majority of cases are genetic, but that the greatest likelihood of gene expression is in the ninth decade. Thus a genetic case may appear sporadic because relatives have died of other causes before the disease becomes clinically apparent. On the other hand, non-genetic cases may appear familial if they cluster in individual families, which is to be expected to occur by chance in such a common disease. It is possible that many cases are the result of an interaction between genetic and environmental influences, as is supported by reports of both concordant (Cook *et al.*, 1981) and discordant (Hunter *et al.*, 1972) identical (MZ) twin pairs.

Little is known about environmental factors which may play an etiological role. One possible risk factor is a high concentration of aluminium in drinking water. In an epidemiological survey of 88 country districts in England and Wales, Martyn *et al.* (1989) estimated rates of Alzheimer's disease in those under 70 years of age from CT scan data. These authors claimed that individuals living in districts with higher mean water aluminium concentrations (measured over the previous 10 years) had a one-and-a-half times greater risk of developing the disease.

Association with Down's syndrome

The association of dementia with Down's syndrome was noted over 100 years ago; more recently Heston (1977) argued from post-mortem data that all those with Down's syndrome who live beyond the age of 35 have the neuro-pathological features of Alzheimer's disease. Furthermore, there is an increased incidence of Down's syndrome in relatives of those with Alzheimer's disease (Heston *et al.*, 1981). These strands of evidence led to the suggestion that the locus for FAD was on chromosome 21 (Oliver and Holland, 1986).

This notion was supported by St. George-Hyslop *et al.* (1987), who found linkage of the disorder to two markers on the long arm of chromosome 21 in four multiply affected families. Although neither marker was on the 'obligate' Down's region (on the distal part of the long arm of chromosome 21), an etiological link between the disorders is still likely, given that most Down's individuals have the whole chromosome in triplicate. In the same year, the A-4 amyloid gene was also localized to this region of the chromosome (Tanzi *et al.*, 1987a). However, the reasonable hypothesis that a defect in the A-4 amyloid gene is responsible for Alzheimer's disease (given that an abundance of cortical amyloid plaques is a histopathological hallmark of the illness) has not been supported by linkage studies (Van Broekhoven *et al.*, 1987; Tanzi *et al.*, 1987b). Owen *et al.* (1990) provided evidence that the FAD locus lies nearer the centromere of chromosome 21 than the A-4 amyloid gene.

Two other studies (Roses *et al.*, 1988; Schellenberg *et al.*, 1988) have failed to replicate the linkage of FAD to chromosome 21, leading to the suggestion that FAD may be genetically heterogeneous (Pericak-Vance *et al.*, 1988). Some (but not all) of the families in these studies are descended from the Volga Germans, a group who migrated from Germany to two small neighbouring towns on the Volga river in the Soviet Union, and subsequently to the United States. Goate *et al.* (1989), amongst others, have argued that data from these studies is consistent with chromosome 21 linkage in the early onset families, if they are considered as a separate group from the Volga German and late onset families.

Affective Disorder

Disturbance of mood is ubiquitous; indeed, one recent community study (Bebbington *et al.*, 1989) claimed that 70% of women and over 40% of men will have experienced clinically significant symptoms of depression by the time they are 65 years of age. It is, of course, highly likely that such a common disorder, with its variable clinical presentation, is etiologically heterogeneous; it might be expected that any genetic influence will be more important in more severe forms of the disorder.

Classical genetic studies

Family studies

Most recent family studies of affective disorder are based on Leonhard's division of the illness into bipolar (BP) and unipolar (UP) subtypes. Generally, the results show an excess of both types of affective disorder in the families of BP probands. Thus the morbid risk of BP illness to first degree relatives of BP probands is nearly 8% and of UP illness is over 11%. On the other hand, relatives of UP probands are at increased risk of UP illness only, with a morbid risk of about 9% overall (McGuffin and Katz, 1986). In comparison, the lifetime risk in the general population for BP disorder is less than 1% and for UP disorder about 3% (Reich et al., 1982). While it is true that the degree of familial aggregation of illness varies widely between studies, this is probably partly due to the use of different diagnostic criteria, and to differences in lifetime risk of affective illness in the populations from which the study samples were drawn.

Twin studies

Most twin studies agree that MZ twin concordance rates are some 2.5–5 times greater than those seen in DZ pairs, thus providing further evidence for an hereditary component (e.g. Gershon et al., 1976; Torgersen, 1986). MZ twins are rarely reared apart, but this form of natural experiment does control for the fact that a 'special twin environment' might contribute to both twins becoming ill. Of the 12 reared-apart pairs with at least one affected twin identified by Price (1968) from the world literature, eight (67%) were concordant for affective illness. This figure agrees so closely with the concordance rates for MZ twins reared together, as to suggest that this specific type of environmental factor contributes little. It also lends validity to the use of the twin method with reared-together twins since it appears that the assumptions of the twin method are not violated (see Sham et al., Chapter 12, this volume).

Adoption studies

Mendlewicz and Rainer (1977) compared illness rates in the biological and adoptive parents of BP adoptees. The biological parents had significantly higher rates of affective illness than the adoptive ones (Table 13.1). The ill biological parents were more likely to suffer from UP than BP illness, a finding confirmed by Wender et al. (1986). These workers found a significant excess of UP disorder and suicide in the biological relatives of affectively ill adoptees, compared with adoptive relatives and the relatives of a control group of normal adoptees.

TABLE 13.1 Rates of affective illness in biological and adoptive parents of bipolar adoptees (Mendlewicz and Rainer, 1977).

Adoptee	Affected biological parents (%)	Affected adoptive parents (%)
Bipolar ($N = 29$)	28	12
Normal ($N = 22$)	5	9

Subtypes of affective illness

Leonhard's original distinction between UP and BP disorder has been widely accepted, but in terms of the genetic component of their etiology, the two partly overlap. Thus, relatives of BP patients have an increased risk of developing both BP and UP illness. Furthermore, in their study of 46 MZ twin pairs concordant for affective disorder, Bertelsen *et al.* (1977) found that, while there was a tendency for proband and co-twin to have the same illness, in 10 pairs one twin had UP and the other BP illness.

These patterns of inheritance have been explained by postulating a continuum of liability to affective disorder (e.g. Taylor *et al.*, 1980; Gershon *et al.*, 1982, and Sham *et al.*, Chapter 12, this volume for an explanation of liability). BP disorder lies at the more severe end of the continuum (in terms of capacity to transmit illness within families). Gershon and colleagues proposed that schizoaffective disorder is a manifestation of the greatest vulnerability of all, on the basis of their findings from a family study of 1254 adult relatives of patients and controls. First degree relatives of probands with schizoaffective disorder had a lifetime prevalence of major affective disorder of 37%. This was greater not only than that found in relatives of normal controls, but also than that in relatives of probands with any other category of affective disorder.

Non-endogenous (neurotic) depression, on the other hand, lies at the opposite end of the continuum. McGuffin *et al.* (1987) reported that, when considering in-patient treatment only, the 7.9% morbid risk of illness in relatives of neurotic cases is only half that observed in relatives of endogenous cases (14.7%). The same authors estimated heritability (see Sham *et al.*, Chapter 12, this volume, for explanations of genetic terminology) at 86% for BP disorders, but only 8% for neurotic depression.

Gene-environment interaction

According to the theory of a continuum of genetic vulnerability, genetic factors are of most importance in schizoaffective (SA) illness and BP disorder, and least so in mild depression.

$\longrightarrow$*Increasing genetic vulnerability*

NORMAL   UP   BP   SA

Of the environmental contributions which might be important, there is now much evidence that significant adverse life-events are associated with the onset of depression (Brown and Harris, 1978).

Pollitt (1972) found that relatives of patients whose illness followed such a life-event have a lower morbid risk of depression than relatives of patients whose illness was 'non-reactive'. This finding was not replicated by McGuffin et al. (1988), who studied the families of 83 depressed patients. Indeed, the prevalence of illness in relatives of both classes of proband was roughly equal. Furthermore, the experience of life-events in these families was much higher than that found in a control sample drawn from the general population, though it was not significantly associated with the experience of a depressive illness in individual relatives. The authors concluded that the association between life-events and depression is more complex than that proposed by sociologists. Whether some predisposition to react to life-events is conferred by genetic means, or by the intra-familial culture, or whether the findings are artifactual, remains to be seen.

Mode of transmission

Given that a genetic basis to the severe forms of affective disorder has been established, considerable efforts have been made to identify its mode of trans-mission. Studies employing complex segregation analysis (see Sham et al., Chapter 12, this volume) have, in the main, been applied to BP probands and their families, but have failed to demonstrate the existence of a single major locus (SML). However, the possibility that such a locus could be operating against a multifactorial background has not been excluded (O'Rourke et al., 1983). Several reports have been made of pedigrees compatible with an incompletely dominant X-linked gene (e.g. Reich et al., 1969). Although the presence of male-to-male transmission excludes this mode of inheritance in most cases, such pedigrees may provide evidence for the existence of genetic heterogeneity in BP illness. For exmaple, Risch et al. (1986) suggested that one-third of cases of BP illness might be X-linked.

Linkage studies

Linkage studies using protein polymorphisms such as ABO groups, the rhesus system, red cell enzymes and histocompatibility antigens as autosomal markers, have not been productive. Application of the new molecular genetic techniques to multiply affected BP families has attracted considerable recent attention, but again, the results have been inconsistent. In 1987 a report was made by Egeland et al. of linkage between manic depression and two markers on the short arm of chromosome 11: the Harvey-ras oncogene and the insulin gene. The authors investigated a large branch of the Old Order Amish in Pennsylvania, USA whose close-knit kindred had the advantages of a lack of assortative mating and strong religious and cultural taboos against drug and alcohol abuse, thus making accurate diagnosis an easier task.

The result could not, however, be replicated in other North American pedigrees (Detera-Wadleigh et al., 1987), Icelandic families (Hodgkinson et al.,

TABLE 13.2   Morbid risk of schizophrenia to relatives.

Relationship	Proportion of genes shared with proband	Morbid risk
MZ co-twin	100%	40–50%
First degree relative (parent, child, sibling)	50%	6–12%
Second degree relative (grandchild, aunt, uncle)	25%	3–4%

1987) or an Irish family (Gill *et al.*, 1988). The initial explanation of this was that genetic heterogeneity of the illness must exist. More recently, however, doubt has been cast on the original Amish results, since reanalysis of the pedigree data after inclusion of further branches of the family, and allowing for changes in diagnosis in two individuals, reduced the final Lod score to below the level generally considered to be statistically significant (Kelsoe *et al.*, 1989).

Linkage of markers to the X chromosome is still a possibility. Evidence to suggest this had long been derived from studies using classical X-linked markers such as colour blindness (Mendlewicz *et al.*, 1972) and glucose-6-phsophate dehydrogenase (Mendlewicz *et al.*, 1980). Two more recent studies have supported the notion. Baron *et al.* (1987) found linkage between these two markers and BP illness in several Israeli families, and Mendlewicz *et al.* (1987) found linkage between the illness and the Factor IX gene, which is known to be on the X chromosome. M. Gill and D. Castle (pers. commun.) have also identified a pedigree in which affective illness and Christmas disease (caused by Factor IX deficiency) appear to co-segregate.

Schizophrenia

Classical genetic studies

Family studies

Almost all family studies have shown that the more closely related an individual is to a patient with schizophrenia, the greater his or her risk of also developing it. Using a broad definition of the illness, the morbid risk in the general population is about 0.8%, but increases to 3% in second degree relatives, and an average of 10% in first degree relatives (Table 13.2). The observed rate is somewhat lower in parents than in siblings, probably due to the fact that many severely affected individuals do not have children. The risk, however, to a child with two affected parents rises to as high as 40%.

In the early 1980s two groups of researchers (Pope *et al.*, 1982; Abrams and Taylor, 1983) challenged the evidence that schizophrenia is familial on the grounds that the older studies failed to make diagnoses 'blind' to the status of the proband, or according to operational criteria. In their studies, both claimed to find no familial aggregation of the illness, but each has in turn been criticized on methodological grounds. Pope *et al.* studied a very small sample and applied DSM-III criteria to family history data only, rather than conducting personal interviews with all relatives (Weissman *et al.*, 1983). Abrams and Taylor, on the other hand, were accused of using very narrow diagnostic criteria and no controls (Kety, 1983).

More recent methodologically sound studies have confirmed the familial aggregation of schizophrenia. Kendler *et al.* (1985), for example, compared rates of illness in 723 first degree relatives of probands and 1056 similar relatives of matched surgical controls. Diagnoses were made blind to the status of the proband, according to DSM-III criteria, and using information from direct personal interviews wherever possible. The risk for schizophrenia was 18 times greater in the relatives of probands than in relatives of controls. This increased risk was not confined to schizophrenia alone, but included schizoaffective, paranoid and atypical psychoses (though the majority were schizophrenic).

Familial aggregation of an illness does not, of course, confirm genetic transmission, and a variety of intra-familial environmental factors have been suggested as contributing to risk. These include the possibility that children learn an abnormal form of behaviour from their schizophrenic parents, or that familial transmission is via an infectious agent such as a virus (Crow, 1983).

Twin studies

Pooled data from five studies of schizophrenia give a concordance rate of 47% for the 261 MZ co-twins, and 14% in 329 same-sexed DZ pairs (Gottesman and Shields, 1982). None of these studies employed the current stringent criteria for diagnosis, but one series of systematically ascertained twins (Gottesman and Shields, 1972) has been reassessed by blind raters, applying a variety of operational criteria (McGuffin *et al.*, 1984; Farmer *et al.*, 1987). Those criteria which include longitudinal features of the illness (such as RDC, DSM-III or Feighner criteria) led to similar MZ and DZ concordance rates to those found in the older studies, and a heritability estimate for the illness of over 70%. Purely symptomatic criteria, i.e. Schneiderian first rank symptoms, on the other hand, were found not to differ significantly between MZ and DZ twins. The latter finding may have been an artifact due to the case summaries having been drawn up before first rank symptoms were considered important, and therefore the relevant information often being excluded.

However, Kendler (1989) has justifiably criticized such studies which attempt to find the 'most genetic' definition of the illness on the grounds that the twin concordance ratios are base rate sensitive; the small sample sizes give rise to large standard errors for the concordance ratio which are not usually reported.

It has been suggested that the higher concordance in identical twins is due to their parents treating them more alike, so making their environment more similar, than non-identical pairs. Although the numbers are small, studies have been made of MZ twins raised apart, thus eliminating this confounding factor (Gottesman and Shields, 1982). These pairs show similar concordance rates for schizophrenia to pairs raised together, which supports the importance of genetic factors in transmission.

Adoption studies

As noted by Sham *et al.* (see Chapter 12, this volume), adoption studies provide a means of controlling for the effects of common family environment by examining morbid risk to children adopted away from ill parents at birth, compared to that found in control adoptees with normal biological parents. One such follow-up study of 47 adopted-away children of schizophrenic mothers found that, by a mean age of 36 years, five had become schizophrenic compared to none in a control group (Heston and Denney, 1968).

Using an alternative approach, Kety *et al.* (1968) identified 33 schizophrenic adoptees and blindly rated life histories of both their biological and adoptive relatives. In the study, 21% of the former, compared with only 5% of the latter, received diagnoses of 'schizophrenia spectrum disorder'; this term covers not only frank schizophrenia but also schizotypal and paranoid personality disorders. The implication is that what is inherited is a vulnerability to a broader category of illness than to schizophrenia alone.

Whilst adoption studies control for post-natal familial effects, they cannot do so for pre-natal, organic ones. It is possible, for example, that the intrauterine environment provided by a schizophrenic mother might differ from the normal in some way that increases the risk to her child of developing schizophrenia. The same would not apply to offspring of schizophrenic fathers. Kety *et al.* (1975) found higher rates of spectrum disorders in the paternal half-siblings of probands (who share on average one quarter of their genes). This result supports the hypothesis of genetic transmission of at least part of the vulnerability to schizophrenia.

Schizophrenia spectrum disorders

It has long been observed that some close relatives of schizophrenics, although not psychotic, are somewhat eccentric. As mentioned above, the Danish–American adoption study by Kety *et al.* (1968) found an increased risk not only of schizophrenia, but of the so-called 'schizophrenia spectrum disorders' in biological relatives of schizophrenic patients. These have now been more accurately characterized, and incorporated into the DSM-III criteria under the term 'schizotypal personality'. Kendler *et al.* (1981) applied DSM-III criteria to the case histories in Kety's study, and found an excess of schizophrenia and schizotypal personality in the biological, but not the adoptive, relatives of probands. The characteristics of schizotypal personality disorder include 'magical' thinking, a preoccupation with parapsychology and similar topics, odd speech patterns, suspiciousness, and poor social skills or difficulty developing a rapport with others, leading to social isolation.

Recent studies provide confirmation that schizotypal personality is genetically related to schizophrenia. In six family studies (Kendler, 1988), the relatives of schizophrenics were found to be at greater risk for schizotypal personality than relatives of controls.

Mode of transmission

In general, schizophrenia does not appear to follow simple Mendelian patterns of transmission. This may be because it is etiologically heterogeneous, a group of illnesses rather than a single disease entity. Alternatively, in most individuals, it may be the result of several interacting factors, both genetic and environmental. Such multifactorial etiology is known to be important in many common medical disorders, such as coronary artery disease and diabetes mellitus.

Some authors (e.g. McGue and Gottesman, 1989) favour the classical polygenic/multifactorial model of inheritance of schizophrenia, in which the disorder is considered to be the result of the additive effects of many genes and environmental effects. However, the results of segregation analysis are also compatible with a single major locus operating against such a multifactorial background. These two models are very difficult to distinguish in practice, as such a single gene would be moderately prevalent, but of relatively low penetrance. Rare multiply-affected pedigrees have been reported, where it appears that a single gene of high penetrance is being inherited along autosomal dominant (Kennedy et al., 1988), or partly dominant (Karlsson, 1988) lines. Since it is in such families that major gene effects are most likely to be detected, they are the most suitable for linkage studies whose aim is to establish the location of the causal gene or genes.

The existence of reduced penetrance (or failure of individuals carrying a genetic vulnerability to the illness to develop the clinical illness) has recently been confirmed in a study of twins discordant for schizophrenia by Gottesman and Bertelsen (1989). They looked at rates of illness in the children of well MZ co-twins, compared to those in the children of their schizophrenic counterparts, and found them to be remarkably similar. Thus it would appear that the well twin need not have developed the clinical illness in order to transmit the genetic vulnerability. Of course, this is also compatible with a multifactorial polygenic model, assuming less influence of precipitating environmental factors in the well co-twin even though his/her genes are identical.

Linkage studies

Several Icelandic and British families multiply affected with schizophrenia were studied by Sherrington et al. (1988), who published evidence suggestive of linkage of schizophrenia to two DNA markers on chromosome 5. The idea that this region might be of interest came from a report by Bassett et al. (1988) of a Chinese family where an uncle and nephew both had a diagnosis of schizophrenia and a partial trisomy of chromosome 5.

Subsequent studies in a large Swedish pedigree (Kennedy et al., 1988), in a number of Scottish families (St. Clair et al., 1989) and in North American families (Detera-Wadleigh et al., 1989) have not replicated the result. This could indicate genetic heterogeneity, but the experience of the Old Order Amish result in manic depression (see above) has taught us that false positive linkage results can occur. The validity of the chromosome 5 result will not be known until either it is replicated in these or other families, or the finding is shown to be false in the same families. Genetic heterogeneity can only safely be assumed to exist once positive evidence of linkage to differing loci is found in two or more independent studies.

Environmental factors in schizophrenia

There is, of course, evidence from CT and MRI studies that a significant proportion of schizophrenics do have structural brain abnormalities (e.g. Johnstone *et al.*, 1976). The abnormalities include enlargement of the cerebral ventricles and widening of the cortical sulci, implying that cerebral damage has occurred at some stage. The changes are already present in young, first-onset patients, and are apparently unrelated to length of illness or treatment (Shelton and Weinberger, 1986). Twin studies have shown that, overall, ventricular size is under a considerable degree of genetic control (Reveley *et al.*, 1982), but that among MZ twins discordant for schizophrenia, the ill twin has larger ventricles than the well twin, implying the operation of some environmental factor. These findings have recently been confirmed by Suddath *et al.* (1990) in an MRI study of 15 pairs of MZ twins discordant for schizophrenia; this study also showed the schizophrenic member of the pair to have a diminished volume of grey matter in the temporal lobe. The most likely causal factor is some form of environmental hazard to the brain at or before birth.

Schizophrenic patients have suffered more obstetric complications (OCs) than their well siblings (McNeil and Kaij, 1978), and almost all recent studies (e.g. Lewis and Murray, 1987) have found that OCs are associated with increased ventricular size in adulthood. This correlation holds true in normal twins and psychiatric patients in general, but is most strongly positive in schizophrenics; it is especially seen in those with a negative family history, but is also present in patients with affected relatives. Schizophrenic patients with enlarged ventricles tend also to be those with poor pre-morbid personalities (Shelton and Weinberger, 1986), and significantly lower than average IQs prior to the onset of the illness (Offord and Cross, 1971). All of these could be consequent on OCs or hypoxic damage at birth. However, both the OCs and the structural brain abnormalities could also be secondary to some earlier but undetectable hazard such as maternal viral infection. Green *et al.* (1987) found that schizophrenics were more likely to have minor physical anomalies, such as a furrowed tongue, curved fingers and low-set ears, which are known to be associated with early fetal insult.

Schizophrenics show a 7–15% excess of births in the late winter and early spring months (Shur, 1982). It has been hypothesized that being born in the colder months of the year is associated with increased risk of 'constitutional damage', such as impaired development of the fetal brain, which might predispose to the development of schizophrenia in adult life. This seasonal effect is more frequently seen in patients with no family history of the illness (Shur, 1982; O'Callaghan *et al.*, 1990). Since viral infections also peak during the winter months, these could be of etiological importance. An epidemiological study by Mednick et al. (1988) in Helsinki claimed that individuals who were in their second trimester of fetal life during the Asian influenza epidemic of Autumn 1957 were at increased risk of developing schizophrenia in later life. A similar risk-increasing effect of the Asian flu epidemic has now been reported by O'Callaghan et al. (1990) in England; the number of schizophrenics who were born 4 months after the epidemic was significantly greater than expected. Presumably, maternal influenza (or some factor associated with it) must cause some subtle impairment of fetal brain development.

Alcoholism

Although a number of socio-environmental factors are known to have a major effect on the prevalence of alcoholism (e.g. occupation and religious belief), it also provides an example of a complex genetically influenced disorder. It has been noted for centuries that alcohol abuse runs in families, and several systematic family studies confirm an average seven-fold increased risk to first degree relatives of probands compared with controls (reviewed by Cotton, 1979). This increased risk is consistently higher in male than in female relatives, regardless of the sex of the proband. The implication is that this finding is due to sex differences in environmental exposure to alcohol, rather than sex differences in the transmission of the genetic risk.

Twin studies have been used in two ways to examine the genetics of alcohol abuse (Marshall and Murray, 1989). First, series of twins drawn from the general population have been studied to estimate the heritability of drinking habits, by comparing the variation in MZ with DZ pairs. Such studies have shown overall consumption (Clifford et al., 1984a; Kaprio et al., 1987), inability to control and cease drinking (Partanen et al., 1966), and the experience of hangovers (Loehlin, 1972) to be subject to modest but significant genetic effects. Second, series of twins from alcohol treatment centres have been studied to establish if there is a genetic contribution to severe abuse by comparing MZ and DZ concordance rates. Three studies found a ratio of 2:1 for concordance rate among male MZ versus DZ twins (Kaij, 1960; Hrubec and Omenn, 1981; Pickens and Svikis, 1988), but a fourth found no difference in concordance rates between MZ and DZ pairs (Gurling et al., 1981).

Adoption studies have also been undertaken. These provide the strongest evidence that the tendency to abuse alcohol is inherited. Three controlled studies (Goodwin et al., 1973; Bohman, 1978; Cadoret and Gath, 1978) have shown that the average relative risk to children raised away from an alcoholic parent of developing alcoholism themselves is 2.4 for men and 2.8 for women. This greater than two-fold increase in risk over controls occurs in the absence of contact with the biological alcoholic parent.

Cloninger (1987) claims to find two types of alcohol abuse, based on data derived from Bohman's (1978) Swedish adoption study. He believes 'Type 1' (milieu-limited) abuse to be a milder, adult-onset form, occurring equally in men and women, and 'Type 2' to be male-limited, associated with teenage onset of severe abuse and serious criminality in the biological fathers. Subsequent studies have not wholly supported the distinction between these two categories, but 'familial' alcoholics tend to have the features said to characterize the second type (Goodwin, 1983) and are also more likely to have antisocial personalities than those without affected relatives (Penick *et al.*, 1978; Hesselbrock *et al.*, 1982). 'Type 2' abuse may, therefore, simply represent the clinical expression of a more genetic kind of alcoholism.

Evidence for single gene effects

It might be expected that a complex phenotype such as alcoholism would be determined polygenically rather than by individual genes. However, it has been claimed that single genes are of major importance in the development of, or protection against, alcohol abuse (Gilligan *et al.*, 1987; Aston *et al.*, 1988).

It is well established that two- to three-fold differences exist in alcohol elimination rate between individuals (Li, 1983), and comparisons of MZ and DZ twins show that about half of this variability is genetically determined (Martin, 1987). The explanation may lie in the fact that different individuals possess different allelic variants of the major alcohol-metabolizing enzymes, alcohol and aldehyde dehydrogenase (ADH and ALDH, respectively). These produce differing protein subunits, which combine to form enzymes of greater or lesser activity.

The ALDH2 gene codes for the enzyme which is responsible for most of acetaldehyde oxidation. About 50% of Orientals have an inactive form of ALDH2 as a result of a single nucleotide base-pair change in DNA (Bosron *et al.*, 1988). Such individuals develop a very high blood acetaldehyde level after the ingestion of low doses of alcohol. Immediately after drinking, they experience a dysphoric reaction including facial flushing and tachycardia, similar to that induced by the ALDH inhibitor drug Antabuse. Japanese alcoholics and sufferers from alcoholic cirrhosis are much less likely to have the inactive ALDH2 variant than the general Japanese population. The influential effect of a single gene is in this case clear, i.e. the possession of the inactive variant leads to high acetaldehyde levels and an unpleasant reaction to alcohol which is a strong protective factor against the development of alcohol abuse (Harada *et al.*, 1980).

Linkage studies

The linkage strategy is beginning to be applied to families multiply affected with alcoholism. As yet, no genetic marker has been clearly shown to be linked to the disorder, though Hill *et al.* (1988) reported a result suggestive of linkage between the MNS blood group locus on chromosome 4 and alcoholism in 30 families. Blum *et al.* (1990) recently described an association between a particular allele of the D2 receptor gene (on the long arm of chromosome 11) and the disorder in a sample of 35 alcoholics. No such association was observed in the control group. The authors suggest that this D2 allotype, or a very closely neighbouring gene, might confer susceptibility to the alcoholism. This finding awaits replication.

Personality and Neurosis

The modern idea that neurotic disorders often occur in the context of a vulnerable personality developed from Eliot Slater's (Slater and Slater, 1944) studies of psychiatric breakdown in soldiers. He observed that the severity of the soldiers' neuroses bore little direct relation to the degree of war stress they had experienced, and that many of those who became ill had a personal or family history of neurotic disorder. A similar model was proposed by Eysenck (1952) who suggested that psychiatric disorders were extremes on a continuous dimensional model, in which the traits of extraversion–introversion, and neuroticism–stability were arranged on two dimensions (derived from factor analytic studies), with varying degrees of each observed in different disorders. For example, those with anxiety states were considered to be introverted neurotics, and those with hysteria extraverted neurotics. Genetic studies of personality and of neurotic disorders have tended to proceed separately, the former examining 'normal volunteer' subjects and the latter clinically ascertained samples. However, for neurosis in particular, the question of whether personality traits are inherited is clearly a pertinent one.

Most studies of the influence of heredity on normal personality have involved the completion of self-report personality questionnaires by twin pairs. Eaves et al. (1989) review 22 such twin studies, conducted prior to 1976, most of which studied fewer than 100 twin pairs; a crude meta-analysis of these studies in terms of extraversion–introversion and neuroticism–stability traits found that the average correlation for MZ twins significantly exceeded that for DZ twins, and suggested that about one-third of the variation in neuroticism within families could be attributable to genetic inheritance.

Subsequently, four large twin studies were carried out; in England (Eaves and Eysenck, 1977), the United States (Loehlin and Nicholls, 1976), Sweden (Floderhus-Myrhed et al., 1980) and Australia (Martin and Jardine, 1986). The results of these have been subjected to extensive model-fitting analyses, and some consistencies emerge. Firstly, the results confirm the importance of heredity. Furthermore, there appear to be sex-specific genetic effects on neuroticism, with some 51% of variation in males being due to additive genetic factors against 45% in females; the remainder in both sexes is obviously due to environmental factors (Martin and Jardine, 1986). Even in such large studies capable of detecting dominance (single gene) effects, neuroticism still fits a polygenic model.

Secondly, shared family environment appears to have little influence on personality dimensions; rather it is non-shared environmental experience specific to each individual twin which seems to be important. Results from studies of other types of relatives also support a lack of influence of shared environmental factors on neuroticism. There is no evidence of increased similarity of spouses which might be a result of living together, or of selecting a mate with a similar personality. Nor is there any noteworthy resemblance in personality between foster-parents and adopted children, who are genetically unrelated but live together and so provide an ideal way of assessing

TABLE 13.3   Family history studies of anxiety neurosis.

Study (proband diagnosis)	No. of probands	Anxiety neurosis in relatives (%)
Brown (1942) (anxiety neurosis)	63	15.5
Cohen *et al.* (1951) (neurocirculatory asthenia)	111	15.6
Noyes *et al.* (1978) (anxiety neurosis)	112	15.5

environmental influences in the absence of the confounding effects of shared genes.

Many will find it surprising that although environmental factors do contribute to personality variability, accounting for 50% or more of the variation, the crucial environmental influences do not seem to be those shared by family members, which have traditionally been assumed to be important, particularly by psychoanalysts. The 'slings and arrows of outrageous fortune' which tend to be specific to individuals, seem more important in forming personality. However, this is still an area of controversy, and the negative findings may be partly due to difficulty in measuring the salient aspects of the shared environment in such studies.

Separated MZ twins show reasonably similar correlations for neuroticism scores to MZ twins reared together (Newman *et al.*, 1937; Shields, 1962; Bouchard and McGue, 1990). Indeed, the correlations are slightly higher. This suggests that in the absence of a shared environment, identical twins may become slightly more alike as they follow their 'nature' more closely; when reared together MZ twins may seek to emphasize their differences! Results for extraversion suggest greater effects of competitive interaction of the twins, i.e. the correlations are considerably higher in reared apart MZ twins than in reared together twins. Shields (1962) obtained a correlation of 0.61 from a sample of reared apart MZ twins while Bouchard and McGue (1990) calculated a correlation of 0.60 on a more recently collected sample. These may be compared with 0.42 for reared together MZ twins in Shields' study. Again, there is an absence of spousal correlations or significant foster parent–adoptee correlations for extraversion. Unlike other traits such as intelligence and social class, it seems people do not select a mate for their similar personality—the cliché that 'like attracts like' is never less true than for personality.

Anxiety Neurosis

Family studies

Many studies have suggested a familial contribution to anxiety neurosis. Two early investigations, and a more recent family history study (Table 13.3) show that 15% of first degree relatives of anxiety neurotics are similarly affected; this compares with general population rates of between 3 and 6%.

Cloninger *et al.* (1981) interviewed the relatives of 66 subjects meeting index and follow-up diagnostic criteria for a primary or secondary anxiety disorder,

TABLE 13.4   Twin studies of anxiety neurosis.

	MZ probands (no.)	DZ probands (no.)	MZ co-twins		DZ co-twins	
			Any anxiety disorder (%)	Any psychiatric disorder (%)	Any anxiety disorder (%)	Any psychiatric disorder (%)
Slater and Shields (1969)	17	28	41	47	4	18
Torgersen (1983a)	32	53	34	53	17	38

comparing them with the relatives of the remainder of a cohort of 500 out-patients whose diagnosis was of a non-anxious type. The results show a positive relationship between severity of illness in the index case and the proportion of affected relatives. Affective disorder was not over-represented in the relatives of anxiety neurotics, in spite of the fact that a very high proportion of the probands had secondary diagnoses of affective disorder.

Twin studies

There are no published adoption studies of anxiety neurosis. Therefore, the studies of Slater and Shields (1969) and Torgersen (1983a) provide the clearest evidence of a genetic component to anxiety neurosis. As shown in Table 13.4, they indicate a higher concordance rate in MZ than in DZ co-twins, suggesting a genetic effect, e.g. 41% versus 4% respectively in Slater and Shields' study.

Slater and Shields' study preceded the development of operationalized criteria, but they noted that the concordance changed depending on the strictness of the diagnosis applied to the co-twin (thus concordance rates were higher when any psychiatric disorder in co-twins was included, e.g. from 41% to 47% in MZ co-twins). Strictly speaking, the same criteria should be used to assess co-twins and index twins, but looser concordance is frequently reported, and generally increases concordance rates of both MZ and DZ pairs and reduces the ratio of MZ/DZ concordance. A lower MZ/DZ concordance ratio is frequently inter-preted as 'less genetic' but because such comparisons are enmeshed in population base rates, which are higher when looser criteria are applied, care must be taken in attaching too much importance to this ratio (Kendler, 1989).

Subtypes of anxiety neurosis

The introduction of DSM-III largely discarded the 'neurosis' umbrella, and categorized anxiety disorders into various hierarchical subtypes (including panic disorder, agoraphobia with and without panic attacks, generalized anxiety disorder, social and simple phobias). A number of investigations of familiality of the subtypes have led to proposals that panic disorder is the 'most genetic' and that it breeds true. Complexities arose for genetic studies from the hierarchical nature of DSM-III categories; for example a subject could not be diagnosed panic

TABLE 13.5 Morbid risk of anxiety and other disorders in relatives of panic disorder, agoraphobic and control probands (from Noyes *et al.* 1986).

Proband diagnoses	Morbid risk in relatives			
	Agoraphobia (%)	Panic disorder (definite and probable) (%)	Alcohol (abuse and dependence) (%)	Affective disorder (%)
Agoraphobia	11.6	8.3	17.0	7.4
Panic disorder	1.9	17.3	8.4	6.3
Controls	4.2	4.2	5.5	10.7

disorder if suffering from major depressive disorder. These difficulties have been partly resolved by the introduction of DSM-III-R, which allows for multiple diagnoses.

Cloninger *et al.*'s (1981) study described the chronology of symptoms in panic disorder probands, with individuals apparently progressing from nervousness to palpitations to panic attacks in their early 20s. This was then followed by depression leading to treatment seeking, and ultimately agoraphobia following panic. These authors seem to regard panic disorder as a 'severe variant' of anxiety neurosis with markedly increased risk in relatives.

A number of family studies comparing the subtypes of anxiety neurosis have been reported by a group in Iowa (e.g. Crowe *et al.*, 1980; Noyes *et al.*, 1978, 1986) using some of the same subjects. Table 13.5 compares the relatives of probands with agoraphobia and panic disorder. The relatives of agoraphobics had higher rates of agoraphobia, and they also had more anxiety and alcohol disorders overall compared with both the relatives of panic disorder probands and the relatives of controls. This suggests that agoraphobia and panic disorder share a fundamental disturbance, panic attacks, and that agoraphobia is a severe variant of panic disorder, a finding which has been taken into account in the modified DSM-III-R classification.

Noyes *et al.* (1987) compared the relatives of the cases in the above study with those of 20 index cases with generalized anxiety disorder recruited through newspaper advertisements. They found a rate of 19.5% for generalized anxiety disorder in relatives of generalized anxiety disorder cases, compared with 5.4%, 3.9% and 3.5% rates of generalized anxiety disorder in relatives of panic disorder, agoraphobic and control probands, respectively. The overall risk of any anxiety disorder in generalized anxiety disorder relatives was 30.1%, higher than the risk to relatives of panic disorder or other proband types, but the diagnoses were distributed differently, resembling the distribution in control relatives except for the excess of generalized anxiety disorder. The probands with generalized anxiety disorder reported frequent psychosocial stressors, and there was a strong association of the diagnosis with personality disorders in both index cases and relatives.

Preliminary data from a recent study of familiality of simple phobias (Fyer *et al.*, 1990) indicated that 31% of relatives of simple phobics received a lifetime diagnosis of simple phobia compared with 11% of control relatives, with no difference between proband and control relatives for risks of other affective disorders. There was no evidence of specificity of type of phobia transmitted (e.g. a parent with snake phobia did not necessarily have an affected relative with snake phobia, but just as likely of heights or cats). Nor was there any evidence of familiality of subclinical fears. The probands in this study were drawn from a clinical population, and therefore probably had relatively severe phobias, and so these results are in accord with Torgersen's (1983b, see below) finding of increased familiality according to severity of proband's disorder.

The only report available of a twin study examining anxiety specifically in DSM-III terms is that of Torgersen (1983a). All probands, selected through the Norwegian state twin register, had been registered for some form of psychiatric treatment. Overall, 34% of MZ and 17% of DZ pairs were broadly concordant. For pairs with an agoraphobic proband, concordance was higher in MZ than DZ twins ($p < 0.025$). If all classes except generalized anxiety disorder were examined MZ concordance increased to 45% versus 15% DZ, a significant difference ($p < 0.02$). However, no MZ co-twins were concordant for exactly the same subtype of anxiety diagnosis. A recent study by Andrews et al. (1990) of neurosis in an Australian volunteer twin sample found a similar lack of specificity in concordant pairs. This tends to support Slater's early view that any genetic predisposition is to a wider neurotic or anxious spectrum, with specific symptoms or subtypes determined by environmental factors.

Carey et al. (1980) have shown that neurosis is subject to widely varying differences in estimations of prevalence, depending not just on the population but on the criteria used. Because of this, the evaluation of familiality is particularly subject to error, and neuroses could appear to be entirely genetic or entirely environmental depending on the choice of prevalence rate or control sample. A graphic illustration of this is provided by Torgersen (1983b), who found that concordance ratios for MZ/DZ twins changed markedly depending on the type of institution at which the proband had been treated for an anxiety disorder and also on the sex of the proband twin. 'Severe' cases who had been in-patients in mental hospitals had higher concordance ratios than out-patients, as did male pairs than female pairs; this is presumably because of the lower prevalences of the severe forms of the disorder, and the lower prevalence rates for comparable disorders in males.

The work of Carey et al. (1980) and Torgersen (1983b) indicates the importance of taking account of such factors when reporting on twin and family studies; the variability in how 'genetic' disorders seem to be according to whence the sample is drawn indicates a danger in attributing too much importance to hospital-based studies showing the apparent importance of genes, without balanced community studies exploring the whole range of anxiety problems. These arguments apply to other diagnostic categories discussed in this chapter, but are especially pertinent for neuroses where diagnostic reliability may be lower, and reported prevalence rates are thus particularly sensitive to variations in syndrome definition.

Single gene effects?

With a lack of any convincing evidence for Mendelian inheritance of any subtype of anxiety disorder, it is only to be expected that there have been no strong positive results from linkage studies. Crowe *et al.* (1987) reported a lod score of 2.3, suggesting weak linkage of panic disorder to the α-haptoglobin locus on chromosome 16q22 in 26 pedigrees. This was not replicated elsewhere and a recent report from the same group (Crowe *et al.*, 1990) on a further 10 pedigrees excludes linkage to this locus. One of the problems with such studies is that linkage analysis relies on making assumptions about the nature of transmission of the disorder; for panic disorder this means that unaffected relatives must either be assumed to be carrying 'the gene' and hence a degree of incomplete penetrance is postulated, or, a 'penetrance free' model must be fitted where unaffected relatives are considered to have an unknown disease phenotype. The results are thus dependent on the validity of the model, which relies on epidemiological data with its attendant problems as discussed above.

To date, the most convincing suggestion that there may be some contribution of single major gene effects to panic disorder comes from a study of 'normal' twins (Martin *et al.*, 1988). When 2903 adult same-sex pairs completed a questionnaire covering symptoms of anxiety and depression in addition to the Eysenck Personality Questionnaire measure of neuroticism, the variation in physical symptoms influencing reporting of 'feelings of panic' seemed to be partly due to non-additive genetic effects, like dominance, particularly in males. This study awaits replication, and the relationship of such questionnaire results on 'normal' samples to family studies of clinically ascertained samples with psychiatric diagnoses is unclear, but represents another useful way of building up a picture of the genetic etiology of neurosis.

Anyone embarking on genetic studies of anxiety disorders faces a considerable challenge. Diagnostic unreliability makes comparison across interviewers and interview schedules difficult. Varying epidemiological data gives rise to spurious heritability estimates, which can make neurosis seem to be strongly inherited or entirely environmental. Operational definitions have changed considerably over the last decade, for anxiety disorder perhaps more than any other, rendering any dogmatic statement about this field impossible. It seems likely that there is a genetic contribution to anxiety; indeed one might expect it on evolutionary grounds, but the specific pattern of transmission and role of environmental factors remains unclear.

Obsessional Neurosis

Varying estimates of prevalence in the general population again prove problematic for attempts to untangle the effects of heredity and environment on obsessional neurosis. The prevalence of obsessional neurosis is commonly taken as 0.05%, obtained by combining a psychiatric hospital prevalence of 0.5% with a psychiatric attendance in the general population of 1%. However, recent epidemiological studies from the USA have suggested a prevalence as high as

TABLE 13.6   Probandwise concordance rates for obsessional twins (from Carey and Gottesman, 1981).

Obsessive-compulsive probands	Probandwise concordance rates		
	Treatment involving obsessional symptoms[a] (%)	Any treatment[a] (%)	Any obsessional features (%)
Monozygotic (n = 15)	33	53	87
Dizygotic (n = 15)	7	33	47

[a]Treatment either by psychiatrist or GP.

3.3% (Karno et al., 1988). Such discrepancies are as much the result of the application of different criteria as of real population differences; the first estimate relies on clinical, and fairly narrow definitions, the second on a lay-administered interview schedule which seems to have very broad diagnostic criteria.

While most family studies of obsessional index cases from hospital populations do show a higher rate of obsessional traits in first degree relatives, the evidence for familiality of narrowly defined obsessional neurosis is equivocal; indeed, the raised rates of psychiatric disorder observed in some studies (Rasmussen and Tsuang, 1986; McKeon and Murray, 1987) are for a broad spectrum of neurotic diagnoses, not obsessional neurosis. Evidence for a genetic contribution to obsessional neurosis has mainly rested on case reports of twins. A number of reports of monozygotic twins concordant for the disorder have been published, while the few reports of dizygotic pairs have been discordant. However, such studies are not systematic and have been justifiably criticized (Rachman and Hodgson, 1980).

Carey and Gottesman (1981) reported a study of obsessional and phobic disorders in 49 pairs of twins ascertained through the Maudsley Hospital Twin Register. Table 13.6 illustrates the probandwise concordance rates for the obsessional twins and shows higher rates for MZ than DZ pairs for obsessional disorders. Once again, concordance rates rose when co-twins not only with obsessional symptoms but also with obsessional personalities were included, e.g. for MZ twins the rates rose from 53% to 87%.

Clifford et al. (1984b) examined the relationship between obsessional traits and symptoms on the self-report Leyton Obsessional Inventory and personality questionnaire measures of neuroticism, in a sample of 404 pairs of twins drawn from the Institute of Psychiatry Volunteer Twin Register. Model-fitting analysis of the responses showed that heredity accounted for 44% and 47% of the variance in obsessional traits and symptoms, respectively. Interestingly, a comparison with the same twins' responses to the Eysenck Personality Questionnaire showed a high genotypic correlation between the obsessional symptom scores and the neuroticism scale scores. This is further support for Slater's model of a polygenic contribution to a general neurotic predisposition, with specific patterns determined by environmental factors.

Hysteria

A study of families of 381 Swedish probands treated for hysterical conversion symptoms by Ljungberg (1957) found that the rate of hysteria was some 2.4% for male first degree relatives and 6.4% for female relatives; these were well above the somewhat uncertain population rate of 0.5% with which these rates were compared. The presence of hysteria in a parent did not increase the rate in sibs of probands, and, therefore, the conclusion of the author that hysteria is under some degree of polygenic control does not accord with polygenic theory.

Slater (1961) attempted to confirm the hereditary nature of hysteria by the systematic study of 12 MZ and 12 DZ twin pairs where the proband had been diagnosed as having hysteria. However, he found no hysteria in any of the co-twins or close relatives. This led Slater to revise his views on hysteria and to state not only that it had no genetic basis but, in a powerful critique (Slater, 1965, 1976), to describe hysteria as a pejorative term for patients neither liked nor understood by clinicians, who gain 'a diagnostic code-sign for each discharge and a black mark on the record'. Slater was scathing about the revival of hysteria under the new title of 'Briquet's Syndrome' by St Louis psychiatrists, and viewed it as 'self-condemned to absurdity' by its restriction to women, and 'a product of male chauvinism'.

In spite of these attacks, the St Louis group's view of hysteria has been influential in America, and several family studies have been published. Guze *et al.* (1986) reported that 6.6% of female relatives of probands with a diagnosis of Briquet's Syndrome also had Briquet's Syndrome versus 2.4% of female relatives of control probands. They also found increased rates of antisocial personality in the relatives of probands and controls, respectively, 18.75% versus 10.48% in male relatives and 8.6% versus 2.6% in female relatives. This accords with their theory that hysteria and sociopathy represent manifestations of the same underlying disorder, the former manifested primarily in females and the latter in males.

Thus, there exist major differences between the prevailing American and British views on the possible role of genes in hysteria, American researchers emphasizing, and their British counterparts dismissing their significance.

Recent observations that 60% of hysterical paraplegics had previous functional disturbance (Baker and Silver, 1987) suggest predisposing personality factors which could be the path for genetic influences. The apparent familial clustering of Briquet's Syndrome, which reflects a rather different concept of hysteria than one covering the range of conversion or dissociative disorders (which Slater studied), may have more to do with a tendency to somatization of neurotic complaints. Such behaviour could be subject to intrafamilial modelling and may well be reinforced by a medical system working in fear of missing some obscure diagnosis.

Anorexia Nervosa

Polygenic influences on height have been long since established, but weight has seemed to be more variable and environmentally influenced. More recently, studies have examined the influences on height-standardized weight (the so-called body mass index; weight in kilograms divided by the square of the height in metres) which provides a measure of 'fatness'. Twin and adoption studies have shown between 64 and 84% of the variation in body-mass index to be attributable to genes, and recent studies of twins reared apart (Stunkard et al., 1990; Macdonald and Stunkard, 1990) further support the conclusion that some 70% of the variability in body-mass index is genetic. In the light of such findings, recent studies which suggest a genetic contribution to eating disorders are perhaps less surprising than they might otherwise be.

Gershon et al. (1984) found that the lifetime risk of eating disorder in first degree relatives of probands with eating disorder was 6%, compared with a risk to control relatives of 1%, the latter being similar to population base rates in the United States. Strober et al. (1985) found that 5% of female first degree relatives of probands with eating disorder had a similar history, and also suggested that severe restricting anorexia may be different genetically from bulimia. Recent twin studies (Holland et al., 1984; Treasure and Holland, 1991) also suggest this. Concordance rates are significantly higher in MZ than DZ twins for anorexia nervosa, implying a genetic effect. However, no such effect is found for bulimia.

Ethical Issues

It is impossible to conclude a chapter on psychiatric genetics without mentioning the tragic events of the 1930s when some of the most notable German psychiatrists became involved in the Nazi campaigns to sterilize psychiatric patients in a horrific (and scientifically absurd) attempt to eliminate mental illness as part of the wider eugenic programme of the holocaust. The complicity of certain psychiatric geneticists cast a pall over the subject for many years. However, one of the consequences has been that those working in the field of psychiatric genetics have been particularly concerned that their work should never again be abused.

Until recently, so little was known about the transmission of psychiatric disorder that genetic counselling had as its main function the dispelling of false beliefs and relief of the consequent anxiety (Foerster and Murray, 1987). However, developments in molecular genetics, and in understanding of the pathogenesis of psychiatric disorders, raises the possibility of more accurate prediction of risk. So far only on Huntington's chorea have careful estimates of risk prediction and counselling been established and provided to relatives of sufferers (see above). It is apparent, however, that even for Huntington's chorea, with its simple mode of inheritance, the issues are extremely complex. They are likely to be even more so for common psychiatric disorders. Consequently, a number of conferences involving those in the field have been held to begin to discuss how to maximize the benefits, and minimize any harm, that the new knowledge may bring. The potential and pitfalls of molecular genetics for psychiatry are summarized in Pelosi and David (1989) and Gill (1991).

References

Abrams, R. and Taylor, M.A. (1983). The genetics of schizophrenia: a reassessment using modern criteria. *Am. J. Psychiat.* **140**, 171–175.

Andrews, G., Stewart, G., Allen, R. and Henderson, A.S. (1990). The genetics of six neurotic disorders: a twin study. *J. Affect. Dis.* **19**, 23–29.

Aston, C.E., Hill, S.Y. and Rabin, B. (1988). Segregation analysis of families of male alcoholic probands. *Am. J. Hum. Genet.* **34** (Suppl.), A210.

Baker, J.H.E. and Silver, J.R. (1987). Hysterical paraplegia. *J. Neurol. Neurosurg. Psychiat.* **50**, 375–382.

Baron, M., Risch, N., Hamburger, R. *et al.* (1987). Genetic linkage between X chromosome markers and bipolar affective illness. *Nature* **326**, 289–292.

Bassett, A.S., McGillivray, B.C., Jones, B.D. *et al.* (1988). Partial trisomy chromosome 5 cosegregating with schizophrenia. *Lancet* **i**, 799–801.

Bebbington, P., Katz, R., McGuffin, P. *et al.* (1989). The risk of minor depression before age 65: Results from a community survey. *Psychol. Med.* **19**, 393–400.

Bertelsen, A., Harvald, B. and Hauge, M. (1977). A Danish twin study of manic-depressive disorders. *Br. J. Psychiat.* **130**, 330–351.

Blum, K., Noble, E.P., Sheridan, P.J. *et al.* (1990). Allelic association of human dopamine D2 receptor gene in alcoholism. *J. Am. Med. Assoc.* **263** (15), 2055–2060.

Bohman, M. (1978). Some genetic aspects of alcoholism and criminality. *Arch. Gen. Psychiat.* **35**, 269–276.

Bosron, W.F., Lumeng, L. and Li, T.-K. (1988). Genetic polymorphism of enzymes of alcohol metabolism and susceptibility to alcoholic liver disease. In: *Molecular Aspects of Medicine*, Vol. 10, pp. 147–158. Oxford: Pergamon Press.

Bouchard, T.J. Jr and McGue, M. (1990). Genetic and rearing environmental influences on adult personality: an analysis of adopted twins reared apart. *J. Personality*, Special Issue: *Biological Foundations of Personality: Evolution, Behavioral Genetics, and Psychophysiology*.

Brandt, J., Quaid, K.A., Folstein, S.E. *et al.* (1989). Presymptomatic diagnosis of delayed-onset disease with linked DNA markers. *J. Am. Med. Assoc.* **261** (21), 3108–3114.

Breitner, J.C., Murphy, E.A. and Folstein, M.F. (1986). Familial aggregation in Alzheimer dementia. II. Clinical genetic implications of age-dependent onset. *J. Psychiat. Res.* **20** (1), 45–55.

Brown, F.W. (1942). Heredity in the psychoneuroses. *J. R. Soc. Med.* **35**, 785–790.

Brown, G.W. and Harris, T. (1978). *The Social Origins of Depression.* London: Tavistock.

Cadoret, R.J. and Gath, A. (1978). Inheritance of alcoholism in adoptees. *Br. J. Psychiat.* **132**, 252–258.

Carey, G. and Gottesman, I.I. (1981). Twin and family studies of anxiety, phobic and obsessive disorders. In: D.F. Klein and J.G. Rabkin (eds) *Anxiety: New Research and Changing Concepts*, pp. 117–136. New York: Raven Press.

Carey, G., Gottesman, I.I. and Robins, E. (1980). Prevalence rates for the neuroses: pitfalls in the evaluation of familiality. *Psychol. Med.* **10**, 437–443.

Clifford, C.A., Fulker, D.W. and Murray, R.M. (1984a). Genetic and environmental influences on drinking patterns in normal twins. In: N. Krasner, J.S. Madden and R.J. Walker (eds) *Alcohol Related Problems*, pp. 115–126. New York: John Wiley & Sons.

Clifford, C.A., Murray, R.M. and Fulker, D.W. (1984b). Genetic and environmental influences on obsessional traits and symptoms. *Psychol. Med.* **14**, 791–800.

Cloninger, C.R. (1987). Neurogenetic adaptive mechanisms in alcoholism. *Science* **236**, 410–416.

294   C.J.A. Taylor et al.

Cloninger, C.R., Martin, R.L., Clayton, P.J. and Guze, S.B. (1981). A blind follow-up and family study of anxiety neurosis: preliminary analysis of the St Louis 500. In: D.F. Klein and J. Rabkin (eds) *Anxiety: New Research and Changing Concepts*, pp. 137–150. New York: Raven Press.

Cohen, M.E., Badal, D.W., Kilpatrick, A., Reed, E.W. and White, D.W. (1951). The high familial prevalence of neurocirculatory asthenia (anxiety neurosis, effort syndrome). *Am. J. Hum. Genet.* **3**, 126–158.

Cook, R.H., Schneck, S.A. and Clark, D.B. (1981). Twins with Alzheimer's Disease. *Arch. Neurol.* **138**, 300–301.

Cotton, N.S. (1979). The familial incidence of alcoholism. *J. Studies Alcohol* **40**, 89–116.

Craufurd, D. (1989). Progress and problems in Huntington's Disease. *Int. Rev. Psychiat.* **1**, 249–258.

Crow, T.J. (1983). Is schizophrenia an infectious disease? *Lancet* **i**, 173–175.

Crowe, R.R., Pauls, D.L., Slymen, D.J. and Noyes, R. (1980). A family study of anxiety neurosis: morbidity risk in families of patients with and without mitral valve prolapse. *Arch. Gen. Psychiat.* **37**, 77–79.

Crowe, R.R., Noyes, R., Wilson, A.F., Elston, R.C. and Ward, L.J. (1987). A linkage study of panic disorder. *Arch. Gen. Psychiat.* **44**, 933–937.

Crowe, R.R., Noyes, R., Samuelson, S., Wesner, R. and Wilson, R. (1990). Close linkage between panic disorder and α-haptoglobin excluded in 10 families. *Arch. Gen. Psychiat.* **47**, 377–380.

Detera-Wadleigh, S.D., Berrettini, W.H., Goldin, L.R. *et al.* (1987). Close linkage of c-Harvey ras-1 and the insulin gene to affective disorder is ruled out in three North American pedigrees. *Nature* **325**, 806–808.

Detera-Wadleigh, S.D., Goldin, L.R., Sherrington, R. *et al.* (1989). Exclusion of linkage to 5q11–13 in families with schizophrenia and other psychiatric disorders. *Nature* **340**, 391–393.

Eaves, L.J., Eysenck, H.J. and Martin, N.G. (1989). *Genes, Culture and Personality: An Empirical Approach*. London: Academic Press.

Eaves, L.J. and Eysenck, H.J. (1977). A genotype-environmental model for psychoticism. *Adv. Behav. Res. Ther.* **1**, 5–26.

Egeland, J.A., Gerhard, D.S., Pauls, D.L. *et al.* (1987). Bipolar affective disorders linked to DNA markers on chromosome 11. *Nature* **325**, 783–787.

Eysenck, H.J. (1952). *The Scientific Study of Personality*. London: Routledge & Kegan Paul.

Farmer, A.E., McGuffin, P. and Gottesman, I.I. (1987). Twin concordance for DSM-III schizophrenia: scrutinising the validity of the definition. *Arch. Gen. Psychiat.* **44**, 634–641.

Floderus-Myrhed, B., Pedersen, N. and Rasmuson, I. (1980). Assessment of heritability for personality based on a short-form of the Eysenck Personality Inventory: a study of 12 898 twin pairs. *Behav. Genet.* **10**, 153–162.

Foerster, A. and Murray, R.M. (1987). Genetic counselling. In: M. Tsuang and J. Simpson (eds) *Handbook of Schizophrenia*, Vol. 3, pp. 563–577 (overall editor H. Nasrullah). Amsterdam: Elsevier.

Fyer, A.J., Mannuzza, S., Gallops, M.S., Martin, L.Y., Aaronson, C., Gorman, J.M., Liebowitz, M.R. and Klein, D.F. (1990). Familial transmission of simple phobias and fears: a preliminary report. *Arch. Gen. Psychiat.* **47**, 252–256.

Gershon, E.S., Bunney, W.S., Leckman, J.F. *et al.* (1976). The inheritance of affective disorders: a review of data and of hypotheses. *Behav. Genet.* **6**, 227–261.

Gershon, E.S., Hamovit, J., Guroff, J.J. *et al.* (1982). A family study of schizoaffective, bipolar I, bipolar II, unipolar, and normal control probands. *Arch. Gen. Psychiat.* **39**, 1157–1167.

Gershon, E.S., Schreiber, J.L., Hamovi, J.R., Dibble, E.D., Kaye, W., Nurnberger, J.I., Andersen, A.E. and Ebert, M. (1984). Clinical findings in patients with anorexia nervosa and affective illness in their relatives. *Am. J. Psychiat.* **141**, 1419–1422.

Gill, M. (1991). Ethics, molecular genetics and psychiatric disorders. In: R.J. Srám, V. Bulyzhenkov, L. Prilipko and Y. Christen (eds) *Ethical Issues of Molecular Genetics in Psychiatry*. Berlin: Springer Verlag.

Gill, M., McKeon, P. and Humphries, P. (1988). Linkage analysis of manic depression in an Irish family using H-ras-1 and INS DNA markers. *J. Med. Gen.* **25**, 634–635.

Gilligan, S.B., Reich, T. and Cloninger, C.R. (1987). Etiologic heterogeneity in alcoholism. *Genet. Epidemiol.* **4**, 395–414.

Goate, A.M., Hardy, J.A. and Owen, M.J. (1989). The genetic etiology of Alzheimer's Disease. *Int. Rev. Psychiat.* **1**, 243–248.

Goodwin, D.W. (1983). Familial alcoholism. *Subst. Alcohol Actions Misuse* **4**, 129–136.

Goodwin, D.W., Schulsinger, F., Hermansen, L. *et al.* (1973). Alcohol problems in adoptees raised apart from alcoholic biological parents. *Arch. Gen. Psychiat.* **28**, 238–243.

Gottesman, I.I. and Bertelsen, A. (1989). Confirming unexpressed genotypes for schizophrenia. *Arch. Gen. Psychiat.* **46**, 867–872.

Gottesman, I.I. and Shields, J. (1972). *Schizophrenia and Genetics: A Twin Study Vantage Point*. London: Academic Press.

Gottesman, I.I. and Shields, J. (1982). *Schizophrenia: The Epigenetic Puzzle*. Cambridge: Cambridge University Press.

Green, M.F., Satz, P., Soper, H.V. *et al.* (1987). Relationship between physical anomalies and age of onset of schizophrenia. *Am. J. Psychiat.* **44**, 666–667.

Gurling, H.M.D., Murray, R.M. and Clifford, C. (1981). Investigations into the genetics of alcohol dependence and into its effects on brain function. In: L. Gedda, P. Parisi and W.E. Nance (eds) *Twin Research*, Vol. 3. pp. 77–87. New York: Alan R. Liss.

Gusella, J.F., Wexler, N.S., Conneally, P.M. *et al.* (1983). A polymorphic DNA marker genetically linked to Huntington's Disease. *Nature* **306**, 234–238.

Guze, S.B., Cloninger, C.R., Martin, R.L. and Clayton, P.J. (1986). A follow-up and family study of Briquet's Syndrome. *Br. J. Psychiat.* **149**, 17–23.

Harada, S., Misawa, S., Agarwal, D.P. *et al.* (1980). Liver alcohol dehydrogenase and aldehyde dehydrogenase in the Japanese: isozyme variation and its possible role in alcohol intoxication. *Am. J. Hum. Genet.* **32**, 8–15.

Hayden, M.R., Robbins, C., Allard, D. *et al.* (1988). Improved predictive testing for Huntington Disease by using 3 linked DNA markers. *Am. J. Hum. Genet.* **43** (5), 689–694.

Hesselbrock, V.M., Stabenau, J.R., Hesselbrock, M.N. *et al.* (1982). The nature of alcoholism in patients with different family histories for alcoholism. *Progr. Neuropsychopharmacol. Biol. Psychiat.* **6**, 607–614.

Heston, L.L. and Denney, D. (1968). Interactions between early life experience and biological factors in schizophrenia. In: D. Rosenthal and S. Kety (eds) *The Transmission of Schizophrenia*, pp. 363–376. Oxford: Pergamon Press.

Heston, L.L. (1977). Alzheimer's disease, trisomy 21 and myeloproliferative disorders: associations suggesting a genetic diathesis. *Science* **196**, 322–323.

Heston, L.L., Mastri, A.R., Anderson, V.E. *et al.* (1981). Dementia of the Alzheimer type: clinical genetics, natural history and associated conditions. *Arch. Gen. Psychiat.* **38**, 1085–1090.

Heyman, A., Wilkinson, W.E., Stafford, J.A. *et al.* (1984). Alzheimer's Disease. A study of epidemiological aspects. *Ann. Neurol.* **15**, 335–341.

Hill, S.Y., Aston, C. and Rabin, B. (1988). Suggestive evidence of genetic linkage between alcoholism and the MNS blood group. *Alcoholism: Clin. Exp. Res.* **12** (6), 811–814.

Hodgkinson, S., Sherrington, R., Gurling, H.M.D. *et al.* (1987). Molecular genetic evidence for heterogeneity in manic depression. *Nature* **325**, 805–806.

Holland, A.J., Hall, A., Murray, R.M., Russell, G.F.M. and Crisp, A.H. (1984). Anorexia nervosa: a study of 34 twin pairs and one set of triplets. *Br. J. Psychiat.* **145**, 414–419.

Holloway, S.M. and Smith, C. (1975). Effects of various medical and social practices on the frequency of genetic disorders. *Am. J. Hum. Genet.* **27**, 614–627.

Hrubec, Z. and Omenn, G.S. (1981). Evidence of genetic predisposition to alcoholic cirrhosis and psychosis: twin concordances for alcoholism and its biological end-points by zygosity among male veterans. *Alcoholism: Clin. Exp. Res.* **5**, 207–215.

Hunter, R., Dyan, A.D. and Wilson, J. (1972). Alzheimer's disease in one monozygotic twin. *J. Neurosurg. Psychiat.* **35**, 707–710.

Johnstone, E.C., Crow, T.J., Frith, C.D. *et al.* (1976). Cerebral ventricular size and cognitive impairment in chronic schizophrenia. *Lancet* **ii**, 924–926.

Kaij, L. (1960). *Alcoholism in Twins.* Stockholm: Almquist & Wiksell.

Kaprio, J., Koskenvuo, M., Langinvainio, H. *et al.* (1987). Genetic influences on use and abuse of alcohol: a study of 5638 adult Finnish twin brothers. *Alcoholism: Clin. Exp. Res.* **11**, 349–356.

Karlsson, J.L. (1988). Partly dominant transmission of schizophrenia in Iceland. *Br. J. Psychiat.* **152**, 324–329.

Karno, M., Golding, J.M., Sorenson, S.B. and Burnam, M.A. (1988). The epidemiology of obsessive–compulsive disorder in five US communities. *Arch. Gen. Psychiat.* **45**, 1094–1099.

Kelsoe, J.R., Ginns, E.I., Egeland, J.A. *et al.* (1989). Re-evaluation of the linkage relationship between chromosome 11p loci and the gene for bipolar affective disorder in the Old Order Amish. *Nature* **342**, 238–243.

Kendler, K.S. (1988). Familial aggregation of schizophrenia and schizophrenia spectrum disorders. *Arch. Gen. Psychiat.* **45**, 377–383.

Kendler, K.S. (1989). Limitations of the ratio of concordance rates in monozygotic and dizygotic twins. *Arch. Gen. Psychiat.* **46**, 477–478.

Kendler, K.S., Gruenberg, A.M. and Strauss, J.S. (1981). An independent analysis of the Copenhagen sample of the Danish Adoption Study of Schizophrenia. II: The relationship between schizotypal personality disorder and schizophrenia. *Arch. Gen. Psychiat.* **38**, 982–984.

Kendler, K.S., Gruenberg, A.M. and Tsuang, M.T. (1985). Psychiatric illness in first degree relatives of schizophrenic and surgical control patients. A family study using DSM-III criteria. *Arch. Gen. Psychiat.* **42**, 770–779.

Kennedy, J.L., Giuffra, L.A., Moises, H.W. *et al.* (1988). Evidence against linkage of schizophrenia to markers on chromosome 5 in a Northern Swedish pedigree. *Nature* **336**, 167–170.

Kety, S.S., Rosenthal, D., Wender, P.H. *et al.* (1968). The types and prevalence of mental illness in the biological and adoptive families of adopted schizophrenics. In: D. Rosenthal and S. Kety (eds) *The Transmission of Schizophrenia*, pp. 345–362. Oxford: Pergamon Press.

Kety, S.S., Rosenthal, D., Wender, P.H. *et al.* (1975). Mental illness in the biological and adoptive families of adopted individuals who have become schizophrenic. In: R.R. Fieve, D. Rosenthal and H. Brill (eds) *Genetic Research in Psychiatry*, pp. 147–165. Baltimore, MD: Johns Hopkins University Press.

Kety, S.S. (1983). Response to Abrams and Taylor. *Am. J. Psychiat.* **140**, 1111–1112.

Klein, D.F. (1981). Anxiety reconceptualised. In: D.F. Klein and J. Rabkin (eds) *Anxiety: New Research and Changing Concepts*. New York: Raven Press.

Lewis, S.W. and Murray, R.M. (1987). Obstetric complications, neurodevelopmental deviance and risk of schizophrenia. *J. Psychiat. Res.* **21**, 413–421.

Li, T.-K. (1983). The absorption, distribution and metabolism of ethanol, and its effects on nutrition and hepatic function. In: B. Tabokoff, P.B. Sutker and C.L. Randall (eds) *Medical and Social Aspects of Alcohol Abuse*. New York: Plenum Press.

Ljungberg, L. (1957). Hysteria: a clinical, prognostic and genetic study. *Acta Psychiat. Neurol. Scand.* **32** (Suppl. 112).

Loehlin, J.C. (1972). An analysis of alcohol-related questionnaire items from the National Merit Twin Study. *Ann. NY Acad. Sci.* **197**, 117–120.

Leohlin, J.C. and Nichols, R.C. (1976). *Heredity, Environment and Personality: A Study of 850 Sets of Twins*. Austin: University of Texas Press.

Macdonald, A.M. and Stunkard, A.J. (1990). The body mass index in British separated twins. *New Engl. J. Med.* **322** (21) 1530.

McGue, M. and Gottesman, I.I. (1989). Genetic linkage in schizophrenia. *Schizophrenia Bull.* **15**, 453–464.

McGuffin, P. and Katz, R. (1986). Nature, nurture and affective disorder. In: J.F.W. Deakin (ed.) *The Biology of Depression*, pp. 26–52. London: The Royal College of Psychiatrists, Gaskell Press.

McGuffin, P. and Murray, R.M. (1991). *The New Genetics of Mental Illness*. Oxford: Butterworth–Heinemann Ltd.

McGuffin, P., Farmer, A.E., Gottesman, I.I. *et al.* (1984). Twin concordance for operationally defined schizophrenia. Confirmation of familiality and heritability. *Arch. Gen. Psychiat.* **41**, 541–545.

McGuffin, P., Katz, R. and Bebbington, P. (1987). Hazard, heredity and depression. A family study. *J. Psychiat. Res.* **21** (4), 365–375.

McGuffin, P., Katz, R. and Bebbington, P. (1988). The Camberwell Collaborative Depression study. III. Depression and adversity in the relatives of depressed probands. *Br. J. Psychiat.* **152**, 775–782.

McKeon, P. and Murray, R.M. (1987). Familial aspects of obsessive-compulsive neurosis. *Br. J. Psychiat.* **151**, 528–534.

McNeil, T.F. and Kaij, L. (1978). Obstetric factors in the development of schizophrenia —complications in the births of preschizophrenics and in reproduction by schizophrenic parents. In: L.C. Wynne (ed.) *The Nature of Schizophrenia*, pp. 401–429. New York: John Wiley & Sons.

Marshall, J.E. and Murray, R.M. (1989). The contribution of twin studies to alcoholism research. In: H.W. Goedde and D.P. Agarwal (eds) *Alcoholism: Biochemical and Genetic Aspects*. New York: Pergamon Press.

Martin, N.G. (1987). Genetic differences in drinking habits, alcohol metabolism and sensitivity in unselected samples of twins. *Prog. Clin. Biol. Res.* **241**, 109–119.

Martin, N.G. and Jardine, R. (1986). Eysenck's contributions to behavior genetics. In: S. Modgil and C. Modgil (eds) *Hans Eysenck: Consensus and Controversy*, pp. 13–61. Lewes, Sussex: Falmer Press.

Martin, N.G., Jardine, R., Andrews, G. and Heath, A.C. (1988). Anxiety disorders and neuroticism: are there genetic factors specific to panic? *Acta Psychiat. Scand.* **77**, 698–706.

Martyn, C.N., Barker, D.J.P., Osmond, C. *et al.* (1989). Geographical relation between Alzheimer's disease and aluminium in drinking water. *Lancet* **i**, 59–62.

Mednick, S.A., Machon, R.A., Huttenen, M.O. *et al.* (1988). Adult schizophrenia following prenatal exposure to an influenza epidemic. *Arch. Gen. Psychiat.* **45**, 189–192.

Mendlewicz, J. and Rainer, J.D. (1977). Adoption study supporting genetic transmission in manic-depressive illness. *Nature* **268**, 327–329.

Mendlewicz, J., Fleiss, J.L. and Fieve, R.R. (1972). Evidence for X-linkage in the transmission of manic depressive illness. *J. Am. Med. Assoc.* **222**, 1624–1627.

Mendlewicz, J., Linkowski, P. and Wilmotte, J. (1980). Linkage between glucose-6-phosphate dehydrogenase deficiency and manic depressive psychosis. *Br. J. Psychiat.* **137**, 337–342.

Mendlewicz, J., Simon, P., Sevy, S. *et al.* (1987). Polymorphic DNA marker on X chromosome and manic depression. *Lancet* **i**, 1230–1232.

Nee, L.E., Polinsky, R.J., Eldridge, R. *et al.* (1983). A family with histologically confirmed Alzheimer's disease. *Arch. Neurol.* **40**, 203–208.

Newman, H.H., Freeman, F.N. and Holzinger, K.J. (1937). *Twins: A Study of Heredity and Environment.* Chicago: University of Chicago Press.

Noyes, R., Clancy, J., Crowe, R., Hoenk, P.R. and Slymen, D.J. (1978). The familial prevalence of anxiety neurosis. *Arch. Gen. Psychiat.* **35**, 1057–1509.

Noyes, R., Crowe, R.R., Harris, E.L., Hamra, B.J., McChesney, C.M. and Chaudhry, D.R. (1986). Relationship between panic disorder and agoraphobia: a family study. *Arch. Gen. Psychiat.* **43**, 227–232.

Noyes, R., Clarkson, C., Crowe, R.R., Yates, W.R. and McChesney, C.M. (1987). A family study of generalized anxiety disorder. *Am. J. Psychiat.* **144**, 1019–1024.

O'Callaghan, E., Gibson, T., Colohan, H. *et al.* (1990). The season of birth effect in an Irish schizophrenic sample—environmental damage or genetic morphism? *Schizophrenia Res.* **3** (1), Special Issue.

O'Rourke, D.H., McGuffin, P. and Reich, T. (1983). Genetic analysis of manic-depressive illness. *Am. J. Phys. Anthropol.* **62**, 51–59.

Offord, D. and Cross, L. (1971). Adult schizophrenia with scholastic failure or low IQ in childhood. *Arch. Gen. Psychiat.* **24**, 431–436.

Oliver, C. and Holland, A. (1986). Down's syndrome and Alzheimer's disease: a review. *Psychol. Med.* **16**, 307–322.

Owen, M.J. and Murray, R.M. (1989). Psychiatry and the new genetics. *Int. Rev. Psychiat.* **1** (4), 217–320.

Owen, M.J., James, L.A., Hardy, J.A. *et al.* (1990). Physical mapping around the Alzheimer disease locus on the proximal long arm of chromosome 21. *Am. J. Hum. Genet.* **46**, 316–322.

Partanen, J., Bruun, K. and Markkanen, T. (1966). Inheritance of drinking behaviour: a study of intelligence, personality and use of alcohol of adult twins. *The Finnish Foundation for Alcohol Studies*, No. 14, Helsinki.

Pelosi, A.J. and David, A.S. (1989). Ethical implications of the new genetics for psychiatry. *Int. Rev. Psychiat.* **1**, 315–320.

Penick, E.C., Powell, B.J., Othmer, E. *et al.* (1978). Subtyping alcoholics by co-existing psychiatric syndromes, course, family history and outcome. In: D.W. Goodwin, K.T. Van Dusen and S.A. Mednick (eds) *Longitudinal Research in Alcoholism.* Boston: Kluwer-Nijhoff.

Pericak-Vance, M.A. Conneally, P.M., Merritt, A.D., Roos, R.P., Vance, J.M., Yu, P.L., Norton Jr, J.A. and Antel, J.P. (1979). Genetic linkage in Huntington's disease. *Adv. Neurol.* **23**, 59–72.

Pericak-Vance, M.A., Yamaoka, L., Haynes, C. *et al.* (1988). Genetic linkage studies in AD families. *Exp. Neurol.* **102** (3), 271–279.

Pickens, R.W. and Svikis, D.S. (1988). The twin method in the study of vulnerability to drug abuse. *NIDA Research Monograph* **89**, 41–51.

Pollitt, J. (1972). The relationship between genetic and precipitating factors in depressive illness. *Br. J. Psychiat.* **121,** 67–70.

Pope, H.G., Jonas, J.M., Cohen, B.M. *et al.* (1982). Failure to find evidence of schizophrenia in first degree relatives of schizophrenic probands. *Am. J. Psychiat.* **139,** 826–828.

Price, J. (1968). The genetics of depressive behaviour. In: A.J. Coppen and A. Walk (eds) *Recent Developments in Affective Disorders,* pp. 37–54. *Br. J. Psychiat.,* Special Publication No. 2. Ashford, Kent: Headley Bros.

Rachman, S.J. and Hodgson, R.J. (1980). *Obsessions and Compulsions.* Englewood Cliffs, NJ: Prentice Hall.

Rasmussen, S.A. and Tsuang, M.T. (1986). Clinical characteristics and family history in DSM-III obsessive–compulsive disorder. *Am. J. Psychiat.* **143,** 317–322.

Reich, T., Clayton, P.J. and Winokur, G. (1969). Family history studies V. The genetics of mania. *Am. J. Psychiat.* **125,** 1358–1369.

Reich, T., Cloninger, C.R., Suarez, B. *et al.* (1982). Genetics of the affective psychoses. In: J.K. Wing and L. Wing (eds) *Handbook of Psychiatry. Psychoses of Unknown Origin,* pp. 147–159. Cambridge: Cambridge University Press.

Reveley, A.M., Reveley, M.A., Clifford, C.A. *et al.* (1982). Cerebral ventricular size in twins discordant for schizophrenia. *Lancet* **i,** 540–541.

Risch, N., Baron, M. and Mendlewicz, J. (1986). Assessing the role of X-linked inheritance in bipolar-related major affective disorder. *J. Psychiat. Res.* **20,** 275–288.

Roses, A.D., Pericak-Vance, M.A., Haynes, C.S. *et al.* (1988). Genetic linkage studies in Alzheimer's disease. *Neurology* **38** (Suppl. 1), 173.

St. Clair, D., Blackwood, D., Muir, W. *et al.* (1989). No linkage of chromosome 5q11–q13 markers to schizophrenia in Scottish families. *Nature* **339,** 305–309.

St. George-Hyslop, P., Tanzi, R., Polinsky, R. *et al.* (1987). The genetic defect causing familial Alzheimer's disease maps on chromosome 21. *Science* **235,** 885–890.

Schellenberg, G.D., Bird, T.D., Wijsman, E.M. *et al.* (1988). Absence of linkage of chromosome 21q21 markers to familial Alzheimer's disease. *Science* **24,** 1507–1510.

Shelton, R.C. and Weinberger, D.R. (1986). CT studies in schizophrenia: a review and synthesis. In: H.A. Nasrallah and D.R. Weinberger (eds) *The Neurology of Schizophrenia,* pp. 205–250. Amsterdam: Elsevier.

Sherrington, R., Brynjolfsson, J., Petursson, H. *et al.* (1988). Localization of a susceptibility locus for schizophrenia on chromosome 5. *Nature* **336,** 164–167.

Shields, J.S. (1962). *Monozygotic Twins: Brought Up Apart and Brought Up Together.* London: Oxford University Press.

Shur, E. (1982). Season of birth in high and low genetic risk schizophrenics. *Br. J. Psychiat.* **140,** 410–415.

Slater, E. (1961). The Thirty-fifth Maudsley Lecture: 'Hysteria 311'. *J. Mental Sci.* **107,** 359–381.

Slater, E. (1965). Diagnosis of 'Hysteria'. *Br. Med. J.* **1,** 1395–1399.

Slater, E. (1976). What is hysteria? *New Psychiat.* **3** (7), 14–15.

Slater, E. and Shields, J. (1969). Genetical aspects of anxiety. In: M. Lader (ed.) *Studies of Anxiety,* pp. 62–71. *Br. J. Psychiat.,* Special Publication No. 3. Ashford, Kent: Headley Bros.

Slater, E. and Slater, P. (1944). A heuristic theory of neurosis. *J. Neurol. Psychiat.* **7,** 49–55.

Strober, M., Morrell, W., Burroughs, J., Salkin, B. and Jacobs, C. (1985). A controlled family study of anorexia nervosa. *J. Psychiat. Res.* **19,** 239–246.

Stunkard, A.J., Harris, J., Pedersen, N.L. and McLearn, G.E. (1990). The body-mass index of twins who have been reared apart. *New Engl. J. Med.* **322** (21), 1483–1487.

Suddath, R.I., Christison, G.W., Torrey, E.F. *et al.* (1990). Anatomical abnormalities in the brains of MZ twins discordant for schizophrenia. *New Engl. J. Med.* **322**, 789–794.

Tanzi, R.E., Gusella, J.F., Watkins, P.C. *et al.* (1987a). Amyloid beta protein gene: cDNA, mRNA distribution, and genetic linkage near the Alzheimer locus. *Science* **235**, 880–884.

Tanzi, R.E., St. George-Hyslop, P.H., Haines, J.L. *et al.* (1987b). The genetic defect in familial Alzheimer's disease is not tightly linked to the amyloid beta protein gene. *Nature* **329**, 156–157.

Taylor, M.A., Abrams, R. and Hayman, M.A. (1980). The classification of affective disorders: a reassessment of the bipolar–unipolar dichotomy. *J. Affect. Dis.* **2**, 95–109.

Torgersen, S. (1983a). Genetic factors in anxiety disorders. *Arch. Gen. Psychiat.* **40**, 1085–1089.

Torgersen, S. (1983b). Genetics of neurosis: the effects of sampling variation upon the twin concordance ratio. *Br. J. Psychiat.* **142**, 126–132.

Torgersen, S. (1986). Genetic factors in moderately severe and mild affective disorders. *Arch. Gen. Psychiat.* **43**, 222–226.

Treasure, J.L. and Holland A.J. (1991). Genes and the aetiology of the eating disorders. In: P. McGuffin and R.M. Murray (eds) *The New Genetics of Mental Illness.* Oxford: Butterworth-Heinemann.

Van Broeckhoven, C., Genthe, A., Vandenberge, A. *et al.* (1987). Failure of familial Alzheimer's disease to segrate with the A4-amyloid gene in several European families. *Nature* **329**, 153–155.

Wasmuth, J.J., Hewitt, J., Smith, B. *et al.* (1988). A highly polymorphic locus very tightly linked to the Huntington's disease gene. *Nature* **332**, 734–736.

Weissman, M.M., Merikangas, K.R., Pauls, D.L. *et al.* (1983). Heritability of schizophrenia. *Am. J. Psychiat.* **140**, 131–132.

Wender, P.H., Kety, S.S., Rosenthal, D. *et al.* (1986). Psychiatric disorders in the biological and adoptive families of adopted individuals with affective disorders. *Arch. Gen. Psychiat.* **43**, 923–929.

Psychology

— 14

Psychology and Psychiatric Symptoms: An Information-Processing Account

C.R. Brewin

Human beings are born with a variety of psychobiological systems to help them adapt and survive to changing circumstances (Gilbert, 1989). Among the most important for psychiatry are the systems that underlie attachment to care-givers and feelings of safety, and those that coordinate responses to social and physical threats and to loss. In all these situations individuals are likely to experience a set of bodily sensations, emotions and motor impulses, linked to different patterns of physiological activity. When separated from care-givers, for example, there is a period of increased arousal and distress, with active behavioural attempts to re-establish contact, followed by a period of despair in which the return of the care-giver appears to have little positive impact. When attacked, either physically or verbally, by someone more powerful, individuals typically make various appeasement gestures, altering their posture and avoiding eye contact. They are likely to experience alternating feelings of shame and rage. With repeated attacks increasing helplessness may ensue, leading eventually to complete passivity and demoralization.

From the regularity of reactions such as these to a small number of well-defined circumstances surrounding physical and social well-being, and from the fact that these reactions may occur early in life, it would seem to follow that people must be equipped at birth with appraisal systems that can recognize information spelling various kinds of danger or safety. Survival may depend on attending to this information and activating the appropriate response. When similar emotional and behavioural reactions occur later in life, apparently without sufficient justification, they are often labelled as psychiatric symptoms and a corresponding diagnosis made. Thus the despair, hopelessness and behavioural retardation that sometimes follow the end of an important relationship may be labelled as depression, and extreme insecurity in intimate relationships, typically accompanied by jealousy, anger, and intrusive thoughts, may be labelled as borderline personality disorder.

Psychotherapists respond to these symptoms by presenting patients with various kinds of new information, using a range of different techniques, to try to convince them that their powerful reactions to the perception of threat or loss are out of proportion to their current situation. Thus behaviour therapists typically have patients carry out assignments in which they try new responses to and test their expectations of problematic situations. Cognitive therapists may

TABLE 14.1   Characteristics of automatic and controlled processing.

Automatic processing	Controlled processing
Parallel	Sequential
Fast	Slow
Effortless	Effortful
Attention not required	Attention required
Inflexible	Flexible
Difficult to modify	Easy to modify

Adapted from Schneider *et al.* (1984).

do this, and in addition get patients verbally to specify and re-evaluate the evidence for their beliefs, testing them against alternative interpretations. Psycho-dynamic therapists present patients with interpretations, and use the experience of the therapeutic situation to correct mistaken assumptions about human relationships. In summary, the issue of how human beings evaluate and respond to information is central to psychiatry and to the understanding of psychiatric symptoms.

Two Cognitive Systems

There is general agreement that people cannot always successfully report how or why they have carried out certain actions. Sportsmen and women are notoriously inarticulate at explaining their skill, and social psychologists such as Nisbett and Wilson (1977) have shown that people are frequently unaware of the causes of their behaviour. Similarly, it is not uncommon for psychiatric patients to show little appreciation of the role of life-events in precipitating their symptoms, and to find it hard to give a satisfactory account of their feelings and reactions. How are we to account for such instances of behaviours that on the one hand are lawful and regular, but do not appear to be under conscious control?

Research in experimental psychology, on such diverse topics as subliminal perception, signal detection, binocular rivalry, selective attention and skill acquisition, strongly suggests that information may be processed in two separate ways, one conscious or 'controlled' and one non-conscious or 'automatic' (Brewin, 1988; Dixon, 1981). Their characteristics are shown in Table 14.1. Sensory inflow is first subjected by the brain to extensive automatic processing that takes into account its physical properties, meaning and emotional significance, and relates it to material stored in memory. The brain appears able to handle a very large amount of information very quickly, almost certainly by processing it in parallel. It operates entirely outside conscious awareness, so that we may become aware of some of the products of this processing when they enter consciousness, but not of the processing itself. In contrast, conscious or controlled processing operates with an extremely limited capacity. We are only able to think consciously about a few items of information at a time, usually one after the other. This form of processing is slow and effortful, and is easily disrupted by stress or other competing demands. It can easily become overloaded with too much information. The advantage of controlled processing, on the other hand, is that it is much easier to modify, and we can readily search for new information and take it into account as we become aware of it. Automatic processing tends to operate in a fairly stereotyped fashion on stimuli which are classified as familiar, and new information typically has less impact upon it unless repeated many times.

It appears that we are all born with the capacity to process certain kinds of stimuli automatically. This confers the evolutionary advantage that as babies we are equipped to learn about regularities in the environment, and also about stimuli associated with reward and punishment. Conditioning experiments indicate that learning in young, pre-verbal children is very similar to that shown by animals. As consciousness and language develop, however, conditioning begins to follow the adult pattern, with children becoming much more influenced by their conscious expectancies of the reinforcement contingencies than by their actual experience of stimulus–reward or stimulus–punishment pairings (Lowe, 1983). Separation of conscious and non-conscious processing can also be demonstrated in patients with various kinds of neurological damage affecting their vision or their memory. Thus some blind patients can detect the location or orientation of stimuli despite being subjectively unable to see the display (Weiskrantz, 1977), and some patients with Korsakov psychosis demonstrate new learning despite profound deficits in short-term memory that eliminate conscious recall or recognition (Schacter, 1989).

If conscious processing depends on a maturational process and is not present at birth, and if non-conscious and conscious processing can be independently measured both in the laboratory and in certain neurological patients, it is tempting to speculate that there may be two separate cognitive systems underlying these two forms of processing. At present it is not clear whether this is the case, or whether there are simply two levels within a single cognitive system. For the purposes of simplicity, and with this caveat in mind, I will talk in the remainder of the chapter as though there were indeed two separate systems.

The likely existence of two cognitive systems raises the question of their relative importance in mediating behaviour. For many years behaviourists have argued that people's actions are shaped by environmental events through processes such as operant and classical conditioning, and that conscious beliefs and feelings are 'epiphenomenal' by-products of these processes rather than causal influences in their own right. These conclusions derived much of their conviction from the study of pathological behaviours over which individuals could exert little conscious control. According to the more recent social learning theorists, on the other hand, conscious goals and plans are among the most important influences on the self-regulation of behaviour. Once aware of their next goal, people adopt what they believe to be the most effective means of achieving it, and adjust these strategies in a flexible way in line with their relative success or failure (Bandura, 1977a). Social learning theory is here espousing the common-sense view that people's actions are not wholly determined by past experiences but are in the service of a being with aims and purposes. It is the fact that behaviour is so often simply a means to an end, and not an end in itself, which permits the great variety and capacity for innovation which characterizes human action.

The differences between the social learning and behaviourist views have been considered by some to reflect a different philosophical position concerning the nature of man, and to amount to little more than a resuscitation of the free will versus determinism debate in a new but no more satisfactory guise. Certainly the behaviourist position that all conscious experience is in some way a product of past learning and has no direct role to play in behaviour mediation is difficult to disprove, but its heuristic value in accounting for complex human behaviour is extremely limited. It is more fruitful to regard the two approaches as having developed to provide an explanation for qualitatively different kinds of behaviour, which we may call regulated and unregulated (Brewin, 1988). The latter is often relatively stereotyped, and occurs in response to well-defined environmental circumstances. If asked, individuals are unlikely to be able to provide a good account of why they are behaving in exactly this way. Indeed, they may be unaware of these actions, or may even report that they performed them against their own volition. Regulated behaviour, on the other hand, is flexible and adaptable to changing circumstances. Individuals typically find no difficulty in accounting for their actions, and are likely to invoke some kind of objective, whether immediate or distant.

The distinction between regulated and unregulated actions is illustrated by research on facial expression. At least five basic emotions (happiness, sadness, fear, anger, disgust) are associated with expressions that are recognized across many different cultures, which suggests that there is an unregulated, evolutionarily-determined component involved in their production. Equally, it has been found that facial expression is more often regulated than body cues or tone of voice, and is subject to cultural display rules that dictate when emotions should be expressed and when they should be concealed. When asked to dissimulate their feelings individuals usually modify their facial expressions rather than postural or vocal cues and, similarly, when people anticipate deception they are most likely to discount facial expression as an accurate index of the other's real attitude. To quote a leading researcher in this area, Paul Ekman:

> The true, felt expressions of emotion occur because facial actions can be produced involun-
> tarily, without thought or intention. The false ones happen because there is voluntary
> control over the face, allowing people to interfere with the felt and assume the false. The
> face is a dual system, including expressions that are deliberately chosen and those that occur
> spontaneously, sometimes without the person even aware of what emerges on his own face.
>
> (Ekman, 1986, p. 123)

Ekman argues that different groups of muscles are involved in the production of spontaneous, unregulated expressions and contrived, regulated ones. He has shown that whereas most people cannot distinguish between 'false' smiles deliberately put on to please and spontaneous 'felt' smiles of pleasure, it is possible to train them to do so by careful observation of the muscles involved in the smile. Spontaneous feelings may also 'leak', for example in the form of micro-expressions. Mary, a 42-year-old housewife with a history of suicide attempts, was filmed telling a hospital doctor that she was feeling much better and would like a weekend pass. Before receiving the pass, however, she confessed that she had been lying and still desperately wanted to kill herself. Close examination of the film in slow motion revealed that, when asked about her plans for the future, a fleeting expression of despair, too brief to be noticed in ordinary conversation, had crossed Mary's face. Micro-expressions typically last for less than one quarter of a second, and are then covered by a different expression. But Ekman suggests that experienced clinicians may be able to spot these clues to people's true feelings, and that even the inexperienced can come to recognise them with an hour's intensive practice.

It is, however, important to bear in mind that most activities will involve some combination of automatic and conscious processing, although the relative balance between the two may be altered. Studies of skill acquisition show that, with repetition, activities that were once conscious, such as learning to operate the controls on a motor car, become automatized and no longer require conscious attention. Similarly, automatic sequences of thoughts and behaviour may be disrupted by paying conscious attention to them. Cognitive therapists attempt to elicit the 'automatic thoughts' that come unbidden into the minds of depressed patients, to focus the patients' attention upon them, and to train patients to question their veracity. This frequently leads to a reduction in the frequency or the intensity of the automatic thoughts. In practice there is a complex interplay between conscious and automatic processing.

Automatic Processing and Psychiatric Symptoms

The characteristics of automatic processing described in Table 14.1 are uncannily similar to the qualities possessed by many psychiatric symptoms. Phobic and obsessional patients typically experience fearful sensations, images, and thoughts without knowing why they do so and in spite of the conscious, 'objective' belief that there is no reason to be frightened. At the same time they may experience powerful impulses to flee or perform a ritualized action such as handwashing. Anxious patients also become hypervigilant for threatening stimuli and can detect these even when they are presented below the threshold for conscious awareness (Mathews and MacLeod, 1986). Similarly, patients with post-traumatic stress disorder often have terrifying 'flashbacks' of the traumatic situation, of such intensity that they can appear real. Bereaved patients may 'see' or 'hear' the person they have lost, and depressed patients frequently have distressing negative thoughts come unbidden into their minds that are compelling in their conviction. Sudden mood swings are another common symptom that appear subjectively inexplicable, occur with frightening unexpectedness, and are difficult to control.

In addition to the rapidity and uncontrollable nature of these experiences, the other feature that suggests the operation of a non-conscious information-processing system is the context in which symptoms occur. Careful interviewing generally elicits that symptoms appear in response to well-defined situational cues. These may be events such as losing a job, environmental cues, such as buses or supermarkets, or internal cues such as thoughts about particularly upsetting experiences. Many patients report that symptoms appear when they are watching television and a certain topic is mentioned. Sometimes the patient is unaware of the cues that trigger symptoms, or may be mistaken about the crucial feature, and the therapist has to establish the cues by questioning and by inference. What seems to be happening is that the sensory input is accessing internal cognitive representations of threatening or painful experiences (it may be helpful to think of these as a kind of 'memory', although not necessarily one that can be consciously recalled). The person then becomes aware to a greater or lesser extent of the feelings, physiological reactions, images, thoughts, and motor impulses that are part of this representation or 'memory' (Brewin, 1989).

Relating these symptoms to automatic processing also enables us to account for the instances when psychiatric patients are unable to locate the origin of their symptoms. One would only have to assume that the person's conscious recollection of events did not correspond to the cognitive representation created by the non-conscious processing system. This might occur for a number of reasons. For example, the critical event or events might have occurred very early in childhood during the period of infant amnesia. There would thus be no conscious recollection of the events, even though learning could have taken place. Other events occurring later in life might have been so distressing that they were defensively excluded from consciousness. Victims of abuse in childhood quite often mention that they deliberately tried to prevent themselves from thinking about what was happening, sometimes by escaping to a fantasy world. Repetition of such a strategy over and over again might result in the original memories becoming harder and harder to recall.

Inability to identify the origin of symptoms might also arise because the non-conscious representation created by the automatic processing system is theoretically based on the full array of sensory input, plus related material in memory, whereas, due to our limited span of attention, the conscious memory would be based on a much smaller amount of information. It is by no means certain that all the relevant causal factors would be consciously perceived by an individual already fearful, in shock, or otherwise distressed. Indeed, there is considerable evidence that anxiety increases attentional selectivity and reduces short-term memory capacity (Eysenck, 1984). Furthermore, social pressures may operate to influence the conscious interpretations that people form of their experience. Children are sometimes deceived about what is really happening in the family, and victims of verbal or physical abuse and humiliation frequently have the experience that others (and not only the perpetrators) deny what has happened to them. Particularly to anyone in a vulnerable position, such suggestions may have the effect of completely distorting their recollections.

The next question to consider is under what circumstances extensive automatic processing is likely to occur. In the experimental psychology literature automatic processing has mainly been seen as arising from repeated experiences with the same set of stimuli. Thus after much practice motor skills such as playing the piano gradually become automatic, and people can learn to search automatically for particular features in a visual display. Repeated experience with complex computer programs can lead to individuals learning the rules by which they operate, even though they cannot state verbally what those rules are. To consider some clinical parallels, it seems likely that repeated experiences of being rejected, or of being told one is incompetent or unlovable, would lead to certain beliefs about oneself becoming deeply entrenched. Related thoughts would tend to come to mind automatically in similar situations encountered later in life, with the result that the person might overreact to slights or other behaviours that fell short of full acceptance. A particularly extreme example of such a pattern is typical of individuals with so-called borderline personality, who frequently have histories of rejection by parental figures. They are characterized by having a very low opinion of their own worth and by being hypersensitive to signs of acceptance or rejection by others. This often leads to intensely dependent relationships with friends, family, and with their doctor or therapist, punctuated by despair and suicidal gestures at any behaviour that appears to signal withdrawal or rejection by the other person. They are subject to intense mood swings and find it very difficult to make sense of or control their reactions.

Research on the family antecedents of depression (Gotlib, 1990) suggests that excessive criticism, indifference or parental control is associated with an increased risk of disorder. These are factors which patients will usually be able to report on being questioned. However, the existence of a non-conscious processing system implies that children may be exposed to repeated situations and learn from them without being necessarily conscious of what they are learning. So a daughter may passively observe many instances of her mother's anger being followed by withdrawal or rejection by her father and later, without knowing why, come automatically to inhibit the expression of her own anger in an intimate relationship. The patterns observed may indeed go completely unrecognized by any of the participants in the drama. An interesting situation arises when a child is consistently being given mixed messages, for example is being told her parents only want what is best for her and yet constantly has the experience that they ignore her needs. Bowlby (1973) and other psychoanalytic writers have suggested that children may develop alternative models of themselves and of their parents, oscillating involuntarily between them according to the situation they find themselves in. From an information-processing perspective it is perfectly possible for mutually contradictory sets of memories to coexist and be accessed by different kinds of cues.

The clinical data indicate that automatic processing also occurs in the context of single traumatic experiences. Post-traumatic stress disorder is a frequent accompaniment of disasters and of individual traumas such as assault and rape. In other words automatic processing of stimuli, mediated by non-conscious perceptual processes, may develop even after single experiences, provided that they involve sufficiently strong emotional arousal. This may be because the hormonal effects of acute stress diminish neural activity in anatomical structures serving conscious processing, devolving control onto non-conscious processing systems (Jacobs and Nadel, 1985). Table 14.2 summarizes the kinds of experience that, according to survey and epidemiological research, are likely to be associated with psychiatric disorder (Harris *et al.*, 1986; Jacobson and Richardson, 1987; Gotlib, 1990). Some involve single and some repeated experiences.

TABLE 14.2   Kinds of experience associated with later psychiatric disorder.

Threats to life or health
Separation and loss
Assault and abuse
Neglect
Rejection or humiliation
Criticism
Excessive parental control

Conscious Processes and Psychiatric Symptoms

Conscious processes are intimately involved in determining how a person responds to psychiatric symptoms and hence how long they last. Their importance is underscored by the fact that the vast majority of symptoms are dealt with by the individual concerned and remain untreated by professionals. The awareness of unwanted or unpleasant symptoms usually leads first to a deliberate search of memory and other available sources of information. Among the aims of this search are to label or classify the experience, to locate the responsible causal agents, and to assess future severity and the individual's future vulnerability. Labelling and classification depend on the person's knowledge of illness and on the subjective probability of different types of illness. Family experiences frequently influence perception, with patients being much more likely to believe their chest pains herald a heart attack if there is someone else in their family with a history of heart trouble. Cultural factors may also exert a strong influence on the definition of illness and on decisions about seeking help.

Causal attribution of symptoms may also affect patients' responses at this stage. Unwanted symptoms such as panic attacks, insomnia, or impotence are frequently attributed to personal defects and inadequacies, a point of view that can only too easily be reinforced by others' reactions. Compared to external attributions, for example to a temporarily stressful situation, such self-attributions are likely to be distressing, to provoke further anxiety, to inhibit disclosure to people who are in a position to help, and to make the problem worse (Storms and McCaul, 1976; Brewin, 1988).

Conscious cognitions are also an important part of the coping process. In most cases there are likely to be a range of more or less effective coping strategies that will spontaneously come to mind, or that other people will suggest, and that people in distress will choose among. Two common types are strategies aimed at altering a problematic situation, such as getting one's doctor to support an application for transfer to better accommodation, and strategies aimed at regulating the person's own emotional response, such as increasing alcohol intake or confiding in a sympathetic friend (Lazarus *et al.*, 1980). In the case of both problem-focused and emotion-focused coping, the sorts of methods people most commonly use are information-seeking, direct action, inhibition of action, and intrapsychic methods such as denial (pretending the problem does not exist) and intellectualization (thinking about the problem in an emotionally detached way).

These coping options are then evaluated by taking into account which is most likely to be effective and the relative balance of benefits and costs associated with each one. The effect of the selected strategy on mood, arousal, or other unwanted emotional reactions can then in turn be consciously monitored. In the short-term, feedback of this kind leads to revisions in the analysis described above and to deliberate alterations in coping strategy. In the longer-term, the consequences of different strategies would be recorded in memory. Successful ones would come more readily to mind, or in certain circumstances might be automatically triggered, whereas unsuccessful ones would become less available to consciousness.

The analysis of people's choice of coping strategy, and what determines the persistence with which they pursue it, comes within the scope of research on motivation. The important factors here are people's views about the cause of the problem, their knowledge and beliefs about the range of appropriate strategies, their estimate of the resources, both personal and environmental, that they think are available to carry out these strategies, and the existence of values and goals that are in opposition to particular coping strategies or coping efforts in general (Bandura, 1977b; Weiner, 1985; Brewin, 1988). Faulty analysis of the cause of a problem, ignorance of an effective strategy, and overestimation of the difficulty involved, could all lead to giving up coping attempts prematurely. It has become recognized that therapeutic strategies are only likely to be helpful if they are compatible with the individual's own analysis of their problem. If therapist and patient have different assumptions there is a high probability that treatment will be prematurely terminated. Therapists therefore need to ensure that they have explored the patient's understanding of the problem and of the reason for the therapeutic tasks.

Causal beliefs also influence the formation of expectancies, for many years a central concept in theories of human motivation. A person's motivation to perform an action has been thought of as the product of two major factors, the value of the goal that the action is designed to attain, and the expectancy that the action will achieve that goal (Feather, 1982). The more important the goal, and the higher the expectancy of success, the more vigorously should the action be performed. 'Unmotivated' patients may therefore attribute their problems to uncontrollable causes and feel there is little hope for the future, an idea captured in Seligman's learned helplessness theory (Seligman, 1975; Abramson *et al.*, 1978). Behavioural and cognitive therapies have developed a number of techniques for overcoming hopelessness, for example by making the problem much more specific, by breaking tasks down into very small steps, and by providing explicit encouragement. Psychodynamic therapies, in contrast, pay much more attention to the possibility that patients have competing goals that undermine their commitment to the therapeutic enterprise (the notion of 'secondary gain'). Many of their techniques are oriented to uncovering these goals and removing resistance to treatment.

Another example of an influential theory based on an expectancy–value framework is the Health Belief Model (Rosenstock, 1966; Becker and Maiman, 1975). Although developed to explain preventive health behaviour and patient adherence to medical regimens in the context of physical disease, it is in principle applicable to the psychiatric domain. According to the HBM, a person's readiness to perform some health-related behaviour is related to three sets of factors: health motivations, such as a general concern about health, willingness to seek medical help, and intention to comply with the suggested action; aspects of perceived threat, such as vulnerability to a particular disorder, and the severity of the symptoms or side effects; and the perceived effectiveness of the actions proposed. The last two sets of factors are clearly estimates of value and expectancy, respectively. A more general theory that has sometimes been applied in the clinical domain is Fishbein and Ajzen's (1975) theory of reasoned action. This states that any attempt to perform some behaviour is preceded by an intention to do so. This intention is in turn a function of two factors, attitude toward the behaviour and the subjective norm. Attitude toward the behaviour is determined by the perceived value of the consequences and by the perceived effectiveness of the behaviour, whereas the subjective norm is a social factor referring to perceived social pressure to carry out the behaviour.

With the exception of learned helplessness, which developed from research with animals, these various motivational theories are characterized by the explicit or implicit role played by conscious intentions. Unlike a behaviourist account of people's actions, they assume that most behaviour is self-generated and that human beings first consciously evaluate and then deliberately attempt to regulate themselves and their environment.

Conclusions

In this chapter the emphasis has been on how the two human cognitive systems are involved in the genesis of and response to neurotic symptoms, but they are also relevant to psychotic symptoms. It has been suggested, for example, that psychosis involves a breakdown of the inhibitory mechanisms that keep automatic processes from entering awareness (Frith, 1979). In this view hallucinations are closely related to the operation of the non-conscious information-processing system, and hence are likely to be related in lawful ways to the individual's past and present experiences. Similarly it has been suggested that delusions represent conscious, essentially rational attempts to make sense of abnormal perceptual phenomena.

From the point of view of the practising psychiatrist a consideration of the different cognitive systems is particularly relevant to patient assessment. Patients are typically expected to give detailed accounts of their feelings, their attempts to manage complicated interpersonal situations, and the causes of salient life-events. In many cases their circumstances will correspond to those least conducive to conscious recall, with a plethora of relevant stimuli past and present, and unexpected reactions in themselves of which they have little understanding. For these reasons there should be an emphasis on collecting a wide variety of data from patients, such as behavioural assessment of their performance in problematic situations and consideration of their response to their therapist ('transference'). Vital clues about the nature of the problem are often likely to be contained in their behaviour, particularly their unregulated behaviour, as well as in their verbal account of themselves.

Understanding psychiatric symptoms ultimately involves drawing on knowledge from a number of different disciplines and appreciating the interplay of social, psychological, and biological factors. In this discussion of symptoms we have invoked many different psychological processes, including memory, attention, appraisal, causal attribution, and coping. Many more could have been included. In studying a particular phenomenon we repeatedly find that we have to draw on the whole of psychology, not just on 'social', 'cognitive', or 'biological' psychology. The field of psychiatry happens to be one where the interplay between conscious and non-conscious processes is especially striking, but it is still only one aspect of a complex whole.

References

Abramson, L.Y., Seligman, M.E.P. and Teasdale, J.D. (1978). Learned helplessness in humans: critique and reformulation. *J. Abn. Psychol.* **87**, 49–74.

Bandura, A. (1977a). *Social Learning Theory.* Englewood Cliffs, NJ: Prentice-Hall.

Bandura, A. (1977b). Self-efficacy: toward a unifying theory of behaviour change. *Psychol. Rev.* **84**, 191–215.

Becker, M.H. and Maiman, L.A. (1975). Sociobehavioural determinants of compliance with health and medical care recommendations. *Medical Care* **13**, 10–24.

Bowlby, J. (1973). *Attachment and Loss,* Vol. 2: Separation. London: Hogarth Press.

Brewin, C.R. (1988). *Cognitive Foundations of Clinical Psychology.* London & Hove: Lawrence Erlbaum.

Brewin, C.R. (1989). Cognitive change processes in psychotherapy. *Psychol. Rev.* **96**, 379–394.

Dixon, N.F. (1981). *Preconscious Processes.* Chichester: Wiley.

Ekman, P. (1986). *Telling Lies.* New York: Berkley Books.

Eysenck, M.W. (1984). *A Handbook of Cognitive Psychology.* London: Lawrence Erlbaum.

Feather, N.T. (ed.) (1982). *Expectations and Actions: Expectancy-value Models in Psychology.* Hillsdale, NJ: Lawrence Erlbaum.

Fishbein, M. and Ajzen, I. (1975). *Belief, Attitude, Intention, and Behaviour: An Introduction to Theory and Research.* Reading, MA: Addison-Wesley.

Frith, C.D. (1979). Consciousness, information processing and schizophrenia. *Br. J. Psychiat.* **134**, 225–235.

Gilbert, P. (1989). *Human Nature and Suffering.* London & Hove: Lawrence Erlbaum.

Gotlib, I.H. (1990). An interpersonal systems approach to the conceptualisation and treatment of depression. In: R.E. Ingram (ed.) *Contemporary Approaches to the Study of Depression.* New York: Plenum Press.

Harris, T.O., Brown, G.W. and Bifulco, A. (1986). Loss of parent in childhood and adult psychiatric disorder: the role of lack of adequate parental care. *Psychol. Med.* **16**, 641–659.

Jacobs, W.J. and Nadel, L. (1985). Stress-induced recovery of fears and phobias. *Psychol. Rev.* **92**, 512–531.

Jacobson, A. and Richardson, B. (1987). Assault experiences of 100 psychiatric inpatients: evidence of the need for routine enquiry. *Am. J. Psychiat.* **144**, 908–913.

Lazarus, R.S., Kanner, A.D. and Folkman, S. (1980). Emotions: A cognitive-pheno-menological analysis. In: R. Plutchik and H. Kellerman (eds) *Emotion, Theory, Research and Experience*, Vol. 1. New York: Academic Press.

Lowe, C.F. (1983). Radical behaviourism and human psychology. In: G.C.L. Davey (ed.) *Animal Models of Human Behaviour*. Chichester: Wiley.

Mathews, A. and MacLeod, C. (1986). Discrimination of threat cues without awareness in anxiety states. *J. Abn. Psychol.* **95**, 131–138.

Nisbett, R.E. and Wilson, T.D. (1977). Telling more than we can know: verbal reports on mental processes. *Psychol. Rev.* **84**, 231–259.

Rosenstock, I.M. (1966). Why people use health services. *Milbank Mem. Fund Quart.* **44**, 94–127.

Schacter, D.L. (1989). On the relation between memory and consciousness: dissociable interactions and conscious experience. In: H.L. Roediger and F.I.M. Craik (eds) *Varieties of Memory and Consciousness*. Hillsdale, NJ: Lawrence Erlbaum.

Schneider, W., Dumais, S.T. and Shiffrin, R.M. (1984). Automatic and control processing and attention. In: R. Parasuraman and D.R. Davies (eds) *Varieties of Attention*. Orlando, FL: Academic Press.

Seligman, M.E.P. (1975). *Helplessness: On Depression, Development, and Death*. San Francisco: Freeman.

Storms, M.D. and McCaul, K.D. (1976). Attribution processes and the emotional exacer-bation of dysfunctional behaviour. In: J.H. Harvey, W.J. Ickes and R.F. Kidd (eds) *New Directions in Attribution Research*, Vol. 1. Hillsdale, NJ: Lawrence Erlbaum.

Weiner, B. (1985). An attributional theory of achievement motivation and emotion. *Psychol. Rev.* **92**, 548–573.

Weiskrantz, L. (1977). Trying to bridge some neuropsychological gaps between monkey and man. *Br. J. Psychol.* **68**, 431–435.

— 15

Perception and Attention

J.A. Weinman and C.D. Frith

In order to respond appropriately to an ever-changing environment, every organism must be able to detect and make sense of any environmental changes. Perception concerns the sensation and interpretation of our environment. It therefore comprises the mechanisms and processes that provide a useful representation of the outside world in our brains. An obvious metaphor is the camera, in which an image of the view appears on the film behind the lens. While this may be analogous with what happens in the eye, it is a totally inadequate model of subsequent representation in the brain. What good would it do to have a detailed reproduction of the outside world somewhere in our brains? The problem of how to interpret and act upon it would remain untouched. As we shall see, perception involves a series of processes of selection, simplification and abstraction, rather than precise reproduction.

Selection begins at the earliest stages of perception. There are many aspects of the environment that we cannot perceive at all, for example infrared and ultraviolet light. For primitive organisms, this is the only mechanism by which selection occurs; but for higher organisms, and for humans in particular, selection is flexible, but still strongly determined by the likely importance of the information to be obtained. We shall turn to the considerable problem of how information is selected for importance, in a later section.

Sensation

Measuring sensory thresholds

First we shall consider the very basic sensitivity of the organism, for the complex processes of selection and interpretation can only begin if the changes in the environment can actually be detected. It would seem to be a simple matter to measure the sensitivity of a person to a simple stimulus, such as a light flash or a tone. We could, for example, find the lowest intensity of the stimulus that could be detected. This is called the *absolute threshold*. It is often determined by gradually increasing the intensity of, say, the light, until the observer says that he can see it. (The 'method of ascending limits'.) We can also investigate difference thresholds by measuring the smallest change in intensity that a person can detect. When this is done we find that, for most sensations, the size of the smallest detectable difference ('just noticeable difference' or JND) increases with the initial intensity. Thus we can detect very small differences at low intensities, but only rather large differences at high intensities. The precise relationship between threshold and intensity is usually a logarithmic one (the Weber–Fechner law).

In all these investigations the relationship between subjective psychological sensations and objective physical changes is being mapped and so the subject has become known as psychophysics (not to be confused with psychophysiology). In this approach the observer is treated as a very simple system, which is investigated by feeding in a known signal and noting the output. The observer's subjective experience is used as a sort of meter from which this output may be read. While this approach to sensation and perception is perfectly adequate for many situations, such as testing for visual and/or auditory acuity, it is of course a gross over-simplification of the human perceptual system. In particular, it does not allow for differences in the state of the observer.

The role of other factors in determining thresholds

The concept of a fixed threshold is that up to a certain intensity the observer perceives nothing, but that at the point of threshold there is a sudden change and from that point upwards all stimuli are perceived. This idea of a sudden change seems intuitively unlikely and can be shown to be false. Around the threshold there is, in fact, a gradual increase in the strength or the likelihood of a sensation. The apparent sudden change occurs because the observer has been instructed to say 'yes' or 'no', according to whether a stimulus has been perceived. In order to make such a response the observer must choose some arbitrary level of sensation (the 'criterion') and only say 'yes' if the actual sensation is above this level. The setting of this criterion may be quite independent of the physical stimulation, but it can dramatically affect the apparent threshold or sensitivity. A major determinant of the criterion is the degree of caution adopted by the observer. A very cautious observer will apparently have a lower sensitivity in terms of threshold than a less cautious observer. This degree of caution can easily be manipulated by varying the consequence of the two types of errors associated with the task. Thus for the civilian radar operator who is having to detect birds in the path of aircraft approaching the runway, it would be better to mistakenly report a flock when there was not one present than to fail to report a flock when there was one present. Hopefully, the opposite is true of a military radar operator watching out for incoming enemy missiles. The important point here is that these two observers will have very different detection thresholds and thus will appear to have very different sensitivities, even though these differences may depend entirely on the different criteria they adopt.

Signal-detection theory

The problem of how to distinguish and measure these two components of detection (i.e. sensitivity and criterion) has been tackled in recent years by signal-detection theory (Green and Swets, 1966). Signal-detection theory proposes that the observer's sensitivity and criterion (or response bias) are independent but will jointly contribute to the detection of stimuli. The sensory component is referred to as 'd'' and provides a measure of the discriminability of a stimulus; the criterion adopted by the observer is referred to as 'beta'. The mathematics of this technique are too complex to go into here, but the methodology is essentially straightforward. To apply signal-detection theory it is necessary to present some trials in which no signal is actually present. The extent to which an observer is prepared to say 'yes' incorrectly to these trials (the 'false positive response') allows an estimation of the strictness or lenience of the criterion adopted. Thus a signal-detection approach implicitly recognizes that the observer does not detect stimuli passively in an 'all or none' fashion, but that a decision has to be made as to whether a stimulus was present.

Attention

In our discussion of thresholds and the sensitivity to simple stimulation, we found it necessary to introduce the concept of a variable criterion that is independent of external stimulation, but which can affect the subject's apparent detection threshold. The term *attention* has often been used to describe this property of the observer. Thus we might say on finding some unexpected result that 'the subject failed to perceive the stimulus because he was not attending'. Perceptual difficulties shown in various pathological states, such as schizophrenia or mental deficiency, are often 'explained' as failure of attention. However, all too frequently this term is used in such a vague and general way that it is not very useful. In particular, it is important to distinguish between attention as an overall state of the observer and as a form of selection.

Levels of attention

It should be clear from the earlier discussion of signal-detection theory that even the simplest aspects of perception do not function in a fixed and predictable way. Over a period of time one's overall level of attention or alertness will fluctuate for all sorts of reasons and, as a result, perceptual efficiency may be affected. There are many factors which determine the level of alertness and these include the motivation of the observer, the degree of monotony involved in the task and even the time of day. These factors can be understood more clearly in relation to the concept of arousal, which is discussed elsewhere in this book (see Chapter 21).

The relationship between the level of attention, in the sense discussed here, and perceptual efficiency is neither linear nor incremental. At low levels of arousal, performance on perceptual tasks is generally poor; it tends to improve exponentially with increasing arousal, until an optimal level is reached. Further increases in arousal may bring about an exponential decrease in performance. Performance may be radically disrupted at very high levels of arousal and there may be changes in the ways information is processed. Thus there may be a narrowing of attention or an attentional bias to selected environmental stimuli which are particularly associated with the source of the arousal (see Eysenck and Keane, 1990, pp. 486–487). The exact nature of the relationship between the level of arousal and performance ultimately depends on the complexity of the task and on the skill of the perceiver.

One of the best known experimental techniques for both monitoring and measuring changes in an observer's level of attention are 'vigilance tasks'. These tasks emphasize the maintenance of alertness and accuracy of perception over long periods of time, during which the observer is required to detect weak and infrequent signals (e.g. small blips on a radar screen). After thirty minutes or more, vigilance performance consistently deteriorates. At first it was thought that this decrement reflected a fatiguing of the sensory system, but more recent signal-detection analyses of vigilance have shown that the sensitivity ('d'') does not usually change significantly over time but that observers may become less certain or more cautious about saying that they have 'seen' a signal. Thus it is possible to understand fluctuations in level of attention more precisely in terms of changes in an observer's criterion or willingness to respond. Recently Baddeley (1990) has proposed that vigilance decrements are more likely to be found on tasks which place particular demands on working memory (e.g. having to make judgements about sequences of items rather than single items).

In addition to these fluctuations in an observer's overall level of alertness, there are also important differences in the mode of attention, which will be discussed later (see focal versus ambient attention and controlled versus automatic attention). These differences are determined by the characteristics of the stimuli, by tasks requiring specific types of response, and by the skill and experience of the observer. They all serve to illustrate that attention is not a fixed property of the observer.

Selective attention

So far we have discussed the observer as if only one type of signal is received but in reality a multitude of signals from many different sources are constantly arriving. The traditional, if now somewhat dated, example of this situation is the cocktail party in which we may be within earshot of a dozen conversations. It is a striking human ability that we can pick out and attend to one of these conversations while ignoring the rest. This is quite a different aspect of attention from the one we have already discussed, since we are simultaneously attending to one signal while ignoring another. A signal of this sort from a single source and extended over time is known as a *channel*.

There are two main problems in achieving selective attention. Firstly, the observer must decide which of the many available signals to be attended to. This is presumably done on the basis of the likely importance of the signal in the current circumstances. Secondly, having chosen the signal to attend to, there must be mechanisms available that enable the observer to focus on that signal and apparently ignore the rest. In addition, for reasons of safety, it must be possible to switch attention to other signals if some event of vital importance occurs on one of the unattended channels (e.g. a fire alarm outside; the mention of a pertinent name in a rival, non-attended conversation).

Dichotic listening

One of the most widely used experimental tasks for investigating selective attention involves the technique of *dichotic listening*. In this, two different messages are presented simultaneously to the listener, usually over headphones, and the task is to pay exclusive attention to one of them. It has been found that subjects can attend to one channel and will report that they are unaware of all but the physical features (e.g. loudness, pitch) of the other 'unattended' message. However, there is ample evidence to show that the 'unattended' message is still being processed, since the listener can switch attention rapidly to it if its contents are more appropriate, behaviourally. Thus if the message being attended to is continued in the unattended channel or if the listener's name appears there, attention will be switched to it automatically (Treisman, 1969).

Limited channel capacity

The ability to attend selectively to one message among many and the consequent difficulty in attending to more than one at any one time has given rise to the notion of the 'limited channel capacity' of the human perceiver. Put simply, this states that we can process, consciously, only a limited amount of information. Once this maximum has been reached, additional processing cannot occur and either existing processing operations must slow down or information has to be ignored. Although it is possible to regard this as a structural limitation of the human brain, it might be more plausible to regard it as a direct consequence of our ability to attend selectively. Furthermore, there is not a fixed limit on the amount of information we can process and attend to at any one time. Information that is familiar or predictable appears to use up less processing capacity and allows some attention to be allocated to other stimuli. Thus it is still possible to attend successfully to this type of information in the presence of competing stimuli. In contrast, attending to unfamiliar information may not only be less efficient but will also be more disrupted by competing stimuli.

Over the years there has been considerable debate as to how early attentional selectivity occurs in processing and, hence, what happens to information which the observer is not conscious of (i.e. to what extent has it been processed?). The current view proposes that the timing of selection and the fate of 'unattended' information will depend on the nature of the task and the skill and intention of the perceiver (see Johnston and Dark, 1986). Some of these factors are discussed in the next section.

Automatic and controlled attention

In the preceding section, it became clear that the way in which a subject attends can depend on the type of information that he is having to process. If the subject is skilled at a task and if, as a result, relatively little conscious effort is required to maintain a high level of performance, then this type of processing is referred to as *automatic*. This mode of processing contrasts with *controlled* processing, in which a great deal of effort or conscious attention is necessary on the part of the subject because he is relatively unskilled on that particular task (see Schneider and Shiffrin, 1977).

Although some researchers have encouraged the view that attention can be dichotomized into either automatic or controlled processes, this is almost certainly misleading. It is probably more realistic to conceive of any particular type of information processing as lying somewhere on a continuum from the highly automatic to the highly controlled, depending on the type of stimuli and the subject's skill. Whereas simple tasks may be processed relatively automatically from the outset, it is also clear that many complex processes are carried out automatically.

An influential theory which addresses the question of levels of automaticity has been proposed by Norman and Shallice (1986), who distinguish between fully automatic processes, partially automatic processes and those involving deliberate control. Automatic processes are usually well-learned skills which can carry on without conscious control but occasionally it may be necessary to decide between two ongoing activities (e.g. driving and talking) in the face of an additional demand (e.g. an unpredictable driver ahead). Here decisions can be made by a relatively automatic decision process known as 'contention scheduling' which uses prior rules to make choices based on importance or utility. In addition to these two systems, Norman and Shallice include a 'supervisory attentional system' which operates as a high level control system capable of interrupting or changing ongoing processes, to deal with changing environmental circumstances. Shallice (1982) has linked this system with the controlling and organizational functions of the frontal lobes and interprets frontal lobe deficits, such as perseveration, as a failure of this system.

Occasionally, automatic processes become so ingrained that they can interfere with a more controlled process. A well-known example of this is the Stroop effect, in which colour names are printed in inks of inappropriate hues. If subjects are asked to name the colours of the inks as quickly as possible, they usually find this much more difficult than reading out each colour name. This is because of a highly learned and overriding response to read out words as soon as we see them, which, in this task, directly interferes with the conscious attempt to name the ink colours. Thus in this task it is very difficult to suppress the automatic process of extracting meaning from a written word, with the result that it interferes with the observer's conscious attention to the surface colour of the words.

Defects of controlled attention and consciousness

It is relatively easy to study defects in automatic processes. In most cases the patient himself is aware of his problems in this area (e.g. difficulties with remembering or reading) and can to some extent describe them. The failure in the automatic process appears to cause the allocation of controlled attention to the problem and results in attempts to find alternative methods of solving it. All this activity will involve some degree of awareness as to what constitutes the problem.

However, if controlled attention fails there is no higher level system to take over. Thus it will be very difficult for the patient to gain any insight into what is going wrong. Furthermore, for an observer of the patient's behaviour, it will appear that failure occurs during various automatic processes, such as memory and orientation. However, the precise nature of the failure will be inconsistent and variable. In particular, it will be difficult to test the functioning of an automatic process, since the defect in controlled attention may result in failure to implement the process correctly even though it is intact. It may well appear that the patient is constantly carrying out a task slightly different from the one intended by the investigator. (Frith, 1981, has speculated that a defect of controlled attention might underlie the symptoms of schizophrenia.)

Attentional biases and mood

Since there is growing evidence that many internal and external factors can determine what aspects of the environment are attended to, it is perhaps not surprising to note recent evidence showing that mood can influence attention. The most striking and consistent findings here are found with highly anxious individuals and patients. Following Beck and Emery (1985) and Eysenck (1988) it is postulated that since anxious individuals feel vulnerable and are concerned about threats or dangers, they are likely to be more vigilant or attentive to possible danger signals. Recent findings demonstrate that highly anxious individuals selectively attend to socially threatening (e.g. humiliation) or physically threatening (e.g. injury) words when these are presented together with more neutral stimuli. In contrast non-anxious subjects will either show no bias or selectively attend to neutral stimuli. Eysenck (1988) also argues that highly anxious inividuals have a reduced attentional capacity since part of this capacity will be used up on attentional processes involved in maintaining a vigilance for threatening stimuli. With other adverse mood states such as depression, an attentional bias to mood-congruent stimuli is not found even though depressed individuals are more likely to show a selective recall of negative memories (see Eysenck and Keane, 1990, Chapter 13, for a more detailed discussion).

Eye Movements

With the senses of sight and touch, we can selectively attend in a very concrete way. Unlike the ears, our eyes are constantly moving, searching and exploring the visual environment. The primary function of these eye movements is to ensure that light information from the environment is directed onto the small foveal region of the retina, which is best suited for the detailed analysis of the visual field. Thus when we are looking at a scene or even a relatively small object, we do not take all the information in at a glance but our eyes scan around in a

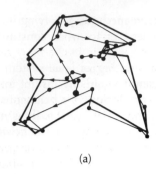
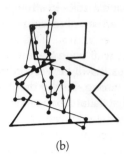

(a)   (b)

FIG. 15.1   Eye movement records for an observer viewing (a) an asymmetrical shape and (b) a symmetrical shape (from Locher and Nodine, 1973).

characteristic and semi-systematic manner. These scanning movements are jerky and ballistic in nature and are made approximately three times per second. Smooth eye movements are only made when the eyes are following a moving stimulus in the environment; they cannot be generated voluntarily.

By studying the sequence of eye fixations made while scanning a scene or object, we can learn a great deal about attention and perception. Figure 15.1 shows typical sequences of fixations associated with two meaningless geometric designs (Locher and Nodine, 1973). The shape shown in Fig. 15.1(a) is asymmetric and fixations have occurred all round its borders, with a slight excess of fixations at or near corners. In such an object the corners can be considered to be particularly important or informative features, since they indicate changes in the direction of the boundary. So here we see evidence that the fixations have been directed to the most important and informative areas. The shape shown in Fig. 15.1(b) is symmetrical. As a consequence half the object is redundant, in the sense that if we know the shape of the left half and the symmetry rule, then the shape of the right half is completely determined. The pattern of eye fixations reflects this redundancy, since they occur only on one side of the object. The perceptive reader will notice an apparent paradox in these results. How does the observer know that he need only look at one side of the figure? Surely he must look at both sides in order to observe the symmetry and thus discover the redundancy? An answer to this apparent paradox follows in the next section, where it will be shown that there appears to be a preliminary analysis of the visual scene which precedes the more detailed processing of information falling on the foveal region.

Two visual systems

In addition to the main visual system, based on the visual pathway from the eye to the visual cortex, there are two, or perhaps more, anatomically distinct systems with complementary functions. Whereas the cortical system resolves fine details of a visual image, a second system appears to carry out an initial primitive analysis of the scene, presumably making use of peripheral vision, which guides the subsequent sequence of eye fixations. In other words peripheral vision is used to pick up areas of probable importance, which can then be focused on for a more detailed investigation. This concept of vision operating in two distinct modes is consistent with recent neurophysiological and neurological evidence.

Neurophysiological recordings of retinal ganglion cells and from the visual pathways have revealed that there are at least two distinct types of neurone that respond to visual information (see Ikeda and Wright, 1974). One type ('x' cells) is found to be triggered predominantly by light falling on the foveal and parafoveal regions of the retina and has a characteristic sustained response (i.e. it continues to fire for some time after it has been triggered). The fibres from cells of this type conduct relatively slowly and project primarily to the visual cortex. In contrast, the more peripheral regions of the retina are responded to by another type of retinal ganglion cell ('y' cells), which has a relatively transient response. Fibres from these cells conduct much more rapidly and project to regions of the midbrain, particularly the superior colliculus, as well as the visual cortex. Thus it has been proposed that the cortical system based on the 'sustained' cells is concerned with the detailed analysis of the visual environment, whereas the superior colliculus plays an important role in a very early pre-conscious phase of processing, which can determine where conscious attention will be allocated.

The results of studies of patients with neurological damage to the visual cortex, but with an intact superior colliculus, are consistent with the idea that there is a second visual system that carries out a preliminary analysis of incoming visual information. These patients seem to have some visual information available at a pre-conscious level. Thus they can 'guess' where a light has flashed on in a blind visual field, even though they have no conscious awareness of the stimulus. However they do not appear to be able to make guesses about any details of a stimulus. These strange visual capacities have been referred to as 'blindsight' and are thought to reflect the residual contribution of the pre-conscious attentional mechanisms mediated by the superior colliculus (see Perenin and Jeannerod, 1975; Weiskrantz, 1986).

Eye movements and complex scenes

Figure 15.2 shows the sequence of fixations shown by an observer studying a complex scene. The small black dots show each eye fixation and the sequence of fixations over time can be easily seen. The example is taken from the work of Yarbus (1967), a pioneer in the study of eye movements. In the various examples the sequences of eye movements are very different. This is a consequence of the question the observer has been asked about the picture. Thus, if he has been asked for the ages of the people in the picture, he concentrates on the faces and makes repeated comparisons of one face with another. If, on the other hand, he has been asked for the social class of the family, he concentrates on the objects in the room and the clothes of the individuals. This is a clear example of selective attention. However, whereas in Fig. 15.1 selection was elicited by the properties of the stimulus, in Fig. 15.2 it has been determined by the requirements of the observer. It is important to remember that perception is never entirely determined by the

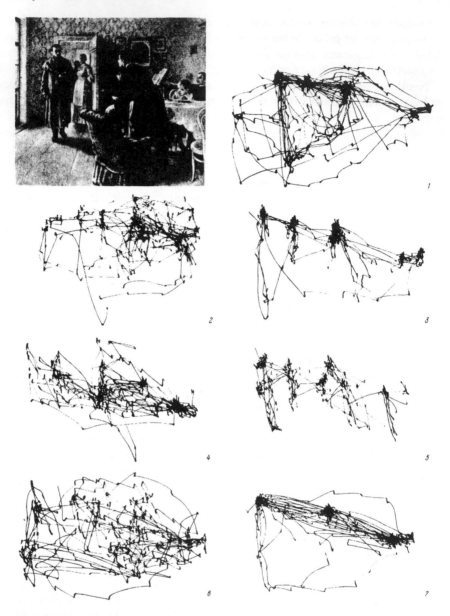

FIG. 15.2   Seven records of eye movements by the same observer. Each record lasted 3 minutes. The observer examined the picture with both eyes. (1) Free examination of the picture. Before the subsequent recording sessions, the observer was asked to: (2) estimate the material circumstances of the family; (3) give the ages of the people; (4) guess what the family had been doing before the 'unexpected visitor' arrived; (5) remember the clothes worn by the people; (6) remember the position of the people and objects; and (7) estimate how long the 'unexpected visitor' had been away from the family (from Yarbus, 1967).

stimulus. It is always an interaction between the stimulus and the observer. These two determinants of perception have been referred to as 'data driven' and 'conceptually driven' respectively.

Feature Detection and Perception

In our discussion of eye movements we introduced the concept of a feature that is considered to be the basic unit of which an object or scene is composed. The use of the term 'feature' was introduced by linguists to describe the properties of phonemes, the basic units of sound in speech. In this case a phoneme either had or did not have certain features, such as voicing and affrication. This model describes the perception of phonemes very well. The term feature is often used in this way so that only two states are possible. However, it can also be used to imply a dimension with many possible states or even a continuous dimension.

Neurophysiological mechanisms for feature analysis

The attraction of a model in which perception is seen as decomposing a scene into its component features is enhanced by the neurophysiological evidence, which has shown that the visual cortex is made up of cells that respond only to very specific visual features, such as small line or edge segments in a particular orientation (Hubel, 1979). This research has also demonstrated the existence of feature-detecting cells for many other elements, including some of considerable complexity. There is currently some debate as to the exact nature of these building blocks of the brain's representation of a visual scene. For example, it is claimed that cortical cells respond to specific spatial frequencies rather than to specific line segments (Maffei and Fiorentini, 1973). Although this debate continues, it is agreed that the cells in the visual cortex do respond to very specific elements of the visual image and that these provide the initial representation, on which more detailed processing must take place.

The neurophysiological evidence of image processing beyond the primary visual cortex shows that there are adjacent cortical areas that appear to carry out separate, parallel analyses of different attributes of the visual scene, such as colour, movement and depth (Zeki, 1978). The output from these separate analyses is re-combined in the inferotemporal regions of the brain, where the complicated process of recognizing whole objects appears to take place. Very little is known about the neurophysiological mechanisms mediating object recognition. Some neurophysiologists have claimed that there are single cells that only respond to the very specific collection of features associated with a particular object (Gross *et al.*, 1972; Perrett *et al.*, 1982). Also, it is known that patients with neurological damage involving this region of the brain can suffer from visual-object agnosia, in which they can see all the component features of an object yet appear to be unable to perceive the object as a whole (see Ratcliff and Ross, 1981). This perceptual disorder can be understood as a failure of a later stage of perceptual processing in the model proposed by Marr (1980) and described below.

Object recognition by features

One of the main problems for an observer is to be able to recognize the objects he is perceiving. One way to do this is by representing an object as a list of features (i.e. an elephant must have a trunk, be grey, be large, have a small tail, have big ears, etc.). By perceiving an object as a list of features it can be recognized by comparing observed features with the store of lists held in long-term memory. This is clearly a fairly simple and economic way of handling complex stimuli. It has the drawback that in a list of features the relationships between them are not retained. Thus it would create problems for perceiving distorted or inappropriately oriented versions of the object. Moreover a number of other important earlier stages are required in object recognition and these are described below.

Hierarchies of features

In this section we have grouped together under the term feature, entities such as redness and lines of a certain orientation, with much higher-level entities such as ears and tails. It is possible to arrive at such high-level features on the basis of a hierarchy of feature detectors such that the detection of a high-level feature depends on the detection of a suitable combination of low-level ones. As we remarked earlier, some neurophysiologists have speculated that such hierarchies of detectors do indeed exist and suggest, if somewhat playfully, that there could be a single cell that responds only to the appearance of one's grandmother. This type of processing may be possible for familiar or predictable stimuli, in which it might also be possible to bypass some of the earlier stages of analysis. This type of processing is an extreme example of how perception, concept formation and object recognition must ultimately come together.

Perceiving Structure

It is clear that perception does not stop at the level of constructing a list of features. There is much evidence for mechanisms that retain the relationships between features. Many stimuli are, in fact, only distinguishable because of relationships and are difficult to recognize from their component features (see later section on face perception, for an example). A great deal more information has to be extracted and organized from the retinal image in order to provide the observer with a usable representation of his visual environment. Firstly, it will be necessary to determine which component features 'go together' to form larger units and to segregate these from the background. Occasionally the reverse process may be necessary, since the component features of a whole object may be so organized that it may be difficult to identify individual subunits. In addition to these basic processing requirements, the observer needs to gain an accurate representation of the distance of, and spatial relationships between objects, as well as having a sensitivity to movement of part or the whole of a visual image. A consideration of some of these higher-level organizational processes follows, preceded by a brief introduction to an influential and useful general model for object recognition.

A model of object recognition

A great deal of current experimental and neuropsychological work on perception has been influenced by the model of object recognition proposed by Marr (1980). Marr has developed a model which assumes that vision involves the computation of efficient descriptions or representations of the retinal image in order to provide usable visual information. He argues that this process involves three stages or types of representation.

For Marr, the basic representation involves a description of the intensity changes in the field of vision. This first representation is referred to as the *primal sketch* and this provides a set of statements about all the edges and features present in the visual image (the raw primal sketch) which is then used to identify the larger structures which are present (the full primal sketch). The next stage involves the production of a viewer-centred representation, which is referred to as the $2\frac{1}{2}$-*D sketch*, and is achieved by an analysis of the depth, movement, shading and other structural information present in the primal sketch. Thus this provides a viewer-centred description of the visual information but the third stage is necessary for object recognition. This is referred to as the *3-D model representation* and is a representation of the seen objects and surfaces which is independent of the viewer's vantage point. It therefore describes the real shape of the objects and surfaces and their relative positions. In doing this it accesses stored descriptions of objects and uses these to identify the scanned objects. Some of these processes were referred to above in the account of feature perception and some of the processes involved in the earlier stages of Marr's model are described in the next section.

Figure–Ground Segregation

A major problem in object perception is to distinguish the object from its background. In most cases there is a clear edge separating the two and so the detection of change is an efficient strategy for achieving separation. The essence of camouflage is to break up this edge both by matching the colours of the two and by creating many false edges which confuse and overload the change detecting system. For example, in Fig. 15.3, it may initially be quite difficult to detect an object as distinct from the background. In this situation all the feature analysers will be working perfectly, providing local feature information, but it is clear that no meaningful perception will occur until an object is perceived and distinguished from the background.

In real life a far more powerful cue for distinguishing an object from its background is movement. When in motion, all the components will move in one way while the background moves in another (common fate). This is an immensely salient aspect of a scene and can arise not only from movement of the object, but also, because of motion parallax, from movement of the observer in relation to his environment.

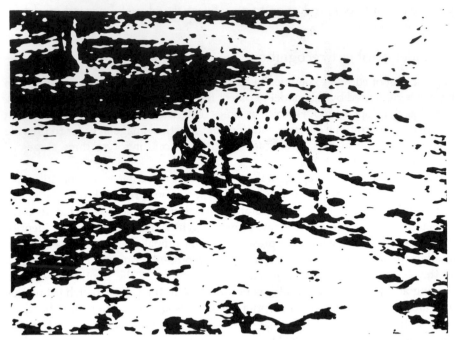

FIG. 15.3 Perceiving the whole object involves more than merely identifying the component features. (Photograph by R.C. James, taken from Thurston, J. and Carraher, R.G. (1966) *Optical Illusions and the Visual Arts*. New York: Litton Educational.)

Movement perception

There are two ways in which movement information is processed by the visual system. Firstly, a moving object can be tracked with smooth, pursuit eye movements, which maintain the image of the object on the foveal region of the retina ('the eye–head system'). Thus the nature of the pursuit movements of the eyes provides direct information about the nature of the movement of an object in the environment. Secondly, a moving image may pass across the retina while the observer is fixating another object ('the image–retina system'). In the latter case, it is the sequential detection of matched features on proximal regions of the retina that gives rise to the experience of movement. It is therefore possible to trick the visual system into perceiving movement by presenting identical stimuli in neighbouring parts of the visual field, with a brief time interval between them ('apparent' or 'phi' movement).

Depth perception

In Marr's model, depth perception also plays an important role in structuring a scene into its important components. Although all the information we get about a visual scene appears upon the two-dimensional retinal surface at the back of our eyes, our perception of the world is fully three-dimensional. This internal view

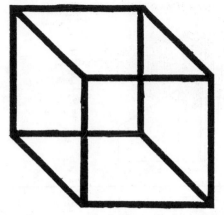

FIG. 15.4   The Necker cube.

is constructed on the basis of the relationships between many component features.

At short distances, the discrepancy between the views of the two eyes is used (stereopsis). For longer distances, cues provided by motion parallax, relative sizes, density gradients and overlapping, are all combined to give a plausible three-dimensional reconstruction of the scene. This is often regarded as an over-simplification. It is probably easier to handle a world in which people are roughly the same size but appear at different distances, than it is to handle one in which they move all over a two-dimensional sheet changing size as they do so. The Necker cube is an extremely simplified example of depth perception, based on the principle of simplification (see Fig. 15.4). By seeing the collection of lines as a cube in depth, their relationships are much simplified. All the lines are the same length and all the angles are 90°. The price we pay for this simplification is that the three-dimensional version is ambiguous. For the Necker cube, two versions are equally plausible. Consequently our perception of the figure spontaneously switches from one version to the other.

Constancies

Although we have a reasonable representation of depth information, we tend to see objects as staying the same size rather than getting smaller as they move away from us. This is called 'size constancy'. Indeed, this perception is so powerful that it is often difficult for an observer to estimate the real retinal size of an object. Few, unless they have tried it, will believe that the moon can be completely covered by a new five pence piece held at arm's length.

There are many other examples of constancy in perception. For example, objects are perceived as having a relatively constant colour and albedo whatever their illumination ('colour constancy') and round tables are perceived as round in spite of an oblique viewpoint ('shape constancy'). All these percepts depend on interpreting many different features and cues. Like all interpretations they can be wrong. An extreme example is the Ames room in which, as a consequence of the

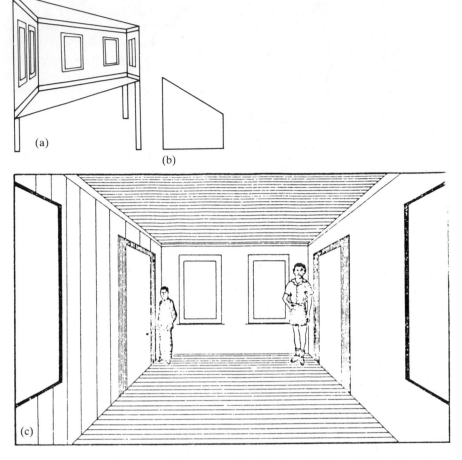

FIG. 15.5   The Ames 'distorted room'. (a) Elevation from the front. (b) Plan from above. (c) The appearance of the room, which we prefer to see as a square room containing people of the wrong size rather than as a distorted room with people of normal size. (From Vernon (1962) *The Psychology of Perception*. London: Penguin Books.)

erroneous interpretation that the room is rectangular, we perceive that people of identical or similar height appear to differ greatly in size when standing in the two opposite corners of the room (see Fig. 15.5).

Recoding

To achieve depth perception we have recoded two-dimensional retinal information into a three-dimensional version. This is clearly very useful when we come to act upon our perceptions and move about in a world that really is three-dimensional. However, recoding seems to be a common principle in perception and is not always so obviously relevant. Conrad (1964) studied the errors that people made when having to remember letters shown briefly on a screen. He found that confusions occurred between the letters X, S, F and between B, T, V. It is difficult to see, at first, why these confusions should occur, since these groups of letters have markedly different appearances. However, when named, the sounds of the letters within those two groups are very similar. This suggests that the subjects first recoded the letters as sounds and based their recall on these sounds rather than on the shapes they had seen. This may seem rather an unnecessary example of recoding. However, it is likely that we are more practised at handling letters as sounds rather than shapes. One reason might be that the shapes of letters vary quite a bit (e.g. a, A, *a*)—whereas the name is the same. It is also possible that short-term memory for sounds is more accessible than short-term memory for shapes. This is consistent with current models of short-term memory which incorporate a speech-based system or 'articulatory loop', capable of coding and storing information (Baddeley, 1986).

Face perception

Of all the different perceptual processes, face recognition is clearly one of the most important in day to day life. Although many of the processes described in earlier sections are also involved in perceiving faces, there is growing evidence that faces are a rather special class of stimuli which may be processed in a number of different ways. A very useful recent account of face recognition has been provided by Bruce and Young (1986), who propose that many component processes are involved, depending on the type of face which is being perceived (e.g. familiar or unfamiliar) and the perceiver's task (e.g. naming; identifying the expressed emotion, etc.). Following Marr (1980), they propose that the initial perception involves a *structural encoding* of the face. Following this a number of other processes can be used and these include: *expression analysis*, in which the emotional state can be identified from the configuration of facial features; *facial speech analysis*, which involves the perception of lip movements for perceiving speech; *directed visual processing*, involving the direction of attention to specific facial features; *assessing facial recognition units* (stored structural information), in the case of previously identified faces; *accessing person identity notes* in order to obtain other information about the owner of the face (i.e. who they are and what they do); and *name generation* in order to name the person perceived. Bruce and Young also suggest that, in addition to making use of all these systems, face recognition must also rely on more general cognitive information. Studies of patients with neurological lesions have shown that occasionally these can involve a selective disruption of face recognition (prosopagnosia), sometimes affecting all of the above systems and sometimes only affecting certain components (see Ellis and Young, 1988—Chapter 4).

In addition to the very specific neurological impairments of face recognition, there is some evidence that schizophrenic patients may have difficulties in processing facial information. Recent evidence indicates that this may involve a problem in integrating perceptual information (Schwartz Place and Gilmore, 1980; Frith, 1981) which may be associated with problems in judging facially-expressed emotions (Gessler *et al.*, 1989).

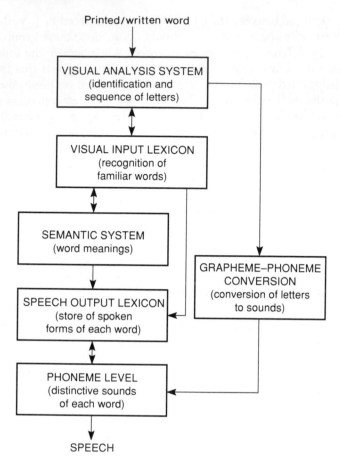

Printed/written word

FIG. 15.6   Routes and processes involved in reading (adapted from Eysenck and Keane, 1990).

Information processing models in reading

Because of its complexity and importance, reading has been studied in detail by experimental psychologists and is one of the few processes for which complete perceptual models have been proposed (see Fig. 15.6). Such models typically involve many of the components that have been discussed in this chapter and would include the following processes. On the basis of their component features, the lines and curves that make up each letter are matched by the reader with known letter shapes. These letters or groups of letters are then recoded into phonemes ('grapheme to phoneme conversion'). Once the transfer from vision to sound has been achieved, the reader can make use of his well-established speech processing system to transform the groups of phonemes into words and then can look up these words in his internal lexicon to discover their meaning (see Allport, 1979).

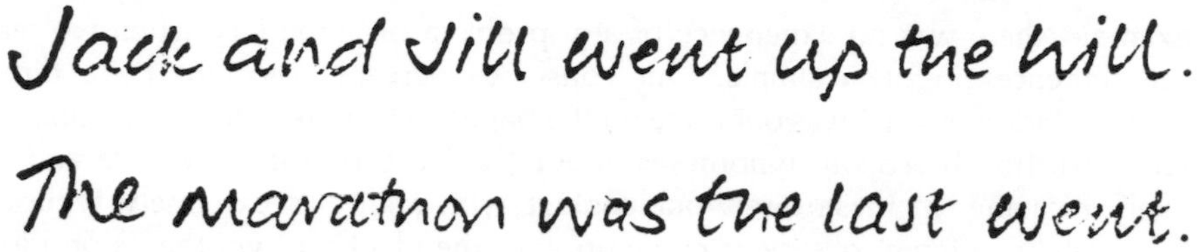

Jack and Jill went up the hill.

The marathon was the last event.

FIG. 15.7   The perception of individual letters and words depends on the meaning of the whole sentence.

It turns out that the reading process is somewhat more sophisticated than this. It is not always necessary to go via sound to get from graphic shapes to identified words, since there is a so-called direct route from graphemes to meaning. This type of process occurs more obviously in the reading of an ideographic orthography such as Chinese, in which (theoretically at least) no specific sound is associated with each character. Certain stroke patients who acquire an inability to read (acquired dyslexia) have apparently lost the ability to use the reading route that depends on recoding to sound, but can still use the direct route from graphemes to meaning. As a consequence, they sometimes read a word wrongly but with the correct meaning (e.g. flower for bloom). In addition, they cannot read new words or nonsense words (e.g. cernalit), since such words can only be 'read' by translating them into sounds (see Coltheart, 1980; Ellis and Young, 1988 —Chapter 8).

Bottom-up/top-down processing

Both these models of reading are essentially linear and 'bottom-up', in that each stage of processing, from the most basic form of detection and recognition, must be completed before going on to the next and higher stage. It is easy to show that such models cannot fully account for reading or any other perceptual process. The two sentences shown in Fig. 15.7 are easy to read and at first sight it may be difficult to see what they are supposed to be demonstrating. However, a closer look will reveal that the graphic shape at the beginning of the words 'went' and 'event' is identical and yet in one word it is interpreted as 'ev' and in the other as 'w'. The linear bottom-up model could not handle this example because it would not be able to decide which interpretation of the ambiguous graphic shape to pass on to the next stage. Indeed, the correct interpretation can only be known after the meaning of each sentence has, to some extent, been worked out.

A successful model of reading (and of perception in general) must therefore allow for feed-back from the later stages of interpretation onto the earlier stages. In other words, hypotheses above what the sentence might mean are used to convert ambiguous graphemes into phonemes. This aspect of perception is known as top-down processing. It is unlikely that either bottom-up or top-down processing operates in isolation, but rather that both are used to varying degrees as the circumstances demand.

All of these complex processes usually occur very rapidly and without any awareness of this complexity or even that any processing is happening at all. For example, there was no experience of any problem or ambiguity when we read the sentences in the example. Our conscious percepts seem to be a direct representation of what was out there on the paper. In fact, they are an imaginative reconstruction based on hypotheses about the basic sensory evidence and its likely meaning. In these terms our contact with reality is extremely tenuous. Fortunately, different observers come up with the identical hypotheses on most occasions.

References

Allport, A. (1979). Word recognition in reading. In: P.A. Kolers, M.E. Wrolstad and H. Bouma (eds) *The Processing of Visible Language*, Vol. 1. New York: Plenum.

Baddeley, A. (1986). *Working Memory*. Oxford: Oxford University Press.

Baddeley, A. (1990). *Human Memory: Theory and Practice*. Hove: Lawrence Erlbaum.

Beck, A.T. and Emery, G. (1985). *Anxiety Disorders and Phobias: a Cognitive Perspective.* New York: Basic Books.

Bruce, V. and Young, A.W. (1986). Understanding face recognition. *Br. J. Psychol.* **77**, 305–327.

Coltheart, M. (1980). Deep dyslexia: a review of the syndrome. In: M. Coltheart, K.E. Patterson and J.C. Marshall (eds) *Deep Dyslexia*. London: Routledge & Kegan Paul.

Conrad, R. (1964). Acoustic confusions in immediate memory. *Br. J. Psychol.* **55**, 75–84.

Ellis, A.W. and Young, A.W. (1988). *Human Cognitive Neuropsychology*. Hove: Lawrence Erlbaum.

Eysenck, M.W. (1988). Anxiety and attention. *Anxiety Res.* **1**, 9–15.

Eysenck, M.W. and Keane, M.T. (1990). *Cognitive Psychology: A Student's Handbook*. Hove: Lawrence Erlbaum.

Frith, C.D. (1981). Schizophrenia: an abnormality of consciousness. In: G. Underwood and R. Stevens (eds) *Aspects of Consciousness*, Vol. 2. London: Academic Press.

Gessler, S., Cutting, J., Frith, C.D. and Weinman, J. (1989). Schizophrenic inability to judge facial emotion: a controlled study. *Br. J. Clin. Psychol.* **28**, 19–29.

Green, D. and Swets, J. (1966). *Signal Detection Theory and Psychophysics*. New York: Wiley.

Gross, C.G., Rocha-Miranda, C.E. and Bender, D.B. (1972). Visual properties of neurons in inferotemporal cortex of the macaque. *J. Neurophysiol.* **35**, 96–111.

Hubel, D.H. (1979). Brain mechanism of vision. *Scient. Am.* **241** (3), 150–162.

Ikeda, H. and Wright, M.J. (1974). Evidence for sustained and transient neurones in the cat's visual cortex. *Vision Res.* **14**, 133–136.

Johnston, W.A. and Dark, V.J. (1986). Selective attention. *Ann. Rev. Psychol.* **37**, 43–75.

Locher, P.J. and Nodine, C.F. (1973). Influence of stimulus symmetry on visual scanning patterns. *Percept. Psychophys.* **13** (3), 408–412.

Maffei, L. and Fiorentini, A. (1973). The visual cortex as a spatial frequency analyser. *Vision Res.* **13**, 1255–1267.

Marr, D. (1980). Visual information processing: the structure and creation of visual representations. *Phil. Trans. R. Soc. (Lond.)* **B290**, 199–218.

Norman, D.A. and Shallice, T. (1986). Attention to action: willed and automatic control of behaviour. In: R.J. Davidson, G.E. Schwartz and D. Shapiro (eds) *Consciousness and Self Regulation: Advances in Research and Theory*, Vol. 4, pp. 1–18. New York: Plenum Press.

Perenin, M.T. and Jeannerod, M. (1975). Residual vision in cortically blind hemifields. *Neuropsychologia* **13**, 1–7.

Perrett, D.I., Rolls, E.T. and Caan, W. (1982). Visual neurones responsive to faces in the monkey temporal cortex. *Exp. Brain Res.* **47**, 329–342.

Ratcliff, G. and Ross, J.E. (1981). Visual perception and perceptual disorder. *Br. Med. Bull.* **37** (2), 181–186.

Schneider, W. and Shiffrin, R.M. (1977). Controlled and automatic human information processing: I. Direction, search and attention. *Psychol. Rev.* **84**, 1–66.

Schwartz Place, E.H. and Gilmore, G.C. (1980). Perceptual organization in schizophrenia. *J. Abnorm. Psychol.* **89** (3), 409–418.

Shallice, T. (1982). Specific impairments of planning. *Phil. Trans. R. Soc. (Lond.)* **B298**, 199–209.

Treisman, A.M. (1969). Strategies and models of selective attention. *Psychol. Rev.* **76**, 282–299.

Weiskrantz, L. (1986). *Blindsight: A Case Study and Implications*. Oxford: Oxford University Press.

Yarbus, A.L. (1967). *Eye Movements and Vision*. New York: Plenum Press.

Zeki, S.M. (1978). The cortical projections and foveal striate cortex in the rhesus monkey. *J. Physiol.* **277**, 227–244.

Further Reading

Bruce, V. and Green, P.R. (1990). *Visual Perception: Physiology, Psychology and Ecology*, 2nd edn. Hove: Lawrence Erlbaum.

Corens, S., Porac, C. and Ward, L.M. (1984). *Sensation and Perception*, 2nd edn. New York: Academic Press.

Frisby, J.P. (1979). *Seeing*. Oxford: Oxford University Press.

Gregory, R.L. (1966). *Eye and Brain*. New York: World University Library.

Humphreys, G.W. and Bruce, V. (1989). *Visual Cognition*. Hove: Lawrence Erlbaum.

Sleep and Activation

A. Steptoe

A dimension of non-specific arousal is considered to underlie all behavioural activities and levels of consciousness. This arousal continuum encompasses both wakefulness and sleep, and ranges from mania through normal alertness to the 'twilight' state on the edge of sleep, and into deep sleep. The degree of activation is determined by structures in the brain stem, while also being sensitive to external stimuli and the actions of higher neural centres. Sleep is therefore just one segment of the larger arousal continuum.

Sleep and Its Stages

Sleep is characterized by physical inactivity together with a loss of awareness and responsivity. It is distinguishable from states such as coma, since the individual can be roused. EEG recording techniques have revealed that sleep is not a unitary state, but that systematic variations in brain activity occur during each episode. Sleep has been categorized into a number of stages and these may be associated with different brain stem mechanisms. The generally accepted scheme consists of five phases.

Stage 1

Mixed frequency, low voltage EEG, with peaks of activity in the α (8–12 Hz) and θ (4–6 Hz) wavebands. This is the lightest sleep stage, and is the first to be entered on falling asleep. It leads to:

Stage 2

A low voltage pattern in which slower frequencies predominate. These are interrupted by bursts of activity in the 12–14 Hz band (sleep spindles), and high amplitude 'k' complexes.

Stages 3 and 4

These stages are characterized by the appearance of high amplitude, low frequency (2 Hz) δ waves. δ waves comprise less than 50% of the record in stage 3, and some sleep spindles persist. In stage 4, δ waves occupy more than 50% of the

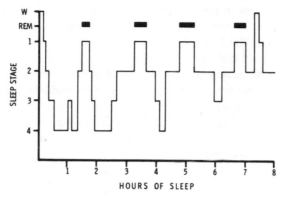

FIG. 16.1   Typical pattern of sleep stages in a healthy young adult.

time, and there are no longer any sleep spindles. Stages 3 and 4 together are referred to as slow wave sleep (SWS) or synchronized sleep. Thus the progression from stages 1 to 4 is marked by an increase in low frequency EEG activity at the expense of the higher frequencies typical of the waking state. However, the pattern of sleep stages is complicated by the existence of:

Rapid eye movement (REM) sleep

This is also known as desynchronized or paradoxical sleep. The EEG indicates cortical activation, with a mixed frequency low voltage spectrum similar to that of the waking brain. It is associated with conjugate rapid eye movements and indices of autonomic arousal (raised O_2 consumption, penile erections, large fluctuations in blood pressure, heart rate and breathing pattern), and a paradoxically low muscle tonus. Moreover, despite the alert EEG, the individual in REM is even harder to wake than when in SWS. REM sleep presents a marked contrast to the other stages, which are therefore collectively referred to as non-REM or orthodox sleep. A connection between dreams and REM has been established. When people are woken from REM the incidence of dream reports varies between 60 and 88% in different surveys, while dreams are only recalled on some 20% of wakings from SWS. There is also some evidence that eye movements during REM are related to dream content, and concurrent stimuli such as noises may be incorporated into dreams.

Patterns of Sleep

The sleep stages recur in a cyclical pattern during the night (see Fig. 16.1). There is an initial progression through stages 1 to 4, followed by a regular oscillation between REM and non-REM. REM phases are repeated at 80–90 minute intervals, and comprise some 20% of the total sleep time. Stages 3 and 4 together take up another 15–20%, but the bulk of time is spent in stage 2. It is interesting to note that SWS is concentrated in the early part of the night, while most REM occurs later in the sleep phase.

Important variations in this pattern occur with age. The proportion of total sleep time spent in SWS and particularly in REM is high in neonates, and a rapid reduction occurs over the first few years of life. At the other end of the spectrum, it is generally assumed that sleep time declines in the elderly. However, studies involving 24-hour monitoring have shown that the shortening of the night-time sleep in people over 60 is compensated by a greater incidence of daytime naps. Nevertheless, there is an increase in the number of awakenings during the night in the elderly, and this may be one reason for their frequent use of hypnotics. It should also be emphasized that even in healthy young adults, there is a wide variation in average sleep times.

Functions of Sleep

Scientific hypotheses about the functions of sleep have conventionally been orientated around the SWS–REM distinction. The association of REM with dreaming and the high levels of REM in infancy have led to the suggestion that REM is important for brain rather than bodily functions. In contrast, SWS has been identified with body restitutional processes and protein synthesis. The proportion of SWS increases after intense physical exercise and with the length of the previous period of wakefulness. Metabolically, the sleep phase of the diurnal cycle is a period of intense activity. Growth hormone is secreted during SWS, while increased amounts of cortisol are released episodically through the early hours of the morning.

Although this distinction between the functions of SWS and REM appears to have been supported by early sleep deprivation experiments, more recent studies have cast doubt on the importance of this pattern. Methodological problems frequently confound studies in which people are selectively deprived of SWS or REM, with disruptions of diurnal patterns and alterations in total sleep time. When specific tests are made of cognitive functioning in REM-deprived individuals, impairments of ability are slight and inconsistent; nor does intense daytime learning increase REM levels. Under normal conditions, REM tends to predominate not in the first few hours when sleep is most necessary (Fig. 16.1), but later in the night and during morning naps. The link between SWS and body restitution has also been disputed. The growth hormone effect may be misleading, since it is not typical of most mammals, and increases in protein synthesis have not been recorded.

Total sleep deprivation studies have also produced inconsistent results, due in part to procedural variations. In the majority of investigations, the biological effects of total sleep deprivation are extremely limited, both in stress-related endocrine systems and in energy conservation or protein synthesis. The psychological effects are also modest, with few mood changes. Perhaps not surprisingly, the main effect is an increase in sleepiness, and this may lead to impairment in vigilance and concentration. The performance deficits of sleep-deprived volunteers can be mitigated by compensatory increases in effort. The longest well-documented episode of sleep deprivation was 264 hours (11 days) in a healthy 17-year-old.

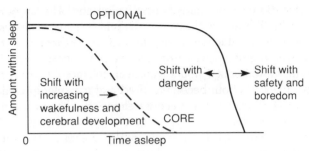

FIG. 16.2   General trends in core and optional sleep over the daily sleep period, showing some of the factors influencing the two types of sleep. (Reproduced with permission from Horne, 1988.)

Bodily functions remained normal, while serious disturbances of concentration, perception, temporal orientation, speech and memory were observed. Nevertheless, there was no loss of contact with reality, and the adverse effects disappeared after sleeping for about 15 hours. The responses that occur under natural conditions of sleep disturbance may be due to breakdown of normal diurnal rhythms rather than sleep loss *per se*. Thus during long intercontinental flights, the regular fluctuations of plasma cortisol are disrupted. Similarly, workers alternating between day and night shifts show alterations in the diurnal pattern of body temperature and catecholamine release. But with prolonged night work, adaptation to the new sleep–waking cycle takes place.

When considering the functions of sleep, it may be useful to invoke the distinction drawn by Horne (1988) between 'core' and 'optional' sleep. This distinction is illustrated in Fig. 16.2. Core sleep occupies the first 4–5 hours of sleep, includes both SWS and some REM sleep, and may be required for the restitution of the central nervous system. Optional sleep occurs in the later hours of a normal sleep period, and stage 2 sleep predominates. Optional sleep can be modified to suit circumstances and may even be dispensed with altogether.

The distinction between core and optional sleep is supported by three phenomena. The first is the pattern of recovery sleep that occurs following a period of sleep deprivation. Although people sleep for longer after they have been sleep deprived, only about 30% of the total sleep lost is recovered. A very high proportion of stage 4 sleep is recovered, together with about one-third of the REM sleep lost. In contrast, little stage 1 or stage 2 sleep is regained. For example, one study involved analysis of EEGs during three nights of recovery from eight nights of total sleep deprivation. SWS sleep was 79% above baseline, while 33% of REM was regained. The time spent in stages 1 and 2 was 11% below baseline, indicating that this sleep was lost permanently.

The second line of evidence comes from studies of natural variations of sleep time. Short sleep times of 5–6 hours are not uncommon, and a few people who claim to sleep regularly for less than 3 hours by preference have also been examined. These short sleepers have similar sleep patterns to those recorded early in the night for long sleepers, so the total time spent in SWS is very similar.

Natural short sleepers lose the stage 2 and REM sleep that occupy the later part of the night. Finally, the notion that some sleep is optional is also supported by studies of gradual sleep reduction. In one investigation subjects were persuaded to reduce total sleep time by 30 minutes every two weeks. Reductions from 8 hour baselines down to about 5 hours were well tolerated, but few people could go below these levels without becoming tired and irritable. Interestingly, some participants did not return to their sleep baselines after the study, but stabilized with 1 to 2 hours less sleep.

It should not be concluded from this perspective that most people sleep too much. People who naturally sleep rather little do not invariably fill their additional waking hours with productive or pleasurable activities. In addition, a number of prospective studies of health-related practices have shown that mortality is greater among people who regularly sleep less than 7 hours than those who sleep from 7–8 hours. The mechanism underlying this phenomenon is not understood. Reduced levels of SWS have been observed in both depression and schizophrenia, but the significance of this pattern is also uncertain.

Mechanisms of Sleep and Activation

Early theories of sleep favoured a passive process, in which sleep resulted from reductions in brain activity following diminished sensory input. But a series of brain stem lesion studies pioneered by Bremer and later by Bertini demonstrated that sleep is an active process governed by intrinsic brain stem mechanisms (see Bloom and Lazerson, 1988). Total brain stem transections at three levels revealed several distinct patterns of sleep and wakefulness, as assessed by EEG patterns and pupillometry. Moving up the brain stem (caudal to rostral), these are:

Encephalé isolé

Separation of the brain and the brain stem from the spinal cord, eliminating all somatosensory inputs. This results in a normal sleep/waking cycle.

Mid-pontine preparation

Transection of the pons, prior to the entry of the trigeminal nerve. The brain is put into a state of permanent wakefulness.

Cerveau isolé

A higher brain stem lesion at the mid-collicular level. This produces the EEG and pupil responses characteristic of permanent sleep.

These studies disprove the passive theory, since wakefulness is maintained (with the mid-pontine section) despite the lack of sensory input. They also imply two distinct functional regions: a lower brain stem sleep-promoting area (isolated by the mid-pontine section), and a rostral arousal area (operative in the mid-pontine preparation but isolated in the cerveau isolé). This pattern is consistent with results from other neurophysiological investigations. Moruzzi and Magoun showed that stimulation of the reticular activating system which arises from the brain stem medulla evoked a wakeful EEG from encephalé isolé animals in the sleep phase. Similarly, sedation of the caudal sleep-promoting region with thiopental arouses sleeping cats.

Unfortunately, the simple picture of cyclical alternation between two regions has been complicated by investigations of the specific brain structures involved. It is likely that different mechanisms underlie SWS and REM sleep. It is also clear that the brain stem alone does not regulate sleep, and that the cerebral cortex is necessary for the development of SWS. Stimulation of the anterior hypothalamus may elicit sleep, while posterior regions of the hypothalamus may promote wakefulness. These mechanisms confirm that the brain stem does not operate autonomously, but that the sleep/wakefulness cycle is the product of integrated central nervous activity.

As far as the waking portion of the arousal continuum is concerned, the most influential brain stem structure is the reticular activating system (RAS). This net-like (reticulated) tract of grey matter ascends from the brain stem into the diencephalon, projecting diffusely to neocortical and subcortical areas alike. Stimulation of the RAS alerts the cortical EEG, while arousing behavioural, autonomic and neuroendocrine mechanisms. It thus has a crucial role modulating the general level of behavioural alertness and efficiency. Two groups of cells that are particularly relevant to brain activation are the noradrenaline-containing neurones in the locus coeruleus and the cells of the dorsal raphe nucleus which secrete serotonin.

Although the RAS has intrinsic activity, it also receives collateral inputs from the ascending somatosensory pathways. These inputs augment the non-specific neural tone of the RAS; thus an unexpected stimulus is not only projected by specific sensory pathways to the cortex for analysis, it also contributes to the general level of arousal. This pattern has led Lindsley (1960) and others to develop an *activation theory* of RAS function. The RAS is said to have a generalized non-specific arousing role in the nervous system, and a reciprocal relationship with behaviour. Thus the RAS enables the organism to respond appropriately to external stimuli, while behaviours are executed in order to restore the equilibrium of arousal. Conditions of extreme sensory stimulation, either high or low, will therefore be avoided.

This theory is in keeping with the disruptive effects of excessive sensory stimulation on behaviour. Less well known is the damage done by low stimulation, which has been investigated in detail during sensory deprivation experiments. In these studies, volunteers are isolated in sound-proof rooms, with their limbs wrapped in padding and opaque goggles over their eyes. These conditions rapidly produce disturbances in thought, concentration and behavioural performance, together with visual and auditory hallucinations. Even well-motivated participants find such low sensory inputs intolerable after a short period.

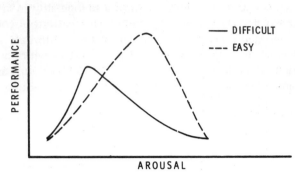

FIG. 16.3   The general relationship between performance efficiency and arousal for behavioural tasks. The optimal level of arousal varies as a function of task difficulty.

Activation theory and the concept of non-specific arousal provide a useful framework for the understanding of the interplay between external and intrinsic sources of activation. They have, however, been criticized on a number of grounds, and these can be illustrated by looking at the link between behavioural efficiency and arousal.

Arousal and Performance

The relationship between arousal and performance has traditionally been assumed to take a curvilinear form, often known as the Yerkes–Dodson or 'inverted U' curve. Performance improves from low to intermediate levels of arousal, but then deteriorates, and for every task there is an optimal level of arousal (see Fig. 16.3). The optimal level of arousal is higher for easy than for difficult tasks.

This pattern can be observed anecdotally in many walks of life. A learner driver may perform correctly in practice, but the additional arousal of a driving test leads to errors. Similarly, musicians and actors may not acquit themselves well at prestigious performances because the pressures of the occasion provoke memory lapses and simple mistakes. The 'inverted U' function has also been documented systematically in the laboratory. For example, the performance of mental arithmetic and reaction time tasks is at its best when heart rate and muscle tension are moderately elevated, but deteriorate when arousal is too high or low. One experiment tested performance of a reaction time task at three levels of difficulty, while activation was manipulated by exercise on a bicycle ergometer. The best performance occurred at high exercise levels on the simplest task, at moderate levels on the two-choice, and at low exercise rates on the more complex four-choice task.

Despite the performance–arousal association being one of the best known theories in psychology, the underlying processes are poorly understood. The relationship seems to operate more consistently for motor tasks than other types of activity, and tends to have been observed when arousal is manipulated artificially by induced tension or exercise. It is probable that the deterioration in performance that occurs at high levels is a result of distraction effects rather than a direct response to over-arousal. Different types of arousing stimulus such as noise, alcohol, sleep loss, amphetamine and anxiety appear to have different effects on performance, and cognitive disturbances are also selective (see Hockey, 1983). Activation is best seen therefore as a patterned state, rather than as a non-specific, unidimensional 'energizing' process.

Measures of Arousal

The problem of measurement is complex, and the poor correlations between different indices have also cast doubt on the existence of a unitary concept of arousal or activation. Subjective, behavioural and physiological qualities are all involved. Several pencil and paper tests have been devised to measure the experience of arousal and alertness (see MacKay, 1980). They range from complex and carefully tested instruments such as Thayer's activation–deactivation–adjective checklist (AD–ACL), to simple analogue scales. Such measures are sensitive to experimental manipulations that influence arousal (demanding tasks, distracting noise, etc.), and are reliable on repeated administration. But their use is limited in many settings, since they are not continuous measures. Moreover, subjective assessment is inevitably distracting, and may interfere with concurrent behaviour. For these reasons, continuous physiological monitoring is frequently employed.

The alertness of the brain can be assessed most directly with recordings of cortical electrical activity. However, EEGs are gross measures of cortical function, responding to the combined activity of many different sites. They may not therefore be sensitive to finer variations in activation. Peripheral psychophysiological measures do not have this limitation. A number of different indices have therefore been used to monitor arousal (see Turpin, 1989).

Cardiovascular measures

These include heart rate, blood pressure, and cutaneous and forearm blood flow. Increases in activation are frequently associated with raised heart rate, probably as a result of sympathetic stimulation and vagal withdrawal. The control of blood pressure is more complex and pressor responses are not necessarily observed, since raised cardiac output may be balanced by peripheral vasodilation. Cutaneous blood flow can be recorded either with a strain gauge or photoplethysmograph (photocell) transducer. Stimulation of the sympathetic nervous system results in cutaneous vasoconstriction, so peripheral pulses diminish with increased arousal, while blood flow to muscle beds is raised.

Electrodermal activity

The activity of sweat glands is under sympathetic nervous control, while also being influenced by local factors. The resistance of the tissue to passage of a low current varies inversely with moisture level, and sympathetic nervous stimulation increases the skin conductance. Experimental investigators generally record either the absolute level of skin conductance, or the small fluctuations in activity (skin conductance responses).

Breathing patterns

These are also sensitive to arousal, with increases in rate occurring in the alert individual. Non-invasive measures can be difficult to quantify, since respiration may vary in depth as well as rate. Hyperventilation may occur in conditions of stress, leading to somatic symptoms that can trigger panic in susceptible individuals.

Muscle tensions

These are also recorded as indices of arousal, using small electrodes attached to the skin surface to measure the electromyogram (EMG), or by monitoring finger tremor. Typically, an individual will generate higher levels of EMG as arousal increases.

Several other measures such as pupil diameter, salivation and genital arousal are used under certain circumstances, while biochemical indices are sensitive to intense levels of arousal.

Despite this diversity of assessment procedures, there are difficulties in using peripheral psychophysiological indices as simple measures of arousal. Responses in the different parameters frequently do not co-vary in a reliable fashion. This may be due to a number of factors. Each of the measures is sensitive not only to autonomic simulation, but to local physiological influences and metabolic demands; the effect of autonomic stimulation may therefore be diluted by environmental factors or concurrent behaviours. In addition, the physiological measures each have their own sensitive ranges. Cutaneous blood flow, for example, is modified even at moderate levels of arousal, while skin conductance level may not alter until arousal is higher.

More important, however, is the possibility that peripheral physiological activation is a differentiated rather than unitary phenomenon. Not only do organ systems respond selectively to particular situations (situational stereotypy), but different individuals may also be specially sensitive in certain measures (individual response specificity or stereotypy). Thus one person may show large heart rate and small skin conductance responses to mental arithmetic while another will produce the reverse pattern. These variations may be significant to the development of psychosomatic disorders. They also imply that no single variable can be confidently employed as an index of arousal.

References

Bloom, F.E. and Lazerson, A. (1988). *Brain, Mind and Behavior*, 2nd edn. New York: W.H. Freeman.

Hockey, R. (1983). *Stress and Fatigue in Human Performance*. Chichester: John Wiley.

Horne, J. (1988). *Why We Sleep*. Oxford: Oxford University Press.

Lindsley, D.B. (1960). Attention, consciousness, sleep and wakefulness. In: J. Field, H.W. Magoun and V.E. Hall (eds) *Handbook of Physiology, Section 1, Neurophysiology, Vol. 3*, pp. 1553–1593. Washington DC: American Physiological Society.

Mackay, C.J. (1980). The measurement of mood and psychophysiological activity using self-report techniques. In: I. Martin and P.H. Venables (eds) *Techniques in Psychophysiology*, pp. 501–562. Chichester: John Wiley.

Turpin, G. (1989). *Handbook of Clinical Psychophysiology*. Chichester: John Wiley.

— 17

Principles of Learning

D. Mackay

Learning theory has traditionally served as an important bridge between experimental psychology and clinical psychiatry. It offers an explanation of the genesis of neurotic disorders in terms of conditioning models, and provides a theoretical basis for certain well established methods which are commonly used in the treatment of anxiety related disorders. However, in recent years, its basic premises have been challenged by academics and clinicians alike. It has proved difficult to replicate many of the basic conditioning experiments with human subjects, its account of the development of neuroses has been shown to be incomplete, and directive therapists have recently begun to look to other models of change in order to elaborate their approach to treatment. This chapter will attempt to review the current status of traditional learning theory, particularly as it applies to psychiatry.

The Learning Process

A widely accepted but deceptively simple definition of learning is that it refers to 'the change in a subject's behaviour or behavioural potential to a given situation brought about by the subject's repeated experiences in that situation' (Bower and Hilgard, 1981). Given that a person can act differently in a particular setting for a variety of reasons (e.g. maturation, fatigue, drug state), the onus is on the observer to exclude these possibilities before inferring a direct link between experience and change. Another potential source of confusion here concerns the relationship between *learning* and *performance*. Thus although a person may learn a specific response as a result of past events, common sense dictates that he may 'choose' to suppress the performance of this response for motivational or emotional reasons. From a strictly behaviourist perspective, it can then become problematical to ascertain as to whether or not the non-responding subject has acquired the propensity to behave in the desired way or has been left unaffected by the particular training experiences he underwent.

This takes us on to a longstanding issue of contention within psychology involving the *stimulus–response* (S–R) theorists (e.g. B.F. Skinner), on the one hand, and the *cognitive* theorists (e.g. A. Bandura) on the other. At the heart of this conflict lies disagreement about the very nature of the learning process. The S–R theorist would argue that the subject acquires a series of habits which collectively form his behavioural repertoire, whereas the cognitivist would claim that the person gains factual knowledge together with an understanding of the 'rules' concerning how his personal environment operates. Although cognitive theory might intuitively appear to be the more relevant model for understanding problems of psychological adjustment, S–R theory in fact has given rise to a particularly powerful set of treatment methods collectively referred to as *behaviour therapy* (or behaviour modification). For this reason, we will focus on the two main S–R models in the body of this chapter and provide a brief cognitive commentary on this material at the end of each section.

Basic Models of Learning

Early behaviourists, such as Skinner, were more concerned to predict and control the observable responses of the individual organism than to account for the underlying processes involved. Consequently, abstract concepts such as motivation, emotions and expectations were considered unnecessary for a true science of behaviour. Of far greater importance to them was the need to exert maximum control over the external variables. For this reason, much of the laboratory work was carried out with animal subjects. According to Skinner, since science advances from the simple to the complex, psychologists should begin by devising laws of animal behaviour which can later be tested out with humans and revised if necessary. The two learning paradigms to emerge from this research are as follows:

1. Classical conditioning.
2. Operant (or instrumental) condition.

Classical conditioning

Although the Russian physiologist, Pavlov, was not strictly a behavioural psychologist, his work is considered to be one of the cornerstones of this scientific approach to learning. In his most celebrated experiment, dogs were trained to salivate to a stimulus which had previously been demonstrated to be neutral. A tone was sounded immediately prior to the presentation of meat powder—a stimulus that reliably elicited this particular response. After a number of pairings of this sort, it was found that the dogs would salivate to the tone itself. Thus by presenting two stimuli close together in time, a new response was learned (see Fig. 17.1). There are two requirements in order for classical conditioning to take place:

1. An established reflex comprising an *unconditioned stimulus* (UCS) and an *unconditioned response* (UCR). The word 'unconditioned' refers to the fact that the stimulus–response connection is not the result of learning. In this experiment, meat powder and salivation serve as the UCS and UCR, respectively.

2. A neutral stimulus which can be paired with the UCS. When, as a result of learning, it acquires response-eliciting properties, it is referred to as a *conditioned stimulus* (CS). In this example, the tone acts as the CS.

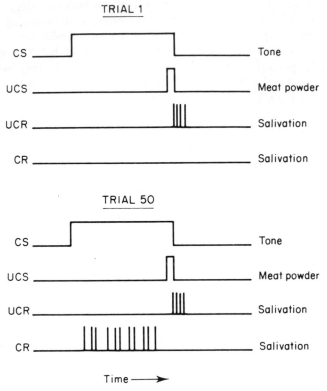

TRIAL 1

FIG. 17.1   The classical conditioning paradigm (from Davey, 1981, p. 22).

It is customary to make a distinction between the responses evoked by the UCS and the CS. Pavlov noted that, even after a large number of trials, the dogs salivated less to the tone than to the meat powder. Moreover, muscular contractions of the stomach—a marked feature of the original UCR—were almost absent when the CS alone was presented. For this reason, the term conditioned response (CR) is used to refer to the newly acquired reaction.

Classical conditioning could not take place were it not for the phenomenon of 'stimulus generalization'. Since it is impossible to replicate experimental conditions exactly on any two occasions, there would be no transfer of learning from one to the other if the stimulus–response connection was an 'all or nothing' affair. Pavlov investigated this and found that dogs would salivate to a tone which was similar, but not identical, to the one originally used. As a rule, the further removed a stimulus is from the CS, the lower the amplitude of the CR.

Another important discovery is that of 'higher-order conditioning'. It proved possible to train dogs to salivate to a light that had been paired with the tone but never with the meat powder. In other words, the tone acted as if it were the UCS and the light became the new CS. This whole procedure could then be repeated with the light serving as the UCS.

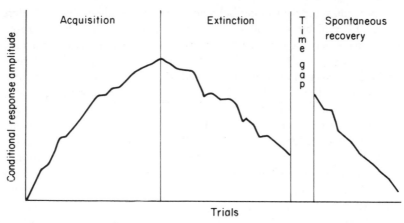

FIG. 17.2 Learning and extinction curves in classical conditioning (from Mackay, 1982, p. 8).

It was implied in the operational definition above that any response that is learnt can be unlearnt. In classical conditioning, this process is called 'extinction'. If the CS is presented on a number of occasions unaccompanied by the UCS, the amplitude of the CR will diminish and eventually disappear. However, if the CS is presented alone at a later stage, the CR will return, although in a weakened form. 'Spontaneous recovery' of the CR is only a temporary occurrence and further presentations of the CS will lead to extinction at a faster rate than before. The three stages of acquisition, extinction and spontaneous recovery are illustrated in Fig. 17.2.

Operant conditioning

A limitation of classical conditioning is that it can only account for the learning of responses that are governed by the autonomic nervous system. Operant conditioning, on the other hand, is primarily concerned with voluntary behaviour. The fundamental principle underlying this model is that behaviour is governed by its consequences. Skinner distinguished between three types of outcome that can affect the learning process:

1. *Positive reinforcement* (reward), which can be defined as the consequence of an act that will lead to an increase in the frequency of that act, under similar circumstances, in the future.

2. *Punishment*, which is an unpleasant outcome that reduces the probability that the response in question will recur.

3. *Negative reinforcement*, which involves the sudden removal of an aversive stimulus following a particular action. Its occurrence will strengthen the avoidance or escape responses that preceded it.

Behaviour modification would be a very time-consuming procedure if the experimenter simply punished undesired responses and waited for the target response to occur so that he could reinforce it. Skinner described a much more effective procedure for controlling behaviour, which he called 'shaping'. Here the change agent begins by rewarding crude approximations to the desired response. Once these have become established, he then raises the criteria for an acceptable response, so that only closer matches are reinforced. This procedure is repeated until the organism is making only the desired response in that particular situation. His behaviour can therefore be said to be under 'stimulus control'.

Although operant conditioning is usually thought of in relation to the skeletal musculature, claims have been made (Miller, 1969) that it is possible to modify specific autonomic responses (e.g. heart rate, systolic blood pressure) directly by means of the behaviour modification paradigm. As a result of this pioneering laboratory work, *biofeedback* was launched as a panacea for a variety of anxiety related disorders including tension headaches, essential hypertension and duodenal ulcers. However, in his comprehensive review of the behaviour therapy literature, Emmelkamp (1986) concludes that biofeedback techniques are not demonstrably more effective than conventional forms of relaxation training so far as the treatment of the neuroses are concerned. Nevertheless, from a theoretical point of view at least, this work is of interest in that it demonstrates that operant conditioning is not restricted to motor responses.

A cognitive perspective

According to the preceding conditioning models, learning can be fully accounted for through a knowledge of the external variables involved, and it is therefore not necessary to speculate about symbolic processes that might mediate between the stimulus and the response. Bandura (1979), for example, argues that behaviour techniques are effective only inasmuch that they provide the patient with evidence of his 'self-efficacy' and thereby cause him to change his beliefs about his competence.

A major weakness of traditional learning theory is that it assumes that the individual must be subjected directly to conditioning procedures if his behaviour is to change. Common sense tells us that this is not the case. People learn by observing the interactions between other people and their environment and may not even need to test out the behaviour themselves. Learning without reinforcement is referred to as 'modelling'. Rosenthal and Bandura (1978) cite a number of studies that demonstrate convincingly that subjects will learn a response after having had an opportunity to watch others (i.e. models) being rewarded for behaving in this way. The sudden emergence of a complete response following an observation experience cannot be accounted for in operant conditioning terms. According to Bandura, learning of this sort takes place through an association of the stimuli that arise through perception of the model, and the images and thoughts to which these stimuli give rise. These images subsequently act as discriminative stimuli for the response in question, in much the same way as external stimuli operate in instrumental conditioning.

It must be emphasized that social learning theorists do not reject the early conditioning work out of hand. Indeed, they acknowledge that, even where awareness of contingencies is ruled out, some degree of learning can take place.

Their main argument is that paradigms that do not include some reference to perceptual and thinking processes cannot account for a vast body of experimental data. Nevertheless, even observational learning can be construed in stimulus–response terms if their definitions are broadened to include covert events.

Learning–Theory Formulations of the Neuroses

Despite the acknowledged shortcomings of the two conditioning models in relation to human learning, behaviourists have used these paradigms to construct useful models of the way in which certain phobias might be acquired and maintained. It is assumed further that, through a process of stimulus generalization and higher order conditioning, phobic anxiety can spread to such a degree that it becomes 'free floating' by the time the patient presents for treatment.

The 'two-process' model, first proposed by Rachman (1977), is generally regarded as the classic behaviourist model of phobia acquisition. The irrational anxiety response first arises through a chance pairing between a neutral object and a noxious stimulus which leads to a persistent classically conditioned emotional response. Then, rather than allow this response to extinguish in time, the patient engages in sundry avoidance and escape behaviours which are negatively reinforced through anxiety relief. It should be noted that alcohol intake, obsessional ruminations and compulsive rituals are examples of phobic reduction behaviours which can be acquired at this time. It follows from this explanation that the treatment of choice should be to expose the patient to the feared object until the anxiety has subsided. However, before looking at the implications of this model for therapy, it is important to examine some of its acknowledged deficiencies.

1. *Phobias comprise a non-arbitrary list of situations and objects.* During any traumatic incident there are a wide variety of stimuli that could emerge as the CS for an anxiety response. If classical conditioning offered a complete explanation of the genesis of phobias, there would be as many patients presenting with fears of grass, curtains, and lampshades as with fears of animals, insects, heights, crowds, and closed-in spaces. This is manifestly not the case. Seligman has proposed a theory of 'preparedness' to account for this. In his view 'phobias are highly prepared to be learned by humans and, like other highly prepared relationships, they are selective and resistant to extinction, learned even with degraded input, and are probably non-cognitive' (Seligman, 1971). This can be seen to be an attempt to preserve the traditional Pavlovian model by integrating it with untestable speculations about deeply buried human instincts.

2. *Phobias often increase in severity.* The fact that many phobias develop slowly, increase in strength, and eventually reach panic proportions, cannot be accounted for by the 'two factor' theory. Eysenck's (1976) theory of 'incubation' is an attempt to account for this phenomenon in physiological rather than cognitive terms. It has long been recognized, particularly in the Russian literature, that enhancement rather than extinction of the CR will occur under certain circumstances. In brief, the conclusion Eysenck reaches is that conditioned responses that

act as drives (e.g. pain avoidance), particularly where a strong UCS is employed, will be subject to the law of incubation. The rationale he provides is as follows: 'Apparently the CS (after conditioning) produces fear/anxiety, i.e. the UCR, even though the UCS may now be absent. This process should set up a positive feedback cycle, with each presentation of the CS only reinforcing itself and thus continuing to increment the CR' (Eysenck, 1976). As will be argued later, if it is accepted that cognitions play a part in all kinds of human learning, it is not necessary to 'invent' further laws of classical conditioning of this kind.

3. *Individuals differ in their susceptibility to phobias.* It is a well-recognized fact that some people develop irrational fears with remarkable ease, while others display no signs of phobic–avoidance behaviour even after having undergone a highly traumatic experience. Eysenck has attempted to account for individual differences in conditionability in terms of his model of personality (Eysenck, 1976). From the results of a number of factor-analytic studies, he postulates that non-cognitive differences between people can be subsumed within two main dimensions of personality: 'extraversion–introversion' and 'neuroticism–stability'. According to this theory, an individual's position on these dimensions reflects certain characteristics of his biological make-up, which are largely inherited. One of the conclusions he reaches from this research is that people who are high on neuroticism and low on extraversion are predisposed to acquire phobias. Although there is no doubt that withdrawn, anxious people are over-represented in the phobic population, it does not necessarily follow that this is due primarily to the functioning of their autonomic and central nervous systems.

4. *Phobia acquisition usually follows a single traumatic event.* In most classical conditioning experiments, the CS has had to be paired with the UCS on a number of occasions before the CR has become established. Yet those phobics who can recall the onset of the disorder attribute it to a particularly distressing incident. One possibility is that if the UCS is sufficiently intense, one-trial learning might be possible. Support for this viewpoint comes from a study (Campbell et al., 1964) in which scoline, a drug which produces momentary motor paralysis without impairing consciousness, was employed as the UCS. A tone, which was paired with it on one occasion only, subsequently elicited a powerful CR, which proved very resistant to extinction. On this point, at least, the classical conditioning model stands firm.

5. *Many phobics do not undergo a traumatic experience.* A major weakness of the conditioning explanation is that it cannot easily account for the fact that many patients do not recall having undergone a traumatic experience that could have triggered off the phobic disorder. Although it is possible that they have repressed the incident, traditional behaviourists would not accept a mentalistic explanation of this kind. Furthermore, it is difficult to see how snake phobia, for example, could be acquired by individuals who have never encountered this species in real life. Even if we accept the concept of preparedness, the role of cognitions in this instance must be acknowledged.

A cognitive perspective

Many of the difficulties that the classical conditioning model has run into can be overcome if it is accepted that symbolic processes have a part to play in learning. For example, modelling can easily account for the fact that phobias can arise in the absence of a traumatic incident. If a child observes avoidance behaviour on the part of a parent, it would be surprising if he did not restructure his cognitions and subsequently his behaviour when he found himself in a similar situation. Even being told that intercourse is painful or that snakes are dangerous will conjure up a powerful image which will be immediately re-evoked when the situation, object, or key word is presented in the future. The image then serves as a covert CS for the anxiety response.

Observational learning can also account for the fact that the range of phobias is so limited, without having to introduce new ethologically-derived concepts. It is perfectly conceivable that the parents who model avoidance and escape behaviour learned it through imitation of their own parents, who in turn acquired it from theirs. In other words, the same few phobias may be being passed on from generation to generation. Even if the observational learning experience is not particularly powerful, one-trial classical conditioning may be sufficient to turn a partially learnt anxiety response into a full-blown phobia.

The problem of individual differences in phobia acquisition is a more difficult one to deal with in cognitive terms, as social learning theorists have always been critical of simple trait and type theories of personality. Bandura (1979) has put forward a theory of 'self-efficacy' to account for the fact that some individuals expect to find solutions to their problems and succeed, whereas others readily give up and fail. Where this theory differs from more behavioural accounts of controllability and helplessness (e.g. Seligman, 1975) is in its emphasis that the repeated experience of non-contingent reinforcement does not necessarily lower self-perceived capability: 'People can give up trying because they seriously doubt that they can realize the required level of performance. Or they may be assured of their capabilities but give up trying because they expect their efforts to produce no results in an environment that is unresponsive or is consistently punishing' (Bandura, 1979).

According to this theory, fear is evoked by events which the individual does not believe himself to be competent to deal with. The fact that he may, in reality, be as effective as others in this situation is irrelevant. It is therefore his low perceived self-efficacy, rather than particularly traumatic occurrences, that makes the individual a phobic (see Chapter 22 for a discussion of individual construct systems).

The question remains as to why the person 'at risk' develops such a low set of expectations about himself. Although Bandura acknowledges the fact that negative past experiences contribute to a lowering of self-efficacy, he naturally places more emphasis on the role played by observational learning. Watching or hearing about how significant others fail in their efforts, serves to decrease one's personal belief in the environmental control.

A cognitive explanation as to why phobias not only persist but can increase in severity has been offered by Meichenbaum (1977). He claims that anxious patients generally use unhelpful self-statements (e.g. 'If I enter that room I know I will panic'), which act as self-fulfilling prophecies. A vicious circle arises, whereby the actual panic reinforces the thinking pattern, which, in turn, becomes a more potent stimulus for eliciting anxiety in the future. This is consistent with Bandura's claim that people who are low on self-efficacy generate negative statements about themselves, which make them less able to cope in situations that are actually controllable.

Clinical Applications of Learning Theory

Although the simple behaviourist model does not provide a convincing explanation of the genesis of even the simple phobia, it has certainly helped to generate a wide range of psychiatric treatment techniques. These are described elsewhere (Mackay, 1982). Recently, however, it has been questioned whether the effectiveness of these methods can be attributed primarily to the learning principles that are presumed to underlie them or whether 'non-specific' factors play at least as important a role. Most of the theoretical and experimental literature in this area has been concerned with *systematic desensitization* (Wolpe, 1958). The standard procedure can be summarized as follows:

1. The patient is trained in muscular relaxation.
2. A hierarchy of feared situations is obtained from him.
3. The patient is presented with the lowest item on the list, either in fantasy or *in vivo*, while he is relaxed.
4. If he experiences no anxiety, the next item is presented, and so on.
5. If he experiences anxiety at any stage, he is exposed to a lower item in the hierarchy.
6. Treatment is terminated when he is able to relax in the most feared situation.

The traditional behaviourist explanation for this procedure is that it enables a maladaptive stimulus–response (S–R) bond to be replaced by a more desirable one. However, later commentators have not been impressed by the evidence for this view. Attempts to isolate the effective components of this procedure have revealed that most of it is unnecessary ritual. According to Marks (1978), neither relaxation training nor carefully graded hierarchies are critical features of the programme. The only essential element appears to be exposure, almost regardless of how this is brought about. Consequently, behaviourists have recently abandoned the counter conditioning model in favour of simple extinction of the feared response.

A cognitive perspective

Bandura (1977) argues that social-learning theory provides a more plausible account of the mechanisms involved. He cites studies that show that it is the opportunity for 'enactive mastery' rather than mere exposure to the feared stimuli, which produces behavioural change. Moreover, he points out that patient reports of efficacy expectations are better predictors of outcome than physiological data related to conditioned autonomic responses. In other words, behaviour therapy works because it mobilizes changes in the patient's attitudes about himself in relation to this problem, rather than because of conditioning mechanisms.

Conclusion

Throughout this chapter it has been argued that the simple conditioning paradigms of Pavlov and Skinner cannot account for human learning experiments. Social learning theory, with its emphasis on the cognitions that mediate between stimulus and response, provides a more plausible, alternative explanation.

What is particularly impressive about the work of Bandura and others is that it demonstrates that it is possible to investigate learning processes, as opposed to the performance of learned responses, with the same degree of rigour as the early behaviourists.

References

Bandura, A. (1977). *Social Learning Theory*. Englewood Cliffs, NJ: Prentice-Hall.

Bandura, A. (1979). Reflections on self-efficacy. In: C.M. Franks and C.T. Wilson (eds) *Annual Review and Behaviour Therapy: Theory and Practice*, Vol. 7. New York: Brunner/Mazel.

Bower, G.H. and Hilgard, E.H. (1981). *Theories of Learning*. Englewood Cliffs, NJ: Prentice-Hall.

Campbell, D., Sanderson, R.E. and Laverty, S.G. (1964). Characteristics of a conditioned response in human subjects during extinction trials following a single traumatic conditioning trial. *J. Abnorm. Social Psychol.* **68**, 627–639.

Davey, G. (1981). *Animal Learning and Conditioning*. London: Macmillan.

Emmelkamp, P.M.G. (1986). Behaviour therapy with adults. In: S.L. Garfield and A.E. Bergin (eds) *Handbook of Psychotherapy and Behavior Change*, 3rd edn. New York: John Wiley.

Eysenck, H.J. (1976). The learning theory model of neurosis—a new approach. *Behav. Res. Ther.* **14**, 251–267.

Mackay, D. (1982). Behaviour therapy techniques. In: R.G. Priest (ed.) *Psychiatry in Medical Practice*, pp. 1–69. Plymouth: Macdonald & Evans.

Marks, I.M. (1978). Behavioural psychotherapy of adult neurosis. In: S.L. Garfield and A.E. Bergin (eds) *Handbook of Psychotherapy and Behavior Change*, 2nd edn. New York: John Wiley.

Meichenbaum, D. (1977). *Cognitive-behaviour Modification: An Integrative Approach*. New York: Plenum Press.

Miller, N.E. (1969). Learning of visceral and glandular responses. *Science (NY)* **163**, 434–445.

Rachman, S. (1977). The conditioning theory of fear acquisition: a critical examination. *Behav. Res. Ther.* **15**, 375–387.

Rosenthal, T. and Bandura, A. (1978). Psychological modeling: Theory and practice. In: S.L. Garfield and A.E. Bergin (eds) *Handbook of Psychotherapy and Behavior Change*, 2nd edn. New York: John Wiley.

Seligman, M.E.P. (1971). Phobias and preparedness. *Behav. Ther.* **2**, 307–320.

Seligman, M.E.P. (1975). *Helplessness: On Depression, Development and Death.* San Francisco: Freeman.

Wolpe, J. (1958). *Psychotherapy by Reciprocal Inhibition.* Stanford: Stanford University Press.

— 18

Human Memory

M.W. Eysenck

Introduction

In general terms, human learning and memory are affected by at least four major classes of factors as follows:

1. The stimulus information presented to the learner.
2. The processing activities engaged in by the learner.
3. The learner's personal characteristics (e.g. his past experience and motivation).
4. The nature of the memory test.

It is probably not overstating the case to argue that accurate prediction of the learner's memory for specific information is only possible when all of these factors are considered together.

Within the compass of this chapter there is insufficient space to consider each of these factors in turn. In particular, the idiosyncratic characteristics of the learner and the nature of the to-be-learned information will only be mentioned briefly; they are dealt with at length by Eysenck (1977) and by Eysenck and Keane (1990).

It has long been recognized that memory depends crucially on the ways in which the learner handles or processes information which he or she wishes to learn; those processing activities occurring at the time of storage help to determine the nature of the memory traces which are stored in the brain. The next section of this chapter deals with processes operating at the time of storage. After that, the third section of this chapter deals with the important role played by the nature of the memory test in determining whether or not previously acquired information is remembered.

Storage

Levels of processing

It is a truism that memory is substantially affected by the cognitive processes occurring during learning. However, it has proved rather difficult to take the next step and identify those encoding operations most advantageous for long-term remembering. A very influential attempt was made by Craik and Lockhart (1972).

They proposed a levels-of-processing theory which they expressed in the following way: 'Trace persistence is a function of depth of analysis, with deeper levels of analysis associated with more elaborate, longer lasting, and stronger traces' (p. 673). 'Depth' was defined in terms of the amount of meaningfulness extracted from the stimulus.

In order to investigate this theory experimentally, we need to use a paradigm that permits control over the learner's processing activities. The typical procedure is to give the subject a shallow or deep task to perform on a list of words under incidental learning conditions. This is followed by an unexpected test for recall. For example, subjects may be presented with a list of words one at a time, and asked to answer questions involving either shallow levels of processing (e.g. 'Does the word rhyme with hare?') or deep levels (e.g. 'Is the word a member of the following category: animals?'). Most researchers have found that semantic encodings (i.e. those based on meaning) are recollected much better than phonemic encodings (i.e. those based on the sounds of words), exactly as predicted by the theory.

Since the various groups of subjects within each study all receive the same list of words, it is clear that the kind of processing during storage is of great importance in determining subsequent retention. However, it is not easy to explain with any precision why this should be so. However, Craik and Lockhart (1972) suggested that deep processing improves retention because it enables the learner to make substantial use of learned rules and past knowledge.

We have focused so far on the notion that memory depends primarily on the qualitative aspects of processing. However, there is also much evidence demonstrating the importance of quantitative aspects (i.e. the amount or elaboration of processing). This was shown at the semantic level by Johnson-Laird, Gibbs and de Mowbray (1978), who varied the number of semantic decisions that needed to be made about words. Recall increased from 32% when only one decision was required to 57% when three decisions were needed.

While retention usually increases *pari passu* with the amount of elaboration, this is not invariably true. In a study by Bransford, Franks, Morris and Stein (1979), learners were presented with sentences, some consisting of minimally elaborated similes (e.g. 'A whale is like a deer because they are both large'), and others of multiply elaborated similes (e.g. 'A whale is like a deer because they both eat, move, and sleep'). Cued recall was better when the amount of elaboration was low than when it was high; thus the kind of elaboration (probably its distinctiveness) must be considered in addition to the sheer amount.

The weakest aspect of the levels-of-processing approach is its emphasis on encoding operations. As was pointed out in the introduction, memory depends jointly on the information contained in the trace produced by encoding processes *and* on the information available in the retrieval environment. The crucial nature of this omission can be seen very clearly in a study by Stein (1978). Words with one letter capitalized were presented; the learner had to determine either whether each word fitted into a sentence frame (deep or semantic processing condition) or whether a particular letter was capitalized (shallow processing condition). On the subsequent unexpected recognition test, list words were presented either among non-list words having the same letter capitalized (semantically-oriented test) or among distractors consisting of a list word but with different letters capitalized (case-oriented test). Here is an example of the latter form of test: chAir (list word); Chair; cHair; chaiR).

On the semantically-oriented test, semantic encodings were better recognized than case encodings (93% correct versus 76% correct, respectively). However, on the case-oriented test, case encodings were better recognized than semantic encodings (45% correct versus 29% correct, respectively). This latter finding disproves the notion that deep levels of processing necessarily lead to greater retentivity than shallow levels of processing. The reason why deep semantic processing led to poor performance on the case-oriented test is straightforward; since the test required only retention of the identity of the capitalized letter, semantic processing was totally irrelevant. Stein's finding also demonstrates that the memorial consequences of different learning activities depend far more than is usually realized on the way in which memory is tested.

Schemata and learning

When we are reading a text and attempting to understand it, it is often necessary for us to use our stored knowledge to draw inferences from what is presented. Consider, for example, the following story taken from Rumelhart and Ortony (1977):

1. Mary heard the ice cream van coming.
2. She remembered the pocket money.
3. She rushed into the house.

In order to make full sense of that story, you probably drew several inferences, such as that Mary wanted to buy some ice cream, that buying ice cream costs money, and that Mary had some pocket money in the house.

Several psychologists (e.g. Bransford, 1979) have claimed that schemata (=integrated chunks of knowledge about the world; the singular is 'schema') are used to facilitate our understanding of text and of the speech of others. It is these schemata which allow us to draw appropriate inferences. Some schemata are in the form of scripts, which deal with knowledge of events and sequences of events. For example, it has been argued that we have a restaurant script (Schank and Abelson, 1977), and this enables us to anticipate that going to a restaurant to have a meal will include several events such as sitting down, ordering from the menu, paying the bill, and so on.

Evidence that schemata influence the storage and retrieval of information was obtained by Bransford, Barclay and Franks (1972). They presented sentences like, 'Three turtles rested on a floating log, and a fish swam beneath them.' They assumed that subjects would draw the inference that the fish must have swum beneath the log as well as the three turtles, and that the subjects would store information about the inference as well as the sentence itself in long-term memory. If those assumptions are correct, then it is reasonable to predict that on a subsequent memory test subjects might mistakenly believe that the inference had actually been presented.

Bransford *et al.* (1972) discovered that subjects on a recognition test were reasonably confident that they had previously heard sentences which had not actually been presented, but which incorporated inferences based on presented sentences (e.g. 'Three turtles rested on a floating log, and a fish swam beneath it'). Indeed, subjects displayed as much confidence in their recognition memory for such inference sentences as for sentences which had actually been presented previously.

One of the limitations of the study by Bransford *et al.* (1972) is that it is not clear whether schematic information produced an inference at the time of comprehension or at the time of retrieval. Clearer evidence was obtained by Bransford and Johnson (1972). They presented a text which was deliberately written so that it was difficult to decide which schemata were relevant to understand it. This is the passage they used:

> The procedure is quite simple. First you arrange items into different groups. Of course one pile may be sufficient depending on how much there is to do. If you have to go somewhere else due to lack of facilities that is the next step; otherwise, you are pretty well set. It is important not to overdo things. That is, it is better to do too few things at once than too many. In the short run this may not seem important but complications can easily arise. A mistake can be expensive as well. At first, the whole procedure will seem complicated. Soon, however, it will become just another facet of life. It is difficult to foresee any end to the necessity for this task in the immediate future, but then, one never can tell. After the procedure is completed one arranges the materials into their appropriate places. Eventually, they will be used once more and the whole cycle will have to be repeated. However, that is part of life. (p. 722.)

When subjects heard this passage in the absence of a title which indicated the appropriate schemata, they rated the passage as incomprehensible, and could remember only 2.8 idea units from it. On the other hand, those who were given the title 'Washing clothes' before hearing the passage were able to make use of the relevant schemata. They reported that the passage was reasonably easy to understand, and they were able to remember an average of 5.8 idea units. It could be argued that the title facilitated the task of retrieving the passage. However, other subjects who were given the title after hearing the passage but before recalling it showed poor comprehension and poor levels of recall (an average of 2.6 idea units).

It has been argued against the findings of Bransford and Johnson (1972) that they used a rather artificial passage, and so it may be unwise to extrapolate their findings to more conventional material. However, confirmatory evidence using normal text was obtained by O'Brien, Shank, Myers and Rayner (reported in Rayner and Pollatsek, 1987). They recorded eye movements during reading, and discovered that the fixation time on a given word (e.g. 'knife') was less when that word had been mentioned previously than when a more general word (e.g. 'weapon') had been used before. However, if the word 'weapon' had been used in a context that permitted the inference to be drawn that it was a knife, then the fixation time was the same as when the word 'knife' had been presented before. This suggests that subjects in the last condition had drawn the inference at the time that the word 'weapon' was presented, and this speeded up their comprehension of the word 'knife' when it was presented.

In sum, there is much empirical support for the central notion of schema theory that schemata often play a central role in the interpretation and storage of information from passages and stories. However, schema theory has been criticized on a number of grounds (see Alba and Hasher, 1983). Firstly, it has proved extremely difficult to pinpoint the characteristics of schemata in any detail. Secondly, and related to the first point, most versions of schema theory are rather low in testability. If the predicted effects of schema use are not observed, it can be (and has been) argued that the subjects simply failed to make use of the schema in question. Thirdly, as in the study by Bransford *et al.* (1972), schema theory predicts that the use of schemata will often lead to memorial distortions. As a consequence, schema theorists sometimes find it difficult to explain why human memory is often relatively accurate and free of error.

Declarative and procedural knowledge

The philosopher Ryle (1949) argued that there is an important distinction between *knowing that* and *knowing how*. So far in this chapter, we have been concerned primarily or exclusively with knowing that (e.g. subjects know that a particular word was presented in a list, or that a specific sentence was presented ten minutes ago). In contrast, knowing how typically refers to the ability to perform skilled actions, such as playing the piano or riding a bicycle.

Ryle's (1949) distinction between knowing that and knowing how corresponds closely to the more modern distinction between declarative and procedural knowledge. The latter terms were defined with some precision by Cohen (1984). He proposed that declarative knowledge is represented 'in a system quite compatible with the traditional memory metaphor of experimental psychology, in which information is said to be first processed or encoded, then stored in some explicitly accessible form for later use, and then ultimately retrieved upon demand' (p. 96). In contrast, procedural knowledge is involved when 'experience serves to influence the organization of processes that *guide* performance without access to the knowledge that *underlies* the performance' (p. 96).

Some of the strongest evidence in favour of the distinction between declarative and procedural knowledge has come from the study of amnesic patients. The original evidence came in anecdotal form in an article by Clarapede (1911). He hid a pin in his hand before shaking hands with one of his patients. Subsequently, he found that she was unwilling to shake hands with him, but could not express the reasons for this. Her motor performance indicated good procedural knowledge, but her complete lack of conscious recollection of what Clarapede had done previously indicated a deficiency in declarative knowledge. Much subsequent research has confirmed the notion that many amnesic patients have a severely impaired ability to store new declarative knowledge, but essentially intact ability to store new procedural knowledge.

While the distinction between procedural and declarative knowing is an important one, it is not always easy to decide whether a task involves primarily procedural or declarative knowledge. For example, one might assume that since learning to play golf involves the acquisition of motor skills, this means that only procedural knowledge is involved. However, most golfers know that they should keep their heads still during the swing, that they should keep their left arm straight, and so on. Making use of these tips facilitates the acquisition of a good golf swing, but the knowledge involved is essentially declarative.

It has sometimes been argued (e.g. by Tulving, 1972) that declarative knowledge should be subdivided into episodic and semantic memory. Episodic memory consists of an experiential record of events and occurrences and is essentially autobiographical in nature. Thus, for example, remembering what you had for breakfast this morning is information which is stored in episodic memory. In contrast, semantic memory is concerned with our knowledge of the world, and was defined by Tulving (1972) in the following terms: 'It is a mental thesaurus, organized knowledge a person possesses about words and other verbal symbols, their meanings and referents, about relations among them, and about rules, formulas, and algorithms for the manipulation of these symbols, concepts, and relations' (p. 386).

It is clear that episodic and semantic memory differ substantially in terms of content, i.e. the information stored in episodic memory is quite different from the information stored in semantic memory. However, it has proved extremely difficult to demonstrate that episodic and semantic memory represent separate memory systems operating with different processes. If there were separate episodic and semantic memory systems, one might anticipate that some amnesic patients would suffer impairment to only one or other system. In fact, the great majority of amnesic patients have impaired ability to form both new episodic and semantic memories. All in all, it remains unclear whether the episodic–semantic distinction is of theoretical importance.

Retrieval

One of the major ways in which memory depends on the conditions of retrieval is familiar to everyone: recognition is usually much easier than recall. For example, even if you could not remember someone's name, you would nevertheless probably recognize it if you were given three or four names to select from.

Two-stage or two-process theory (see Watkins and Gardiner, 1979) provides one way of attempting to account for the superiority of recognition over recall. In essence, it is assumed by the theory that recall involves two separate stages. The first of these stages involves a search through long-term memory for items, and the second stage involves making a decision as to whether each item retrieved in the search process is appropriate. In contrast, recognition memory involves only the second of these two stages. Therefore, the reason that recognition memory is better than recall is because there are two fallible stages in recall, against only one fallible stage in recognition.

Two-stage theory provides a much better account of recall than of recognition. It is certainly the case that the processes involved in recall sometimes resemble those described by the theory. For example, if we are trying to remember someone's name, we will sometimes think of a number of names, rejecting the first few and then finally accepting a subsequent one. However, the theory is flawed in some ways, and is not consistent with all of the relevant evidence. It will be remembered that two-stage theory predicts that recognition will always be better than recall. In fact, however, there are circumstances in which this prediction is not supported. Watkins (1974) asked people to learn paired associates such as 'SPANI-EL' and 'EXPLO-RE'. Subsequently, there were tests of recognition (e.g. 'EL' and 'RE') or of cued recall (e.g. 'SPANI-?' and 'EXPLO-?'). Recall was substantially superior to recognition memory (67% versus 9%). Presumably the to-be-remembered item (e.g. 'EL') and its context (e.g. 'SPANI') formed a cohesive totality (e.g. 'SPANIEL'), and this totality was more readily evoked by the retrieval cue used for recall than that used for recognition.

Tulving (e.g. 1983) has proposed a very different theoretical account of retrieval phenomena. According to his *encoding specificity principle*, 'A to-be-remembered (TBR) item is encoded with respect to the context in which it is studied, producing a unique trace which incorporates information from both target and context. For the TBR item to be retrieved, the cue information must appropriately match the trace of the item-in-context' (Wiseman and Tulving, 1976, p. 349).

The reason that the encoding specificity principle does not refer explicitly to either recall or recognition is because it is intended to be equally applicable to both kinds of memory test. One of the interesting implications of the encoding specificity principle is that it is possible for recall to be higher than recognition. If the context at the time of learning differs greatly from the context on the subsequent recognition test, whereas the context at the time of learning is very similar to that on a recall test, then recall could be better than recognition. The study by Watkins (1974) illustrates clearly how such manipulations of context can produce this result.

Tulving's encoding specificity principle has proved reasonably successful in accounting for the findings from numerous studies of recall and recognition. However, one of the major limitations of the principle is the notion that the matching of the information available at the time of retrieval with the information stored in memory occurs in a very simple and direct fashion. This seems unlikely in some circumstances. For example, answering a question such as 'What did you do last Wednesday?' usually requires a time-consuming attempt to reconstruct the events of the last few days, and very rarely happens in the simple fashion envisaged by the encoding specificity principle.

Schema theory was discussed earlier in the chapter, because there is good evidence that schemata influence the comprehension and storage of information. There is also evidence that schemata can affect the processes involved in retrieval. For example, Anderson and Pichert (1978) asked their subjects to read a story either through the eyes of a potential buyer of a house or someone interested in burgling from a house. They were then asked to recall the story as accurately as possible. After that, they were instructed to shift to the alternative perspective (i.e. from buyer to burglar or vice versa), and try to recall the story again. This led to the recall of information relevant only to the second perspective which had not been recalled on the first recall. In the words of one of the subjects in this experiment, 'When he gave me the homebuyer perspective, I remembered the end of the story, you know, about the leak in the roof. The first time through I knew there was an ending, but I couldn't remember what it was. But it just popped into my mind when I thought about the story from the homebuyer perspective' (p. 10).

There is a growing realization that recall and recognition can both involve a number of different strategies. According to Jones (1982), recall can occur by means of a direct route, in which the information presented at the time of test permits direct accessing of the to-be-remembered information. There is also an indirect route, in which the information available at the time of test produces recall by means of inferences and search processes. In essence, the direct route corresponds to what is envisaged by the encoding specificity principle, whereas the indirect route corresponds to that described by the two-stage theory. Jones's (1982) theoretical position appears to be an advance on both of the earlier theories we have considered.

According to Mandler (1980), recognition memory can occur on the basis of either the *familiarity* of the stimulus or on *identification*, which involves a retrieval process. If the stimulus on a recognition memory task appears very familiar, then the subject decides rapidly that he recognizes the stimulus. If the level of familiarity is low, then a rapid decision is made that the stimulus is not a to-be-remembered item. If the level of familiarity is intermediate, then there is reliance on identification, in which there is a search for additional relevant information to assist the recognition decision. This theory appears to be on the right lines, but unfortunately the familiarity and retrieval processes are very vaguely and inadequately specified.

Implicit memory

Until comparatively recently, nearly all experimental studies of retrieval had made use of recall and/or recognition as the measures of memory performance. The limitations of such research have now become apparent, and can be seen if we consider the conceptual distinction between explicit and implicit memory. According to Graf and Schachter (1985), 'Implicit memory is revealed when performance on a task is facilitated in the absence of conscious recollection; explicit memory is revealed when performance on a task requires conscious recollection of previous experiences' (p. 501). Traditional recall and recognition tests involve use of direct instructions to retrieve information about specific experiences, and thus qualify as measures of explicit memory.

One of the earliest studies to provide good evidence for a distinction between explicit memory and implicit memory was reported by Jacoby and Dallas (1981). They used recognition memory as their measure of explicit memory and word identification as their measure of implicit memory (word identification involves deciding on the identity of a briefly presented word). Prior to these memory tasks, subjects were presented with words and had to process them in terms of their meaning, their sound, or whether they contained a particular letter. Explicit memory was highest for those words whose meaning had been processed, and lowest for those words which had been processed for a particular letter. In contrast, implicit memory was unaffected by the processing task which had been performed. The differential effect of question type on explicit memory suggests that different processes are involved in the two kinds of memory.

The distinction between explicit and implicit memory has proved especially useful in accounting for the memory performance of amnesic patients suffering from Korsakoff's syndrome (see Chapter 8, this volume). In essence, amnesic patients typically show great impairments of long-term memory when tests of explicit memory are used, but small or non-existent impairments in implicit memory. Such evidence strengthens the view that separate processes are involved in explicit and implicit memory.

The explicit–implicit memory distinction suffers from some limitations. The most important was identified by Schachter (1987), who pointed out that explicit and implicit memory 'are *descriptive* concepts that are primarily concerned with a person's psychological experience at the time of retrieval' (p. 501). In other words, it is not clear as yet what processes are involved in explicit and implicit memory.

References

Alba, J.W. and Hasher, L. (1983). Is memory schematic? *Psychol. Bull.* **93**, 203–231.

Anderson, R.C. and Pichert, J.W. (1978). Recall of previously unrecallable information following a shift in perspective. *J. Verb. Learn. Verb. Behav.* **17**, 1–12.

Bransford, J.D. (1979). *Human Cognition: Learning, Understanding and Remembering.* Belmont, CA: Wadsworth.

Bransford, J.D. and Johnson, M.K. (1972). Contextual prerequisites for understanding: Some investigations of comprehension and recall. *J. Verb. Learn. Verb. Behav.* **11**, 717–726.

Bransford, J.D., Barclay, J.R. and Franks, J.J. (1972). Sentence memory: A constructive versus interpretive approach. *Cognitive Psychol.* **3**, 193–209.

Bransford, J.D., Franks, J.J., Morris, C.D. and Stein, B.S. (1979). Some general constraints on learning and memory research. In: L.S. Cermak and F.I.M. Craik (eds) *Levels of Processing in Human Memory.* Hillsdale, NJ: Lawrence Erlbaum.

Clarapede, E. (1911). Recognition et moiite. *Arch. de Psychol.* **11**, 75–90.

Cohen, N.J. (1984). Preserved learning capacity in amnesia: Evidence for multiple memory systems. In: L.R. Squire and N. Butters (eds) *Neuropsychology of Memory.* New York: Guilford Press.

Craik, F.I.M. and Lockhart, R.S. (1972). Levels of processing: a framework for memory research. *J. Verb. Learn. Verb. Behav.* **11**, 671–684.

Eysenck, M.W. (1977). *Human Memory: Theory, Research, and Individual Differences.* Oxford: Pergamon Press.

Eysenck, M.W. and Keane, M.T. (1990). *Cognitive Psychology: A Student's Handbook.* London: Lawrence Erlbaum.

Graf, P. and Schachter, D.L. (1985). Implicit and explicit memory for new associations in normal and amnesic subjects. *J. Exp. Psychol.: Learn. Mem. Cogn.* **11**, 501–518.

Jacoby, L.L. and Dallas, M. (1981). On the relationship between autobiographical memory and perceptual learning. *J. Exp. Psychol.: Gen.* **110**, 306–340.

Johnson-Laird, P.N., Gibbs, G. and de Mowbray, J. (1978). Meaning, amount of process-ing, and memory for words. *Mem. & Cogn.* **6**, 372–375.

Jones, G.V. (1982). Tests of the dual-mechanism theory of recall. *Acta Psychol.* **50**, 61–72.

Mandler, G. (1980). Recognising: the judgement of previous occurrence. *Psychol. Rev.* **87**, 252–271.

Rayner, K. and Pollatsek, A. (1987). Eye movements in reading: a tutorial review. In: M. Coltheart (ed.) *Attention and Performance XII: The Psychology of Reading.* London: Lawrence Erlbaum.

Rumelhart, D.E. and Ortony, A. (1977). The representation of knowledge in memory. In: R.C. Anderson, R.J. Spiro and W.E. Montague (eds) *Schooling and the Acquisition of Knowledge.* Hillsdale, NJ: Lawrence Erlbaum.

Ryle, G. (1949). *The Concept of Mind.* London: Hutchinson.

Schachter, D.L. (1987). Implicit memory: history and current status. *J. Exp. Psychol.: Learn. Mem. Cogn.* **13**, 501–518.

Schank, R.C. and Abelson, R.P. (1977). *Scripts, Plans, Goals and Understanding.* Hillsdale, NJ: Lawrence Erlbaum.

Stein, B.S. (1978). Depth of processing re-examined: the effects of the precision of encoding and test appropriateness. *J. Verb. Learn. Verb. Behav.* **17**, 165–174.

Tulving, E. (1972). Episodic and semantic memory. In: E. Tulving and W. Donaldson (eds) *Organisation of Memory.* London: Academic Press.

Tulving, E. (1983). *Elements of Episodic Memory.* Oxford: Oxford University Press.

Watkins, M.J. (1974). When is recall spectacularly higher than recognition? *J. Exp. Psychol.* **102**, 161–163.

Watkins, M.J. and Gardiner, J.M. (1979). An appreciation of generate-recognize theory of recall. *J. Verb. Learn. Verb. Behav.* **18**, 687–704.

Wiseman, S. and Tulving, E. (1976). Encoding specificity: relation between recall superiority and recognition failure. *J. Exp. Psychol.: Hum. Learn. Mem.* **2**, 349–361.

— 19

Intelligence

J. Freeman, M.P.I. Weller and M.W. Eysenck

Intelligence is an abstraction that stresses the differences between individuals. It is intertwined with the concepts of cognitive psychology, that emphasize the similarities of processing procedures. Intelligence is not a single function but a constellation of separable cognitive functions. By substituting a single global concept for the parcel of abilities we have invented a shorthand notation which can be as misleading as it is convenient. The structure of intelligence and the scaling of the separate components, is a similar problem to the description of personality (see Chapter 22, this volume).

At the beginning of this century psychologists began to use the developing statistical technique of factor analysis to investigate the structure of the intellect. The original mathematical meaning of the term 'factor' was given a new psychological interpretation by assigning a numerical value to measured aspects of intellectual activity. The level of statistical agreement (correlation) between these new numerical values, when compared in different combinations, seemed to promise a deeper, scientific measure of mental processes.

Years of further research on these lines have clouded that promising picture by exposing the limitations of factor analysis as a research tool. The main problem is the necessarily subjective, psychological interpretation of essentially mathematical concepts like factors. Initially, the research design itself must affect the quality of the resultant factors, and then the factors themselves have to be interpreted as abstractions from the statistical matrix. Spearman's 'g' for general intelligence was calculated, for example, by an early form of factor analysis (Spearman, 1904). This means that it can be viewed, not only as a psychological construct, but also as a statistical factor or even an artifact, resulting from psychometric operations. In a hierarchical fashion Spearman put his 'g' factor superordinate to his 's' or 'verbal', 'numerical', 'visuospatial', 'memory' and so on.

Using similar methods, Thurstone (1931) described a range of 'primary' mental abilities, which provided a profile style of intelligence. More recently, Cattell (1963) partialled out two primary intellectual abilities. 'Fluid ability' was described as the basic biological capacity of the individual and was measured on non-verbal tests; 'crystallized ability' was the effect of acculturation in intellectual ability and was measured by most standardized tests of intelligence which include verbal and achievement measures. Lately he has subdivided these factors and added a personality measure to his test of intelligence. Hebb (1949) also bisected intelligence: type 'A' was genetically-based potential, and type 'B' was effective intelligence. A third type 'C' was later added by Vernon, who described it as 'the intelligence which the intelligence tests measure' (Vernon, 1955).

In an attempt to break out of the hierarchical mode, Guilford (1967) used factor analysis to confirm, rather than to discover, his pre-structured model. He proposed no less than five types of mental operation, resulting in six types of products and four types of content on which the operations were performed. In all 120 abilities were proposed, which were presented as a subdivided, rigid, cube-shaped model which has not, however, been empirically successful.

Jean Piaget struck out a new course by rejecting all these ideas of fixed, linear causal explanations of intellect. Instead, he based his idea of intellectual activity on a self-righting system, which accepts new information and adapts to it by a feedback system. He saw intellectual activity as continuously functioning in a similar way to biological systems, using the principle of homeostasis, so that a cumulative building up of complex and flexible mental 'schemata' is always taking place. The developing intelligence is not then a passive recipient of input, but from infancy a person positively constructs his own reality and goes on doing so for the rest of his life. This dynamic intellectual model is based on his three key notions of 'wholeness, transformation and self-regulation' (Piaget, 1971), meaning that the intellect is always complete within itself and adapts and accommodates in its constant restructuring, so keeping its balance and order (see Chapter 21, this volume).

Conventionally measured, intelligence increases during childhood but plateaus at about 16 and declines, very gradually, from around 25, the rate of decline slowly accelerating. Nevertheless, many creative people have accomplished their greatest work in the senium; men such as Michaelangelo, Verdi and Shakespeare were at the height of their powers at the end of a long life.

Most discussions of intelligence focus on logico-deductive reasoning, so-called convergent tests of ability. Creative abilities also depend on divergent abilities, e.g. how many uses can you think of for a brick? Creativity, foresight and flexibility of mind are important for achievement, as are motivation and persistence (cf. Hudson, 1966). All these characteristics are dependent on the integrity of the frontal lobes, a relatively silent area for neuropsychological testing (Hebb and Penfield, 1940).

Sternberg (1985) developed a theory of intelligence derived from information theory which addresses this problem by laying emphasis on contextual intelligence, made up of adaption, selection and shaping. These terms all refer to the individual's interactions with the environment. Sternberg posited two other aspects of intelligence, component intelligence and experiential intelligence. Component intelligence is dependent on verbal reasoning and deductive ability, used for planning and execution of tasks. This is the component stressed in conventional tests. Experiential intelligence is the ability to automate familiar tasks, freeing attention and processing capacity for novel problems. This concept is related to Horn and Cattel's (1966) notion of fluid and crystallized intelligence, distinguishing between potential and actual abilities.

Gardner (1983) has identified six factors in intelligence, which include bodily-kinaesthetic and personal intelligence, as well as the more conventional factors of linguistic, musical, logico-mathematical and spatial intelligence. Bodily-kinaesthetic intelligence relates to fluency and elegance of movement, as highlighted by dancers. Such abilities can be well developed in mentally impaired children (Illingworth, 1970). Personal awareness refers to the ability to identify correctly others' feelings, as well as one's own, prerequisites to social accomplishment.

In spite of the many differences between the theoretical positions of Sternberg and Gardner, the two theorists agree that intelligence has traditionally been treated in too narrow a fashion. The traditional view is that intelligence is concerned with intra-individual cognition. In contrast, Sternberg and Gardner both argue that intelligence has an important inter-individual component. In other words, intelligence involves coping successfully with other people and with the cultural context, as well as being able to think convergently. This conceptualization has the advantage over the traditional one that it is considerably richer and more comprehensive. It also has the potential disadvantage that it blurs somewhat the distinction between intelligence and personality. For example, individuals with certain personality characteristics (e.g. high sociability) get on better with other people than those with different personality characteristics (e.g. low sociability).

At present there is no definitive, universally-accepted solution to the problem of the dimensionality of intelligence, though considerable agreement can be detected under the veneer of different models and theoretical constructs. The single pervasive factor may be considered as inadequate to describe the wealth of mental activity. Intelligence can most usefully be considered as a collection of intellectual faculties such as reasoning, critical judgement, flexibility of mind, thinking and memory, which work together.

The Measurement of Intelligence

The search for 'g' continues. The most popular tests are those which offer a single numerical description of intelligence such as an IQ or a percentile score. But different tests can produce different IQs for the same child, so that more flexible, wider-ranging types of mental ability tests are advocated. For example, the British Intelligence Scales (Elliot *et al.*, 1978) offers wide profiles of abilities for children, with 24 scales of measurement and a new form of construction. Unfortunately, though, this makes the technical details of make-up and delivery more complicated. In Edinburgh, Brand and Deary (1981) found a close relationship between measured intelligence and perceptual reaction time—a technique which might bypass the constant problem of environmental influences on testing and be particularly useful with brain-damaged patients. Eysenck is investigating new means of testing what he considers to be the three major components of intelligence—speed, accuracy and persistence.

Eysenck (e.g. Barrett and Eysenck, in press) has argued that intelligence is fundamentally biological in nature and can be assessed by means of the evoked potential. In essence, the argument is that individuals of low intelligence display many errors of transmission which lead to a smooth, undifferentiated average evoked potential. In contrast, those of high intelligence transmit information in a more consistent and error-free fashion, leading to a much more differentiated average evoked potential.

It was claimed in some of the early research that differentiation or complexity of the average evoked potential correlated up to approximately +0.8 with intelligence as conventionally assessed by intelligence tests. This would imply that the evoked potential provided an almost pure measure of intelligence. However, subsequent research has suggested that the typical correlation is approximately +0.3. This is of some theoretical significance, but it is too low to allow the evoked potential to be regarded as more than a very indirect measure of intelligence.

There are dozens of IQ tests, based on various population norms, and designed to follow the statistical, normal curve of distribution, with a mean of 100 and a standard deviation usually of 15. Thus, IQ is not an absolute measure, like height or weight, but is always relative. The tests are based on questions of increasing difficulty, which can be oral, written or manipulative. The level that each child reaches on the test is known as his mental age, which is his chronological age associated with about a 68% chance of answering correctly. IQ is calculated by dividing mental age by chronological age and multiplying by 100, to round off any decimal points thus

$$IQ = \frac{Mental\ age}{Chronological\ age} \times 100$$

The two most popular measures of IQ are the Stanford–Binet Intelligence Scale (Terman and Merrill, 1961) and the several Wechsler Intelligence Scales designed for different age groups—including adults (Wechsler, 1949, 1955, 1958). The Wechsler scales are not built up item by item, like the Stanford–Binet, but each of the 11 subscales is a 'whole' test in itself. They fall into two major categories —verbal and performance—and can jointly produce a single IQ. The Stanford–Binet and Wechsler IQ tests correlate highly, though they have different upper IQ limits.

The Wechsler scales are often preferred by psychologists, since the Stanford–Binet is not only more cumbersome to give, but its subtest scores, which make up the final IQ, are in different combinations for different ages, so that there may be discrepancies between them. Even so, the Stanford–Binet scale is so widely used that other measures of intelligence are often validated against it during their construction. Thus there are many IQ tests that are remarkably like the Stanford–Binet in make-up and scoring. This means that whatever type of test measures, it is likely to be the same as its model.

Raven set out to tap 'observation and clear thinking' in his very popular set of matrix tests of different age groups, including adults. The subject is asked to select a pattern piece, which is the missing part of a matrix, and his raw score is expressed as a percentile. As there is no recall of learned information, poorly educated people and those with communication problems can do well on them. Correlations between the matrices and IQ scores are usually of the order of 0.7 to 0.9. Although the test has been standardized on British subjects, norms may be unstable for different parts of the country and at the extremes of ability. But the test is easy to use, and suitable for research or as a screening device for general intellectual ability.

A test can only take a sample of intellectual behaviour at a specific time. During the test, the subject gives evidence of how well he has accepted and understood the processes of learning offered to him—all tests, even the non-verbal, involve experience and from that result performance is assessed. The benefit of intelligence measures is that they can enable children and adults who would otherwise be regulated only by social or random pressures, in for example a selective system, to function at around their own level. A test is an objective measure in a sea of opinion, but its value depends on the discretion and understanding with which it is used.

Psychobiological Influences

A full understanding of psychobiological influences on intelligence would involve knowledge of both genetic and environmental matters, but unfortunately both are always indirect and confused.

The normal development of intelligence involves a constant interaction between developmental and environmental factors. Sandra Scarr-Salapatek, writing on genetics and intellect, explained that 'as the CNS matures, previously irrelevant aspects of the environment become relevant, learning occurs—the CNS develops' (1976). But such healthy progression can be disrupted by specific pathogenic factors in the environment such as disease, drugs, radiation or severe undernutrition; this last, when prolonged, can cause a permanent deficit of developing cells (Brasel, 1974), with persisting differences between malnourished and well-nourished groups (Winick *et al.*, 1975; Weber *et al.*, 1981). Another example is the intellectually destructive effect of the accumulation of phenyl-alanine in phenylketonuria (see Chapter 21, this volume).

Environmental factors undoubtedly affect intellectual development. A considerable and progressive fall in measured IQ was recorded in educationally deprived gypsy children and in children brought up on canal boats (Gordon, 1923). In the latter group there was an inverse correlation between age and measured IQ of 0.8, accounting for 64% of the variance, but this negative relationship was reversed in the gypsy group by school attendance. Skeels and Dye (1939) describe a loss of 21 IQ points over 4 years in children in a deprived orphanage in Iran. This contrasts with a gain of 32 points in children moved from the orphanage to a well provided mental impairment hospital.

In a population survey of roughly 400 000 19-year-old men in the Netherlands, there is an inverse correlation between intelligence, measured on the Raven matrices, and family size, and intelligence and birth order, with a tendency for a gradient, so that first borns showed better ability than second borns, who in turn were superior to third borns, and so on. Because birth order and family size are interrelated, each variable was examined within the context of the other. In general the results indicated separate effects of birth order and family size on intellectual performance. However, there was no systematic relationship between intellectual performance and family size in a farm group and the effect was less marked in a non-manual group and most marked in a manual group. In contrast, the effect of birth order position on intellectual performance within each family size was relatively consistent across social groups. The effect of birth order was regular and systematic in two- through four-child families, less consistent in five- and six-child families, and present but inconsistent in large families (Belmont and Marolla, 1973).

Evidence for the inheritance of intelligence, as well as its modification by environmental factors, can be found in both animals and man. Two strains of rats were specially bred, one of which was made up of rats which were adept at maze running ability, while the other consisted of rats poor in this ability (Tyrone, 1963). Testing the progeny of both groups many generations later, the same divergence in ability was noted (Rosenzweig, 1969). Skodak and Skeels (1949) have shown a substantial correlation (0.44) between the intelligence measured at the age of thirteen years of children adopted before the age of six months and the intelligence of their natural mothers. Moreover, Honzik (1957) has shown that this correlation tends to increase with age.

Intelligence and Mental Disorder

There is some relationship between diagnosed psychiatric illness and intellectual functioning, though this is not entirely reliable. Both the diagnostic method used and the emotional ambience during testing can affect the test results of mentally disturbed people. Problems of attention and motivation make interpretation difficult in severe disorders, but performance tests are more impaired than verbal in depression. Neurotic disorders seem to produce little intellectual impairment: any which does occur is most probably the product of decreased speed of functioning, since most tests are timed.

Intelligence tests cannot diagnose specific brain damage accurately, but they do identify some of the consequences of brain damage, usually as a pattern of defects. Such damage may produce widespread deterioration, linked effects, or very specific effects; it may be acute or chronic, temporary or permanent, but of course, measured cognitive impairment is common to a number of psychotic conditions. Though intellectual impairment indices will indicate impaired cognitive functioning, they cannot localize cerebral dysfunction. However, the Wechsler tests do show up some specific defects, for example in aspects of dyslexia, which can indicate a locus of brain damage, though cerebral dominance for language is not well established in very young children. The Stanford–Binet cannot be used in this way, but has other advantages, such as being the better measure of very high level intellectual abilities.

Brain damage often results in impairment of one's ability to understand new ideas and to make judgements, of language function and possible abstract reasoning, in addition to general intellectual impairment. Such damage can be more devastating in children than in adults, particularly in the frontal lobes, as it affects a developing intelligence, rather than a sustained one, though in other areas the earlier in life the damage occurs the better the chances may be for recovery, especially with good motivation, as the brain has functional and anatomical plasticity (see Chapter 9, this volume).

Intelligent behaviour is affected by the normal processes of ageing such as arteriosclerosis deterioration in cerebral perfusion. A form of psychological disengagement may also occur—a gradual reduction in a person's range and involvement with outside matters—accompanied by lowered motivation. It is probable that old people are hampered in tests of intelligence by a reduction in what Cattell called 'fluid', or innovative style of intelligence, rather than by their 'crystallized' or well used intelligence. These tests are not, after all, reflections of full mental activity in everyday life involving experience and so may seem to discriminate against the old. However, a 'terminal drop' has been noted by Riegel and Riegel (1972) which refers to a sudden decrement in IQ up to 5 years before death.

A measurement of mental deterioration in old age was devised by Wechsler using his Adult Intelligence Scale or W-B1 which has norms up to 80 years (Wechsler, 1955). The most difficult clinical problem is to identify a change in intellectual function, as the patient is unlikely to have had a comparable psycho logical examination before and differences between present and expected performance, based on educational history, are unreliable. Intellectual deterioration should be measurable before it becomes patently obvious (Wechsler, 1958).

Preservation of function: 'hold' tests

Wechsler (1958) argues that as certain abilities hold up better overall than others, rates of decline can be measured using the differences between them. The test scores of abilities which are the least likely to deteriorate—'hold' tests—such as vocabulary and comprehension, are used as indicators of previous intelligence levels, which are rarely available. The test scores of abilities which are most likely to deteriorate such as substitution, similarities and memory span—'don't hold' tests—are used as indicators of present levels of intelligence. Both the 'hold' and 'don't hold' batteries have the same number of verbal and performance tests. Deterioration is assessed by comparison between the two batteries thus:

$$\text{Deterioration loss} = \frac{\text{Hold} - \text{Don't hold}}{\text{Hold}}$$

This quotient may be used as part of the clinical diagnosis of mental deterioration, along with other indices, independently of the chronological age factor. Though the test can sometimes be tiresome for old people to take, used judicially it can be helpful in the assessment of possible brain damage.

Two other useful tests for old people are 'The Kendrick Battery' (Gibson and Kendrick, 1979) and 'The Clifton Assessment Procedures for the Elderly' (Pattie and Gilleard, 1979). Both have the advantage of rare refusal by poorly motivated people and are based on British norms. The first has two quick tests of memory and speed, the second helps with placement as it includes both a brief cognitive scale for the subject and a behaviour rating scale to be filled in on his behalf by the care-giver. It also provides a grade, from A (no impairment or dependency) to E (severe impairment and maximum dependency).

Mental retardation implies a disorder involving the development of intellectual functioning, rather than an inability to cope at any specific point in time (Mackay, 1975) (see Chapter 21, this volume). Although physical causes, such as birth trauma, brain injury, thyroid deficiency or chromosomal abnormalities are often presumed to have been present, in the vast majority of cases no such cause can be found. The label of mental retardation is heavily loaded with social/educational criteria and is especially vulnerable when an IQ cut-off point is used in its definition (Kamin, 1974). But low intelligence is usually accompanied by other abnormalities of psychological functioning, such as lack of curiosity, slowness in response, and poor muscular coordination, which provide support for the validity of the diagnosis.

IQ Controversies

Some sort of social and moral values are often implied when one person measures another. This applies not only to the standards of measurement, but to the reason for doing it. After over a century of use, the concept of intelligence and its measurement are still in a state of paper-war.

The heritability of IQ is a particularly contentious issue. Research on this has involved separated twins, siblings, foster parents and wider kinship studies. Generally, the closer the biological relationship, the closer the resemblance in IQ, though only 25% of offspring variance is directly related to parent IQ (McAskie and Clarke, 1976). Criticism of the evidence is three-fold; firstly, the estimate of heritability is so simplified as to disregard many potent environmental influences, secondly the IQ tests are not measuring what they are supposed to measure, and thirdly, most of the data are flawed. Eysenck and Kamin have put forward their well-referenced, opposing consideration on this matter in *Intelligence: The Battle for the Mind* (1981).

The concern which threads through the controversies about IQ tests is about what exactly they are measuring. Arguably, it is not only intelligence, but also the roots of achievement such as educational experience and social background. For example, an item in the Stanford–Binet shows two drawings of a woman; one is neat, the other untidy. Question: Which is the prettier? Answer: The tidy one. Even supposedly 'culture-free' intelligence test results relate positively to children's socioeconomic levels. As intelligence is subject at all times to environmental influence, including the testing situation, it is impossible to avoid this influence in measurement (Clarke and Clarke, 1976). Such influences may be largely responsible for the different performances of racial and minority groups in IQ tests and the recognized effect of birth order and family size on test scores. Children's IQ scores do not always predict adult behaviour; the measurement of children's intelligence is largely concerned with school-type learning, but adults' lives require many different attainments and abilities.

Childhood IQ predicts adult IQ much better than it predicts adult educational and occupational attainment (McCall, 1977). Opportunity and encouragement are important and educational attainment has a complex relationship with family background, varying with epoch and sex (Heath *et al.*, 1985).

A number of variables which affect children's IQ test scores have been isolated (Freeman, 1979, 1981). The non-verbal Raven's test scores of 210 children of above average ability were compared with their Stanford–Binet IQ scores and note taken of their personalities and environments. Aspects of their lives which appeared to be most highly effective in promoting the children's IQ scores were: their levels of perseverance, their home life-styles and their educational provision. IQ scores were found to be heavily loaded with environmental influences, which gained in strength progressively up the IQ scale. These influences were not directly related to socioeconomic class or parental aspirations, but rather to an appropriate educational input. It was concluded that the IQ score provided a fair measure of children's achievement on a basis of intelligence rather than their native intellectual ability alone, particularly at its higher levels.

On the other hand, as previously mentioned in connection with canal boat and gypsy children, educational factors undoubtedly affect intellectual development (Gordon, 1923). Similarly, the decline in measured IQ of 21 in a deprived Iranian orphanage and a gain of 32 points on removal to a well provided environment (Skeels and Dye, 1939) demonstrate the importance of environmental factors.

There has been a lack of consistency in the results of research studies, which have compared adults of the two sexes for intelligence. Certainly, it is not possible to conclude that one sex is more intelligent than the other in the present state of measurement development, but there is evidence for a greater range of intelligence among boys. This means that there are, relatively speaking, both more low ability and more gifted boys than girls, which appears to fit in with the 'common sense' observation that men are greater achievers and that schools for the mentally retarded contain a relative excess of boys. Reproductive casualty is higher in males, who have an earlier age of onset of schizophrenia and are more prone to neurodevelopmental disorders. However, there are many and varied socio-cultural reasons for these sex disparities, which undermine the apparent meaning of what is perceived. For example, among the reasons why more boys than girls are institutionalized for mental retardation may be that girls are in general more likely to be kept at home than boys. Eysenck and Wilson (1976) have described how intelligence testing in mental subnormality institutions have found individuals with quite high IQs (up to IQ 125) who are 'nearly always male'. It is probable that similar underlying social reasons are responsible for the relative lack of recognized genius in women, such as a drive to achieve, which is likely to be encouraged for boys and possibly even discouraged in girls.

Differences in intelligence test results have been seen clearly and regularly when normal boys and girls are compared at different ages. Female superiority in IQ is notable in childhood, but this is followed by changes in levels of specific abilities which bring about male equality of IQ and for some actual male superiority. Probably the best known attribute at which girls excel is linguistic ability, though curiously not vocabulary. Older boys are better at mathematical skills and at skills involving spatial relations (Maccoby, 1966). This can be seen in their relatively high scoring on the subtest of the Wechsler Intelligence Scale for Children, called the 'performance scale', which measures practical and mathematical ability (Hitchfield, 1973). Girls do relatively better on the 'verbal abilities' subscale. These levels of abilities appear to be stable characteristics of either sex, as they show up no matter which test is used, according to Maccoby and Jacklin (1974). Clearly, using a test of verbal abilities or a maths test in school as an intelligence test would distort the results between boys and girls.

Since boys and girls have different rates and types of intellectual development, results on tests will be affected by the age at which they are measured. The future adult intelligence level of girls can be predicted between three and six years of age, due to girls' speedy rate of intellectual growth during this time. However, boys' measurable intellectual growth takes place later—between six and ten years of age. During this later period, almost twice as many boys as girls show increases in intellectual measurement (Kagan and Moss, 1962). The measurement of IQ in boys and girls respectively is affected by their different rates of mental growth. As the method of calculation of IQ involves a division of mental age by chronological age, the latter will remain constant for both sexes, but mental age will not. It is particularly notable on the Wechsler scale that girls' IQs begin to decline in late childhood, while those of boys increase. These later types of development seem to be those of the 'male' computational abilities (Kipnis, 1976). For girls, it seems that their mental age results from items which have been accomplished for some time, while boys' rates of development are slower.

At present the IQ tests we have available do not encompass the wide theoretical range of intelligence. This latter would subsume both the IQ test and an adaptive functioning in one's own environment. It is probable that there is constant reciprocal feedback operating between ability and the means with which it can be exercised. Among less advantaged children improved achievement, by virtue of special education, seems to improve IQ scores, while constant deprivation is associated with a cumulative decrease (Jensen, 1977; Clarke and Clarke, 1981). Social effects on the IQ score are probably even more effective than psychologists had realized until now.

References

Barrett, P.T. and Eysenck, H.J. (in press). Brain electrical potentials and intelligence. In: A. Gale and M.W. Eysenck (eds) Handbook and Individual Differences: Biological Perspectives. Chichester: Wiley.

Belmont, L. and Marolla, F.A. (1973). Birth order, family size, and intelligence. Science 182, 1096–1101.

Brand, C. and Deary, I.J. (1981). Intelligence and inspection time. In: J.J. Eysenck (ed.) Models of Intelligence, pp. 133–148. New York: Springer.

Brasel, J.A. (1974). Cellular changes in intra-uterine malnutrition. In: M. Winick (ed.) Nutrition and Fetal Development. New York: Wiley.

Cattell, R.B. (1963). Theory of fluid and crystallized intelligence: a critical experiment. J. Ed. Psychol. 54, 1–22.

Clarke, A.M. and Clarke, A.D.B. (1976). *Early Experience: Myth and Evidence*. London: Open Books.

Clarke, A.M. and Clarke, A.D.B. (1981). Intervention and sleeper effects: a reply to Victoria Seitz. (Personal correspondence.)

Elliot, C., Murray, D.J. and Pearson, L.S. (1978). *British Ability Scales—Manuals*. Windsor: NFER.

Eysenck, H.J. and Kamin, L. (1981). *Intelligence: The Battle for the Mind*. London: Pan Paperbacks.

Eysenck, H.J. and Wilson, G.D. (eds) (1976). *A Textbook of Human Psychology*. Lancaster: MTP Press.

Freeman, J. (1979). *Gifted Children: Their Identification and Development in a Social Context*. Lancaster: MTP Press; Baltimore: University Park Press.

Freeman, J. (1981). The intellectually gifted. In: K.I. Abroms and J.W. Bennett (eds) *Primer in Genetics and Exceptional Children*, pp. 75–86. San Francisco: Jossey–Bass.

Freeman, J. (1983). Environment and high IQ—a consideration of fluid and crystallised intelligence. *Person. Indiv. Diff.* **4**, 307–313.

Gardner, H. (1983). *Frames of Mind*. New York: Basic Books.

Gibson, A.J. and Kendrick, D.C. (1979). *Kendrick Battery for the Detection of Dementia in the Elderly*. Slough: NFER.

Gordon, H. (1923). *Mental and Scholastic Tests among Retarded Children*, Pamphlet no. 144, London Board of Education.

Guilford, J.P. (1967). *The Nature of Human Intelligence*. New York: McGraw-Hill.

Heath, A.C., Berg, K., Ves, L.J. et al. (1985). Education policy and the heritability of educational attainment. *Nature* **314**, 734–735.

Hebb, D.O. (1949). *The Organisation of Behaviour*. New York: Wiley.

Hebb, D.O. and Penfield, W. (1940). Human behaviour after extensive bilateral removal of the frontal lobes. *Arch. Neurol. Psychiat.* **44**, 421–438.

Hitchfield, E.M. (1973). *In Search of Promise*. London: Longman.

Honzik M.P. (1957). Developmental studies of parent–child resemblance in intelligence. *Child Dev.* **28**, 215–228.

Horn, J.L. and Cattel, R.B. (1966). Refinement and test of fluid and crystallized ability intelligence. *J. Ed. Psychol.* **57**, 253–270.

Hudson, L. (1966). *Contrary Imaginations*. London: Methuen.

Illingworth, R.S. (1970). *The Development of the Infant and Young Child: Normal and Abnormal*. London and Edinburgh: E. and S. Livingstone.

Jensen, A.R. (1977). Cumulative deficit in IQ of blacks in the rural south. *Dev. Psychol.* **13**, 184–191.

Kagan, J. and Moss, H.A. (1962). *Birth to Maturity*. London: Wiley.

Kamin, L.J. (1974). *The Science and Politics of IQ*. London: Wiley.

Kipnis, D.M. (1976). Intelligence, occupational status and achievement orientation. In: J. Archer and B. Lloyd (eds) *Exploring Sex Differences*, pp. 95–122. New York: Academic Press.

McAskie, M. and Clarke, A.M. (1976). Parent–offspring resemblances in intelligence: theories and evidence. *Br. J. Psychol.* **67**, 243–273.

McCall, R.B. (1977). Childhood IQ's as predictors of adult educational and occupational status. *Science* **197**, 482–483.

Maccoby, E.E. (1966). Sex differences in intellectual functioning. In: E.E. Maccoby (ed.) *The Development of Sex Differences*, pp. 25–55. Stanford: University Press.

Maccoby, E.E. and Jacklin, C.S. (1974). *The Psychology of Sex Differences*. Stanford: University Press.

Mackay, D. (1975). *Clinical Psychology: Theory and Therapy*. London: Methuen.

Pattie, A.H. and Gilleard, C.J. (1979). *Clifton Assessment Procedures for the Elderly*. Sevenoaks: Hodder & Stoughton.

Piaget, J. (1971). *Structuralism*. London: Routledge & Kegan Paul.

Riegel, K.R. and Riegel, R.M. (1972). Development drop and death. *Dev. Psychol.* **6**, 303–319.

Rosenzweig, M.R. (1969). Effects of heredity and environment on brain chemistry, brain anatomy and learning ability in the rat. In: M. Manosevitz, G. Lindzey and D.D. Thiessen (eds) *Behavioural Genetics*. New York: Appleton-Century-Crofts.

Scarr-Salapatek, S. (1976). An evolutionary perspective on infant intelligence. In: M. Lewis (ed.) *Infant Intelligence*. New York: Plenum.

Skeels, H.M. and Dye, H.B. (1939). A study of the effects of differential stimulation on mentally retarded children. *Proc. Am. Ass. Ment. Defic.* **44**, 114–136.

Skodak, M. and Skeels, H.M. (1949). A final follow-up study of one hundred adopted children. *J. Genet. Psychol*, **75**, 85–125.

Spearman, C. (1904). General intelligence, objectively determined and measured. *Am. J. Psychol.* **15**, 201–293.

Sternberg, R.J. (1985). *Beyond IQ: A Triarchic Theory of Human Intelligence*. Cambridge: Cambridge University Press.

Tanner, J.M. (1978). *Foetus into Man*. London: Open Books.

Terman, L.M. and Merrill, M.A. (1961). *Stanford–Binet Intelligence Scale*. Third revision Form L-M. Manual for the third revision. London: Harrap.

Thurstone, L.L. (1931). Multiple factor analysis. *Psychol. Rev.* **38**, 406–427.

Tyrone, R.C. (1963). Experimental behavioral genetics of maze learning and a sufficient polygenic theory. *Am. Psychol.* **18**, 442.

Vernon, P.E. (1955). *The Assessment of Children*. Studies in Education No. 7. London Institute of Education.

Wechsler, D. (1949). *Wechsler Intelligence Scale for Children*. New York: Psychological Corporation.

Wechsler, D. (1955). Manual for the WAIS. New York: Psychological Corporation.

Wechsler, D. (1958). *The Measurement and Appraisal of Adult Intelligence*, 4th edn. Baltimore: Williams & Wilkins.

Winick, M., Meyer, K.K. and Harris, R.C. (1975). Malnutrition and environmental enrichment by early adoption. *Science* **190**, 1173–1175.

— 20

Emotion and Stress

A. Steptoe and C. Vögele

Emotions are complex and subtle phenomena, involving reactions in three distinct components.

Feeling or affect

The subjective aspect of emotion is a private experience that cannot be observed directly. Feelings of joy, anger, sadness or fear can only be assessed introspectively, or by inference from verbal reports. Unfortunately, our language is ill-equipped to capture the quality and intensity of feeling. In empirical investigations, the subjective component is generally monitored through ratings on mood scales, or questionnaires designed to tap particular experiences.

Behaviour

The range of activities reflecting emotional states varies widely between species and even individuals. A broad distinction can however be made between unlearned and acquired emotional behaviours. Defaecation and freezing are taken as indices of fear in the rat, while smiling or laughing may be unlearned signs of happiness in man. Acquired behaviours are more complex, including all those activities motivated by emotion: escape, avoidance, fighting, sexual activity, etc.

Physiological responses

Emotional states tend to be associated with changes in both central and peripheral physiological activity. The indices of activation detailed in Chapter 16 (heart rate, blood flow to muscle beds and skin, electrodermal activity, breathing patterns and muscle tension) are all sensitive to variations in emotion. Catecholamine and corticosteroid output may also increase, due to stimulation of the adrenal glands. The circulating catecholamines reinforce the effects of sympathetic nervous stimulation.

All three components contribute to the experience of emotion. In some emotional states, subjective, behaviour and physiological responses parallel each other closely. For example, a state of fear might result in facial pallor, trembling, tachycardia, attempts at escape, feelings of terror and cries for help. Nevertheless, correlations between the components are frequently poor. Each response has its own time course. For instance, verbal ratings of anger or exhilaration may return to baseline long before physiological reactions subside. A special problem with the measurement of acquired emotional behaviours is that responses may persist in the absence of subjective or physiological disturbances. Thus avoidance behaviours may be motivated by fear, but are executed without discomfort; the claustrophobic person does not become frightened when avoiding a small space, but only when avoidance is prevented. This variability means that it is extremely difficult to evaluate emotions as unified responses.

Emotional expression

An additional aspect of emotion that can be distinguished is emotional expression. There is a strong cultural influence on expression, so that people from some backgrounds are much more open and extravagant in their displays of feeling than others. Cross-cultural studies, however, show that observers recognize facial expressions in a similar way, regardless of their cultural background. The members of many different cultures show similar facial expressions when experiencing similar emotions, unless there is interference from display rules specific to the particular culture. Research by Ekman and co-workers has identified distinctive physiological correlates of different facial expressions. The 'facial feedback' hypothesis developed by Izard and others suggests that emotional expressions may have an impact on the emotional experience itself through an afferent feedback process. The expression of emotion within the family has implications for psychopathology. The term 'expressed emotion' has been used to characterize relatives of schizophrenics who are overtly critical of the patient and show marked levels of emotional involvement or hostility. High levels of expressed emotion from relatives have been associated with greater risk of relapse in schizophrenic patients following discharge from hospital.

Theories of Emotion

Any theory of the development and mechanisms of emotion must account for two basic observations.

1. Insults to subcortical areas of the brain affect emotional state and responsivity. Numerous stimulation and lesion studies have demonstrated the involvement of the hypothalamus and limbic system in emotion (see Plutchik and Kellerman, 1986). Papez suggested that a subcortical circuit involving transmissions between hippocampus, hypothalamus, cingulate gyrus and anterior thalamus mediated emotional activities, while the experience was registered in the frontal cerebral cortex. Subsequently the importance of the amygdala was highlighted by Klüver and Bucy. They observed that bilateral ablation of the temporal lobes (including the amygdalae) turned their experimental monkeys into calm, docile and fearless animals. On the other hand, the decorticate animal (with the diencephalon intact) exhibits 'sham rage', a directionless non-specific irritability.

It might be argued from this perspective that emotions are products of specific neural circuits. Some investigators have argued that there are five fundamental emotions—happiness, sadness, anxiety (or fear), anger and disgust—and that other emotions are mixtures of this basic set. However, the pattern of emotional behaviour following subcortical interventions is not consistent. Both placidity and ferocity have been observed in studies of amygdala lesions. Such effects may be due in part to the presence of excitatory and inhibitory areas within subcortical structures. The environmental context must also be taken into account. This was elegantly demonstrated by Pribram in a series of bilateral amygdalectomies performed on dominant animals in a colony of rhesus monkeys. Following the operation, the dominant monkey either lost its position in the hierarchy, becoming timid and submissive, or else retained its status with heightened ferocity. These variations were not accounted for by differences in lesion site, but the social network. The animals that lost their positions were challenged by eager competitors, while those that successfully maintained their status had placid subordinates who did not attempt to usurp the dominant post.

2. Emotional behaviours and experiences tend to be associated with peripheral physiological arousal. The pattern of physiological response results from activation of the various pathways described above. For example, the sudden appearance of a feared object may elicit tachycardia, cutaneous vasoconstriction, increased sweat gland activity and catecholamine release, together with reduced salivary flow and gastrointestinal motility. This set of responses, known as the emergency or 'fight or flight' reaction, is organized subcortically, and can be reproduced by electrical stimulation of appropriate brain regions.

Taking account of these patterns, William James and Carl Lange almost simultaneously put forward important theories of emotion in the late nineteenth century, attempting to integrate feelings with physiological reactions. They proposed that emotional experience results from the awareness of visceral sensation generated in response to an emotional stimulus. The presence of a feared object, for instance, might elicit rapid, automatic bodily changes (trembling, palpitations, etc.), which would be perceived as fear. They therefore reversed the common sense notion that the subjective experience of fear causes a physical response.

Criticisms of the James/Lange theory focused on the prediction that different emotional states would result from the perception of different patterns of visceral response. Cannon raised a series of objections concerning the sensitivity of peripheral physiological mechanisms, suggesting that these processes could not be responsible for the subtlety and speed of fluctuations in subjective emotion. However, the question of physiological response pattern in different emotions remains controversial. Studies by Ax and Funkenstein supported the hypothesis that anger and fear were differentiated at a neuroendocrine and cardiovascular level, but these have been criticized on methodological grounds. On the other hand, Levi observed similar patterns of catecholamine excretion when volunteers watched films that evoked feelings of anger, joy or fear; the level of catecholamine output varied with the intensity rather than quality of emotion. Yet more recently, studies employing imagery and simulated emotional displays again suggest small variations in pattern of cardiovascular response with different emotions. Emotional experiences may also occur in the absence of detectable physiological arousal, perhaps as purely cognitive activity mediated by emotional memory. The cognitive appraisal of physiological responses may be more significant than the bodily state itself. In recent years, interest has therefore shifted towards understanding the cognitive and situational aspects of the emotion.

Cognitive Processes in Emotion

Much of the variation between individuals in emotional experience appears to depend on differences in their perception of the environment. Some people will consider a snake to be frightening or an incident humorous, while others may not. This suggests that the individual's perception or 'appraisal' of the environment modulates the emotional experience. The relevance of such factors has been investigated by Richard Lazarus and co-workers. One typical study required volunteers to watch a stressful film. Instructions to reappraise the distressing scenes with denial or intellectualization strategies lead to reductions in physiological responses that were interpreted as modifications in emotion. Thus cognitive factors apparently mediate between environmental (situational) cues and emotional responses. These results, however, have only been partially replicated, and the appraisal manipulations may have operated through distracting attention away from the threatening aspects of the situation.

The interaction between cognitive and physiological factors was explored by Schachter (1975). He argued that people utilize cues from the environment to label the physiological arousal (visceral sensations) they experience. The quality of the emotion itself depends on the interpretation of the environment. Although these experiments have been criticized on methodological grounds, they help to emphasize the interactive nature of emotion and cognitions.

The question of whether cognitive processes are central to emotional experience has been the object of an interesting debate between Zajonc and Lazarus (see Leventhal and Scherer, 1987). Zajonc asserts that emotional responses are reflex-like, occurring too rapidly for the involvement of significant cognitive mediation in many cases. Lazarus on the other hand has argued that emotions cannot occur without cognition, even though the appraisal mechanisms may be only fleeting. Part of the problem in this debate is definitional, and concerns the level of information processing that might be defined as cognition. There are a wide range of emotional reactions, and although simple responses may occur without cognitive instigation, cognitive processes must be involved in more complex experiences. Leventhal and Scherer have argued that basic sensory-motor processes develop into complex emotional patterns through the activation of cognitive schemas and conceptual processes.

The relevance of cognition to emotion has been elaborated in recent years through the discovery that basic information processing may be influenced by mood and vice versa (see Williams et al., 1988). For example, anxiety is associated with an attentional bias towards threatening aspects of the environment. When exposed to a large array of stimuli or to ambiguous situations, people with anxiety disorders or high trait anxiety attend to potential sources of danger even when they are not relevant to the task at hand. Depression by contrast appears to be linked with memory biases, and selective retrieval of negatively-valenced material. These patterns may be relevant to the development and maintenance of emotional disorders, and provide support for the cognitive therapeutic approach.

The Concept of Stress

Stress is one of the most overworked terms in the vocabulary. It is invoked to account for most of the ills of modern existence, from truancy and crime to divorce and disease. This proliferation has devalued the concept, and it is all too easy to provide glib explanations of complex behavioural, social or psychophysiological phenomena in terms of stress. Such explanations add little to understanding, and may actually discourage more detailed analyses (see Steptoe, 1980).

There is considerable disagreement about the definition of stress. Hans Selye, the founder of modern stress research, defined stress in response terms as a complex pattern of physiological activation characterized by the release of corticosteroids through stimulation of the pituitary–hypothalamic–adrenocortical axis. Selye emphasized that the stress response was non-specific and could be elicited by any stressor, and that it was a universal defensive adaptation serving to protect and preserve the biological integrity of the organism. He further postulated that the stress response progresses through three distinct phases as the individual is exposed to continual or repeated threat. On initial exposure to the stressor, an alarm reaction occurs and the level of resistance is reduced. If the stressor is sufficiently severe, resistance may collapse and death results. If not, the person might enter the second stage in which continued exposure to stimulation leads to adaptation and increased resistance. The third phase is one of exhaustion and possible death through depletion of resistance following continued exposure. Selye described this cascade of responses as the General Adaptation Syndrome, being adaptive in its early phases but potentially damaging in the long term.

Selye's model has been criticized on many grounds. The emphasis on physiological responses overlooks reactions in the cognitive, emotional and behavioural domains. Physiological stress responses are not non-specific, but are patterned according to the demands on the organism and the nature of the coping behaviours elicited. There are wide individual differences in the experience of stress. Contemporary theorists tend to favour transactional definitions, in which stress may arise from certain interactions between organism and environment. For example, Cox and Mackay consider that stress is the result of an imbalance between the perceived demands on people and their perceived resources or capabilities. The imbalance may lead to a subjective experience of distress, together with behavioural disruption and physiological responses. This type of definition emphasizes the crucial role of individual differences in response, for what is seen by one person as stressful may be challenging for another. It also indicates that stress reactions can arise from under- as well as over-stimulation.

If people perceive demands on them that are slight and do not match up to their capabilities, the effects may be as severe as in cases of excessive demand (see Cox, 1978). Such models give cognitive appraisal mechanisms a major role in mediating stress reactions.

Psychobiological Response Patterns

The multi-faceted pattern of psychobiological responses to stress is outlined in Table 20.1 (see Steptoe, 1990). It is important to emphasize that not all components will be stimulated to a comparable extent under every circumstance, and that there are important variations depending on the nature and efficacy of coping responses deployed in the situation.

The reaction pattern is organized through two basic pathways. The first is the sympathetic nervous system, which operates in tandem with catecholamines secreted from the adrenal medulla to prepare the organism for physical work. Thus blood is diverted towards skeletal muscle at the expense of visceral beds, while stored energy supplies are released. Even the electrodermal responses (see Chapter 16, this volume) are thought to have a residual functional role, since moisture may improve traction and grip in some animal species, improving their mobility. The sympathetic nervous component is an elaboration of the emergency reaction described earlier in relation to emotional responses.

The second pathway involved in stress responses is the pituitary–adrenocortical axis. This promotes release of mineralocorticoids and glucocorticoids, which have a number of biologically significant functions in the maintenance of fluid balance, kidney function, the suppression of inflammatory responses and the facilitation of free fatty acid production. Other substances thought to play a minor role include insulin, prolactin, β-endorphin, thyroid hormone and growth hormone.

The relationship between psychological stress and immune function has become an exciting field of research in recent years. Most work has focused on cell mediated immunity. It has been found that under many stressful conditions, mitogen-induced lymphocyte proliferation is suppressed and natural killer cell activity may be modified. Humoral immunity can also be affected, and studies of salivary immunoglobulins have shown changes under stressful conditions. The mechanisms responsible for these responses are not clear, but may involve corticosteroids, catecholamines and endogenous opioid pathways.

Some of these responses are biologically adaptive in preparing the organism for survival and the avoidance of acute danger. They operate rapidly to mobilize the body for exertion, and to protect against wounds. However, prolonged stimulation may lead to exhaustion and damage arising from the physiological responses themselves. Episodes of immunosuppression may reduce the body's natural resistance to infection, and may also permit more rapid proliferation of malignancies.

Numerous studies have been carried out on humans and other animals demonstrating how these mechanisms can be stimulated under laboratory and natural conditions. The pattern of response is influenced by situational demands. For

TABLE 20.1 Acute physiological stress reactions.

Principal effector pathways	Pituitary–adrenal cortex (releases glucocorticoids, mineralocorticoids)		Sympathetic nervous system–adrenal medulla (releases adrenaline, noradrenaline)				
Target organs and tissues	Fat stores	Kidney	Heart	Blood vessels	Digestive system	Immune system	Other tissues
Reactions	Free fatty acid mobilization ↑ Plasma triglyceride ↑	Fluid retention Plasma renin activity ↑	Heart rate ↑ Myocardial contractility ↑	Vasoconstriction in viscera and skin Vasodilatation in muscle beds	Motility ↓ Salivation ↓	Immunosuppression Inflammatory reactions ↓	Platelet aggregation and blood coagulation ↑ Sweat gland activity ↑

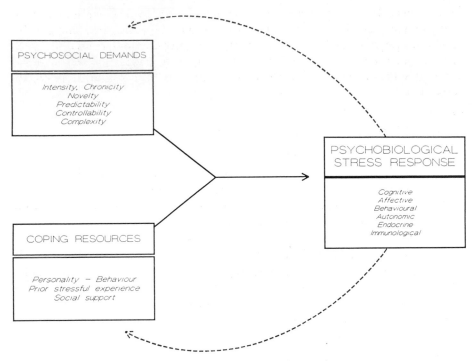

PSYCHOSOCIAL DEMANDS

Intensity, Chronicity
Novelty
Predictability
Controllability
Complexity

COPING RESOURCES

Personality — Behaviour
Prior stressful experience
Social support

PSYCHOBIOLOGICAL
STRESS RESPONSE

Cognitive
Affective
Behavioural
Autonomic
Endocrine
Immunological

FIG. 20.1   Factors contributing to psychobiological stress responses.

instance, a pattern of active behavioural coping is frequently elicited when the person is confronted by challenging tasks requiring alert and effective behavioural responses. At the physiological level, this is associated with sympathetic nervous stimulation and catecholamine release. In contrast, conditions in which the organism is faced with uncontrollable overwhelming stimulation or with helplessness and defeat, may be associated with corticosteroid release.

Factors Moderating Stress Responses

The physiological, subjective and behavioural reactions to distressing conditions may be exacerbated or blunted by a number of factors, illustrated in Fig. 20.1.

Intensity and chronicity

In terms of the demands on the person, the most obvious parameters to affect psychobiological reactions are the intensity and chronicity of the stressor. In humans, it is difficult to investigate 'dose–response' relationships, although research on life-events indicates that associations with ill-health depend on the severity of the experience. Systematic studies of people involved in major industrial accidents have shown that the prevalence of post-traumatic stress disorder is linked with proximity to the event. It is difficult to draw a firm distinction between acute and chronic stressors. Many acute events (such as bereavement) have long-term consequences (exposure to new social and living environments). Acute events such as surgery may be anticipated uneasily for weeks or even months. Nevertheless, persistent threats or high levels of demand, such as are experienced in certain occupations or in people looking after the chronically sick, are especially likely to be associated with severe psychobiological responses.

Predictability

A series of studies was carried out by Weiss, in which rats were administered electric shocks in either predictable or unpredictable fashion. The duration and intensity of shock was equated for the groups, but in the predictable condition each shock was preceded by a 10-second tone. It was found that plasma corticosterone responses were greater in the unpredictable condition, while these animals also developed larger stress-induced gastric lesions.

Predictability is an important element in modulating human reactions as well. For example, comparisons have been made between loud jarring bursts of noise presented in predictable or unpredictable fashion. Although performance of behavioural tasks during the noise was unaffected, subjects exposed to unpredictable noise later showed impaired efficiency (poor task performance and low tolerance to frustration).

Novelty

The physiological reactions to environmental demands tend to be greater when conditions are novel. In some animal experiments, the largest neuroendocrine reactions have been observed on initial exposure to apparatus, even before the imposition of experimental stressors. Familiarity is clearly related to predictability, but also to the knowledge people have about their ability to cope, and the possible outcome of the situation. For example, physiological examinations of parachutists indicate higher levels of plasma renin activity, heart rate and catecholamines just prior to jumps in novices compared with practised subjects, while responses in the latter also subside more rapidly. The novelty/familiarity factor has practical implications in the preparation of patients for hospitalization, surgery and other medical procedures. Several studies indicate that the provision of information about procedures and likely experiences can alleviate distress, and in some circumstances reduce analgesic requirements and hasten recovery.

Behavioural control over stressors

The literature concerning personal control over stress is complex. On the one hand there is considerable evidence that exposure to stressors with no possibility of control or escape leads to a state of helplessness, and exacerbates gastric lesions, immunosuppression and myocardial pathology. Loss events have been associated with depression, while experimentally induced states of helplessness may even parallel human depression (the 'learned helplessness' theory). Yet on the other hand, physiological reactions may actually be magnified when the individual can with difficulty exert some control over the source of stress. The important element may be the nature of the coping response. When the individual has to engage in active coping, and remain alert in order to carry out difficult responses with an uncertain outcome, then autonomic and subjective distress is heightened. The confidence that people have in their abilities to control stressful events (efficacy expectations) also influences response magnitude.

Psychological Coping Resources

Psychological coping refers to the cognitive and behavioural responses displayed by people when attempting to avert or reduce the impact of potentially stressful events. Many taxonomies of psychological coping have been put forward. A broad distinction can be made between 'problem-focused' coping, directed at the stressful situation itself, and 'emotion-focused' coping. The latter is concerned with the regulation of emotional responses to the experience, and not to the stressor. Coping responses can involve overt acts or cognitive processes without behavioural correlates. An example of a behavioural problem-focused response is an active attempt at problem-solving, while emotion-focused coping behaviours might involve displacement activities such as drinking and smoking. An example of a cognitive coping response directed at the problem would be attempting to redefine the situation in a positive fashion, while an emotional-focused cognitive response might be denial or repression of the event.

An important consequence of this perspective is that coping responses are not necessarily effective, and that some coping attempts may even be maladaptive. The most appropriate form of coping will also depend on the situation. When faced with an academic examination, active problem-solving will be beneficial, but little may be gained from this approach when the stressor is a recent bereavement.

A number of factors have been shown to influence the coping responses available to the individual.

Personality and behaviour patterns

Several personality factors and patterns of habitual behaviour influence psycho-biological stress responses. They include general factors such as neuroticism or anxiety proneness, and specific factors that might be associated with particular disorders. It has been argued, for example, that the suppression of hostile feelings during stressful transactions may be associated with increased risk for hypertension. Type A coronary-prone behaviour may be regarded as a pattern of response to challenging events that is detrimental to health. On the other hand, a sense of optimism and belief in personal control may be protective. The concept of a 'hardy' personality, involving a sense of personal control, commitment or involvement in activities and the perception of events as opportunities rather than as threats, has been developed by Kobasa. There is limited evidence that hardy individuals are less likely to become ill following life stress than are less hardy people.

Prior experience

The evidence linking previous stressful experience with ability to tolerate later stress is mixed. On the one hand early experience may mitigate the subsequent effects of aversive events, leading to a toughening of resistance. On the other hand, experiences such as premature maternal separation or early malnutrition have been shown to diminish adult immune competence. Studies of life-events in humans also indicate that early traumatic experiences may render people more vulnerable to later events. The after-effects of prior stressful experience presumably depend on the severity of the early trauma and the extent to which it was resolved emotionally.

Social support

One of the most important factors moderating the impact of distressing incidents in everyday life is the availability of social support. People with firmly supportive families, or those belonging to closely knit social and religious communities, have been found to suffer less after major disasters or personal crises. Conversely, those in socially isolated positions, or who are placed in conflicting roles due to social mobility, may sustain a higher incidence of disorders such as ischaemic heart disease and depression. In the Alameda County Study, for example, a social network index was developed through assessments of marriage, contacts with extended family and friends, church and other group affiliations. Over a nine year period, the all-cause death rate was two to three times greater in those with poor as opposed to good social network scores. Social support may have a series of functions, such as the provision of material assistance, information and services, and emotional intimacy and empathy. It is not clear at present which processes are most significant for health.

Although social support is frequently regarded as a factor buffering the effects of adverse life stress, it may in fact have a direct effect on health irrespective of the prevailing level of environmental challenge. At an operational level, it is often difficult to distinguish stressors from support, since many negative life-events involve the severing of social ties and the disruption of relationships.

Conclusions

Stress reactions can be seen as exacerbations of the pattern of responses observed during emotional experiences. In both cases, the impact of environmental stimuli is modified by cognitive appraisal and coping mechanisms. The autonomic and neuroendocrine components of the reaction pattern mobilize the body for vigorous physical exercise, but may lead to pathological disturbances if sustained or repeatedly elicited. The concept of stress is vague and poorly defined, and is being replaced by more precise hypotheses relating social, environmental and personal factors to physical and psychiatric disorders.

References

Cox, T. (1978). *Stress*. London: Macmillan.

Leventhal, H. and Scherer, K. (1987). The relationship of emotion to cognition: A functional approach to a semantic controversy. *Cognition & Emotion* **1**, 3–28.

Plutchik, R. and Kellerman, H. (1986). *Emotion: Theory, Research, and Experience. Volume 3: Biological Foundations of Emotion*. New York: Academic Press.

Schachter, S. (1975). Cognition and peripheralist-centralist controversies in motivation and emotion. In: M.F. Gazzaniga and C. Blakemore (eds) *Handbook of Psychobiology*, pp. 529–564. New York: Academic Press.

Steptoe, A. (1980). Stress and medical disorders. In: S.J. Rachman (ed.) *Contributions to Medical Psychology*, Vol. II, pp. 55–78. Oxford: Pergamon Press.

Steptoe, A. (1990). Psychobiological stress responses. In: M.J. Johnston and L. Wallace (eds) *Stress and Medical Procedures*, pp. 3–24. Oxford: Oxford University Press.

Williams, J.M.G., Watts, F.N., Macleod, C. and Mathews, A. (1988). *Cognitive Psychology and Emotional Disorders*. Chichester: Wiley.

— 21

Some Biological, Psychological and Social Factors in Development

M.P.I. Weller, T. Fundudis and I. Kolvin

Development presupposes change and continuity. In effect, however, it can also be discontinuous, as in the development of the embryo, there are certain post-natal periods when development is particularly sensitive to outside influences. The human infant undergoes a long period of gestation, but emerges vulnerable and incomplete. Thus the potential for developmental disturbance is greatest in infancy. Although adaptation implies corrective forces, recent neurological findings indicate that, ironically, some adaptations can themselves cause problems. Initially we are dominated by reflexive responses, like the innate mass-action startle reaction of the infant. These responses are gradually refined, but the earlier, primitive reflexes are unmasked if the brain is damaged, indicating that these reflexes are suppressed rather than lost. Some functions, like locomotion, seem to develop through practice, but on closer scrutiny, appear to be the result of maturation. Although the response is later lost, a pre-programmed organization is indicated by the fact that a neonate will make stepping movements if its weight is supported and will take ascending steps on stairs.

The complex biological system of human development was thought to be expressed through a hierarchically organized process in terms of different levels of function involving genes, cells, cytoplasm, organs, organ systems, behaviour and ultimately personality, and the outcome of the individual's development and adjustment was thought to depend on the interaction between biological and experiential influences.

However, two variations of the above-mentioned developmental sequence merit comment. First, the view that suggests that the structures subserving psychological development invariably show a sequential continuity (Kagan, 1980), in that changes follow directly from previous structures, is the postulated basis of the continuity of psychological development. However more modern evidence suggests that in a number of circumstances changes in development are 'characterized by replacement of an old structure . . . by a new one' (Brim and Kagan, 1980). Second, learning theory has been applied widely to explain the development of intelligence, language and other complex aspects of psychological development. But Chomsky (1959) has rejected the Skinnerian viewpoint concerning the 'sufficiency of the learning theory explanations even though it is accepted that learning in some form is important' (Berger, 1985). For instance, it is argued that reinforcement principles are inadequate to explain the basis of psychological attachments in infancy (Sroufe, 1979).

Further, Scarr and McCartney (1983) have proposed a theory which links genetic differences between individuals and the responses elicited from care-takers. Thus it is suggested that new psychological structures are partially determined by genes. Such matters are discussed further in the next section.

Influence on Development

Genetic factors

Certain individual characteristics seem to be set very early in life, if not *in utero*, and certain behavioural dimensions measured by separate, independent raters have been shown to persist from shortly after birth to school age (Thomas *et al.*, 1977; see Chess and Thomas, 1984). There is some support for the findings in the observation that recurrent problems with feeding, bathing and dressing, together with loud crying, protest at novelty and tantrums are over-represented in those who subsequently developed conduct disorders (Rutter *et al.*, 1964), which seem to start earlier than other psychiatric conditions (Behar, 1982), and a history of childhood conduct disorder is often found to be significantly related to criminality in adulthood (Robins, 1978).

Thus it is not surprising that a variety of authorities are in broad agreement in arguing for neurobiological correlates for specific traits, such as harm avoidance, novelty seeking and reward seeking (see Rutter, 1987) and also for heritability of aggressive behaviour (Rushton *et al.*, 1986), which seems consistent over time (see Olweus, 1979). However aggression and distractability do not show as strong a genetic loading as other behavioural characteristics (Plomin and Foch, 1980). There is an heritable component in crimes against property (see Weller, 1986) and further information on a biological substrate is accumulating —in one prospective study, Raine, Venables and Williams (1990) have shown that four independent measures of central arousal were all reduced in 101 15-year-olds who subsequently went on to receive criminal convictions in the following nine years.

Lange, and later Rosanoff and his colleagues (1941), showed that monozygotic (MZ) twins, separated early in life, generally have surprisingly similar lives with much greater concordance than dizygotic (DZ) twins. A recent, remarkable single case study is extremely compelling (see Chapter 22, this volume). Adopted children develop physical and mental diseases, including schizophrenia (see Chapter 12, this volume) and alcoholism (Goodwin, 1976; see Chapter 13, this volume), which correspond to their natural rather than their adopted parents.

Evidence for the inheritance of intelligence as well as its modification by environmental factors have been the subject of much debate. In developed countries twin and adoption studies have emphasized that polygenic factors account for up to 60% of the variance of behaviour (Anderson, 1974), but where there is serious environmental disadvantage, a more substantial proportion of the variance is accounted for by environmental influences (Rutter, 1985). Thus both nature and nurture contribute to individual differences in intelligence. Skodak and Skeels (1949) have shown a moderate correlation ($r = 0.44$) between the intelligence measured at the age of thirteen years of children adopted before the age of six months and the intelligence of their natural mothers. Moreover, Honzik (1957) has shown that this correlation tends to increase with age (see Chapter 19, this volume). Although the correlation between monozygotic twins is somewhat reduced if they are reared apart, the correlation coefficient is still 0.74 (Rowe and Plomin, 1978).

A wide variation of individual characteristics seems to be established very early in life (Thomas *et al.*, 1963; Chess and Thomas, 1984). For instance, it has been observed that babies differ from one another in temperamental qualities —with the above-mentioned authors describing nine of these—activity, intensity, quality of mood, approach/withdrawal, adaptability, rhythmicity of biological functions, threshold of responsiveness, distractibility and persistence. Three syndromes of temperament were defined subsequently — the 'easy child', the 'difficult child' and the 'slow to warm-up child'. There are four additional important issues which merit comment. The first concerns the genetic contribution to temperament. It is undeniable that there is a genetic contribution to temperament—for instance, greater similarities have been demonstrated in monozygotic than in dizygotic twins for some of these characteristics (Scarr and Kidd, 1983). But the crucial question concerns the extent of this similarity in comparison with environmental influences (Plomin, 1982, 1983). Hence it is not surprising that some experts view temperamental characteristics as inherited personality traits, whilst others see them as potentially modifiable by environmental opportunities and expectations (Goldsmith *et al.*, 1987). Second, there is the question of the conceptual relationship between early temperamental style and later personality. Despite much theorizing and some research, the association still remains unclear (Berger, 1982; Goldsmith, 1983). Third, there is the question of stability—the evidence is that some temperamental traits appear more stable than others, at least over early and mid-childhood. Finally, there are some important cross-cultural differences—for example USA-born Chinese and white babies respond differently to minor frustrations (Kagan *et al.*, 1986).

Both twin and adoption studies support a genetic contribution to adult criminality (Mednick *et al.*, 1986), but such a contribution is of lesser magnitude in juvenile delinquency and petty criminality (Cloninger *et al.*, 1982).

Aggression in early childhood mainly affects boys and tends to persist, often being a precursor of antisocial behaviour and delinquency in later childhood. This trend towards stability over time of severe or persistent aggressive behaviour has ominous implications, and one cannot assume that such children will improve spontaneously (Robins, 1978). High serum levels of male sex hormones in aggressive adolescent boys suggest an important likely mediating mechanism (Olweus, 1986).

The evidence for a genetic basis of serious childhood psychopathology is quite strong, especially when based on twin studies—for instance 56% of MZ twins and 7% of DZ twins are concordant for anorexia nervosa (Holland *et al.*, 1984);

68% of MZ twins and 36% of DZ twins concordant for enuresis (Baldwin, 1971); and 36% of MZ and 0% of DZ concordant for autism (Folstein and Rutter, 1977).

Perinatal insults

Impulses in nerve pathways exert an organizing influence on the extent of synaptic connections. Certain environmental events must occur at circumscribed times for normal development. In the same manner neural connections must be intact for these experiences to be effective. If the normal connections are disturbed inappropriate connections are formed, while others fail to degenerate (e.g. Movshon and Van Sluyters, 1981; Archer et al., 1982; Perry and Cowey, 1982). Since deliberate lesions at an early age produce persisting anomalies in neural organization in mammalian brains, perinatal damage and damage in utero may have the same effect and may be further compounded by disconnection syndromes. Just such damage seems to occur in schizophrenia, which would be consistent with neuropsychological and neurophysiological findings.

The long-term effects of early developmental hazards depend on the quality of the care-giving environment. A paradigm for this is the subject of 'premature children', who are technically of two kinds—those who are premature by virtue of being born too soon, and those who are too small for their gestational age (Neligan et al., 1976). Any findings may be difficult to explain because often there are close links between such perinatal experiences and relatively poor social environments. Thus once an abnormality in a baby is excluded the premature children appeared to 'catch up' spontaneously, but the small-for-dates babies subsequently showed poorer intellectual and behavioural development. Even so, any poor performance is mainly determined by social rather than biological factors (Neligan et al., 1976); furthermore, recent work clearly demonstrates that now, with modern neonatal paediatric care, even very low birth weight children, if free of serious defect at birth, mostly show an unremarkable outcome (Hawdon et al., 1990).

A high incidence of infant deaths and congenital malformations was reported in the offspring of schizophrenic mothers (Sobel, 1961) and has been confirmed in a controlled prospective study (Reider et al., 1975). There are more birth complications in children born in a group at high risk for schizophrenia (e.g. Mednick and Schulsinger, 1968; McNeil and Kaij, 1973—certain aspects of the work were retracted later (Mednick et al., 1973), but this point remains unaffected).

A larger proportion of schizophrenic patients was small for gestational age at birth (McNeil and Kaij, 1973; Mednick et al., 1973; McNeil and Person Blennar, 1975) and significantly lower in birth weight than their siblings (Lane and Albee, 1966). In those schizophrenic patients with little genetic loading the evidence of birth injury was greater than with those who had a strong family history of schizophrenia (Kinney and Jacobsen, 1978).

Marked anoxia at birth in one of two twins is often associated with schizophrenia in that twin (Pollin and Stabenau, 1968). In monozygotic twins discordant for schizophrenia the affected twin is likely to be left-handed (Boklage, 1977), suggesting specific left-hemisphere damage. More left-handed schizophrenic patients have enlarged cerebral ventricles than right-handed schizophrenic patients (Andreasen *et al.*, 1982), suggesting cerebral damage in this group. This finding is in accord with a number of neurological, psychological and physiological findings (see Gruzelier, 1979, for review).

The normal, regular, cellular architecture of the hippocampus is disrupted in the post-mortem brain specimens of some schizophrenic sufferers. This may provide an underlying neurobiological substrate for the disorder. The orderly array is dependent on glial tissue and it is believed by some that the glial-dependent guidelines may be disorganized by intrauterine and perinatal damage, as might occur through viral infections and anoxic damage (Falkai *et al.*, 1988; see Roberts, 1991).

Early developmental hazards

Humans and chimpanzees reared for a period in darkness are indistinguishable from the congenitally blind if the visual deprivation occurred early. A review of this work is given in an interesting paper on double lesions to the visual cortex (Dru and Walker, 1975). Recovery does not occur if visual experience is withheld between the two lesions. However, if visual experience is permitted, it must be accompanied by self-produced locomotion for recovery to take place. Gregory (1977) has described a case of congenital cataract removed in maturity. There had been a preservation of the retinal mechanisms, since diffused light could enter the eye. Touch was often necessary for visual perception in this patient and Gregory reports how after running his hands over a piece of equipment the patient exclaimed 'Oh, now I see it!'

At a critical age birds are peculiarly sensitive to visual stimulation. Whatever visual stimulus is presented at this circumscribed period becomes irresistibly attractive (see Chapter 25, this volume). Following exposure to strong stimuli in several modalities, labelled amino acids are incorporated into specific brain regions, demonstrating protein synthesis at this critical period. The phenomenon known as imprinting can be demonstrated only if this protein synthesis occurs (Horn, 1979). Some aspects of this phenomenon can be observed in human infants, who spend more time looking at a familiar mobile suspended over their cot than they do at a novel one (Hunt and Uzgiris, 1964) and, in earlier times, used to be more attracted to their wet nurse than to their natural mother.

The concept of the critical period when applied to humans implies that children deprived of certain stimulatory experiences, including proper parenting, are at risk for deficiency of personality, language and educational achievements, which will not/cannot be compensated for by later experiences. However, this rather rigid concept has been replaced by the notion of the sensitive period during which we are more ready, eager and able to learn and acquire specific skills than before or after that period. Thus it is well known that language and musical skills are best learnt in early life—and so too bladder control (Kolvin *et al.*, 1973). The notion of the sensitive period does not imply that such deficiencies are inevitable.

This notion of even limited stability of deficit is not fully accepted by developmental theorists, some of whom claim recovery of intellectual and language skills from even the most adverse life circumstances is possible, provided there is a sufficiency of emotional and stimulatory input (Clarke and Clarke, 1976), but recovery is difficult and may be incomplete (Wolff, 1989).

The caring environment

The impact of the early environment on adult behaviour has been documented in man and animals: the detrimental effects of separation and inappropriate surrogate motherhood on monkeys (Harlow and Griffin, 1965), the taming effect of handling rodents, with an associated better stress tolerance (e.g. Weininger, 1953; Zarrow et al., 1972), the noxious effects of disruptive family environments, and the early loss of a parent (Brown et al., 1973, 1977) all may influence adult behaviour. However, the lack of specificity of the effects of inconsistent parenting, leading in Western man to higher incidences of all mental illnesses rather than any specific illness (Oltman and Friedman, 1967), indicates that there are often, modifying factors.

Early loss of a parent leaves an individual vulnerable to psychiatric illness (Hill and Price, 1967; Brown et al., 1973, 1977). This effect is particularly strong if the loss was of a disruptive type, such as prolonged disharmony at home. The severity of subsequent psychiatric problems is also related to parental loss (Birtchnell, 1970; Brown et al., 1977) with an increased rate of attempted suicide (Greer, 1966).

Attachments

Attachment behaviour can be defined as behaviour which maintains proximity of the infant to care-givers and reciprocally elicits attention and care from them. These attachments are believed to have survival value in that they maintain the proximity of the care-giver to the child and in this way reduce distress in strange situations or illness. It is not possible here to explore these notions in any depth, but this has been done elsewhere (Bretherton and Waters, 1985).

It has been argued that an attachment system is a psychological structure that is hypothesized to exist within a person (Bretherton, 1985). This system regulates infant behavioural patterns and those behaviours evoked from key care-givers (particularly the mother) which are designed to maintain the infant's proximity to and contact with this care-giver, referred to as the attachment figure (Bowlby, 1982). The implication is that the system is biologically determined, the main aim being to enhance security (Bischoff, 1975) while the baby is immature. Bretherton (1985) emphasizes the dual component of the operation—from the observer's viewpoint, the maintenance of proximity; and from the internal perspective of the infant, the achievement of security. Attachment behaviour is most evident when the infant is psychologically or physically stressed, protecting the infant from harm. Bowlby (1973) argues that an attachment system has distinctive internal motivation (Bretherton, 1985), the purpose of which is to achieve homeostasis between a child and his environment. Thus the attachment system maintains the child in a familiar environment which balances any fear of the novel and the strange—and this allows the child to explore his/her environment under reasonably safe circumstances. The attachment system becomes operationalized in the second six months of life. Bowlby's concept of attachment was of a system that functions in relation to a small hierarchy of familiar individuals that resists re-programming (Bretherton, 1985).

When external threats are minimal, exploratory behaviour can be extensive; with greater degrees of threat the child will prudently return to the secure base. But if the safe base is less than fully responsive, the attachment behaviour will become anxious (Bretherton, 1985); and where the external threats are perceived as maximal, the child may not know how to respond—he may seek clues by checking the mother's face—a phenomenon known as social referencing (Campos and Stenberg, 1981). By continuous monitoring of the environment the child will be able to construct internal working models of the environs, and the significant people in it; over time these become increasingly complex.

The above concepts have been the subject of fruitful research, some of the most creative work being that by Ainsworth and colleagues (Ainsworth *et al.*, 1978). Infants were observed in a *strange situation*, which consisted of being with an unfamiliar adult in a naturalistic laboratory, initially with mother absent. The mother then returned. The responses of the children to their mothers' absence depended on the prior evidence of the mothers' sensitivity to their infants. Responsive mothers tended to have securely attached children who greeted their mothers positively and warmly after the brief absence. Two other reactions were notable—a group of infants who were less positive in their greeting or who actually *avoided* their mothers; and a group who showed angry resistance combined with contact-seeking behaviour. Avoidant behaviour was related to prior insensitivity of the mother to infant signals. The resistant pattern of behaviour related to inconsistency of mothers' responses in the first year of life. It is important to note that early attachment patterns are predictive of nursery behaviour, with more securely attached children subsequently showing better social functioning, including being less dependent on their teachers and more actively involved with peers (Sroufe *et al.*, 1983).

. Thus the environment strongly influences attachments. Secure attachments are facilitated by stimulating interpersonal interactions and other forms of affection and attention and by consistent sensitive response to the infant's needs. In fear or illness the infant is likely to become attached to whoever brings comfort. The converse is true in that attachments appear to be impeded by a non-responsive under-stimulating or insensitive environment.

Cognitive Development

Cognitive behaviour or intelligence may be broadly defined as a process of mental functioning which includes abilities such as perception, memory, reasoning and logical thought. Cognitive development is intricately related to the dynamic interplay between biological, maturational, environmental, experiential and motivational factors (Lerner, 1978). These interactions, as Piaget's theory of cognitive development shows (Miller, 1983; Piaget, 1977) are central to the emergence of what he regards as psychological 'structures' of thinking, the latter of which proceed through four main stages. These are as follows:

(1) The sensorimotor stage (from birth to two years of age). This is dominated by 'action-ridden' learning through the relationship between the child's use of sensori-perceptions (touching, pulling, holding, looking, tasting, etc.), bodily activity and physical objects. A particularly important achievement during this period is the development of the concept of object permanence which entails the child's ability to appreciate that objects and persons continue to exist even when these are not within immediate sight of the child (Piaget, 1954). The development of this concept which begins to establish itself from about six months of age has important implications for attachment behaviours and it also reflects the beginning process of internal representation (Dunst et al., 1982) which only becomes fully developed during the next, pre-operational stage.

(2) The pre-operational stage. During this stage (2–6 years) language assumes a central role and enables the child to deal symbolically with the environment. This is also the period during which symbolic play—e.g. pretending to drink from an imaginary cup—and imaginative play—e.g. using a toy telephone to engage in a conversation with an imaginary other person—reflect the integral relationship between cognitive, environmental and speech behaviours (Shore, 1986).

(3) The concrete operational stage (6–11 years). This sees a progressive upward shift in the capacity for reasoning in terms of abilities such as classifying, number/mathematical concepts and ordering information in a logical manner. These various conceptual abilities are still often dependent on the presence of observable referents and concrete cues, although much less so than in the previous two stages.

(4) The formal operations stage (11 years onwards). The development of truly abstract reasoning and conceptual abilities involving operations such as probability, hypothetical considerations and proportionality become established during the final stage.

The qualitative and quantitative changes in cognitive functioning which occur during these stages are, in Piaget's view, associated with the process of adaptation which is mediated by two further important processes—assimilation and accommodation. Assimilation is the taking in of sensory information into existing organized patterns of experiences and responses that have already been learned —so-called schemata. Accommodation is the process whereby existing response patterns (schemata) are modified to take account of new experiences and information. For example, in the absence of a toy car, a child may use a wooden block as a substitute play object to represent the sounds and movements of a toy car. In other words, the child's knowledge and experience of play (schema) with proper toy cars which he has previously gained (assimilation) enables him to use a different toy object in an appropriate manner (accommodation) to good effect. Assimilation and accommodation are reciprocal processes and the balance

between the two varies from situation to situation. The notion of schema/
schemata in Piaget's theory is viewed as highly important. It represents basic
actions, ideas and memories—functional elements of cognitive structure—that
are built upon and expanded in the course of time and experience and are an
integral part of the processes of accommodation and assimilation through which
learning occurs.

Piaget's theory remains one of the most influential and productive in the field
of developmental psychology (Miller, 1983) and has been applied to the area of
psychopathology (e.g. Lane and Schwartz, 1987). However, it is not without
criticism. For example, the rate at which different children achieve certain levels
of skills and ranges of different skills at each of the stages varies to a much greater
degree than Piaget led us to believe. Similarly, children often develop the
rudiments of more complex thinking earlier in their development than Piaget
thought. Piaget's theory also argues the view that children's thinking tends to
change in structure or form when progressing from one stage to another, instead
of which the evidence suggests that children's thinking achieves a new or higher
level of thought which is a step-up in the sequence of attainment rather than a
change (Miller, 1983).

A different theoretical viewpoint on cognitive development has emerged in
more recent years, the information-processing model (Baylor and Gascon, 1974;
Baylor and Lemoyne, 1975; Swanson, 1985; Borkowski, 1985) which is mentioned only briefly here. It sets out to describe the kinds of intellectual processes
(e.g. memory, speed of mental response, control of attention, mental strategies)
that are involved when children are receiving, attending, discriminating, storing
and recalling information. The strengths of this approach are considered to lie in
its ability to highlight the complexity of thought and its specificity concerning
different areas of performance (e.g. rules and strategies that may be involved in
memory and problem-solving) and in finding out how children arrive at solutions
and how they achieve understanding in the course of learning. On the other hand,
the information-processing approach derives from the computer model with the
shortcomings of such a model. It also has yet to take into fuller account the effects
of social environmental influences within the context of a cohesive developmental perspective (Miller, 1983).

From a more general point of view, the expansion of interest and research in
children's cognitive development has become quite prolific over the past two
decades and we refer to only a few of the numerous areas of study. Within the
domain of social cognition, the concepts of fairness, social rules and conventions
represent an important aspect of moral development which has exercised the
interest of Kohlberg (1980, 1981; Kohlberg and Elfenbein, 1975), a keen follower
of Piaget's work. He has identified three main levels: the pre-conventional level
which is characterized by self-interest and obedience to avoid punishment or gain
reward, rather than by valuing social conventions. This level of reasoning prevails
among young children, especially pre-schoolers, and continues up to about 6 or
7 years of age. The second, so-called conventional level is typified by an
appreciation of the importance of conforming to social rules, family obligations
and considering other people's point of view. This develops over a much wider

age range, from about 6 years through into young adulthood. The third, post-conventional level is the highest and most sophisticated form of moral reasoning. It involves awareness that most values and rules are relative and an appreciation of ethical principles. A longitudinal study of 58 boys over a 20-year period (Colby *et al.*, 1983) revealed that conventional reasoning emerges as important in adolescence and remains the most common form of moral reasoning in adulthood.

Clearly, moral development is linked to increasing age, cognitive maturity and experience, but these factors do not necessarily guarantee the expression of these values and principles. Indeed, the longitudinal study of Colby *et al.* (1983) found that post-conventional reasoning was not very common at any age.

With the growing concerns over the numbers of children being identified as having been abused or suspected of having been abused, memory—as a preservation of experience—among young children has come to assume an important part of the psychological assessment (Ceci *et al.*, 1987). A review of findings on children's memory with specific reference to child sexual abuse (Fundudis, 1989) shows the following: the cognitive abilities of three-year-olds is often sufficiently well-developed for them to be able to recognize the difference between pretence and reality and this has important implications for ability to recall concrete information, such as facial recognition. Memory ability of both younger and older children is better in relation to recognition (concrete details) than to free recall. Even in older children memory is inclined to be poor in relation to specific details involving times, dates and locations (episodic memory). What children remember does not differ in essence from what adults remember. How much children remember depends on age, language and conceptual level of development and on the form in which their memory is questioned, as well as on the style and manner of the interviewer's use of his or her authority.

Cognitive aspects of depression among children have attracted considerable interest in recent years (Kazdin *et al.*, 1986; Asarnow *et al.*, 1987; Kazdin, 1990). Related to this is the child's concept of death. An understanding of the concept of death as final or irreversible is usually achieved some time after the seventh birthday, during the period referred to in Piagetian terms as the concrete operations stage (6–11 years) (Speece and Brent, 1984). In as much as the concept of death in terms of suicidal behaviour is concerned, it has been found that the fuller understanding of this concept develops with the acquisition of abstract thinking abilities. In Piagetian theory this coincides with the stage of formal operations (11 years onwards), which is when the emotions of self-despair, self-hate and anger are more easily recognized as motivating forces behind thoughts and acts of self-destruction (Carlson *et al.*, 1987). This of course does not mean that younger children do not have suicidal thoughts or engage in suicidal behaviour; rather, it is that the frequency of such behaviour is much lower and the motivating factors less clear cut (Fundudis, 1990).

In summary, the increasing cognitive skills that children develop are part of an emerging process of 'multiple learning' (Maccoby, 1984) based on the interaction between biological and experiential factors. These skills imply mainly intellectual expressions of behaviour. However, in many ways they also involve other aspects of reasoning which are part of but extend beyond mere intellectual capacity. These include, for example, moral judgement; thoughts and attitudes about suicide and death; and memory in relation to traumatic experiences. Therefore, in psychiatry and clinical psychology it is important that the assessment of the patient's mental functioning allows for the teasing out of which aspects of the individual's cognitive abilities and related thoughts and attitudes are relevant to the fuller understanding of that patient's psychological problems. Such clarification often has important implications for treatment and management of the patient's problems.

The assessment of these factors has to take account of the child's stage of development. As we have seen, this, in turn, is dependent on genetic, pre-natal and perinatal factors which interact with the family and wider social environment.

References

Ainsworth, M.D.S., Blehar, M.C., Waters, E. and Wall, S. (1978). *Patterns of Attachment: A Psychological Study of the Strange Situation.* Hillsdale, NJ: Lawrence Erlbaum.

Anderson, V.E. (1974). Genetics and intelligence. In: J. Wortis (ed.) *Retardation and Developmental Disabilities,* Annual Review 6, pp. 22–43. New York: Brunner Mazel.

Andreasen, N.C., Dennert, J.W., Olsen, S.A. and Damasio, A.R. (1982). Hemisphere asymmetries and schizophrenia. *Am. J. Psychiat.* **139,** 427–430.

Archer, S.M., Dublin, M.W. and Stark, L.A. (1982). Abnormal development of kitten retino-geniculate connectivity in the absence of action potentials. *Science (NY)* **217,** 743–745.

Asarnow, J.R., Carlson, G.A. and Guthrie, D. (1987). Coping strategies, self-perceptions, hopelessness and perceived family environments in depressed and suicidal children. *J. Consult. Clin. Psychol.* **55,** 361–366.

Baldwin, H. (1971). Enuresis in twins. *Am. J. Dis. Child.* **121,** 222–225.

Baylor, G.W. and Gascon, J. (1974). An information processing theory of aspects of the development of weight seriation in children. *Cognitive Psychol.* **6,** 1–40.

Baylor, G.W. and Lemoyne, G. (1975). Experiments in seriation with children: towards an information processing explanation of the horizontal decolage. *Can. J. Behav. Sci.* **7,** 4–29.

Behar, D. (1982). Aggressive conduct disorder in children. *Acta Psychiatr. Scand.* **65,** 210–220.

Berger, M. (1982). Personality development and temperament. In: R. Porter and G.M. Collins (eds) *Temperamental Differences in Infants and Young Children,* pp. 176–186. London: Pitman.

Berger, M. (1985). Temperament and individual differences. In: M. Rutter and L. Hersov (eds) *Adolescent Psychiatry,* pp. 3–16. Oxford: Blackwell.

Birtchnell, J. (1970). Early parent death and mental illness. *Br. J. Psychiat.* **116,** 281–288.

Bischoff, N. (1975). A systems approach toward the functional connections of attachment and fear. *Child Dev.* **46,** 801–817.

Boklage, C.E. (1977). Schizophrenia, brain asymmetry development and twinning: cellular relationship with aetiological and possibly prognostic implications. *Biol. Psychiat.* **12,** 19–35.

Borkowski, J.G. (1985). Signs of intelligence: strategy generalization and metacognition. In: S.R. Yussen (ed.) *The Growth of Reflection in Children*, pp. 105–144. Orlando, Florida: Academic Press.

Bowlby, J. (1973). *Attachment and Loss*, Vol. 2, Separation. New York: Basic.

Bowlby, J. (1982). *Attachment and Loss*. New York: Basic.

Bretherton, I. (1985). Attachment theory: retrospect and prospect. In: I. Bretherton and E. Waters (eds) *Growing Points of Attachment Theory and Research*, Monograph of the Society for Research in Child Development, Vol. 50, nos 1–2.

Bretherton, I. and Waters, E. (eds) (1985). *Growing Points of Attachment Theory and Research*, Monograph of the Society for Research in Child Development, Vol. 50, nos 1–2.

Brim, O.G. Jr. and J. Kagan, (1980). Constancy and change: a view of the issues. In: O.G. Brim Jr. and J. Kagan (eds) *Constancy and Chance in Human Development*, pp. 1–25. Cambridge, MA: Harvard University Press.

Brown, G.W., Harris, T.O. and Peto, J. (1973). Life-events and psychiatric disorders. Part 2: Nature of causal link. *Psychol. Med.* **3**, 159–176.

Brown, G.W., Harris, T.O. and Copeland, J.R. (1977). Depression and loss. *Br. J. Psychiat.* **130**, 1–8.

Campos, J.J. and Stenberg, C.R. (1981). Perception appraisal and emotion. The onset of social referencing. In: M.E. Lamb and L.R. Sherrod (eds) *Infant Social Cognition*, pp. 273–314. Hillsdale, NJ: Lawrence Erlbaum.

Carlson, G., Asarnow, J.R. and Orbach, I. (1987). Developmental aspects of suicidal behaviour in children. *J. Acad. Child Adolesc. Psychiat.* **26**, 186–192.

Ceci, S.J., Toglia, M.P. and Ross, D.F. (1987). *Children's Eyewitness Memory*. New York: Springer-Verlag.

Chess, S. and Thomas, A. (1984). *Origins and Evolution of Behaviour Disorders*. New York: Raven Press.

Chomsky, N. (1959). Review of verbal behaviour. *Language* **36**, 26–58.

Clarke, A.M. and Clarke, A.D.B. (1976). *Early Experience: Myth and Evidence*. London: Open Books.

Cloninger, C.R., Sigvardsson, S., Bohman, M. and Von Knorring, A.L. (1982). Predisposition to petty criminality in Swedish adoptees. *Arch. Gen. Psychiat.* **39**, 1242–1249.

Colby, A., Kohlberg, L., Gibbs, J. and Lieberman, M. (1983). A longitudinal study of moral judgement. *Monogr. Soc. Res. Child Dev.* **48**, (1–2 Whole No. 200).

Dru, D. and Walker, J.B. (1975). Self-produced locomotion restores visual capacity after striate lesions. *Science* (*NY*) **187**, 265–266.

Dunst, C.J., Brooks, P.H. and Dorsey, P.A. (1982). Characteristics of hiding places and the transition to Stage IV performance in object permanence tasks. *Dev. Psychol.* **18**, 671–681.

Falkai, P., Bogerts, B., Roberts, G.W. and Crow, T.J. (1988). Measurement of the alpha-cell-migration in the entorhinal region: a market for the developmental disturbances in schizophrenia? *Schizophrenia Res.* **1**, 157–158.

Folstein, S. and Rutter, M. (1977). Genetic influence and infantile autism: a genetic study of ZI twin pairs. *J. Child Psychol. Psychiat.* **18**, 297–321.

Fundudis, T. (1989). Children's memory and the assessment of possible child sex abuse. *J. Child Psych. Psychiat.* **30**, 337–346.

Fundudis, T. (1990). Mood disorders, suicide and suicide behaviour. *Curr. Opinion Paediatr.* **7**, 700–704.

Goldsmith, H.H. (1983). Genetic influence on personality from infancy to adulthood. *Child Dev.* **54**, 331–335.

Goldsmith, H.H., Buss, A.H., Plomin, R. *et al.* (1987). Round table: what is temperament? Four approaches. *Child Dev.* **58**, 505–529.

Goodwin, D. (1976). *Is Alcoholism Hereditary?* Oxford: Oxford University Press.

Greer, S. (1966). Parental loss and attempted suicide: a further report. *Br. J. Psychiat.* **112**, 465–470.

Gregory, R.L. (1977). *Eye and Brain*, 3rd edn., pp. 194–198. London: Weidenfeld & Nicolson.

Gruzelier, J. (1979). Synthesis and critical review of the evidence for hemisphere asymmetries of function in psychopathology. In: J. Gruzelier and P. Flor-Henry (eds) *Hemisphere Asymmetries of Function and Psychopathology*, pp. 647–672. Amsterdam: Elsevier/North-Holland Biomedical.

Harlow, H.F. and Griffin, G. (1965). Induced mental and social deficits in rhesus monkeys. In: S.P. Osler and R.E. Cooke (eds) *The Biosocial Basis of Mental Retardation*. Baltimore: Johns Hopkins Press.

Hawdon, J.M., Hey, E., Kolvin, I. and Fundudis, T. (1990). Born too small. Is outcome still affected. *Dev. Med. Child Neurol.* **32**, 943–953.

Hill, O.W. and Price, J.S. (1967). Childhood bereavement and adult depression. *Br. J. Psychiat.* **113**, 743–751.

Holland, A.J., Hill, A., Murray, B.F. *et al.* (1984). Anorexia nervosa: a study of 34 twin pairs and one set of triplets. *Br. J. Psychiat.* **145**, 414–419.

Honzik, M.P. (1957). Developmental studies of parent–child resemblance in intelligence. *Child Dev.* **28**, 215–228.

Horn, G. (1979). Imprinting—in search of neural mechanisms. *Trend. Neurosci.* **2**, 219–222.

Hunt, J. McV. and Uzgiris, I.C. (1964). Cathexis from recognition familiarity: an exploratory study in a volume of studies honouring J.P. Guilford (cited Hunt, J. McV., 1977). Traditional personality theory in the light of recent evidence. In: I.L. Janis (ed.) *Current Trends in Psychology*. Los Altos, CA: Kaufmann.

Kagan, J. (1980). Perspectives in continuity. In: O.G. Brim and J. Kagan (eds) *Constancy and Change in Human Development*, pp. 26–74. Cambridge, MA: Harvard University Press.

Kagan, J., Reznick, J.S. and Suidman, N. (1986). Temperamental inhibition in early childhood. In: R. Plomin and J. Dunn (eds) *The Study of Temperament*. London: Lawrence Erlbaum.

Kazdin, A.E. (1990). Evaluation of the automatic thought questionnaire: negative cognitive processes and depression among children. *Psychol. Assessment: J. Consult. Clin. Psychol.* **2**, 73–79.

Kazdin, A.E., Rodgers, A. and Colbus, D. (1986). The hopelessness scale for children: psychometric characteristics and concurrent validity. *J. Consult. Clin. Psych.* **54**, 241–245.

Kinney, D.K. and Jacobsen, B. (1978). Environmental factors in schizophrenia: new adoption study evidence and its implications for genetic and environmental research. In: L.C. Wynne, R.L. Cromwell and S. Matthysse (eds) *The Nature of Schizophrenia*, pp. 38–51. New York: Wiley.

Kohlberg, L. (1980). *The Meaning and Measurement of Moral Development*. Worcester, MA: Clark University Press.

Kohlberg, L. (1981). *Essays on Moral Development, Vol. 1. The Philosophy of Moral Development*. New York: Harper & Row.

Kohlberg, L. and Elfenbein, D. (1975). The development of moral judgements concerning capital punishment. *Am. J. Orthopsychiatry* **54**, 614–640.

Kolvin, I., MacKeith, R.M. and Meadow, S.R. (1973). *Bladder Control and Enuresis*. London: Heinemann Spastics International Medical Publications.

Kolvin, I., Charles, G., Nicholson, R., Fleeting, M. and Fundudis, T. (1990). Factors in prevention in inner city deprivation. In: D. Goldberg and D. Tantan (eds) *The Public Health in Fact of Mental Disorder*. Stuttgart: Hougrese and Huber.

Lane, E.A. and Albee, G.W. (1966). Comparative birth weights of schizophrenics and their siblings. *J. Psychol.* **64**, 227–231.

Lane, R.D. and Schwartz, G.E. (1987). Levels of emotional awareness: a cognitive developmental theory and its application to psychopathology. *Am. J. Psychiat.* **144**, 133–143.

Lerner, R.M. (1978). Nature, nurture and dynamic interactionism. *Human Dev.* **21**, 1–20.

Maccoby, E.E. (1984). Socialization and developmental change. *Child Dev.* **55**, 317–328.

McNeil, T.F. and Kaij, L. (1973). Obstetric complications and physical size of offspring of schizophrenic, schizophrenia-like and control mothers. *Br. J. Psychiat.* **123**, 341–348.

McNeil, T.F. and Person Blennar, I. (1975). Offspring sex and degree of active maternal disturbance near reproduction among female mental patients. *Compreh. Psychiat.* **16**, 69–76.

Mednick, S.A. and Schulsinger, F. (1968). Some premorbid characteristics related to breakdown in children with schizophrenic mothers. In: D. Rosenthal and S.S. Kety (eds) *The Transmission of Schizophrenia*. Oxford: Pergamon Press.

Mednick, S.A., Mura, E., Schulsinger, F. and Mednick, B. (1973). Erratum and further analysis—perinatal conditions and infant development in children with schizophrenic parents. *Social Biol.* **20**, 111–112.

Mednick, S.A., Moffitt, T., Gabrielli, W. and Hutchings, B. (1986). Genetic factors in criminal behaviour: a review. In: D. Olsweus, J. Block and M. Radke-Yarrow (eds) *Development of Antisocial and Prosocial Behaviour: Research, Theories and Issues*, pp. 33–55. Orlando, Florida: Academic Press.

Miller, P.H. (1983). *Theories of Developmental Psychology*. San Francisco: W.H. Freeman & Company.

Movshon, J.A. and Van Sluyters, R.C. (1981). Visual neural development. *Ann. Rev. Physiol.* **32**, 477–522.

Neligan, G.A., Kolvin, I., Scott, D. McI. and Garside, R.F. (1976). Born too soon or too small. *Clinics in Developmental Medicine*, No. 61. London: Heinemann.

Oltman, J. and Friedman, S. (1967). Parental deprivation in psychiatric conditions. *Dis. Nerv. System* **28**, 298–303.

Olweus, D. (1979). Stability and aggressive reaction patterns in males: a review. *Psychol. Bull.* **86**, 852–875.

Olweus, D. (1986). Aggression and Hormones: Behavioural relationship with testosterone and adrenaline. In: D. Olweus, J. Block and M. Radke-Yarrow (eds) *Development of Antisocial and Prosocial Behavior: Research Theories and Issues*, pp. 51–72. Orlando, FL: Academic Press.

Perry, V.H. and Cowey, A. (1982). A sensitive period for ganglion cell degeneration and the formation of aberrant retino-fugal connections following tectal lesions in rats. *Neuroscience* **7**, 583–594.

Piaget, J. (1954). *The Construction of Reality in the Child*. New York: Basic Books.

Piaget, J. (1977). *The Development of Thought: Equilibration of Cognitive Structures*. New York: Viking Press.

Plomin, R. (1982). Behavioural genetics and temperament. In: R. Porter and G.M. Collins (eds) *Temperamental Differences in Infants and Young Children*, pp. 155–162. London: Pitman.

Plomin, R. (1983). Developmental behavioural genetics. *Child Dev.* **54**, 253–259.

Plomin, R. and Foch, T.T. (1980). A twins study of objectively assessed personality in childhood. *J. Personal. Social Psychol.* **39**, 680–688.

Plomin, R., Fries, J.C. and McClearn, G.E. (1980). *Behavioural Genetics: A Primer.* San Francisco: W.H. Freeman.

Pollin, W. and Stabenau, J.R. (1968). Biological, psychological and historical differences in a series of monozygotic twins discordant for schizophrenia. In: D. Rosenthal and S.S. Kety (eds) *The Transmission of Schizophrenia*, pp. 317–332. Oxford: Pergamon Press.

Raine, A., Venables, P.H. and Williams, M. (1990). Relationships between central and autonomic measures of arousal at age 15 years and criminality at age 24 years. *Arch. Gen. Psychiat.* **47**, 1003–1007.

Reider, R.O., Rosenthal, D., Wender, P. and Blumenthal, R. (1975). The offspring of schizophrenia. *Arch. Gen. Psychiat.* **32**, 200–213.

Roberts, G.W. (1991). Schizophrenia: a neuropathological perspective. *Br. J. Psychiat.* **158**, 8–17.

Robins, L.N. (1978). Sturdy childhood predictions of adult antisocial behaviour: replications from longitudinal studies. *Psychol. Med.* **8**, 611–622.

Rosanoff, A.J., Handy, L.M. and Plesset, I.R. (1941). The aetiology of child behaviour difficulties, juvenile delinquency and adult criminality with special reference to their occurrence in twins. *Psychiatric Monographs I.* Sacramento.

Rowe, D.C. and Plomin, R. (1978). The Burt controversy: a comparison of Burt's data on IQ with data from other studies. *Behav. Genet.* **8**, 81–84.

Rushton, J.P., Fulker, D.W., Neale, M.C., Nias, D.K.B. and Eysenck, H.J. (1986). Altruism and aggression: the heritability of individual differences. *J. Personal. Social Psychol.* **50**, 1192–1198.

Rutter, M. (1981). Stress, coping and development. Some issues and some questions. *J. Child Psychol. Psychiat.* **22**, 323–351.

Rutter, M. (1985). Family and school influence on cognitive development. *J. Child Psychol. Psychiatr.* **26**, 683–704.

Rutter, M. (1987). Temperament, personality and personality disorder. *Br. J. Psychiatr.* **150**, 443–458.

Rutter, M., Birch, H.G., Thomas, A. and Chess, S. (1964). Temperamental characteristics in infancy and the later development of behavioural disorders. *Br. J. Psychiat.* **110**, 651–661.

Scarr, S. and Kidd, K.K. (1983). Developmental behaviour genetics. In: M.M. Haith and J.J. Campos (eds) *Infancy and Developmental Psychobiology II*, pp. 345–433. New York: Wiley.

Scarr, S. and McCartney, K. (1983). How people make their own environment: a theory of genotype–environmental effects. *Child Dev.* **54**, 424–435.

Shore, C. (1986). Combinatorial play, conceptual development and early multiword speech. *Dev. Psychol.* **22**, 184–190.

Skodak, M. and Skeels, H.M. (1949). A final follow up study of one-hundred adopted children. *J. Genet. Psychol.* **75**, 85–125.

Sobel, D.E. (1961). Infant mortality and malformation in children of schizophrenic women. *Psychiat. Quart.* **35**, 60–61.

Speece, M.W. and Brent, S.B. (1984). Children's understanding of death: a review of three components of a death concept. *Child Dev.* **55**, 1671–1686.

Sroufe, L.A. (1979). Socio-emotional development. In: J.D. Osotsky (ed.) *Handbook of Infant Development*, pp. 462–516. New York: Wiley.

Sroufe, L.A., Fox, N.E. and Pancake, V.R. (1983). Attachment and dependency in developmental perspective. *Child Dev.* **54**, 1615–1627.

Swanson, H.L. (1985). Assessing learning disabled children's intellectual performance: an information processing perspective. In: K.D. Gadow (ed.) *Advances in Learning and Behavioural Disabilities*, Vol. 4, pp. 225–272. Greenwich: JAI Press.

Thomas, A., Chess, S., Birch, H.G. *et al.* (1963). *Individuality in Early Childhood*. New York: New York University Press.

Weininger, O. (1953). Mortality of albino rats under stress as a function of early handling. *Can. J. Psychol.* **7**, 111–114.

Weller, M.P.I. (1986). Medical concepts in psychopathy and violence. *Med. Sci. Law* **26**, 131–143.

Wolff, S. (1989). *Childhood and Human Nature. The Development of Personality*. London and New York: Routledge.

Zarrow, M.X., Campbell, P.S. and Denenberg, V.H. (1972). Handling in infancy: increased levels of the hypothalamic corticotropin releasing factor (CRF) following exposure to a novel situation. *Proc. Soc. Exp. Biol. Med.* **141**, 356–358.

— 22

Personality

M.P.I. Weller and D.F. Peck

The Nature of Personality

The concept of personality is rather hazy and confusing in psychiatry, and there have been many different approaches to its study. In psychology, the concept is used to describe a class of enduring characteristics which differentiate individuals from each other. Thus some people are extraverted, and therefore have certain characteristics in common; others are introverted, who also have characteristics in common, but these characteristics are different (or at least differ in degree) from those of extraverts. In psychiatry, however, the concept is often used quite differently, to describe a relatively enduring pattern of abnormal behaviour, which does not easily fit into a more traditional psychiatric category. Some attempts have been made to marry these two notions of personality, with limited success.

Personality Traits

The four main lines of approach are: trait theory, psychodynamic theory, phenomenological approaches, and behavioural approaches. Most approaches to personality assume that there is an enduring pattern of characteristics, which is consistent across place and over time, and which is therefore capable of predicting certain behaviours. The behavioural approach places less emphasis on enduring characteristics, and more on how past experiences and the immediate environment (or 'situational' factors) can influence behaviour; indeed it may be regarded as an alternative to, rather than as an example of, personality theory. Similarly, phenomenological approaches are less firmly rooted in the notions of consistency and continuity in behaviour (see later). Accordingly, the emphasis in this chapter will be on personality traits, psychodynamic or otherwise.

Psychologists disagree about the number or fundamental factors of personality. Eysenck (1970) suggests that there are three (neuroticism, extraversion and psychoticism); Cattell (1965) maintains that there are 16, but that at a different level of analysis, these can be reduced to two which are almost identical to Eysenck's neuroticism and extraversion. A recent addition to this debate is the

407

theory of McCrae and Costa, in which there are five personality factors: neuro-ticism and extraversion (as Eysenck), plus openness, agreeableness and conscien-tiousness. Promising applications have been reported in a variety of clinical areas including self-esteem in the elderly (McCrae and Costa, 1988) and coronary-prone behaviour (Dembroski and Costa, 1988).

Prediction and Personality

Attempts to predict specific behaviour from formally assessed personality measures have generally not been successful. Shank et al. (1981) compared formal measures of personality with ratings of the quality of the marital relationship, and found that the latter was more predictive of the marital sexual relationship. Similarly, Feifel et al. (1987) found that coping in the face of life-threatening illness was more determined by immediate situational factors, than by general coping style. Finally, in a recent review, Cohen and Edwards (1989) concluded that 'From a practical perspective, research on personality factors as buffers of stress-induced pathology has not been very successful' (p. 275).

Partly because of the frequent finding of weak relationships between person-ality and everyday behaviour, many theorists take an immediate position of 'interactionism', in which it is considered that it is the *interaction* of disposition and environment which influences specific patterns of behaviour, in a synergistic fashion, such that the interaction accounts for more of the variation in behaviour than disposition or environment alone or summed. Mischel (Mischel, 1981) is a longstanding advocate of this approach; he notes that the debate is confounded by the fact that few situations are arbitrary, and are at least partially the result of individual selection, reflecting personality dispositions.

A number of authors (e.g. Ajzen, 1988) have attempted to resolve the issue of disposition versus situation by arguing that although dispositional traits do not strongly predict specific behaviours, they are more strongly related to general classes of behaviours, aggregated over occasions. For example, the trait of being energetic may not strongly predict whether a person takes the lift or climbs the stairs, but may predict individuals' activity levels averaged over stair climbing, participation in sports, walking to work, weight training, getting up early and so on. In clinical practice however, it is probably the case that prediction of specific behaviour (e.g. 'Will this patient keep a job if discharged?') is what is required.

Consistency and Continuity in Personality Traits

Block (1971) argued that there was undeniable and impressive evidence for consistency and continuity, citing as evidence his own careful longitudinal study, in which he regularly followed up large numbers of subjects from early school years to middle adulthood. For example, of the numerous personality variables examined from Senior High School to adulthood (an interval averaging nearly 20 years) approximately 30% of the variables correlated at least +0.35. Although

Block's studies may therefore provide evidence of temporal consistency, one could also argue that they provide evidence of variability in that most of the variation between adults was not predictable from Senior High School measures. In addition, in Block's research, the measures were based on self-report and ratings by observers, rather than on specific behaviour patterns.

The issue of consistency remains a contentious issue in normal personality. There is, however, some evidence to show that in non-normal populations, a higher degree of consistency is found (Mariotto and Paul, 1975). There is support for the observation of Chess *et al.* (1968) that recurrent problems with feeding, bathing and dressing, together with loud crying, protest at novelty, and trantrums, are over-represented in those who subsequently develop conduct disorders.

Constitutional Factors

There is some evidence that people are born with enduring temperamental features, such as activity level, rhythmicity, adaptability, approach, withdrawal, intensity of reaction, quality of mood, sensory threshold, distractibility, persistence and attention span, all of which appear to be constitutional (Chess *et al.*, 1968). However, there are several methodological difficulties in establishing these findings and the meaning of the dimensions may change with age; for example, pacificity in early childhood presages non-competitiveness in adult life (Kagan and Moss, 1962) and physical adventurousness correlates with adult sexual behaviour (Ryder, 1967).

Identical twins are more alike than dizygotic (DZ) twins on many behavioural characteristics, such as general activity level, shyness and sociability, anxiety, emotionality and helpfulness (e.g. Plomin, 1981; Daniels and Plomin, 1985; Rushton *et al.*, 1986). Studies by Lange on identical twins separated early in life, and studies by Rosanoff and his colleagues (1941), showed that monozygotic twins generally have surprisingly similar lives with much greater concordance than DZ twins. One pair of American male twins, separated at five weeks of age, met 39 years later. Both had divorced a woman named Linda and remarried a woman named Betty, had sons named James Allan and dogs named Toy, had served as sheriff's deputies, drove Chevrolets, had a white bench around a tree in their gardens, chain smoked the same brand of cigarette and enjoyed similar hobbies (Bernstein *et al.*, 1988).

Several authors (see Magnusson and Endler, 1977) have argued for the further investigation of neurobiological correlates of specific traits, an approach which has proved valuable in the study of schizophrenia; for example Mathews *et al.* (1982) observed a correspondence between hallucinatory experiences and regional cerebral blood flow patterns. An extension of such methods into the study of personality traits may be profitable. At the biochemical level, Shekim *et al.* (1989) have noted small but significant correlations between platelet monoamine oxidase (MAO) activity and sensation-seeking; many such findings have been reported, but generally the results have proved difficult to replicate and any consistently reported effects tend to be of small magnitude.

Cultural and Social Factors

The impact of the early environment on adult behaviour has been documented extensively in animals and humans. Separation and inappropriate surrogate motherhood has detrimental effects on development of young monkeys (Harlow and Suomi, 1970); handling rodents produces subsequent improved stress tolerance (Weininger, 1953). A clear example with humans is the effects of the early loss of the parent (Brown et al., 1977). The effects of inconsistent parenting do not, however, lead irrevocably and invariably to particular psychiatric disorders, although the relationship between inconsistent parenting and psychiatric problems in general is well established. Clearly other modifying factors are involved.

Cultural and anthropological effects on behaviour have also been extensively documented; for example, cultural factors can effect stress and pain tolerance (Lambert et al., 1960), and sexual stereotypes (Stevenson-Hinde and Hinde, 1986). Further discussion of such social influences is outside the scope of this chapter, except to note a close correspondence between sociological approaches and psychodynamic approaches (Erickson, 1973; Weller, 1986). However, before leaving this section, it is important to note the contributions of social psychology to the study of personality; in particular the work of Jones and Nisbett (1971) who have emphasized that in judging the behaviour of others, we are prone to adopt the hypothesis that the observed behaviour reflects enduring characteristics; whereas we tend to ascribe our own behaviour to situational factors. Thus if a colleague breaks a glass, we may describe him as 'a clumsy person'; if, however, you break a glass yourself, you may attribute it to having slept badly the night before. Such influences may operate in psychiatric diagnosis where, for example, a limited sub-sample of a patient's behaviour may be seen as indicative of an obsessional personality, affecting subsequent impressions by influencing the way in which further information is sought and processed.

Phenomenological and Cognitive Approaches

Cognitive style and personality are interwoven in Kelly's (1955) system of personal constructs of analysing the world within a cognitive framework. These constructs can best be elucidated with the technique of the Role Construct Repertory Test, extended to the technique of Repertory Grids (Bannister and Fransella, 1967). Kelly's view of man is of an active scientist and ever-changing creator of hypotheses and a player of multiple roles, rather than a victim of his history, impulses and defences. Kelly's system has some similarities to Vaihinger's (1967) view that behaviour is affected by beliefs which form part of an inner dialogue. Similarities to aspects of analytic theory can be drawn, in that Kelly's system accepts that some constructs may be non-verbal and inaccessible.

In Personal Construct Theory, the constructs are organized hierarchically; they are the dimensions along which each individual interprets his own behaviour and that of others. Constructs are based mainly on a person's previous experiences, and as such are changeable, and specific to each individual. Core or superordinate constructs are relatively stable, and provide a sense of self-identity and con-tinuity; changing core constructs is highly disruptive to a person's psychological life. However, less central or subordinate constructs are more flexible and changes in them have no major untoward consequences. Personal Construct Theory is less firmly rooted in the notion of enduring characteristics, putting more emphasis than trait theory on people's ability to determine their own destiny.

Of particular interest to psychiatry is the current debate concerning the enduring cognitive characteristics of individuals prone to depression. Depressed people are alleged to have automatic and generally self-deprecating thoughts, which remain even when the depressed person is well. In addition there is evidence that people prone to depression have selectivity of memory, in that unpleasant memories are easily evoked, but pleasant memories or those leading to positive self-evaluations are relatively inaccessible (Williams *et al.*, 1988). Parry and Brewin (1988) argue that negative cognitive style alone is unlikely to account for all depressions, and that stressful life-events can also be important triggers.

The idea that cognitive style and perceptual organization are functions of personality bears upon the concept of mental illness as being along a dimension (Claridge, 1985), and upon the relationship between personality disorder and neurotic disorder (Tyrer *et al.*, 1983).

In clinical practice, psychiatric disorder often seems to extend from the previous personality, so that a cyclothymic character, if unwell, seems most likely to develop a manic-depressive disorder. Similarly, relationships have been noted between asocial personality disorder, and schizophrenia (Lowing *et al.*, 1983; Kendler *et al.*, 1984), and drug and alcohol abuse have been related to particular forms of personality disorder (Henn *et al.*, 1977; Reich and Thompson, 1987). However, there seems to be little in the way of a consistent link between formal personality measures such as the 16PF, and psychiatric disorder (Presly and Walton, 1973).

When there are discrepancies between personality and psychiatric disorder, these may arise from the multitude of divisions in nomenclature, in that the most significant classes may not have been clearly identified, and the breakdown of personality types into a paranoid, schizoid, borderline and schizotype, for example, may be going further than clinical discrimination and prognosis warrants. In clinical practice, people often seem to be described best in a conventional way, rather than squeezing them into unsatisfactory, limiting and somewhat arbitrary psychiatric categories. Categories for construing personality seem to be inherently arbitrary; for example, the forthcoming International Classification of Diseases (ICD 10) categories do not overlap with the DSM IIIR categories; the number of items and cut-off points in the criteria are inconsistent across diagnosis; and we are abjured in the ICD to attend to the most prominent characteristics, because the overall categories seldom apply unequivocally.

Psychosomatic Illness

It has been suggested that different personality structures may determine res-ponse to stress (Bridges and Jones, 1968), and differing psychophysiological and immunological responses (Baker, 1987). Personality differences may, to a limited degree, account for differing propensities to develop diseases such as hypertension, myocardial infarction, and cancer (Jenkins *et al.*, 1967; Thomas and Greenstreet, 1973), as well as to develop mental illness and commit suicide. However, these relationships are the subject of much debate. Where such relationships exist, the nature of the causative links is often obscure; characteristics like extraversion may be associated with lifestyles and activities such as smoking, that themselves exert an influence on disease (Lloyd and Cawley, 1980).

Concluding Remarks

It is clear that substantial groundwork is being prepared for a psychological understanding of personality, with widespread implications for psychiatry, but more needs to be done. Traditional psychometric measures of personality have been extensively investigated in relation to psychiatric disorders, and have been found wanting. They need to be supplemented by some of the more recent developments rooted in modern personality theory, as exemplified in the important work of Livesley and his colleagues on personality disorder (Livesley, 1987). They described a systematic multistage development of a scale for assessing personality disorders, based on clinical observation, but supplemented by behaviourally-defined items and careful descriptions, with a detailed analysis of factorial structure and other psychometric properties.

References

Ajzen, I. (1988). *Attitudes, Personality and Behavior*. Milton Keynes: Open University Press.
Baker, G.H.B. (1987). Psychological factors and immunity. *J. Psychosom. Res.* **31**, 1–10.
Bannister, D. and Fransella, F. (1967). *Grid Test of Schizophrenic Thought Disorder Manual*. London: Barnstaple Psychology Test Publication.
Bernstein, D.A., Roy, E.J., Srull, T.K. and Wickens, C.D. (1988). *Psychology*. Boston: Houghton Mifflin.
Block, J. (1971). *Lives Through Time*. Berkeley: Bancroft Books.
Bridges, P.K. and Jones, M.T. (1968). Relationship of personality and physique to plasma cortisol levels in response to anxiety. *J. Neurol. Neurosurg. Psychiatry* **31**, 57–60.
Brown, G.W., Harris, T.O. and Copeland, J.R. (1977). Depression and loss. *Br. J. Psychiatry* **130**, 1–8.
Cattell, R.B. (1965). *The Scientific Analysis of Personality*. Harmondsworth: Penguin.
Chess, S., Thomas, A. and Birch, H.G. (1968). Behavioural problems revisited: Findings of an anterospective study. In: S. Chess and A. Thomas (eds) *Annual Progress in Child Psychiatry and Child Development*. New York: Brunner-Mazel.
Claridge, G. (1985). *Origins of Mental Illness: Temperament, Deviance and Disorder*. Oxford: Basil Blackwell.
Cohen, S. and Edwards, J.R. (1989). Personality characteristics as moderators of the relationship between stress and disorder. In: R.W.J. Neufeld (ed.) *Advances in the Investigation of Psychological Stress*. New York: Wiley.
Daniels, D. and Plomin, R. (1985). Origins of individual differences in infant shyness. *Dev. Psychol.* **21**, 118–121.

Dembroski, T.M. and Costa, P.T. (1988). Assessment of coronary-prone behavior: A current overview. *Ann. Behav. Med.* **10**, 60–63.

Erickson, E.H. (1973). *Childhood and Society*. Harmondsworth: Penguin.

Eysenck, H.J. (1970). *The Structure of Human Personality*. London: Methuen.

Feifel, H., Strack, S. and Tong Nagy, V. (1987). Degree of life threat and differential use of coping modes. *J. Psychosom. Res.* **31**, 91–99.

Harlow, H.F. and Suomi, S.J. (1970). Nature of love—simplified. *Am. Psychol.* **25**, 161–168.

Henn, F.A., Herjanic, M. and Vanderpearl, R.H. (1977). Forensic psychiatry: anatomy of a service. *Compr. Psychiatry* **18**, 337–345.

Jenkins, C.D., Rosenman, R.H. and Friedman, M. (1967). Development of an objective psychological test for the determination of the coronary-prone behaviour pattern in employed men. *J. Chronic Dis.* **20**, 371–379.

Jones, E.E. and Nisbett, R.E. (1971). *The Actor and Observer: Divergent. Perceptions of the Causes of Behaviour*. New York: General Learning Press.

Kagan, J. and Moss, H.A. (1962). *Birth to Maturity*. New York: Wiley.

Kelly, G.A. (1955). *The Psychology of Personal Constructs*. New York: Norton.

Kendler, K.S., Masterson, C.C., Ungaro, R. *et al.* (1984). A family history study of schizophrenia-related personality disorders. *Am. J. Psychiatry* **141**, 424–427.

Lambert, W.E., Libman, E. and Poser, E.G. (1960). The effect of increased salience of a membership group on pain tolerance. *J. Pers.* **28**, 350–357.

Livesley, W.J. (1987). A systematic approach to the delineation of personality disorders. *Am. J. Psychiatry* **144**, 772–777.

Lloyd, G.G. and Cawley, R.H. (1980). Smoking habits after myocardial infarction. *J. R. Coll. Physicians* **14**, 224–226.

Lowing, P.A., Mirsky, A.F. and Pereira, M.A. (1983). The inheritance of schizophrenia spectrum disorders. A reanalysis of the Danish adoptee study data. *Am. J. Psychiatry* **140**, 1167–1171.

McCrae, R.R. and Costa, P.T. (1988). Age, personality, and the spontaneous self-concept. *J. Gerontol.* **43**, S177–S185.

Magnusson, D. and Endler, S. (1977). *Personality at the Crossroads: Current issues in Interactional Psychology*. Hillsdale: Erlbaum.

Mariotto, M.J. and Paul, G.L. (1975). Persons versus situations in the real life functioning of chronically institutionalised mental patients. *J. Abnorm. Psychol.* **85**, 483–493.

Mathews, R.J., Meyer, J.S., Francis, D.J. *et al.* (1982). Regional cerebral blood flow in schizophrenia. *Arch. Gen. Psychiatry* **39**, 1121–1124.

Mischel, W. (1981). *Introduction to Personality*. New York: Holt Rinehart and Winston.

Parry, G. and Brewin, C.R. (1988). Cognitive style and depression: symptom-related, event-related or independent provoking factor? *Br. J. Clin. Psychol.* **27**, 23–35.

Plomin, R. (1981). Behavioural genetics and personality. In: R.M. Liebert and R. Wicks-Nelson (eds) *Developmental Psychology*. Englewood Cliffs, NJ: Prentice-Hall.

Presly, A.S. and Walton, H.J. (1973). Dimensions of abnormal personality. *Br. J. Psychiatry* **122**, 269–276.

Reich, J. and Thompson, W.D. (1987). DSM-III Personality disorder clusters in three populations. *Br. J. Psychiatry* **150**, 471–475.

Rosanoff, A.J., Handy, L.M. and Plesset, I.R. (1941). The aetiology of child behaviour difficulties, juvenile delinquency and adult criminality with special reference to their occurrence in twins. *Psychiat. Mono.* **1**.

Rushton, J.P., Fulker, D.W., Neale, M.C., Nias, D.K.B. and Eysenck, H.J. (1986). Altruism and aggression: The heritability of individual differences. *J. Pers. Soc. Psychol.* **50**, 1192–1198.

Ryder, R.G. (1967). Birth to maturity revised: A canonical re-analysis. *J. Person. Soc. Psychol.* **7**, 168–172.

Shank, J., Pfrang, H. and Rausche, A. (1981). Personality traits versus the quality of the marital relationship as the determinants of marital sexuality. *Arch. Sex. Behav.* **15**, 449–456.

Shekim, W.O., Bylund, D.B., Frankel, F. *et al.* (1989). Platelet MAO activity and personality variations in normals. *Psychiatry Res.* **27**, 81–88.

Stevenson-Hinde, J. and Hinde, R.A. (1986). Changes in associations between characteristics. In: R. Plomin and J. Dunn (eds) *The Study of Temperament: Changes, Continuities and Challenges.* Hillsdale: Lawrence Erlbaum.

Thomas, C.B. and Greenstreet, R.L. (1973). Psychological characteristics in youth as predictors of five disease states: suicide, mental illness, hypertension, coronary heart disease and tumour. *Johns Hopkins Med. J.* **132**, 14–43.

Tyrer, P., Casey, P. and Gall, J. (1983). Relationship between neurosis and personality disorder. *Br. J. Psychiatry* **142**, 404–408.

Vaihinger, H. (1967). *The Philosophy of "As If".* London: Routledge and Kegan Paul.

Weininger, O. (1953). Mortality of albino rats under stress as a function of early handling. *Can. J. Psychol.* **7**, 111–114.

Weller, M.P.I. (1986). Medical concepts in psychopathy and violence. *Med. Sci. Law* **26**, 131–143.

Williams, J.M., Watts, F.N., Macleod, C. and Mathews, A. (1988). *Cognitive Psychology and Emotional Disorders.* Chichester: Wiley.

Social Processes

— 23 ————————————

The Development of the Psychotherapies:
A Brief Historical Overview

W. Ll. Parry-Jones

Psychotherapy comprises a variety of psychological methods, utilizing both verbal and non-verbal interaction and the therapist–patient relationship, for bringing about emotional, behavioural and cognitive changes, thereby relieving symptoms of distress and improving personal functioning. This broad definition allows discussion of the historical development of the principal supportive, re-educative and reconstructive approaches employed in Western psychotherapy. Systems of individual psychotherapy are considered in this chapter in three broad categories, namely psychoanalysis, behavioural psychotherapy and humanistic– existential psychotherapy; the group therapies and family therapy are discussed separately.

The Pre-history of Psychotherapy

Ways of relieving suffering, allaying fears and influencing behaviour based on the healer's personality, on wise counsel or diverse forms of punishment, have been employed over the centuries and explained according to the prevailing philosophies and beliefs, differences in psychological assumptions and the chang-ing concepts of man's self-understanding (Ellenberger, 1970; Ehrenwald, 1976). In Greco-Roman culture, philosophical dialogue fulfilled a verbal therapeutic func-tion with regard to irrationality, in contrast to the non-verbal techniques of contemporary religion and medicine (Gill, 1985). Studies of primitive healing, like shamanism, reveal how themes such as exorcism and other expulsory measures recur both historically and transculturally. A gradual change from supernatural explanations to those involving personal and interpersonal psychological processes can be identified. The sixteenth century treatment recommendations made by R. Burton in his *Anatomy of Melancholy*, for example, included supportive, comforting approaches, with 'an emphasis on confiding in a trusted listener, reflecting the traditions of both humane physicians and clergymen' (Jackson, 1989). Two broad categories of psychotherapy emerge, derived from different traditions of pre-scientific healing, the religio-magical therapies, based on a supernatural explanation of suffering, and the empirical–scientific therapies (Frank, 1961). The latter were used continuously in Western society from the mid-eighteenth century. A century later, the term 'psychotherapeia' had been

417

introduced (Dendy, 1853), referring to the remedial effects of 'psychical influence' and the concept of 'psychotherapeutics' was soon fashionable, applied initially to treatment by hypnosis and suggestion.

The 'discovery' of the unconscious mind and the birth of dynamic psychiatry happened slowly, chiefly during the two centuries 1700–1900 (Whyte, 1962), contributed to by many individuals and movements and influenced by social, cultural and political changes. For example, in late eighteenth and early nineteenth century Germany, a psychodynamically orientated movement emerged as part of the cultural trend of romanticism in philosophy and literature, the pioneers being J.C. Reil and J.C.A. Heinroth. Heinroth described degrees of consciousness of the mind, illustrating, incidentally, the way in which Freudian ideas were anticipated by others (Riese, 1958). But, at this stage, no comprehensive theory of personality, conflict and treatment emerged and romantic psychiatry was soon eclipsed by the organicist, antipsychological views of mid-nineteenth century neuropsychiatrists like W. Griesinger and H. Maudsley. The great lunacy reformers, P. Pinel, the Tukes, J. Conolly and D. Dix powerfully influenced the humanitarian movement in the treatment of the insane in the first half of the nineteenth century. The accent of this movement was on non-restraint and the occupation and physical environment of patients, but the need for a personal relationship between doctor and patient was largely unrecognized. Moral treatment altered the climate of patient care, but, as the century progressed, it became submerged by the growing institutionalization of the asylum era and systematic psychotherapy in asylums remained undeveloped.

It was the therapeutic use of hypnotic phenomena by F.A. Mesmer (1734–1815) that marked the introduction of empirical psychotherapy. Mesmer attributed the curative value to 'animal magnetism' and his theories reflected lingering astrological and mythical beliefs. However, he was discredited and his 'magnetic' theory was undermined by J. Braid, a Manchester doctor, who coined the term hypnotism in 1843. Thereafter, interest in mesmerism declined until hypnosis flourished again as a therapeutic technique around 1880 as part of a new dynamic movement characterized by interest in dreams, sexual pathology, mysticism and exploration of the unconscious. At this time, two influential schools of hypnosis emerged in France led by J.-M. Charcot at the Salpêtrière in Paris and by H.-M. Bernheim and A.-A. Liébeault at Nancy. Charcot believed that hypnosis was a pathological state associated with hysteria, which he regarded as an organic disease of the nervous system, whereas Bernheim believed that it was a psychological process due to suggestion. Liébeault used hypnotic suggestion and É. Coué extended this to suggestion with hypnosis and to autosuggestion. Treatment by persuasion and suggestion lost ground despite such developments as the extension of autosuggestion to autogenic training (Schultz and Luthe, 1959), a form of self-hypnosis which survives as a component of relaxation therapy. P. Janet (1859–1947) was influenced by Charcot and preceded Freud in recognizing unconscious factors in hysteria. He formulated important ideas about the nature of subconscious processes and his work was one of the chief resources for Freud, Adler and Jung. But he was not a psychotherapeutic systems builder (Janet, 1925) and his work had little long-term influence (Ellenberger, 1970).

In 1882, Freud was impressed by J. Breuer's use of hypnosis in treating Anna O., a woman who had various neurotic symptoms. He visited Charcot briefly in 1885, Bernheim in 1899 and, later, he used hypnosis to gain access to patients' reminiscences. Opinions differ about Charcot's influence on Freud, but it appears that it was at the Salpêtrière that he recognized the role of unconscious ideas in hysterical disorders and that this was the source of subsequent theories (Parry-Jones, 1987). Later, Freud abandoned hypnosis in favour of mental catharsis and then free association. But the study of hysteria and the move from primitive healing by 'magnetism' to healing by hypnotism proceeding to more abstract psychological processes, suggestion and early psychoanalysis, were crucial in the development of dynamic psychotherapy.

Psychoanalysis

The central task of psychoanalysis is the uncovering of unconscious conflicts and repressed experiences. The key techniques developed by Sigmund Freud (1856–1939) were free association by the patient, the formation and analysis of transference and the use of interpretation by the therapist. Freud's chief work occurred between 1895 and 1939 (Jones, 1953, 1955, 1957; Freud, 1957; Alexander and Selesnick, 1967). The first decade was formative and early publications included *Studies in Hysteria* with Breuer in 1895, *The Interpretation of Dreams* in 1900 and *The Psychopathology of Everyday Life*, in 1901. The International Psychoanalytic Association was formed in 1910 with Jung as its first president. In 1912, E. Jones, who founded the British Psychoanalytic Society, and B. Hart first presented psychoanalysis systematically in the United Kingdom and J. Putnam and G.S. Hall introduced it to American psychiatry. The resignation from the Association in 1910 of E. Bleuler, professor of psychiatry at the Burgholzi Hospital, Zurich, contributed to the separation of psychoanalysis from academic psychiatry in Europe. In the 1920s and 1930s, prominent analysts left Europe for the United States, including Horney, Fromm, Alexander and Rank, becoming leading figures clinically and academically. Consequently, in the United States, psychoanalysis evolved within academic psychiatry.

At the end of the nineteenth century, when the organic model of mental illness was proving to be of limited therapeutic value, psychoanalysis offered the promise of explaining and treating mental disorders in a radically new way, based on a comprehensive theory of personality. Freud's concept of unconscious motivation had the most profound effect on psychiatric and popular thought. He did not 'discover' the unconscious, but forced 'the attention of the Western world to the fact that the unconscious mind is of importance in every one of us, by giving dramatic illustrations of the way in which it works, particularly when its spontaneous formative processes are deformed by inhibition' (Whyte, 1962). His theories have been challenged, principally because they cannot be proved or disproved (Fisher and Greenberg, 1977). Freud's impact on twentieth century thought is waning with, in recent years, systematic questioning of the validity of his data and his use of the scientific paradigm (Masson, 1984; Fine, 1985;

Stepansky, 1986, 1988a,b). Nevertheless, psychoanalysis remains a comprehensive conceptualization of personality and psychopathology and the most complete system of psychotherapy. The model of verbal self-exploration is still the format of many diverse approaches and derivative links can be recognized between all forms of dynamic psychotherapy and the ideas of Freud.

Dissenters and neo-Freudians

Some of Freud's early followers broke away, setting the future pattern for successive schisms in the psychoanalytic movement (Roazen, 1979). The dissenters were not as influential as Freud and no fundamentally new system has emerged, but amongst his former pupils, Adler, Jung, Rank, Ferenczi and Reich made major contributions. A. Adler (1870–1937) challenged Freud's view of sex as the prime mover of human behaviour and broke away in 1911, to establish 'individual psychology' (Ansbacher and Ansbacher, 1957). He proposed that inferiority feelings were the creative force since they led to striving for superiority and neurotic symptoms were a form of compensation for physical or mental weaknesses. The treatment focus was understanding the individual's 'life-style', followed by re-education in establishing healthier patterns and goals. The long-term influence of Adler's psychology has been considerable. His ideas, particularly the emphasis on social relationships, survive in Rogerian psychotherapy, in counselling, in some group and family therapies, in child guidance and specific techniques such as social skills training. C.G. Jung (1875–1961) parted from Freud in 1913 and developed his own system of 'analytical psychology'. His writing tended to be obscure and mystical and, consequently, his contribution to psychotherapy has not been acknowledged fully (Storr, 1973). His most important concepts were the collective unconscious, archetypes and individuation, an innate striving for self-realization. The aim of analysis was releasing the creative potential of the collective unconscious. O. Rank (1884–1939), who seceded in 1929, examined separation anxiety and experimented with short-term therapy. His concept of birth trauma as the precursor of all later anxiety has a modern counterpart in A. Janov's theory of neurosis as a symbolization of primal pain, due to the denial of primal needs. W. Reich (1897–1957) developed character analysis, exploring the relationship between bodily tension and posture, 'character armour' and psychological defences. Reichian therapy continues in modified form as 'bio-energetics'.

Psychoanalytic concepts have been constantly elaborated and revised in response to sociocultural influences and changes (Greenson, 1969). In the 1920s and 1930s, a group of psychoanalysts emerged concerned that the sociocultural determinants of human behaviour had been neglected. K. Horney, for example, stressed the individual's basic need for security and the cultural and situational factors in the neuroses. H.S. Sullivan developed a system of psychotherapy centred on the interpersonal relations of the patient and the psychiatrist's participant observation, a significant alternative to the Freudian paradigm. E. Fromm emphasized interaction between man and his society, the outcome of stress in industrial society and the effects of existential loneliness.

E. Erikson introduced the concepts of identity and developmental stages in psychosocial development. Another group, the 'ego-psychologists' including Anna Freud, H. Hartmann and D. Rapaport, challenged Freud's emphasis on the unconscious and postulated the existence of an autonomous ego. F. Fromm-Reichmann was one of the first psychoanalysts to apply intensive psychotherapy to overtly psychotic patients. In the English school of psychoanalysis Anna Freud, W.R.D. Fairbairn and Melanie Klein (Segal, 1964) stressed the importance of early relationships. Fairbairn formulated the object relations theory of personality, later elaborated by H. Guntrip. Bowlby worked on maternal deprivation, attachment and loss. More recently, the American self psychologists, O. Kernberg and H. Kohut, developed the ideas of Fairbairn and the Kleinians, with particular interest in disturbance of self-formation that may underlie many neurotic disorders.

As it developed, psychoanalysis became lengthier and the therapist more passive, particularly due to the attention given to resistance and transference. S. Ferenczi and O. Rank tried to reverse this process by adopting a more active style and, in the 1960s, D. Malan, building on the work of M. Balint and co-workers at the Tavistock Clinic, London, developed psychoanalytically-based brief psychotherapy, using more direct interpretation and focal techniques. The brief treatment approach was also taken by P.E. Sifneos and H. Davanloo. Forms of crisis intervention were developed by C. Caplan and others on the basis of abbreviated psychoanalytic techniques.

Child psychotherapy

The specific treatment of children received little attention until the late nineteenth century and prevailing views about disorders were biological and weighted by evolutionary doctrines. Freud's speculations about the influence of early family life added an entirely new dimension. His theories about childhood neurosis were presented in 1905 and, later, in 1909, in his *Analysis of a Phobia in a Five-Year Old Boy*, he described his treatment using the father as an intermediary. H. Von Hug-Hellmuth first treated children by psychoanalytic methods but M. Klein actually introduced modified psychoanalytic techniques for treating the child (Klein, 1963). Difficulties in using free association led to the use of play materials to encourage communication and expression and to play therapy, which became popular in child guidance clinics. These had been established in the 1920s and 1930s as part of the mental hygiene movement. Anna Freud further clarified the differences between child and adult analysis. Her approach was flexible, with less emphasis on transference than Klein and with greater contact with parents. D. Winnicott furthered understanding of early mother–infant relationships and, in an institutional setting, B. Bettelheim applied psychoanalytic ideas to the treatment of maladjusted children. Gradually, child psychoanalysis became distinguished from other psychotherapeutic techniques, adapted to the needs of children, including a non-directive approach developed by Y.M. Axline.

Behavioural Psychotherapy

Techniques derived from the concepts of classical (Pavlovian) and operant or instrumental (Skinnerian) conditioning constitute the most important recent development in psychotherapy and progress has been rapid. Theoretically, disorders are not construed in terms of underlying unconscious processes, but as maladaptive patterns of learned behaviour, so that manifest behaviour becomes the focus of attention. In practice, however, techniques may be quite loosely related to learning theory. Central to the approach is the procedure of behavioural analysis. Significant improvement in abnormal behaviour can be achieved, without the development of substitute symptoms, and in this way, the theories and methods of behaviour therapy have challenged psychoanalysis as a treatment method.

J.B. Watson (1878–1958) founded the school of behaviourism (Watson, 1930), aiming at a new science of psychology discarding concepts of introspection and consciousness, in which the objectivity of data would be accepted by science. In the 1920s, Watson and Raynor reported experimental treatments using these principles and Janet described a method of treating agoraphobia. In 1938, Mowrer and Mowrer described the bell and pad technique for enuresis. In the 1950s, impetus was given to behaviour therapy by the development of the theory and therapeutic method of systematic desensitization based on the neurophysiological model of reciprocal inhibition (Wolpe, 1958; Lieberman, 1986) and the resurgence of interest in aversion therapy, first used in the 1930s and 1940s. Later developments employed operant conditioning techniques developed by B.F. Skinner. The wide application of behavioural methods included social skills training, token economies, marital and family therapy.

Cognitive therapy

Cognitive therapy is concerned with the individual's interpretations of internal and external events and their crucial role in understanding behaviour. It has behavioural, existential and Adlerian roots and takes several forms (Mahoney and Arnkoff, 1978), including the rational–emotive approach of A. Ellis, in which irrational interpretations of reality are regarded as the cause of the disorder. The integration of cognitive and behavioural approaches emerged at a time of growing dissatisfaction with the mechanistic aspects of behaviour therapy and the need to add a cognitive component to established techniques. From the early 1970s two cognitive approaches had major influence. The first was D. Meichenbaum's 'self-instructional training' and the second was A.T. Beck's innovative approach to the treatment of depression, after becoming dissatisfied with the effects of psychoanalytic psychotherapy. His approach was derived from the notion that negative thinking had a central role in both the generation and maintenance of depression. Later, Beck extended his ideas and techniques to a much wider range of disorders.

Humanistic–Existential Psychotherapy

Humanistic psychology has a brief history (Buhler and Allen, 1972), but has been called a 'third force' in addition to psychoanalysis and behaviourism. It emphasizes man as a person and his unique subjective experiences and problems. The principal humanistic theorists were A. Maslow and C. Rogers. There is no single form of humanistic–existentialist psychotherapy, instead it refers to a number of systems of which the best known are those of C. Rogers, L. Binswanger, V.E. Frankl and F. Perls. Other similarly orientated systems are G.A. Kelly's 'personal construct' approach and those focusing on interpersonal transactions, notably 'transactional analysis', founded in the 1960s by E. Berne.

Client-centred psychotherapy

Between 1938 and 1950, C. Rogers developed a non-directive form of counselling, later called client-centred psychotherapy (1961). Freudian, Rankian, gestalt and existential ideas were influential but, from the outset, it was essentially non-psychoanalytic in that insight was not emphasized and transference not employed. Attention was given to the feelings of participants, and diagnosis, interpretation and direction were avoided. Evolving Rogerian therapy became more clearly existential in its orientation. Characteristics of the effective therapist were postulated, such as capacity for unconditional positive regard and accurate empathic understanding (Rogers, 1957). Personal analysis was not a training requirement and the simplified technique and the lack of complex theories encouraged its widespread adoption by lay-therapists, contributing to the interruption of the medical domination of psychotherapy. This approach has had considerable influence in counselling, management and in the encounter group movement.

Existential psychotherapy

This school is less concerned with techniques than with a philosophical view of man and the subjective experience of 'being-in-the-world'. European existential psychology began in the 1940s, spreading a decade later into the United States (May *et al.*, 1958), combining psychoanalysis with the existentialist philosophy of Kierkegaard, Heidegger, Jaspers, Buber and Sartre (Boss, 1963). Heidegger's views, in particular, derived from the 'philosophical anthropology' tradition, were influential on the epistemological foundation of psychiatry and psychotherapy (Chessick, 1986). No unique existential psychotherapy exists; its distinctive technical feature is the therapist's attempt to enter the individual's inner world. L. Binswanger, originally a Freudian, developed existential analysis, concerned with the individual's subjective experiences and with his 'existential modes', the therapeutic objective being the development and utilization of capacities for existence. Logotherapy, developed by V.E. Frankl, focused on man's striving to understand the meaning of his existence and the consequences when this is frustrated. Frankl introduced the technique of 'paradoxical intention'. The writings of the existential psychotherapists tend to be obscure and unscientific, but their humanistic appeal has been considerable at a time of existential crisis in contemporary culture (Yalom, 1980).

Gestalt therapy

Gestalt psychology originated about 1910, derived from the ideas of Wertheimer, Koffka, Kohler, Lewin and Goldstein, and is concerned with the interrelationship of all aspects of the perceptual field. Gestalt therapy was developed by F. Perls from gestalt psychology and from psychoanalysis modified by W. Reich. Its focus is the interplay between the individual and his surroundings; 'here-and-now' existence, self-actualization and responsibility for one's actions are emphasized. Like other humanistic–existential therapies it centres on contemporary experiences, not on the unconscious, historical experiences used in classical psychoanalysis, and its hedonistic appeal emerged clearly in the 1960s and 1970s. The approach is concerned with bodily signs of tension and with changing the experience of bodily processes and, in this respect, it resembles other emotive release therapies or 'body therapies' like bio-energetics or those of the catharsis–abreactive kind like A. Janov's 'primal therapy'.

Group Therapies

The grouping together of people for mutual support is an ancient tradition, although group therapy only came into widespread use after World War II and now comprises very disparate activities. Freud did not work with groups although he wrote about group psychology and, J.H. Pratt (1906), a Boston physician, is credited with first recognizing the therapeutic use of group methods, in the treatment of patients with chronic tuberculosis. His psycho-educational approach was tried out unsuccessfully with psychiatric patients and it was the pioneering work of psychoanalysts treating patients in groups that led to further progress. The 1930s witnessed the burgeoning of the group therapy field, influenced particularly by the work of T. Burrow and J.L. Moreno (1932) in the United States. Moreno introduced sociometry and psychodrama, which he invented in 1921; subsequently, related techniques like role-playing came to be used widely. Concurrently, K. Lewin's field theory approach as a development from gestalt concepts and the introduction of the notion of group dynamics laid the groundwork for the sensitivity training group movement which began in 1947. T-groups were concerned with training in human relations skills, obtained by observing group processes and becoming aware of the effects of interpersonal behaviour. In the United Kingdom experiments with groups in the rehabilitation of hospitalized soldiers during World War II, at the Northfield Military Hospital, were reported by W.R. Bion and J. Rickman and by S.H. Foulkes in the 1940s. This experience led to exploration of group dynamics, to the development of the group-analytic approach by Foulkes and 'the therapeutic community' movement in mental hospital treatment (Taylor, 1958). Innovation in the field of social or milieu therapy was made by T. Main, Maxwell Jones, R.N. Rapoport and D. Clark, but by the 1970s early enthusiasm has not led to wide support for therapeutic community techniques, due in part to the lack of evidence of their effectiveness. Some of the pioneer work in groups was undertaken with adolescents by A. Aichhorn and S.R. Slavson (Rachman and Raubalt, 1984).

The encounter group movement originated largely outside conventional psychiatric services and it spread widely, mainly in the United States. This expansion revealed a widespread quest for personal growth, mutual support and intimacy in contemporary urban society, and reflected a major departure from established psychotherapy with a shift from talk to action and from the authority of the therapist to the power of the peer group. The 'here-and-now' aspects of human feelings and relationships are emphasized and encounter groups may take numerous forms, such as marathon groups and body-awareness groups. The 'human potential movement' drew chiefly upon the procedures of sensitivity training, gestalt therapy, transactional group therapy and, above all, the philosophy of Rogers (1970).

Family therapy

The idea of treating the family as a group only began in the 1950s and the field of family therapy is still in a state of transition. Freud and his followers had recognized the psychological significance of the family for its members and the importance of the child's relationship with its parents was acknowledged, but analysts were cautious about involving the parents. However, growing recognition of the connection between the child's disturbance and parental pathology led to the treatment of both, although not together. Emphasis, initially, was on the mother alone, setting the style for early child guidance and social case-work, before the need to include fathers was recognized. The major shift from individual analysis to family therapy began in the late 1940s and the 1950s. Early family therapists treated families containing severely disturbed individuals and, later, they were joined by those who were disillusioned with traditional individual approaches of treatment. In this way, the groundwork for conjoint family treatment was laid by concurrent psychoanalytic work with marital pairs by B. Mittelman, J. Bowlby's experimental joint sessions with children, J. Howells' family treatment and H. Dicks' conjoint marital techniques.

The major impetus to family work, however, was given by research studies of communication in families of schizophrenic patients by a group of workers at the National Institute of Mental Health including M. Bowen, L. Wynne and T. Lidz. This work generated entirely new concepts about family interaction, such as 'double binding' and the schizophrenogenic mother described by the anthropologist G. Bateson and co-workers, including J. Haley, D. Jackson and J. Weakland, in California. Numerous innovations extending the theoretical models and styles of clinical intervention followed, the key figures being N. Ackerman, J. Bell, J. Haley, D. Jackson, V. Satir and S. Minuchin. In particular, ideas from general systems theory, formulated by the biologist L. von Bertalanffy, cybernetics, and social psychological concepts of role and interaction were incorporated, together with techniques derived from operant conditioning. In the 1960s and 1970s (Zuk, 1971) the accumulating ideas began to be collated into a number of general theories of family interrelationships of which that based on general systems theory has provided the most comprehensive framework. The theoretical base has remained incomplete, experimental work has been open to ambiguous interpretation and there has been no general agreement about the most effective use of the diverse treatment techniques, principally structural therapy (Minuchin) strategic therapy (e.g. Haley and S. Palazzoli) and behavioural methods. The initial schism between the psychoanalytic and interactional models has become consolidated.

Marital counselling developed earlier than family therapy. In the United Kingdom, The National Marriage Guidance Council (now renamed Relate), founded by Mace in 1948, relied largely on Rogerian techniques, whilst accepting, at a later stage, the Masters and Johnson programme for brief sexual therapy. Both psychoanalytic ideas and behavioural principles have been influential in the development of marital or couple therapy.

Conclusion

There has been an ever-changing relationship between psychotherapy, medicine and psychiatry. The assumption of medical responsibility for psychiatric treatment occurred in the mid-nineteenth century, as mental disorder began to be attributed to natural forces. Psychotherapy was received cautiously by psychiatrists and the psychiatric monopoly of psychotherapy did not occur till the late 1930s, associated with substantial medical control of psychoanalysis. Subsequently, it persisted until the last 30 years, when it began to decline due to developments in psychopharmacology, the impact of clinically-applied learning theory and behaviourism and the emergence of the community mental health movement. The social function of psychotherapy became clearer and newer techniques have emphasized a pedagogic rather than a medical function. A wide range of clinical psychologists, social workers and counsellors have entered the field, so that psychotherapy is not the exclusive province of medicine or of any single professional group. Concurrent with the popularization of help-giving, psychotherapies have proliferated for a range of social ills and maladjustments as well as the removal of symptoms.

Over-optimism about its benefits has characterized the history of psychotherapy. It evolved by therapeutic experimentation and clinical observation, but evaluative research was very slow to develop, the first serious outcome study being that of O. Fenichel in 1930. Eysenck's attack on psychotherapy in 1952 was a watershed (Eysenck, 1952) and, subsequently, an extensive body of research on psychotherapy has been established (Garfield and Bergin, 1978), suggesting that these treatment methods have potential value. Psychotherapy is not a unitary process and the emphasis may be more or less on insight and attitude change, modifying emotional states or behaviour. Consequently, studies of outcome across techniques and patient types have proved less informative than investigations of those techniques which are most efficacious in specific disorders. Interest has been focused on the common factors present in different forms of psychotherapy, such as the personality of the therapist and the patient and the cultural context. Success in psychotherapy appears to be related to the therapist's mobilization of the patient's expectations of help. Explanations given need to be culturally meaningful to the patient and Tseng and McDermott (1975) suggested that 'No matter what kind of therapeutic activities are performed, the treatment tends to reinforce the socio-culturally sanctioned coping mechanisms, even though such coping mechanisms may vary greatly in different cultural settings'. The predominant use of directive or non-directive approaches, therefore, may be related chiefly to sociocultural factors. Client-centred psychotherapy, for example, reinforces notions of learning to solve one's own problems, an approach of particular appeal in recent American society.

No convincing evidence exists of the superiority of any single form of psychotherapy in its immediate or long-term benefits. Choice of approach may be a dilemma, although it is likely to be fortuitous, little influenced by an appraisal of competing theories and systems. However, most psychotherapists are eclectic and studies of theory and practice reveal many similarities between schools. For example, psychoanalysts, client-centred and Adlerian therapists have much in common (Fiedler, 1950) and there is clear similarity between 'role playing' in psychodrama and 'behaviour rehearsal' (Garfield, 1980). Attempts to collate and build upon the common features of divergent approaches, particularly dynamic psychotherapy and behavioural–cognitive approaches, and the growing spirit of experimentation, collaboration and eclecticism augur well for the future.

References

Alexander, F.G. and Selesnick, S.T. (1967). *The History of Psychiatry: An Evaluation of Psychiatric Thought and Practice from Prehistoric Times to the Present.* London: Allen & Unwin.

Ansbacher, H.L. and Ansbacher, R.R. (eds) (1957). *The Individual Psychology of Alfred Adler.* New York: Harper & Row.

Boss, M. (1963). *Psychoanalysis and Daseinanalysis.* New York: Basic Books.

Buhler, C. and Allen, M. (1972). *Introduction to Humanistic Psychology.* Monterey, CA: Brooks/Cole.

Chessick, R.D. (1986). Heidegger for psychotherapists. *Am. J. Psychother.* **40,** 83–95.

Dendy, W.C. (1853). Psychotherapeia, or the remedial influence of mind. *J. Psychol. Med. Ment. Pathol.* **6,** 268–274.

Ehrenwald, J. (ed.) (1976). *The History of Psychotherapy: From Healing Magic to Encounter.* New York: Aronson.

Ellenberger, H.F. (1970). *The Discovery of The Unconscious. The History and Evolution of Dynamic Psychiatry.* London: Allen Lane.

Eysenck, H.J. (1952). The effects of psychotherapy: an evaluation. *J. Consult. Psychol.* **16,** 319–324.

Fiedler, F.E. (1950). A comparison of therapeutic relationships in psychoanalytic, non-directive, and Adlerian therapy. *J. Consult. Psychol.* **14,** 436–445.

Fine, R. (1985). The anti-Freudian crusade continues. *J. Psychohist.* **12**, 395–410.

Fisher, S. and Greenberg, R.P. (1977). *The Scientific Credibility of Freud's Theories and Therapy.* Hassocks, Sussex: Harvester.

Frank, J.D. (1961). *Persuasion and Healing.* Baltimore: Johns Hopkins University Press.

Freud, S. (1957). *On the History of the Psychoanalytic Movement,* papers on metaphysical psychology and other works. The Standard Edition of the Complete Psychological Works of Sigmund Freud, Vol. 14. London: Hogarth Press and Institute of Psychoanalysis.

Garfield, S.L. (1980). *Psychotherapy. An Eclectic Approach.* New York: Wiley.

Garfield, S.L. and Bergin, A.E. (eds) (1978). *Handbook of Psychotherapy and Behaviour Change.* New York: Wiley.

Gill, C. (1985). Ancient psychotherapy. *J. Hist. Ideas* **46**, 307–325.

Greenson, R.R. (1969). The origin and fate of new ideas in psychoanalysis. *Int. J. Psychoanal.* **50**, 503–515.

Jackson, S.W. (1989). Robert Burton and psychological healing. *J. Hist. Med.* **44**, 160–178.

Janet, P. (1925). *Psychological Healing.* London: Allen & Unwin.

Jones, E. (1953, 1955, 1957). *Sigmund Freud. Life and Work,* Vols. I, II, III. London: Hogarth Press.

Klein, M. (1963). *The Psychoanalysis of Children* (trans. by A. Strachey). London: Hogarth Press.

Lieberman, S. (1986). Psychotherapy by reciprocal inhibition: Joseph Wolpe. *Br. J. Psychiat.* **149**, 518–519.

Mahoney, M.J. and Arnkoff, D. (1978). Cognitive and self-control therapies. In: S.L. Garfield and A.E. Bergin (eds) *Handbook of Psychotherapy and Behaviour Change.* New York: Wiley.

Masson, J.M. (1984). *The Assault on Truth: Freud's Suppression of the Seduction Theory.* London: Faber & Faber.

May, R., Angel, E. and Ellenberger, H.F. (eds) (1958). *Existence: A New Dimension in Psychiatry and Psychology.* New York: Basic Books.

Moreno, J.L. (1932). *Group Method and Group Psychotherapy,* Sociometry Monograph No. 5. New York: Beacon House.

Parry-Jones, W. Ll. (1987). 'Caesar of the Salpêtrière'. J.M. Charcot's impact on psychological medicine in the 1880s. *Bull. R. Coll. Psychiat.* **11**, 150–153.

Pratt, J.H. (1906). The 'home sanatorium' treatment of consumption. *Boston Med. Surg. J.* **154**, 210–216.

Rachman, A.W. and Raubalt, R.R. (1984). The pioneers of adolescent group psychotherapy. *Int. J. Group Psychother.* **34**, 387–413.

Riese, W. (1958). The pre-Freudian origins of psychoanalysis. In: J. Masserman (ed.) *Science and Psychoanalysis.* New York: Grune & Stratton.

Roazen, P. (1979). *Freud and His Followers.* Harmondsworth, Middx: Penguin.

Rogers, C.R. (1957). The necessary and sufficient conditions of therapeutic personality change. *J. Consult. Psychol.* **21**, 95–103.

Rogers, C.R. (1961). *On Becoming a Person.* London: Constable.

Rogers, C.R. (1970). *Encounter Groups.* New York: Harper & Row.

Schultz, J.H. and Luthe, W. (1959). *Autogenic Training. A Psychophysiologic Approach in Psychotherapy.* New York: Grune & Stratton.

Segal, H. (1964). *An Introduction to the Work of Melanie Klein.* London: Heinemann.

Stepansky, P.E. (ed.) (1986, 1988a, 1988b). *Freud: Appraisals and Reappraisals. Contributions to Freud Studies,* Vols 1, 2, 3. New Jersey: Analytic Press.

Storr, A. (1973). *Jung.* London: Fontana.

Taylor, F.K. (1958). A history of group and administrative therapy in Great Britain. *Br. J. Med. Psychol.* **3**, 157–173.

Tseng, W. and McDermott, J.F. (1975). Psychotherapy: historical roots, universal elements and cultural variations. *Am. J. Psychiat.* **132**, 378–384.

Watson, J.B. (1930). *Behaviourism.* London: Routledge & Kegan Paul.

Whyte, L.L. (1962). *The Unconscious Before Freud.* London: Tavistock.

Wolpe, J. (1958). *Psychotherapy by Reciprocal Inhibition.* Stanford: University Press.

Yalom, I. (1980). *Existential Psychotherapy.* New York: Basic Books.

Zuk, G.H. (1971). Family therapy during 1964–1970. *Psychother.: Theory, Res. Practice* **8**, 90–97.

— 24

The Family and Social Origins of Antisocial Behaviour

I. Kolvin and T. Fundudis

Introduction

The 1940s saw two landmarks in the attempts to unravel the psychosocial origins of antisocial behaviour and delinquency in childhood: the first consisted of clinical research and linked separation from mothers with juvenile delinquency (Bowlby, 1946); the second was based on multivariate analyses and this gave rise to a suggested association between different types of antisocial behaviour with different kinds of family patterns (Hewitt and Jenkins, 1949). Both, while preliminary, were seminal exercises which generated a multitude of questions and provoked widespread research. Subsequent advances were dependent on more precise definitions, diagnosis and the development of classifications which had a sounder scientific basis.

Description and Definition

Mischievous behaviour in childhood is not uncommon and is of greater concern to parents and teachers than to the children themselves. Nevertheless, only a small proportion of such behaviour is sufficient to impair relationships with peers or adults or is seen as contravening social norms. Such disorders of conduct include behaviour which is non-delinquent such as bullying, lying, disruption in classroom, etc. and which may also include truancy and stealing. Inevitably, such behaviour will overlap with what is viewed officially as delinquent behaviour. Delinquency is a common and major problem, especially amongst disaffected youth of the inner neighbourhoods of industrialized cities. It is one variety of conduct disorder in which the children enact potentially illegal behaviours, with some of the acts being known to legal agencies, while others are known only through self-reports (Farrington, 1973).

In this chapter we confine ourselves to school-age delinquent and non-delinquent conduct disorders. As to diagnosis, there is general agreement about the range of symptoms which are subsumed under the category of conduct disorder such as lying, stealing, truancy, disobedience, destructiveness, aggression, poor relationships and wandering. But there has been a lack of agreement about the

430

level or threshold of severity and duration of such symptoms (Offord *et al.*, 1986). The question arises as to when the constellation of symptoms should be considered as a disorder. The answer is, if the behaviour handicaps the child himself or his social or family environment. Furthermore, such behaviours may reveal themselves in either the *home* (1) or the *school* (2), or *both* (3) with the former (i.e. 1 or 2) being labelled *situational* and the latter (i.e. 3) *pervasive.*

Classification

One of the main subclassifications of antisocial behaviour disorders derives from multivariate approaches; factor analysis of child behaviour data invariably has demonstrated emotional and conduct disturbance patterns (Peterson, 1961; Wolff, 1971; Kolvin *et al.*, 1975). Such patterns emerge at all ages but it is only the classic endeavour by Hewitt and Jenkins (1949) that gave rise to a distinction between the so-called unsocialized aggressive behaviour and socialized group delinquency. This distinction has formed the basis of the scheme employed in the DSM-III, which defines a conduct disorder as a persistent pattern of conduct in which the basic rights of others and also major age-appropriate societal norms or rules are violated. Criteria for diagnosis include disturbance of at least six months' duration. In the DSM-III, a number of broad categories of conduct disorder are described. The first is the *under-socialized aggressive type*. This includes manifestations of such behaviours as physical violence against persons or property and theft outside the home. In addition, there is failure to establish a normal degree of affection, empathy or bond with others, as evidenced by no more than one of five indicators of social attachment (for instance, one or more lasting peer group friendships). The duration of such conduct disorder is defined as at least six months. The behaviour of youths over 18 can be labelled as conduct disorder provided that the behaviour does not meet the criteria for antisocial personality disorder.

The *second* category is conduct disorder of the *under-socialized non-aggressive type*. The diagnostic criteria consist, first, of repetitive and persistent patterns of non-aggressive conduct: these include chronic violation of a variety of social rules, repeated running away from home overnight and consistent serious lying and stealing not involving confrontation with the victim. Secondly, there is a failure to establish a normal degree of affection, empathy or bond with others. Thirdly, again there is a duration of at least six months.

A *third* category consists of conduct disorder, of the *socialized aggressive* type. In some ways, this overlaps with the previous category, but the main features are a repetitive and persistent pattern of aggressive conduct. On this occasion, there is evidence of social attachment to others as indicated by at least two of five patterns relating to social attachments.

The *fourth* category consists of conduct disorders that are *socialized non-aggressive*. This again overlaps with the others and has three main diagnostic criteria: first, a persistent pattern of non-aggressive conduct; secondly, evidence of social attachment to others; third, duration of at least six months; the youth must be below the age of 18 if the conduct disorder is to fulfil the criteria for antisocial personality disorder.

There is a *further* category of atypical conduct disorder that is a rag-bag of antisocial behaviours which cannot be included under the specified subtypes of conduct disorder.

Unfortunately, the validation of the above classification has proved difficult, so it is not surprising that the DSM-III-R suggests modifications—for instance conduct disorder is subdivided into three types: (1) a group type, in which most of the above behaviours occur in the company of peers; (2) a solitary, aggressive type, in which there is predominantly aggressive behaviour that is initiated by the child or adolescent alone; and (3) an undifferentiated type, for those children or adolescents with a mixture of clinical features that are not easily classified into any previous two subcategories. However, in addition, conduct disorders are assessed on a scale running from mild through moderate to severe, according to the number of problems in excess of those needed to make the diagnosis (i.e. over three) and the degree of general handicap or actual physical injury that is inflicted on the environment. It is not surprising that these amendments have been made, as Hewitt and Jenkins had based their research on a clinical population that was heavily weighted for delinquency. However, the details of these distinctions have not been widely replicated (Field, 1967).

The ICD-9 offers a variation of the above classifications (Rutter *et al.*, 1976). It defines conduct disorders as those mainly involving aggressive and destructive behaviours, and disorders involving delinquency. It is used at any age for abnormal behaviour that is not part of any other psychiatric condition. To be included, the behaviour needs to be frequent and severe, and it must be abnormal in its context. Such disorders differ from personality disorder in the absence of deeply ingrained maladaptive patterns of behaviour present from adolescence or earlier. The ICD-9 describes four subcategories: unsocialized disturbance of conduct; socialized disturbance of conduct; compulsive conduct disorder; and finally mixed disturbance of conduct and emotions.

The relationship of attention-deficit disorders and hyperkinetic disorders to conduct disorders merits clarification: there is, undoubtedly, a degree of overlap with conduct disorders but longitudinal research (Schacher *et al.*, 1981) suggests differences in outcome that would support such a distinction.

However, there is as yet no good evidence that non-delinquent and delinquent conduct disorders can be differentiated adequately in terms of behavioural features, family and social background and outcome (Moore *et al.*, 1979). Nor, indeed, is there as yet good evidence to support the division of conduct disorders into those with and without aggression. Nevertheless, the strength of the work of Hewitt and Jenkins was that behavioural patterns were found to be associated with family patterns similarly derived from multivariate analysis: unsocialized behaviour correlated with broken homes and family rejection; socialized delinquency correlated with parental neglect and social disadvantage, rather than rejection. But so far this work has not been replicated or validated adequately.

Origins

The origins of delinquency have been of central interest to psychologists and sociologists alike. Sociologists have been interested in the delinquent subculture and the fact that delinquents tend to be concentrated in the poorer areas of the inner city—areas with their own 'subculture'. One of the main advocates of the sociological theories which abounded in the mid-1950s stated that it was not sufficient to understand the delinquent subculture in negative terms as due to disorganization or even culture conflict, but rather that the delinquent feels that he has an inferior status in the wider community and when he meets others who are similarly afflicted, he acquires a new sense of self-esteem which allows the rejection of the values of a wider community (Cohen, 1956). One of the influential views advanced was one which suggested that delinquent acts reflected frustration generated by inequality in material goods. Other theories suggested that living in disadvantage gave rise to a belief that different social norms were permissible within a delinquent subculture (Cloward and Ohlin, 1960).

In summary, such theories suggest that the origins of delinquency reside mainly in endeavours to compensate for the influences of society that deny them equality in the social and material sense. Joining groups allows individuals to identify with group values and thus satisfy their needs by illegitimate means (West, 1985). West points out that such theories have become highly politicized.

On the other hand, one of the psychological explanatory theories advances the view that it is important to distinguish between the individual who has a psychological motivation or basis for becoming delinquent and the so-called 'sociologic delinquent' (Johnson, 1959). However, there has been a reaction against this position by those who consider that such theories lend support to the tendency to label those who are social rebels as psychologically ill or deviant.

Earlier research concentrated on single-factor theories, seeking factors which seemed to be of predominant importance; these included maternal separation, family criminality and other family patterns. However, the specificity of identified patterns has not been validated and further there is a consensus that this approach was far too simplistic. More often than not it has been found that there are multiple factors operating simultaneously; and it has proved difficult to pull apart those variables that usually act in concert (Rutter and Wolkind, 1985). Thus in the last decade the trend has been to appreciate that few factors operate in isolation and to view delinquency as being multifactorially determined and to attempt to highlight the relative importance of these family and parental factors. It is these themes that this chapter addresses. They include personality and criminality; the possibility of a genetic basis; social deprivation and inequality; family disruption; inadequate or weak family relationships; questionable quality of care; questionable child-rearing practices; and, finally, the question of models of conduct.

Family criminality

There is a striking link between a child's delinquency and parental criminality or social deviance (Farrington and West, 1981, Offord, 1982); for instance, 40% of the sons of recidivist fathers also proved to be recidivist (West, 1985). These are important studies but need to be supplemented by twin and adoption studies when trying to explore the possibility of genetic influence (Shields, 1977; Hutchings and Mednick, 1977; Bohman, 1978): such studies report only a small genetic influence regarding juvenile delinquency. However, it would seem that parental criminality is not the decisive factor, as the association applies as well to persistent parental personality and social difficulties, often represented by drinking problems and a poor work record. In these circumstances, it is not surprising that more recent reviews suggest that both heredity and environment influence delinquency and that genetic factors act by making the individual more vulnerable to adverse environmental influences.

Disadvantage and poverty

Conduct disorders, including delinquency, occur more frequently in the lower social strata (West and Farrington, 1977). At least a moderate link is often reported between low social status and delinquency: the Newcastle Study (Kolvin et al., 1988, 1990) reveals a close relationship between offences and occupational status of the family breadwinner, rising from 5% of males from Class I to 26% from Class III and 42% from Class IV and V and lower strata. In their review of the evidence, Rutter and Giller (1983), conclude that the relationship resides mainly at the extremes of the social scale; they question, as well, the extent to which the differences can be accounted for in terms of the differential attitudes to treatment of working class juveniles by the legal system. However, the Newcastle figures relate to more serious delinquency where there is less possibility of variations in legal management and hence such associations are less likely to be explicable in terms of attitudinal and management differences by legal agencies. Furthermore, an even stronger association is found for family deprivation and delinquency, which suggests at least some direct effect of adverse family influences. Indeed, this research links antisocial behaviour more closely with environmental deprivation than with social class (Kolvin et al., 1989).

The question therefore arises of whether poverty has a direct bearing on deliquency (Rutter and Giller, 1983). They note that the major increase in the standard of housing this century does not seem to have been accompanied by a corresponding reduction in crime. However, this is a superficial observation as it would appear that more people are living in poor conditions than are exhibited in the face of official statistics and that community expectations have risen with changing patterns of experience (Townsend, 1979). These factors, taken together, suggest that it is inequality in income rather than overall level of wealth, that may predispose to crime.

Deprivation

This gives rise to the question of the relationship between deprivation and offending. Such issues need to be examined in longitudinal studies. In the Newcastle Study, the proportion of males who offended varied according to the degree of deprivation, ranging from one in six males from non-deprived families to six in ten from families in multiple deprivation. Thus, offending appears to be 'dose-related', i.e. related to the degree of severity of family deprivation in the pre-school years. The above research suggests that some forms of family deprivation appeared less harmful than others; for instance, the criminality rate was relatively lower in the case of parental illness than where there was poor quality of parenting and poor care of the home and children. Moreover, there were significant correlations between the two latter criteria of deprivation, which implies that they are not independent of each other and it is not easy to estimate the relative importance of such explanatory factors in the genesis of delinquency.

Family and parenting variables

A wide number of parenting variables correlate with delinquency. The question arises as to which of these are causal or are most of them a reflection of a third factor common to all (Rutter and Giller, 1983)? With the complexity of such family interactions, care must be taken to avoid *a priori* assumptions regarding the significance of any particular variable. A good example of this is *family size*, where West (1985) revealed that 42% of persistent delinquents came from families with more than seven children. However, as Rutter and Giller (1983) have pointed out, the fall in the fertility rate over the past two decades does not seem to have induced a corresponding fall in crime, which suggests that any assumed link between large families and delinquency is indirect. The crucial link may not be the family size itself but associated factors such as overcrowding, socioeconomic disadvantage, less intensive family interactions, poor child discipline and supervision—all of the above may be underpinned by a lack of parental skills, foresight or planning.

Other factors can be examined in a similar way (Rutter, 1985). For instance, at one time, *family disruption or broken homes* were seen as central to delinquency, but Rutter (1971) quite rightly pointed to the alternative explanation, that the underlying determinant may be pre-existing and continuing family discord and quarrelling. Rutter and Giller (1983) advance evidence that divorce and separation are strongly associated with delinquency, whereas death is only weakly associated. They also point out that discord in both broken and unbroken homes appears to be strongly associated with delinquency and conclude that discord is more important than family breakdown.

They also go on to pose the question of why divorce is still associated with the continued increased risk of delinquency and point out that divorce does not necessarily mean resolution of marital conflict (Wallerstein and Kelly, 1980). Thus, children are particularly vulnerable if they live in homes where divorce has been preceded by seriously discordant family relationships (Rutter and Giller, 1983).

Family relationships

One key theoretical issue has been the subject of the effects of separation from parents on a child (Bowlby, 1946, 1951, 1969). Rutter (1980) suggests that it is the context and circumstances of separation rather than the mere fact of separation that are important—it is the quality of the relationship prior to the separation as well as the quality of care subsequent to the separation. Disturbances of emotions and behaviour are more evident when separations arise because of family discord and disruption (Rutter, 1971). Thus, the persistent effects of separation stem from the prior chronic family discord rather than from the separation experience, *per se*; or it could be a consequence of the subsequent poorer quality of child care (Yarrow and Klein, 1980). In addition, admission to foster care is associated with an increased rate of psychiatric disorder when such admissions occur with children from disharmonious and disadvantaged families (Wolkind and Rutter, 1973). A single admission to hospital has not been shown to be related to later psychiatric difficulties, but when there are multiple hospital admissions (and such circumstances are more likely to be related to family disadvantage), then there is a significant increase in subsequent conduct disorder and delinquency (Quinton and Rutter, 1976; Douglas, 1975). A major question is the subject of affectionless psychopathy, originally described by Bowlby (1946, 1951). More recent evidence concerning this derives from Roy (1983), Wolkind (1974), Tizard and Tizard (1971), Tizard and Reese (1975) and Tizard and Hodges (1978), all relating to institutionalized children. The balance of evidence from the above researches implicates disturbed social behaviour of the exposed children which, although different from the controls, especially in their school settings, does not amount to the type of behaviour originally described as affectionless psychopathy. This has given rise to the conclusion that early lack of bonding experiences did not inhibit these children from making true attachments in later childhood but did appear to influence other social relationships (Rutter and Wolkind, 1985). This brings us back to the question of attachments and relationships which are crucial issues in child psychiatry and psychology.

There is good evidence (Campos *et al.*, 1983; Sroufe, 1983) that securely attached infants are more sociable with adults and show greater competence with peers, more positive affect and a higher self-esteem (Rutter and Wolkind, 1985). There remains the issue of whether the quality of attachments in infancy predicts adult relationships and adult psychological functioning. In a review of the evidence, Rutter and Wolkind (1985) point out that discordant family relationships in early life, including a lack of parental affection, are associated with a greater likelihood of emotional and personality disorders in adult life (Brown *et al.*, 1986; Quinton and Rutter, 1985; Wolkind and Kruk, 1984). Furthermore, at any point in time, an individual's social behaviour is likely to reflect both current social circumstances and previous social experiences (Rutter and Wolkind, 1985).

Moving away from attachments in early life, Rutter (1985) points out that weak family relationships are often found to be associated with delinquency. He goes on to point out that it is important to make a distinction between family discord and weak family relationships. One setting in which there is a lesser amount of discordant and quarrelsome interactions is institutional; but here the children are less likely to form close attachments with their care-takers. All the evidence suggests that conduct disorders are commoner amongst children reared from infancy in such institutional settings (Rutter *et al.*, 1983; Wolkind, 1974).

Rutter therefore concludes that 'Weak family relationships are important in their own right, quite apart from their association with discord'. It is not only that children who lack secure attachments in infancy are going to have impaired social relationships in adolescence, but also that the development of internal controls appears to depend on an affectional identification with parents. Evidence in support of such notions is moderately strong.

One of the more influential theories about the origins of delinquency was Hirschi's (1969) control theory which asserts that lack of attachment to parents, peers and school gives rise to a lack of conventional attitudes and eventually juvenile delinquency. Aspects of this theory have been examined in a number of large-scale studies in senior schools the United States utilizing self-administered, self-report delinquency measures and usually self-report measures of parent–child relationships. Three important findings emerge. First, closeness to father (rather than to mother) may be a better predictor of delinquent behaviour, especially amongst males (Johnson, 1987). Second, that parental and school attachment, conventional beliefs and involvement in youth subculture activities contribute to only low levels of variance of delinquency (Wiatrowski and Anderson, 1987). However, this poor explanatory power of the data in the last study may well be due to an insufficiency of variation of delinquent behaviour, especially at extremes when using a population of high school sophomores. For instance, when combining high school and juvenile correctional institution data Hirschi's model was only supported when delinquent companions were included as an additional explanatory factor in the causal path analysis (Thompson *et al.*, 1984). Furthermore, the latter authors contend that the findings are more consistent with a social learning than a control theory. However, irrespective of whether the findings are construed within a control or a learning theory model, the contribution of positive attachments in protecting children from delinquent behaviour is again confirmed.

Quality of parenting

Another theme concerns quality of parenting. The Newcastle research highlights the importance of poor-quality parenting, especially poor mothering (Kolvin *et al.*, 1990). However, it is not only quality of care that is likely to be important: parental supervision has a particularly strong influence as well (Farrington and West, 1981; Patterson, 1982). West and Farrington (1973, 1977) speculate that poor parental supervision and the associated freedom from restraint, together with police practice, are contributory factors in the determination of levels of delinquency, with poor family and social circumstances playing some part, however marginal, in police decisions to prosecute. Patterson (1982) suggests four ways in which the behaviour of children may be influenced by family rearing patterns: there may be, first, no clear expectations of acceptable child behaviour; second, a lack of monitoring of child behaviour; third, a lack of strategies for following through disciplinary plans in a logical way; fourth, lack of problem-solving techniques in the face of family crises. Thus, some families do not appear to know what their children are doing and their disciplinary management techniques are not very efficient (Rutter, 1985).

Models of behaviour

Here, the implication is that parents of children with antisocial behaviour often have provided a model of antisocial attitude and conduct with which the children can identify or which they can copy (Rutter, 1985; Kelvin, 1969).

Evidence from longitudinal studies

The plethora of ideas which have emerged from cross-sectional studies reflect the difficulties of separating the contribution of different types of family influences. However, longitudinal studies have proved more fruitful. For instance, changes in family circumstances may influence a delinquent outcome—improvement in family relationships (Rutter, 1971) or reduction in family deprivation (Kolvin et al., 1990) is associated with a reduced rate of conduct disturbance in the case of the former and of delinquency in the case of the latter. Such fluctuations become even more impressive if it can be demonstrated that increases and decreases in family pathology are associated with changes in subsequent offending. In the Newcastle Study (Kolvin et al., 1990) if families moved into deprivation, there was a 50% increase in the rate of subsequent offending by their male offspring; if they moved out of deprivation, there was a 40% decrease. This suggests that there are certain factors which serve to counter the motivation to crime, despite youths coming from high-risk backgrounds. In the Newcastle Study, resilience in the face of deprivation was characterized by a number of factors operating on the junior school years. Most prominent amongst these was a good care-giving environment and hence it is argued that good parenting protects youths against the acquisition of a criminal record, irrespective of poverty or other forms of social deprivation. Other studies suggest close personal supervision of boys by parents is similarly protective and beneficial (West and Farrington, 1973, 1977).

Statistical analyses

Modern methods of analysis address themselves to the converse of pulling apart of those variables which usually act in concert and consist of putting them together in order to ascertain any identifiable patterns on the one hand or important predictors within any set of predictors of conduct disorder or delinquency on the other. Finally there are attempts to ascertain pathways to antisocial behaviour, which may contribute to identifying relevant processes and mechanisms. Let us start with predictions. Earlier attempts to develop formulas that would give reasonably accurate predictions of delinquency have not fulfilled the anticipated promise (Glueck and Glueck, 1950, 1964) as subsequent attempts to use the indices that were developed have shown poor predictive performance (Dootjes, 1972). Furthermore, in these early studies, much of the original data was retrospective and therefore the claims about predictive utility must be viewed with caution. Unfortunately, more modern research suggests that multiple regression techniques give, if anything, worse prediction than the simpler methods originally utilized (Farrington, 1983). It is likely that this relatively poor prediction has more to do with the insensitivity of the predictor measures than the statistical techniques employed. The limitation of prediction studies has been well summarized by Rutter and Giller (1983), who draw two conclusions: first, that many youths theoretically at high risk do not necessarily become delinquent; second, that a substantial minority not at high risk do become delinquent. Nevertheless, some researchers have demonstrated the potency of prediction analysis utilizing early life psychosocial data: for instance, the Newcastle Study (Kolvin *et al.*, 1990) report that some two-thirds of boys coming from multiply deprived homes subsequently become delinquent. In addition, in the Cambridge Study, only two behavioural measures and five background measures were found to be independently predictive of delinquency: delinquents tended to be among those boys who were rated troublesome and daring at school; boys who were at risk coming from poorest or largest families; had criminal parents or parents who supervised them poorly or who had low IQs (West and Farrington, 1973, 1977). Further, the Newcastle group (Kolvin *et al.*, 1990) report that the only measure representing family environment that made an independent significant contribution to prediction of criminality was poor child care and mothering. Factors that failed to make a significant independent contribution were marital disruption, parental illness, those representing adverse social circumstances, parental personality, mother's age at marriage, occupational status and neighbourhood influences. However, an index of deprivation derived from the summing of scores of deprivation proved to be a good predictor of subsequent criminality. So too, was family size, which probably directly reflects poor home circumstances. Furthermore, in a series of analyses, prior juvenile delinquency proved to be the most powerful predictor of later criminality.

Finally, there is some evidence of specificity in relation to two types of family experiences. First, whereas marital disruption and parental illness were predictive of offences committed during the school years only, poor mothering was a significant predictor of criminality after the age of 15 years (Kolvin *et al.*, 1990). In the United States, McCord (1979) reported that, whereas home atmosphere was reliably related to criminal behaviour, parental absence failed to distinguish the criminal from the non-criminal, which again supports the notion that mere separation, or absence of parents, on its own does not have a significant effect on antisocial behaviour.

Summary

Although some of the evidence is conflicting, a number of facts have become established and these in turn have given rise to a diversity of theories to explain the associations between offending, antisocial behaviour and family and social influences. Certain theories have social and family and others psychological bases, yet others seek genetic explanations. However, previously fashionable single factor theories are now considered too simplistic and have given way to multi-factorial explanations. Furthermore, while longitudinal approaches have helped to clarify a number of the important issues, as have the application of multivariate analyses, the correlations that are found account for an important but not a substantial proportion of the variance.

References

Bohman, M. (1978). Some genetic aspects of alcoholism and criminality, *Arch. Gen. Psychiat.* **35**, 269–276.

Bowlby, J. (1946). *Forty-Four Juvenile Thieves: Their Characters and Home-Life.* London: Baillière, Tindall and Cox.

Bowlby, J. (1947, 1951). *Maternal Care and Mental Health.* Geneva: World Health Organisation.

Bowlby, J. (1969). *Attachment and Loss: I. Attachment.* London: Hogarth Press.

Brown, G.W., Harris, T. and Bifulco, A. (1986). Long-term effects of early loss of parent. In: M. Rutter, C. Izard and P. Read (eds) *Depression in Childhood: Developmental Perspectives*, New York: Guilford Press.

Campos, J.J., Barrett, K.C., Lamb, M.E., Goldsmith, H.H. and Stenberg, C. (1983). Socio-emotional development. In: M.M. Haith and J.J. Campos (eds) *Infancy and Developmental Psychobiology*, Vol. 2, Handbook of Child Psychology, 4th edn, pp. 783–915. New York: Wiley.

Cloward, R.A. and Ohlin, L.E. (1960). Differential opportunity and delinquent sub-cultures. In: *Delinquency and Opportunity: A Theory of Delinquent Gangs.* New York: Free Press.

Cohen, A. (1956). *Delinquent Boys.* London: Routledge & Kegan Paul.

Dootjes, I. (1972). Predicting juvenile delinquency, *Austral. NZ J. Criminal.* **5**, 157–171.

Douglas, J.W.B. (1975). Early hospital admissions and later disturbances of behaviour and learning. *Dev. Med. Child Neurol.* **17**, 456–480.

Farrington, D.P. (1973). Self-reports of deviant behaviour: productive and stable? *J. Crim. Law Criminol.* **64**, 99–110.

Farrington, D.P. (1983). Offending from 10 to 25 years of age. In: K. van Dusen and S.A. Medrick (eds) *Prospective Studies of Crime and Delinquency.* Boston: Kluwer-Nijhoff.

Farrington, D.P. and West, D.J. (1981). The Cambridge study in delinquent development. In: S.A. Medrick and A.E. Baert (eds) *Prospective Longitudinal Research: An Empirical Basis for the Primary Prevention of Psychosocial Disorders*, pp. 137–145. Oxford: Oxford University Press.

Field, E. (1967). *A Validation of Hewitt and Jenkins' Hypothesis.* Home Office Research Unit Report No. 10. London: HMSO.

Glueck, S. and Glueck, E. (1950). *Unravelling Juvenile Delinquency.* Cambridge, MA: Harvard University Press.

Glueck, S. and Glueck, E. (1964). Potential juvenile delinquents can be identified: What next?, *Br. J. Criminal.* **4**, 215–226.

Hewitt, L.E. and Jenkins, R.L. (1949). *Fundamental Patterns of Maladjustment: The Dynamics of Their Origin.* Springfield, IL: Michigan Child Guidance Institute.

Hirschi, T. (1969). *Causes of Delinquency.* San Francisco, CA: University of California Press.

Hutchings, B. and Mednick, S. (1977). Criminality in adoptees and their adoptive and biological parents. In: R.O. Christianson and S. Mednick (eds) *Biosocial Basis of Criminal Behaviour*, pp. 127–141. New York: Gardner Press.

Johnson, A.M. (1959). Juvenile delinquency. In: S. Arieti (ed.) *American Handbook of Psychiatry*, pp. 840–856. New York: Basic Books.

Johnson, R.E. (1987). Mothers versus Father's role in causing delinquency. *J. Adolescence* **22**, 305–315.

Kelvin, P. (1969). *The Bases of Social Behavior: An Approach in Terms of Order and Value.* London: Holt, Rinehart and Winston.

Kolvin, I., Wolff, S., Barber, L.M., Tweddle, E.G., Garside, R., Scott, D.M. and Chambers, S. (1975). Dimensions of behaviour in infant school-children. *Br. J. Psychiat.* **126**, 114–126.

Kolvin, I., Miller, F.J.W., Fleeting, M. and Kolvin, P.A. (1988). Social and parenting factors and offending. *Br. J. Psychiat.* **152**, 80–90.

Kolvin, I. *et al.* (1989). Parent, child, grandchild, the transmission of deprivation. In: E.J. Anthony and C. Chilland (eds) *The Child in His Family.* New York: Wiley.

Kolvin, I., Miller, F.J.W., Scott, D., Gatzanis, S. and Fleeting, M. (1990). *Continuities of Deprivation? The Newcastle 1000 Family Study.* Aldershot: Avebury.

McCord, J. (1979). Some child-rearing antecedents of criminal behaviour in adult men. *J. Personal. Social Psychol.* **9**, 1477–1486.

Moore, D.R., Chamberlain, P. and Mukai, L.H. (1979). Children at risk for delinquency. *J. Abnorm. Child Psychol.* **1**, 345–355.

Offord, D.R. (1982). Family backgrounds of male and female delinquents. In: J. Quinn and D.P. Farrington (eds) *Abnormal Offenders, Delinquency and The Criminal Justice System*, pp. 129–151. Chichester: Wiley.

Offord, D.R., Alder, R.J. and Boyle, M.H. (1986). Prevalence and sociodemographic correlates of conduct disorder. *Am. J. Social Psychiat.* **6**, 272–278.

Patterson, G.R. (1982). *Coercive Family Process.* Eugene, Oregon: Castalia.

Peterson, D.R. (1961). Behaviour problems of middle childhood. *J. Consult. Psychol.* **25**, 205–209.

Quinton, D. and Rutter, M. (1976). Early hospital admissions and later disturbances of behaviour: an attempted replication of Douglas' findings, *Dev. Med. Child Neurol.* **18**, 447–459.

Quinton, D. and Rutter, M. (1985). Parenting behaviours of mothers raised "In Care". In: A.R. Nicol (ed.) *Longitudinal Studies in Child Psychology and Psychiatry: Practical Lesson from Research Experience.* Chichester: Wiley.

Roy, P. (1983). *Is continuity enough?: Substitute care and socialization.* Paper presented at Spring Scientific Meeting, Child and Adolescent Psychiatry Section, Royal College of Psychiatry, March 1983.

Rutter, M. (1971). Parent–child separation: psychological effects on the children. *J. Child Psychol. Psychiat.* **121**, 233–260.

Rutter, M. (1980). Attachment and the development of social relationships. In: M. Rutter (ed.) *Scientific Foundations of Developmental Psychiatry*, pp. 267–279. London: Heinemann.

Rutter, M. (1985). Family and school influences: meanings, mechanisms and implications. In: R. Nicol (ed.) *Longitudinal Studies in Child Psychology and Psychiatry.* London: Wiley.

Rutter, M. and Giller, H. (1983). *Juvenile Delinquency: Trends and Perspectives.* Harmondsworth, Middx: Penguin.

Rutter, M. and Wolkind, S. (1985). Separation, loss and family relationships. In: *Child and Adolescent Psychiatry—Modern Approaches.* London: Blackwell.

Rutter, M.L., Shaffer, D. and Sturge, C. (1976). *A Guide to Multi-axial Classification Scheme for Psychiatric Disorders in Childhood and Adolescence.* London: Institute of Psychiatry.

Rutter, M., Quinton, D. and Liddle, C. (1983). Parenting in two generations. Looking backwards and looking forwards. In: N. Madge (ed.) *Families at Risk.* London: Heinemann.

Schacher, R., Rutter, M.L. and Smith, A. (1981). The characteristics of situational and pervasively hyperactive children: implications for syndrome definition. *J. Child Psychol. Psychiat.* **22**, 375–392.

Shields, J. (1977). Polygenic influences. In: M. Rutter and L. Hersov (eds) *Child Psychiatry: Modern Approaches* pp. 22–46. Oxford: Blackwell Scientific.

Sroufe, L.A. (1983). Wariness of strangers and the study of infant development. *Child Dev.* **48**, 731–746.

Thompson, W.E., Mitchell, J. and Dodder, R.A. (1984). An empirical test of Hirschi's control theory of delinquency. *J. Deviant Behav.* **5**(1–4), 11–22.

Tizard, B. and Hodges, J. (1978). The effect of early institutional rearing on the development of eight-year-old children. *J. Child Psychol. Psychiat.* **19**, 99–118.

Tizard, B. and Rees, J. (1975). The effect of early institutional rearing on the behaviour problems and affected relationships of four-year-old children. *J. Child Psychol. Psychiat.* **16**, 61–74.

Tizard, J. and Tizard, B. (1971). The social development of two-year-old children in residential nurseries. In: H.R. Schaffer (ed.) *The Origins of Human Social Relations*, pp. 147–163. New York: Academic Press.

Townsend, P. (1979). *Poverty in the United Kingdom*. Harmondsworth, Middx: Penguin.

Wallerstein, J.S. and Kelly, J.B. (1980). *Surviving the Breakup: How Children and Parents Cope with Divorce*. New York: Basil Books; London: Grant McIntyre.

Wiatrowski, M.D. and Anderson, K.L. (1987). The dimensionality of the social bond. *J. Quant. Criminol.* **3**(1), 65–81.

West, D. (1985). Delinquency. In: M. Rutter and L. Hersov (eds) *Child and Adolescent Psychiatry—Modern Approaches*. London: Blackwell.

West, D.J. and Farrington, D.P. (1973). *Who Becomes Delinquent?* London: Heinemann Educational.

West, D.J. and Farrington, D.P. (1977). *The Delinquent Way of Life*. London: Heinemann.

Wolkind, S. (1974). The components of 'affectionless psychopathy' in institutionalized children. *J. Child Psychol. Psychiat.* **15**, 215–220.

Wolkind, S.N. and Kruk, S. (1984). From child to parent: early separation and the adaption to motherhood. In: A.R. Nicol (ed.) *Longitudinal Studies in Child Psychology and Psychiatry: Practical lessons from research experience*. Chichester: Wiley.

Wolkind, S. and Rutter, M. (1973). Children who have been 'In Care'—an epidemiological study. *J. Child Psychol. Psychiat.* **14**, 97–105.

Wolff, S. (1971). Dimensions and clusters of symptoms in disturbed children. *Br. J. Psychiat.* **118**, 421–427.

Yarrow, L.J. and Klein, R.P. (1980). Environmental discontinuity associated with transition from foster to adoptive homes. *Intern. J. Behav. Dev.* **3**, 311–322.

— 25

Ethology

M.P.I. Weller and R.G. Priest

Ethology is *part* of the study of behaviour, but one that developed at first independently of psychology from observations of animals in their natural habitats. It contrasts with the animal observations carried out by the 'learning theory' school of psychology, studying rodents running through mazes or pigeons pecking at the right time and being rewarded with pellets (see Chapter 17, this volume). Ethology is particularly concerned with the process of development in young animals, including a positive bond between members of the same species: courtship, sexual behaviour and care of the young and bonding of the young to their mother. It also involves aggressive reactions: territorial dispute, competition for a mate, and social dominance. For the purpose of this chapter we shall take the following definition:

> Ethology is the biological study of behavioural processes, often social, that are not explained by 'learning theory'.

We are tempted to say that ethology is the study of *instincts*. However, this term fell into disuse during the 1930s and 1940s with the growth of behaviourism. The behavioural scientists found the term objectionable, implying that animals and humans were acting out, like automata, behaviour patterns that are laid down in the genes. Some went so far as to say that instincts, not depending on learned behaviour, just do not exist. However, songs and nest-building activity in birds hatched and reared in isolation illustrate an interaction, at critical periods, between innate patterns and modifying factors. Subtle dialects have been observed as chaffinches pick up the nuances of local song in infancy (Thorpe, 1965). Because of their brief sensitivity to acquiring song the process is open to corruption, and some birds have been observed to have learnt telephone ringing sounds, which no doubt will cause many mating difficulties! On the other hand, the cuckoo is remarkable in preserving its species-specific song in an alien environment.

Recognizing that the term 'instinct' carries overtones that are not necessarily accurate, attempts have been made to find an alternative term. One approach concentrates on the fact that what we would normally think of as an instinct would probably be a complicated piece of behaviour. When we gave examples just now we chose nest-building and bird song. By contrast, elementary actions like standing, walking, eating and so forth would not really be what people mean by instinct. Soon after birth most young mammals can breathe, move their limbs, see and suck. To contrast with these simple activities, Harlow and Griffin (1965) provide the term *late maturing complex behaviour* for what might otherwise be called instincts, and human development follows certain sequences in the development of these behaviours (see Chapter 21, this volume).

The second way of finding an alternative term to instinct is that of Hilgard and his colleagues (1971), who used the term *species-specific behaviour*. Whether or not we accept these two alternative expressions instead of the word instinct, there is no doubt that ethology is much occupied with complex, species-specific social behaviour, which exhibits stereotyped, *fixed-action patterns* (though not always particularly 'late maturing').

Imprinting

Until recent decades, it was possible to regard ethology dismissively as scarcely a serious scientific activity and more like the hobby of nature study. The change in attitude has been reflected in the ethologists Tinbergen, von Frisch and Lorenz being awarded a Nobel prize for their contributions to science. We shall come back to the work of Tinbergen later. Karl von Frisch achieved the remarkable success of decoding the message that bees pass on when they return to the hive. The curious figure-of-eight dance that they perform tells the other bees not only the direction in which they have to fly to find the nectar, but also the distance (von Frisch, 1974).

Lorenz is noted for many discoveries but typical is his work with geese. Geese and ducks lay their eggs in nests built at ground level. The young are *nidifugous* (nest-fleeing), able to leave the nest shortly after hatching. Characteristically, they follow their mother closely wherever she goes, whether walking or swimming. Lorenz (1970) clarified the way in which this comes about. He observed that soon after they hatch the young of nidifugous birds, including the greylag goose, 'begin to follow the first relatively large moving object they see, whether this be the natural mother, some other kind of animal, or Lorenz himself. During subsequent development . . . their sexual behaviour may also become limited to it'. He called this phenomenon *imprinting* (Ambrose, 1968) and believed that this special form of learning was different from ordinary conditioning, distinguishable by the fact that: '(a) it is limited to a very brief period, fixed soon after birth, and (b) it is irreversible'.

If the first moving object to catch their eye after hatching was Lorenz himself, then they followed him. He gives an amusing description (1970) of one occasion on which he was waddling around his front garden, wagging his bent arms and quacking, enjoying the fact that the goslings were dutifully following after him. He then caught sight of the astonished glance of the passers-by. It must have been a remarkable enough sight anyway, but what increased their perplexity was the fact that since the grass was long they could see Lorenz but not the goslings. In fact it is not necessary to waddle and quack. Baby geese will follow even a moving box if that is presented at the crucial time.

Once the goslings have been imprinted by a particular object (Lorenz, a box, or the mother goose) they remain imprinted on it—the procedure is generally irreversible. Since animals showing this phenomenon often tend to choose a mate that is similar in appearance to their adoptive 'parent', this phenomenon may explain why animals in captivity will make sexual overtures to the human keeper that has reared them and, more seriously, spurn animals of their own species. Imprinting is the basis of one theory designed to explain the difficulty of getting pandas to mate in the London Zoo.

A human example of the phenomenon was often seen when wet-nursing was common and babies became more attached to their wet nurse than their mothers. (The question of the reinforcement of the milk is discussed in the section on maternal deprivation.)

Imprinting can take place only over a very brief period (Ambrose, 1968), known as the 'critical period' but because it can be influenced to a certain extent by environmental factors, the less dramatic term 'sensitive period' is preferred by some ethologists (Bateson, 1973). The process is associated with protein synthesis in specific brain areas (Horn, 1979).

Pair bonding, whether in animals or man, is another example of imprinting, occurring in conjunction with sexual maturation. The specific attributes of the beloved become the essential trigger to powerful emotions. (Such specific triggers are known as releasers, discussed in more detail below.) As Henry Kissinger remarked 'I am an acquired taste!' After a complex, ritualized courtship, which tends to prevent animals breeding with other species, the pair faithfully unite and share in the tasks of rearing and defending their young and their communal territory. Lorenz has argued, persuasively, that the joint defence of territory by the bonded pair provides the basis, in microcosm, of human territorial disputes, xenophobia and war.

In human encounters, the approach, greeting and termination are ritualized. Initially an element of threat is intertwined but rapidly attenuated. The practice of removing one's gloves before shaking hands probably takes its origin from the removal of the gauntlet, which increases the vulnerability of the knight, but is also the potential prelude to a challenge (throwing down the gauntlet). The stereotyped enquiries into health and comments about the weather are part of an appeasement ritual that combines solicitude and non-contentious statements designed to elicit ready agreement. The parting too is ritualized with a careful avoidance of abrupt, rejecting cut-off, universally signalled by gaze avoidance and pouting. Although most aspects of the rituals have cultural variants, the basic structure is very similar and exists in all societies that have been studied (Eibl-Eibesfeldt, 1979).

Parental reactions in birds and mammals are also governed by specific stimuli (releasers) such as distress calls and in human parents by eye contact and the infant's smile. Western mothers display a stereotyped behaviour in their typical greeting response towards the newborn, beginning with a slight retroflexion of the head, raised eyebrows, widely opened eyes and slightly opened mouth, followed by a smile or verbal greeting. Following this, the mother mirrors the baby's facial expressions, often exaggerating these (Papousek and Papousek, 1977). The interaction is reinforced for the mother and her baby by synchronous body movements (Fogel, 1977) which can be observed with vocal interactions with neonates (Condon, 1977). The effect is enduring, so that Japanese orphans, who lived as Chinese for most of their lives, retained Japanese facial expressions, gestures and mannerisms allowing them to be easily and accurately identified by biculturally oriented observers, a fact confirmed by the subjects' spouses (Tseng *et al.*, 1990).

Maternal Deprivation in Monkeys

Harlow and his colleagues (1965) advanced our understanding of behavioural development in monkeys, particularly under abnormal conditions. The earlier experiments were concerned with the nature of the bonds between the infant and its mother. The normal infant rhesus monkey clings to its mother's fur, front to front, from time to time sucking at the teats. The question arises, does the body 'love' its mother because that is where the milk comes from?

Harlow designed an experimental situation in which the infant was provided with a choice of artificial or surrogate mothers. The monkey could choose a wire-frame mother-substitute with a milk supply available from a conveniently implanted teat. Alternatively he could choose a surrogate with no milk supply but, to compensate, a soft surface of terry-cloth towelling.

The baby monkeys consistently selected the terry-cloth version. They spent much of the time clinging to this pleasant textured parent substitute. Occasionally they would venture away to explore the surrounding territory. When scared, they would run back and cling to the surrogate once more—a pattern of behaviour very reminiscent of other infant–parent patterns, including the human equivalent of the attachment young children sometimes develop for a 'comfort' blanket. The infant monkey would sometimes go to the wire-frame substitute, but seemed not to spend much more time than was necessary to take the amount of milk appropriate for its needs.

Harlow had done two things. Firstly, he had convincingly demonstrated that, whatever made the infant rhesus monkey keep close to its mother, it was not the milk supply. Secondly, he had raised a cohort of monkeys in isolation from their biological mothers. This cohort of monkeys grew up to demonstrate quite deviant behaviour, the more so if they had access only to the wire-frame substitute.

As they are developing, normal monkeys seem to enjoy being with other young of their kind. They will play and gambol and interact together (cf. 'the best present you can give children is other children'). The maternally deprived monkeys remained isolated, curled up and apparently uninterested in participating.

In adult life, the animals reared in isolation showed abnormalities in the direction of their aggression. If a stranger passes a normally reared monkey's cage, for instance, the animal will hiss and spit at the intruder, making aggressive and hostile gestures. The warped animals behaved differently. They would retreat to the back of the cage, and bite their own arms and legs, sometimes even lacerating themselves and drawing blood.

The maternally deprived animals were also incompetent sexually. The males would show no interest in the females, or fail to complete copulation. The females did not present sexually to the males and, even when at the most approachable phase of the oestrus cycle, would reject a male's courtship as if it were a hostile attack.

Under these circumstances it is not surprising that the adults showed a low fertility. However, it was sometimes possible to impregnate such a female, and then a further behavioural abnormality was revealed. These females made very bad mothers. The normal monkey mother is very tolerant of her infant, allowing it to hang from her own ventral fur, sometimes with the infant glancing sideways, still tugging at the nipple. The maternally deprived females, when they produced their offspring, seemed to have no time for them. They would even keep the youngster conveniently immobilized on the floor by planting a callous maternal foot on it, apparently reluctant to allow more intimate access.

A common threat uniting these abnormal responses is the fact that monkeys raised in isolation have difficulty in correctly interpreting the emotions of their fellows. A monkey will rapidly learn to operate a lever to avoid a shock a few seconds after a signal. Two normally reared monkeys will successfully cooperate if one can see the other monkey but not the signal, and is required to operate the lever to avoid a shock to both of them. Monkeys reared in isolation cannot learn to respond successfully more than 10% of the time when cued only by the facial expressions of another monkey, although they can be used as effective detectors of the impending shock (Miller *et al.*, 1967).

The persisting effects of early experience is demonstrated by the fact that morphological changes occur in the neurones of socially isolated monkeys (Floeter and Greenhough, 1979), which have more dendritic spines and branches, while rats that have enjoyed a stimulating environment showed analogous but converse changes (Volkmar and Greenhough, 1979).

An emotionally deprived environment can produce physiological and morphological changes, including changes in brain weight (Bennett *et al.*, 1969) and neuronal structure (Volkmar and Greenhough, 1972; Floeter and Greenhough, 1979), and general growth, biochemical and endocrinological changes in humans (Powell *et al.*, 1967a,b; Money, 1977; Chesney and Brusilow, 1981).

Maternal Deprivation in Humans

Early loss of a parent leaves an individual vulnerable to psychiatric illness and suicide, particularly if the loss was of a disruptive type, such as prolonged disharmony at home (see Chapter 21, this volume).

Young children become intensely miserable when separated from their mothers, going through the stages of protest, rejection and finally apathy and dejection, termed 'anaclictic depression' (Spitz and Wolf, 1946). When maternal deprivation is maintained, as in some unsatisfactory institutions, there is a failure to thrive with growth retardation (Patton and Gardner, 1963), which is accompanied by biochemical and endocrinological changes

(Powell *et al.*, 1967a,b), and long-lasting emotional scars are likely (Goldfarb, 1945).

The importance of maternal deprivation in pathological human personality development has been emphasized, notably by Bowlby (1973) (see Chapters 21 and 24, this volume). It is now widely accepted that securely attached infants are more sociable as adults and show greater competence with peers, more positive affect and higher self-esteem. On the other hand, children who are deprived of such secure attachments, as may easily happen in harsh and loveless institutions, are more likely to have psychopathic (or sociopathic) personalities, and indulge in delinquent or criminal behaviour. The majority of prisoners in jail in fact do have a history of some abnormality or deficiency in their early unbringing; conflict and disruption are common in the home, where ill-defined and inconsistent standards prevail. Attending these malign influences, poor school achievement, compounded by truancy and an erratic working career are common sequelae. It is not essential that a child is brought up by its biological mother. An adoptive parent may be equally satisfactory, as long as the mothering is benign and consistent. Particularly damaging is the situation in which the young child is passed rapidly from one foster parent to another, or where the household is wracked by conflict and festering relationships.

Some observations on clinical conditions

In clinical experience, in addition to egotism, immaturity, aggressiveness, low frustration tolerance and inability to learn from experience, the main behavioural associations with psychopathic personality are with unusual sexual preferences and drug abuse. Although we believe that minority sexual practices do not necessarily entail any unusual character traits, amongst those persons complaining to doctors about their sexual problems an unusually high proportion *seem* to have a more general abnormality of personality make-up.

With common forms of drug dependence, such as alcoholism, it is possible for a well adjusted person to get into a situation in which he or she suffers from physical dependence of a degree requiring treatment. Nevertheless, an unusually high proportion of patients seeing doctors because of drug dependence are regarded as suffering from personality disorder. In the case of narcotic drugs (opiates) the proportion is extremely high.

Another problem with drugs is that of overdose. The psychiatric diagnosis of patients brought to hospital after a drug overdose commonly lies between a depressive illness, a personality disorder, and normality, i.e. no psychiatric diagnosis. In patients who go on to take repeated overdoses, the proportion who are found to exhibit gross immaturity or a pervasive character problem rises and the risk of an eventual consummated suicide is 10%.

To our mind, the personality disorders that are commonly seen clinically bear a strong behavioural resemblance to Harlow's monkeys. Shallow, damaged, interpersonal relationships are a characteristic feature of personality disorders and, if such patients are not so strikingly withdrawn and isolated as the monkey that refuses to play, their social relationships certainly do not seem to display normal ease and warmth. Sexual problems include frigidity and impotence, and satisfactory heterosexual intercourse is often absent. These patients are often poor parents, and frequently one finds that their own children are in care, fostered out, or being looked after by someone else.

Among those persons with personality disorders who present clinically, it is striking how their high levels of aggression are not channelled solely towards other people (extrapunitive hostility) but are also turned in on the patient's own self (intropunitive hostility). This can be demonstrated scientifically (Foulds, 1965) and is evident in many subtle ways. They become pathologically depressed and, under circumstances in which other persons would get angry and lash out at those around them, these patients typically injure themselves by cutting or taking an overdose of drugs. Alcoholism and other chronic forms of drug abuse can be seen as intropunitive or self-damaging behaviour maintained over a longer period of time. It seems that both drug overdose and drug dependence are forms of human behaviour that have a strong resemblance to Harlow's monkeys biting their own arms.

Displacement Activity

Konrad Lorenz was mentioned earlier when describing imprinting in geese. In his book, *King Solomon's Ring*, he also describes the fights of sticklebacks, based on the principle that 'my home is my castle'. The farther away a stickleback is from his nest, the more his courage deserts him. 'At the nest itself he is a raging fury and with a fine contempt of death will recklessly ram the strongest opponent, or even the human hand.' 'When two sticklebacks meet in battle . . . the one which is further from his nest will lose the match' (Lorenz, 1970).

At the border of the two territories, the sticklebacks are equally impelled to fight or fly, and adopt a vertical posture, in which position they have little to do but dig at the bottom of the fish tank—'executing a ritualized version of the activity normally used in nest-digging'. The term used for this is *displacement activity—an instinctive movement used as an outlet for energy bottled up when some action is blocked by a conflicting drive*. In humans scratching and lighting cigarettes would often seem to serve a similar function. When animals are stressed (or exposed to dopamine agonists), they groom themselves excessively, and this can also often be observed in humans.

The restless pacing and endless cigarettes of expectant men, waiting for their wives to deliver a child, is another example of displacement activity, which at its extreme is converted into the couvade syndrome, where the pains of childbirth are experienced by the husband. Students waiting for an examination perform a wide variety of behaviour that is irrelevant to the approaching task. It is almost as though the flight and fight forces are nearly equally balanced! Similar behaviour occurs when a captive population of students is enclosed in a lecture theatre. Observation shows that a high proportion of the audience will be scratching their faces, rubbing their noses or doodling, unless they are sleeping!

Other types of activity that have been suggested as examples of displacement activity in humans, are inappropriate eating, traumatic scratching, fidgeting, thumb-sucking and smoking. Among pathological forms of behaviour obsessions, such as trichomania, are also candidates for inclusion.

Social Hierarchy

The term *pecking order* (or *peck order*) is a well-known term now in everyday speech. Leyhausen (1965) referred to this type of dominance as *'absolute social hierarchy'*. He quotes Schelderup-Ebbe's discovery, forty years earlier, that:

> the hens of a barnyard do not have equal rights, but establish among themselves a 'peck-order' in which each individual is allocated a definite place on the social ladder which it is normally unable to alter. Usually a subordinate does not even try to fight a superior animal even if grossly provoked . . . Quarrelling usually occurs only between individuals separated by not more than one step of the social ladder; an inferior animal never dares so much as to look straight at an animal two or more steps its superior.

In Whyte's (1965) study of American street corner society, the scores in bowling correlated highly with the social status of the members of the gang, who by their appropriate encouragement and denigration reinforced the existing social order. 'Sides were chosen several times each Saturday night, and in this way a man was constantly reminded of the value placed upon his ability by his fellows and of the sort of performance expected of him.'

This absolute social hierarchy contrasts with the situation described earlier in sticklebacks, where the hierarchy, or dominance, depended on the individual's location in space. Such dominance, dependent on territory, rather than *relative social hierarchy*, is also found in robins. The robin will guard a plot of land and display aggressive behaviour towards a rival robin.

Does the same apply to human behaviour? An inspection of the results of Association Football (soccer) matches in the United Kingdom is illuminating. Looking at the results of matches played in the Football League (e.g. Rollin, 1979) the ratio of home wins to away wins varies to some degree from division to division and from year to year but generally lies between 2:1 and 3:1. It is not clear to what extent this is due to attitudinal factors and it could be argued that, in part, success at home depends on knowing the slope of the pitch, the direction of wind currents and other valuable pieces of local information. However, the phenomenon of the home team wins has its counterpart in human behaviour in other situations in that individuals are more dominant and influential on their own territories than others' territories.

The popular stereotype of British behaviour too has certain similarities with Leyhausen's hens. It is as if, cooped up tightly on a small island, the population conserves its aggressive energies by adopting an absolute social hierarchy, in which people are preoccupied with the question of whether a newly met stranger is higher or lower in social status, and particularly whether just above or just below. People do not speak to each other on railway trains (you do not know if the other individual is more than one rung away from you on the social ladder) but there are few fights. In order to avoid indiscriminate interactions, gaze avoidance is steadfastly maintained in crowded lifts.

The stereotype of American behaviour has more resemblance to the relative social hierarchy of robins. One can suggest that the American male, with a tradition of open spaces and equality, is prepared to exhibit aggression more liberally. Nevertheless some degree of 'peck-order' can be detected in most cultures. Margaret Mead in her book *The American Character* describes how the frontier culture is in conflict with maternal admonitions to avoid fights, and traces the tradition of a literal 'chip on the shoulder', with an implicit invitation to dare to knock it off. She draws a parallel between this strutting and posturing as an invitation to battle with the necessity of Pearl Harbor to induce America to fight the Japanese.

Space is important in many ways, for example morbidity is higher and medical visits fewer on the higher floors of high-rise flats (Richman, 1976). Coleman (1986) has studied the effect of architecture on behaviour in 4000 houses and 4000 blocks of flats in two London boroughs. Using criteria of bad design, including large numbers of flats per block, she showed positive correlations with vandalism, juvenile crime and children in care. Arrest for juvenile crime was seven and a half times greater in the crowded conditions. She cites a Japanese study with similar relationships.

Symbolic boundaries are constantly being erected. Minor features are seized upon to create geographic boundaries in estates and residents create imaginary lines for inclusion or exclusion into neighbourhood cliques if such natural boundaries do not already exist (Whyte, 1961). Experimental intrusions in libraries, by occupying facing or adjacent seats when distant seats were available, result in books and rulers being erected to demarcate spatial boundaries (Felipe and Sommer, 1966). There are some subtle sex differences. This behaviour is most frequently encountered in males when the opposite sex intruder sits facing, and in females when the opposite sex intruder takes up a side by side position (Fisher and Byrne, 1975).

Aggressive display forms part of the complex male behaviour in animal courtship. The female does not flee from this display of dominance, and her staying and presentation has a submissive element. In enforced proximity in a confined space, male birds (Noble *et al.*, 1938; Morris, 1955; Stokes, 1960) and fish (Morris, 1952; Barraud, 1956) adopt homosexual practices. In addition to the prevention of heterosexual contact, the facilitation of homosexual practices amongst prisoners may have common elements with these observations.

The need for personal space is greater amongst violent prisoners than in a group of non-violent individuals (Kinzel, 1974; Curran *et al.*, 1978). In psychiatric wards, aggressive behaviour has territorial components as it does amongst emotionally disturbed children (Esser, 1971; Esser and Deutsch, 1977). These points may be relevant to the inescapable crowding in football stadia at important matches. Although controversial, Newman's (1972) work on crime suggests that clearly demarcated territorial boundaries and 'defensible space' are associated with lower crime rates.

Amongst some animals, defeat in agonistic encounter results in persistent signals, such as a change of colour. One is found in the mimic fish, *Lambroides dentate*, which resembles the cleaner wrasse, whose feeding is dependent on successful mimicry. Another is the pale colour that replaces the normally bright blue scrotum of defeated vervet monkeys (Gartlan and Brain, 1968). These unequivocal signals of defeat, like the bedraggled appearance of a defeated cock's comb and feathers, imply biochemical changes, which include increased vasopressin, ACTH and cortisol secretion. Vasopressin and ACTH increase submissiveness and increase grooming in male mice (Roche and Leshner, 1979). Cortisol, which is elevated in humans under unpleasant stress, is driven by ACTH. The biochemical mechanisms help avoid persistent territorial contests between the same adversaries. More obvious indicators of dominance and submission can be seen in human behaviour when opponents 'square up' to one another, with increased swallowing, downcast eyes, nervous shuffling and other displacement activities in the loser, a calm, level gaze and relaxed posture signalling dominance.

Death is much more likely after defeat, and defeated male grouse in the breeding season have seven to nine times the mortality of territorially successful birds, increased disease being one of the principal causes of death (Jenkins *et al.*, 1963). The increased, non-suicidal, mortality after loss of a spouse (Parkes *et al.*, 1969), during depression (Avery and Winokur, 1976), in anxious states (Coryell *et al.*, 1982), and at times of social stress (White, 1903; Brenner, 1981; Moser *et al.*, 1987) provide striking human analogies.

The incontrovertible signs of defeat limit intraspecies aggression, the defeated animal being limited in its ability to launch any fresh challenges. The higher mortality in the defeated animals, for example in grouse (Jenkins *et al.*, 1963) acts as a mechanism for controlling population density in the competition for scarce resources, particularly those connected with mating and breeding territory. The increased rate of depression and suicide in humans in the spring may be an atavistic remnant of these phenomena, as may be the increase in non-suicidal mortality in depression (see Chapter 30, this volume) and the correlation of depression with population density (White, 1903). The situation is quite subtle, as illustrated by the endocrine profile of wild baboons. Low basal cortisol levels are related to dominance, but within the dominant group also to high levels of social skill, control over the environment, predictability, outlets for frustration and social affiliations. The dominant males with low basal cortisol levels are perceptive and pick the 'right' fights, i.e. fights that they win (Sapolsky, 1990), so that they exhibit a particular style of dominance, that succeeds over long periods.

Several species of birds will group and attack a predator, such as a hawk or owl, and chaffinches will also attack carnivorous mammals, such as dogs and cats. This response is appropriately termed *mobbing* (Hinde, 1970). The response partially depends on novelty, the birds invariably responding to a live owl but becoming erratically habituated to a stuffed one. Although the response is elicited by predators, strange objects and novel conditions can also induce it. The mobbing call acts as an irresistible stimulus to all the birds, whether or not they have seen the danger, and the sound can induce birds to attach non-threatening objects, such as a detergent bottle, if a situation is contrived whereby they cannot

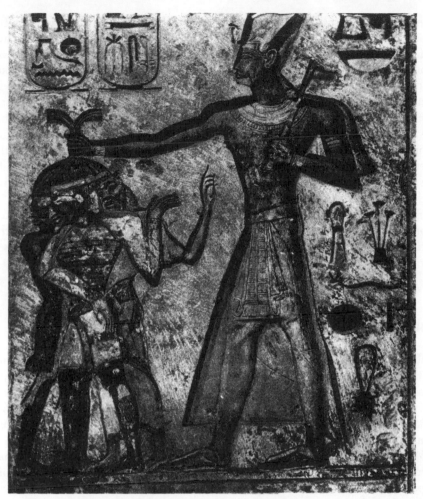

FIG. 25.1 An example of the timeless characteristics of dominance and submission. Note the increased height used to depict the Pharaoh. (Painted relief from the Temple of Ptah at Memphis, XIXth Dynasty.)

see the owl eliciting the mobbing vocalization of a nearby, but visually isolated, group.

Grouping of animals can be advantageous for predation as well as defence. The hunting success of canine packs, as with wolves, or a pride of lions, illustrates this advantage.

In animal communities, the herd distracts the attention of predators from particular animals and discourages them from attack. Fish catch fewer flies as the number of flies in the same area is increased (Lorenz, 1963), in the same manner that it is easier to catch one tennis ball than two or three at a time, when it is more likely that all will be dropped. There are several examples of defence strategies which depend on specific stimuli (releasers). If one of a group of certain primates is startled by a snake, it utters a characteristic cry, which induces the others to climb trees. Vocalizations, in other non-threatening circumstances, have different characteristics which do not elicit this flight response. Dominant vervet monkeys band together and do their best to surround the immature and weaker animals when under attack. The startle response of flocks of birds when one of their number takes flight is a common observation. The alarm calls of many finches, buntings and thrushes are very similar and it is thought probable that they have evolved towards one another so that they provide a common sign-stimulus to which they all respond (Manning, 1979, p. 69). The white tail of the fleeing rabbit likewise provides an irresistible danger signal to other rabbits. With the various advantages of animal groupings, the gregarious tendencies in human society may have phylogenetically early origins.

Symbiotic groupings of different animals is common, for example short-sighted zebras associate with long-sighted ostriches, wildebeest and giraffes on the African plains. This antipredatory device was replicated in the World War II when ship conveys were successful against U-boat attack.

Releasers

Tinbergen has investigated the behaviour of young herring gulls (Manning, 1972). The chick pecks on its mother's beak, and the mother regurgitates food into the chick's mouth. What triggers off the chick's activity? It is the sight of a red spot located on the mother's yellow beak. Here the red spot is the releaser. It has been found that artificial beaks with bigger and more spots are yet more alluring than the natural beak.

What is it that triggers off the robin's aggressive territorial behaviour? It has been found that the main feature of the rival robin that stimulates the hostile response is the colour of the breast feathers. Even a bunch of red feathers dangled in the gaze of the resident robin will do it. The red feathers act as a *releaser*. A releaser is the code combination in the environment, which is purposefully sought by the animal, that triggers the species-specific complex behaviour.

These critical stimuli are generally only a particular characteristic and the colour red is frequently encountered. An analogous situation to the red robin feathers is the red belly of the male stickleback, which elicits aggressive behaviour in another male. On the other hand, the swollen belly of the gravid female stickleback elicits a characteristic zig-zag courtship dance prior to fertilization of the female's eggs (Tinbergen, 1951). The complete neuronal pathway from sensory input to rhythmic motor output that underlies the avoidance swimming of leeches to noxious stimulation has been unravelled (Brodfuehrer and Friesen, 1986a,b,c,d) and arouses expectations for the elucidation of further neuronal mechanisms in releaser behaviour.

A possible human equivalent of a releaser is the raised eyebrows. Look at two men talking. From time to time, one will raise his eyebrows and the other will then nod, signalling entrance and exit points for the discourse. It is quite difficult to avoid nodding in this situation, but conscious control soon causes an interlocutor to 'dry up', according to the taciturn President Calvin Coolidge. He won the admiration of his colleagues by his ability to see a remarkable number of people in a day, which, he explained, he achieved by adopting the expedient of keeping 'dead still'. The nodding is the species-specific behaviour, and one can postulate that the eyebrow raising is the releaser.

In addition to punctuating a conversation with agreement, scepticism, incredulity or calls for information can be signalled by particular movements of the brow or forehead, emphasized by the eyebrows. We are unsure how widespread the conversational response is in different parts of the world. However, in a film allegedly of the first contact between a tribe in the Amazonian rain forest and Caucasian man, conducted through an interpreter, we observed that the head nodding behaviour was very similar in both groups.

The emotional facial expressions of sadness, fear, surprise, anger or distress, signalled by the combined movements of the brow or forehead, are coherent, organized and systematic in their occurrence earlier than most conversational signals (Elkman, 1979). Despite culturally imposed masking when under conditions of known observation, there is excellent cross-cultural concordance in facial expressions for different emotions (Fridlund *et al.*, 1983), and blind children's expressions are very similar to sighted ones (Izard, 1971). Body signals often provide leakage of information when subjects attempt to mask their facial expressions (Elkman and Friesen, 1974). Non-verbal behaviour is certainly an area in which knowledge is rapidly growing (see Chapter 26, this volume) and is a legitimate area for the study of *human ethology*.

Man and Other Animals Compared

Ethological models have attracted contemptuous comment from a psychoanalyst (Kubie, 1963) but favourable interest has also been expressed (McKinney, 1974; Serban and Kling, 1974) and psychotropic drug research is reliant on strategies for modifying animal behaviour (e.g. Suomi *et al.*, 1978; Hrdina *et al.*, 1979; Roche and Leshner, 1979). In any event, the aggressive propensities of mankind, their containment in social encounters and their function in maintaining alliances, including pair bonding, mesh with psychoanalytic views that aggression and destructive tendencies are universal and can be discerned in earliest infancy (Klein, 1932); 'the further back one pursues the phantasy life of childhood the more aggression does one find' (Storr, 1964).

Accounts of ethology vary from the entertaining and anthropomorphic stories especially designed for the lay public to dry and sober academic accounts that carefully avoid any conclusion that goes beyond the experimental evidence presented. Both versions have their advantages and disadvantages. The latter examples are necessary for careful scientific progress, but can be stodgy reading and are not always inspiring. The former may produce enthusiasm and creative ideas in the reader but can easily lead to unjustified conclusions. For instance, analogies are often drawn between a piece of complex behaviour in particular species and some human action. The biological gulf between man and the species may be enormous, and the similarity spurious. Indeed, sometimes the particular complex behaviour pattern in the animal may not be found in a closely related species in the same genus.

Nevertheless, we now recognize man as a social organism, within the family and in the wider society, operating in a social order with a system of social signals, in alignment with other animals. This comprehensive ethological view contrasts with the view of Thomas Hobbes that 'there are no Arts: no Letters; no Society; and which is worst of all, continual fear, and danger of violent death; and the life of man is solitary . . .' Ethology has contributed to this change in attitude and emphasized particular avenues of therapeutic approach in psychiatric care. The importance of detailed attention to the therapeutic environment is increasingly being recognized. Families and the emotional climate can be maladaptive. The experience of emotions such as pride, guilt and anger might be appropriate in certain circumstances and adaptive. Helping patients to appreciate this may be helpful. The need for approval may be frustrated because of over-assertiveness or excessive reticence. Unfulfilled needs may exaggerate maladaptive behaviour rather than reduce it, and patients may be helped by efforts to reduce motivation and techniques of behavioural modification. Ethology is a fascinating field of study, which, until recently, has been relatively neglected by psychiatrists, but which, in time, should prove a fruitful source of new ways of understanding and helping our patients.

References

Ambrose, A. (1968). The comparative approach to early child development: the data of ethology. In: E. Miller (ed.) Foundation of Child Psychiatry, pp. 183–232. London: Pergamon Press.

Avery, D. and Winokur, G. (1976). Mortality in depressed patients treated with electroconvulsive therapy and antidepressants. Arch. Gen. Psychiat. 33, 1029–1037.

Barraud, E.M. (1956). Notes on the territorial behaviour of captive ten-spined sticklebacks (Pygosteus pungitius L.). Br. J. Anim. Behav. 3, 134–136.

Bateson, P.P.G. (1973). The imprinting of birds. In: S.A. Barnett (ed.) Ethology and Development. Clinics in Developmental Medicine No. 47, pp. 1–15. London: Heinemann.

Bennett, E.L., Rosenzweigh, M.R. and Diamond, M.C. (1969). Rat brain: effects of environmental enrichment on wet and dry weights. Science (NY) 163, 825–826.

Bowlby, J. (1951). Maternal Care and Mental Health, WHO Monograph Series No. 2. Geneva: World Health Organization.

Bowlby, J. (1973). Attachment and Loss, Vol. 2. London: Hogarth Press.

Brenner, M.H. (1981). Unemployment and health (letter). Lancet ii, 874–875.

Brodfuehrer, P.D. and Friesen, W.O. (1986a). Initiation of swimming activity by trigger neurons in the leech subesophageal ganglion. 1. Output connections of Tr1 and Tr2. J. Comp. Physiol. (A) Sensory, Neural Behav. Physiol. 159, 489–502.

Brodfuehrer, P.D. and Friesen, W.O. (1986b). Initiation of swimming activity by trigger neurons in the leech subesophageal ganglion. II. Role of segmental swim-initiating interneurons. J. Comp. Physiol. (A) Sensory, Neural Behav. Physiol. 159, 503–510.

Brodfuehrer, P.D. and Friesen, W.O. (1986c). Initiation of swimming activity by trigger neurons in the leech subesophageal ganglion. III. Sensory inputs to Tr1 and Tr2. *J. Comp. Physiol. (A) Sensory, Neural Behav. Physiol.* **159**, 511–519.

Brodfuehrer, P.D. and Friesen, W.O. (1986d). Control of leech swimming activity by the cephalic ganglion. *J. Neurobiol.* **17**, 697–705.

Chesney, R.W. and Brusilow, S. (1981). Extreme hypernatremia as a presenting sign of child abuse and psychological dwarfism. *Johns Hopkins Med. J.* **148**, 11–13.

Coleman, A. (1986). Buildings and behaviour. Biosocial Society Conference London, reported in Medical News. *Br. Med. J.* **293**, 890.

Condon, W.S. (1977). A preliminary phase in the organization of infant responding behaviour. In: H.R. Schaffer (ed.) *Studies in Mother–Infant Interaction*. London: Academic Press.

Coryell, W., Noyes, R. and Clancy, J. (1982). Excess mortality in panic disorders. *Arch. Gen. Psychiat.* **39**, 701–703.

Curran, S.F., Blatchley, R.J. and Hanlon, T.E. (1978). The relationship between body buffer zone and violence as assessed by subjective and objective techniques. *Criminal Justice Behav.* **5**, 53–62.

Eibl-Eibesfeldt, I. (1979). Ritual and ritualization from a biological perspective. In: M. von Cranach, K. Foppa, W. Lepenies and D. Ploog (eds) *Human Ethology*, pp. 3–55. Cambridge: Cambridge University Press.

Elkman, P. (1979). About brows: emotional and conversational signals. In: M. von Cranach, K. Foppa, W. Lepenies and D. Ploog (eds) *Human Ethology*, pp. 169–202. Cambridge: Cambridge University Press.

Elkman, P. and Friesen, W.V. (1974). Detecting deception from body or face. *J. Personal. Social Psychol.* **29**, 288–298.

Esser, A.H. (1971). *Behaviour and Environment. The Use of Space by Animals and Man*. Proceedings of an international symposium held at the 1968 meeting of the American Association for the Advancement of Science in Dallas, Texas. New York: Plenum Press.

Esser, A.H. and Deutsch, R.D. (1977). Private and interaction territories on psychiatric wards. Studies on non-verbal communication of spatial needs. In: M.T. McGuire and L.A. Fairbanks (eds) *Ethological Psychiatry—Psychopathology in the Context of Evolutionary Biology*. New York: Grune and Stratton.

Felipe, N.J. and Sommer, R. (1966). Invasions of personal space. *Social Problems* **14**, 206–214.

Fisher, J.D. and Byrne, D. (1975). Too close for comfort: sex differences in response to invasions of personal space. *J. Personal. Social Psychol.* **32**, 15–21.

Floeter, M.K. and Greenhough, W.T. (1979). Cerebellar plasticity: modification of Purkinje cell structure by differential rearing in monkeys. *Science* **206**, 227–231.

Fogel, A. (1977). Temporal organisation in mother–infant face-to-face interaction. In: H.R. Schaffer (ed.) *Studies in Mother–Infant Interaction*. London: Academic Press.

Foulds, G.A. (1965). *Personality and Personal Illness*. London: Tavistock.

Fridlund, A.J., Ekman, P. and Oster, H. (1983). Facial expression of emotion: review of literature, 1970–1983. In: A. Siegman (ed.) *Nonverbal Behaviour and Communication*. Hillsdale, NJ: Lawrence Erlbaum.

Frisch, K. von (1974). Dialects in the language of the bees. In: D.R. Griffin (ed.) *Animal Engineering*, pp. 109–113. New York: Freeman.

Gartlan, J.S. and Brain, D.K. (1968). Ecology and social variability in *Cercopithecus aethiops* and *C. mitis*. In: P. Jay (ed.) *Primates*. New York: Holt Rinehart and Winston.

Goldfarb, W. (1945). Effects of psychological deprivation in infants and subsequent stimulation. *Am. J. Psychiat.* **102**, 18.

Harlow, H.F. and Griffin, G. (1965). Induced mental and social deficits in rhesus monkeys. In: S.F. Osler and R.E. Cooke (eds) *The Biosocial Basis of Mental Retardation*, pp. 87–106. Baltimore, MD: Johns Hopkins University Press.

Hilgard, E.R., Atkinson, R.C. and Atkinson, Rita L. (1971). *Introduction to Psychology*, 5th edn. New York: Harcourt Brace Jovanovich.

Hill, O.W. and Price, J.S. (1967). Childhood bereavement and adult depression. *Br. J. Psychiat.* **113**, 743–751.

Hinde, R.A. (1970). *Animal Behaviour*, pp. 278–288. New York: McGraw-Hill.

Horn, G. (1979). Imprinting—in search of neural mechanisms. *Trends Neurosci.* **2**, 219–222.

Hrdina, P.D., Von Kulmiz, P. and Stretch, R. (1979). Pharmacological modification of experimental depression in infant macaques. *Psychopharmacologia* **64**, 89–93.

Izard, C.E. (1971). *The Face of Emotion*. New York: Appleton-Century-Crofts.

Jenkins, D., Watson, A. and Miller, G.R. (1963). Population studies on red grouse. *Lagopus lagopus scotius* (Lath.) in North East Scotland. *J. Anim. Ecol.* **32**, 317–376.

Kinzel, A.F. (1974). Syndromes resulting from social isolation. 3. Abnormalities of personal space in violent prisoners. In: J.H. Cullen (ed.) *Experimental Behaviour: A Basis for the Study of Mental Disturbance*. Dublin: Irish University Press.

Klein, M. (1932). *The Psycho-analysis of Children* (trans. A. Strachey, revised H.A. Thorner, 1975). London: Hogarth Press.

Kubie, L.S. (1963). The concept of normality and neurosis. In: M. Heimen (ed.) *Psycho-analysis and Social Work*. New York: International Universities Press.

Leyhausen, P. (1965). The sane community—a density problem? *Discovery* (September) 27–33.

Lorenz, C. (1963). *On Aggression*, p. 26, and *Anonymity of the Flock*, Ch. VIII, pp. 119–127. Reprinted London: Cox and Wyman, 1972.

Lorenz, K. (1970). *King Solomon's Ring*. London: Methuen.

Manning, A. (1972). *An Introduction to Animal Behaviour*, 2nd edn. London: Arnold.

Manning, A. (1979). *An Introduction to Animal Behaviour*, 3rd edn. London: Edward Arnold.

McKinney, W.T. Jr. (1974). Animal models in psychiatry. *Persp. Biol. Med.* **17**, 529–541.

Miller, R.E., Caul, W.F. and Mirsky, I.A. (1967). Communication of affects between feral and socially isolated monkeys. *J. Personal. Social Psychol.* **7**, 231–239.

Money, J. (1977). The syndrome of abuse dwarfism (psychosocial dwarfism or reversible hypomatotropism). *Am. J. Dis. Child.* **131**, 508–513.

Morris, D. (1952). Homosexuality in ten-spined sticklebacks (*Pygosteus pungitius* L.) *Br. J. Anim. Behav.* **4**, 233–236.

Morris, D. (1955). The causation of pseudofemale and pseudomale behaviour: a further comment. *Behaviour* **8**, 46–56.

Moser, K.A., Goldblatt, P.O., Fox, A.J. and Jones, D.R. (1987). Unemployment and mortality: comparison of the 1971 and 1981 longitudinal study census samples. *Br. Med. J.* **294**, 86–90.

Murphy, J.M., Olivier, D.C., Sobol, A.M., Monson, R.R. and Leighton, A.H. (1986). Diagnosis and outcome: depression and anxiety in a general population. *Psychol. Med.* **16**, 117–126.

Newman, O. (1972). *Defensible Space*. New York: Macmillan.

Noble, G.K., Wurm, M. and Schmidt, A. (1938). The social behaviour of the black-crowned night heron. *Auk J. (Washington)* **55**, 7–40.

Papousek, H. and Papousek, M. (1977). Mothering and cognitive headstart: psycho-biological considerations. In: H.R. Schaffer (ed.) *Studies in Mother–Infant Interaction.* London: Academic Press.

Parkes, C.M., Benjamin, B. and Fitzgerald, R.G. (1969). Broken heart: a statistical study of increased mortality among widowers. *Br. Med. J.* **i**, 740–743.

Patton, R. and Gardner, L.I. (1963). *Growth Failure in Maternal Deprivation.* Springfield, IL: C.C. Thomas.

Powell, G.F., Brasel, J.A. and Blizzard, R.M. (1967a). Emotional deprivation and growth retardation stimulating idiopathic hypopituitarism. 1. Clinical evaluation of the syndrome. *New Engl. J. Med.* **276**, 1271–1278.

Powell, G.F., Brasel, J.A. and Blizzard, R.M. (1967b). Emotional deprivation and growth retardation simulating idiopathic hypopituitarism: 2. Endocrinological evaluation of the syndrome. *New Engl. J. Med.* **276**, 1279–1283.

Richman, N. (1976). Depression in mothers of preschool children. *J. Child Psychol. Psychiat.* **17**, 75–78.

Roche, K.E. and Leshner, A.I. (1979). ACTH and vasopressin treatments immediately after a defeat increases future submissiveness in male mice. *Science* **204**, 1343–1344.

Rollin, J. (ed.) (1979). *Rothmans Football Yearbook 1979–80.* London: Queen Anne Press.

Rutter, M. (1981). *Maternal Deprivation Reassessed,* 2nd edn. Harmondsworth, Middx: Penguin.

Sapolsky, R.M. (1990). Adrenocortical function, social rank, and personality among wild baboons. *Biol. Psychiat.* **28**, 862–878.

Serban, G. and Kling, A. (eds) (1974). *Animal Models in Human Psychobiology.* New York: Plenum Press.

Spitz, R.A. and Wolf, K.M. (1946). Anaclitic depression: an inquiry into the genesis of psychiatric conditions in early childhood. *Psychoanalytic Study of the Child,* Vol. 2, p. 313. New York: International Universities Press.

Stokes, A.W. (1960). Nest site selection and courtship behaviour of the blue tit (*Parus caeruleus*). *Ibis* **102**, 507–519.

Storr, A. (1964). *Sexual Deviation,* p. 42. Harmondsworth, Middx: Penguin.

Suomi, S.J., Stephen, F., Jonathan, K., Lewis, M.S., DeLizio, R.D. and McKinney Jr, W.T. (1978). Effects of imipramine treatment of separation-induced social disorders in rhesus monkeys. *Arch. Gen. Psychiat.* **35**, 321–325.

Thorpe, W.H. (1965). The ontogeny of behaviour in ideas. In: J.A. Moore (ed.) *Modern Biology.* New York: Natural History Press.

Tinbergen, N. (1951). *The Study of Instinct.* Oxford: Clarendon Press.

Tseng, W.-S., Ebata, K., Miguchi, M., Egawa, M. and McLaughlin, D.G. (1990). Trans-ethnic adoption and personality traits: a lesson from Japanese orphans returned from China to Japan. *Am. J. Psychiat.* **147**, 330–335.

Volkmar, F.R. and Greenhough, W.T. (1972). Rearing complexity affects branching of dendrites in the visual cortex of the rat. *Science (NY)* **176**, 1445–1447.

Volkmar, F.R. and Greenhough, W.T. (1979). Rearing complexity affects branching of dendrites in the visual cortex of the rat. *Science* **176**, 1445–1447.

White, A. (1903). The geographical distribution of insanity in the United States. *J. Nervous Mental Dis.* **30**, 257–279.

Whyte, W.H. (1961). *The Organization Man,* pp. 308–322. Harmondsworth, Middx: Penguin.

Whyte, W.F. (1965). *Street Corner Society: The Social Structure of an Italian Slum,* pp. 16–25. Chicago and London: University of Chicago Press.

— 26 ——————————————————

Group Process and Non-verbal Communication

A.B. Summerfield

What is a Group?

The conception of a group held by most members of the general public is more diffuse than that found in the psychological literature. Consider seven or eight people sitting in the waiting room of a hospital out-patient clinic. One or two are reading magazines, several sit quietly, a woman is trying to calm the child sitting on her lap. Occasionally someone asks a question of the receptionist. Compare that situation to that of a group of nurses who are sitting together having coffee after coming off duty. One of them is telling the others about the film she saw the previous night, another is showing a magazine to her neighbour, someone asks whether anyone would like another cup of coffee.

The patients in the waiting room may be physically present in the same place but in psychological terms they constitute a pseudo-group, a collection of people without common aims and with no communication between them. The nurses, however, meet Berkowitz's (1980) definition of a group as 'a collection of people who react to each other in some way, however indirectly'. Some social psychologists would regard this as too cautious a definition and would suggest that a collective goal and the communication needed to achieve it are necessary conditions for categorizing a number of people as a group. In either case, interaction is a critical minimum condition.

Who Belongs?

The initial membership of a group is likely to have a significant influence on its subsequent development. Berne (1963) noted that membership may be voluntary or compulsory. Most studies reported in the psychological literature have been carried out with volunteer subjects, often students, but group membership in institutions such as mental hospitals or prisons may be effectively compulsory, even if it is presented to participants as a matter of choice. Group members who have been coerced into attendance by threats of being labelled as non-cooperative if they opt out, have a somewhat different orientation to the group from those who have freely chosen it.

The other important way of classifying group membership is as to whether qualifications are needed for it or not. Thus a study group may admit only people who are doctors, a tennis club may require members to be experienced players and a therapy group may be restricted to patients with a certain diagnosis such as alcoholism or agoraphobia. Many groups have some kind of restriction on membership and the stricter it is, the less the heterogeneity of the members and probably the more limited the range of interpersonal behaviours which can be expected. Real heterogeneity is possibly found in groups such as British juries which simply impose the qualification of being a registered voter within a certain age-range. Even this wide criterion for membership will necessarily exclude some.

Membership of a particular group may be of value in enhancing the status of the individual, or conversely it may detract from it (Ellemers *et al.*, 1990). In a high status group the members may therefore be more identified with the group than they would be if it were less valued. In a series of papers, Tajfel (1974 and elsewhere) has outlined the processes by which this occurs, indicating that people make considerable efforts to join valued groups.

Social Facilitation in Groups

Irrespective of the degree of social interaction in a group, the very presence of others significantly affects how people behave. In reviewing this work, Zajonc (1965) notes that being able to see and hear others, even without talking to them, is sufficient to influence the individual's degree of physiological arousal and thence his cognitive and social functioning. Such an increase in arousal is adaptive for the performance of simple tasks because it reduces attention paid to intrusive peripheral cues, but it is less valuable in relation to a task, when taking such cues into account may be important for performing it correctly. Zajonc goes on to say that a student taking an examination should do so preferably on stage and in the presence of a large audience—providing of course that his material is well-learnt!

The Development of Cohesiveness

If a newly constituted group is to persist as a psychological entity it must achieve some degree of cohesiveness in its functioning. In other words, group members must come to interact smoothly with each other, must value and like at least some of the other members and must obtain some rewards for their continued presence and participation. In general, people who are similar are more disposed to start off by liking each other (Lott and Lott, 1965), and this gives homogeneous groups an initial advantage. Group cohesiveness will only be maintained, however, if the group develops some distinctive group norms at a relatively early stage. Such group cohesiveness is likely to be paralleled by differentiation from other groups, with possible hostility to them occurring (Kelly, 1988). However, as Hinckle, Taylor, Fox-Cardamone and Crook (1990) have pointed out, this is not inevitable, particularly when the group is one without clear comparisons.

Norm Formation

Kelvin (1970) defines a social norm as a shared expectation about behaviour. A group may develop shared expectations about the physical arrangements for their meeting, such as the place and the length of time it will take, about the style of interaction such as whether interruptions are permitted, and about the types of activities in which they engage. Such norms have a value in ordering the social environment and in preventing the information overload which would result from having continually to make decisions about matters of these kinds. Not all norms are automatically adaptive, though. Some norms which have originally developed from simple expediency may persist in a rigid way to the eventual detriment of group functioning. Kelvin also observed that norms are often prescriptive. In other words, they carry the implication that such behaviour is right and that members who do not conform to it should be punished in some way, such as by the withdrawal of social approval. Prescriptive norms may grow up from the simple frequency of a behaviour, which in time comes to be regarded as the only acceptable way to behave.

Conformity in Groups

The pressures which groups exert on members to conform have been studied extensively. Deutsch and Gerard (1955) note that not all pressures are socially coercive. Some are simply informational, as when other members have access to factual information which was unknown to a particular individual. However, many investigators since Asch (1952) have reported that unanimous group pressure may lead people to agree with opinions which they would be unwilling to accept in other circumstances. Asch asked his subjects to take it in turns to state which line out of three was the same length as a standard line. All but one of each group were in fact stooges who had been briefed to give the same wrong answer. A substantial minority of the unwilling subjects yielded to this pressure for reasons which they had some difficulty in explaining afterwards. This result has been supported in many other studies, although the exact amount of yielding is influenced by such facts as the individual's personality, the type of items under discussion and the importance placed on achieving an accurate answer. More recently, Hogg and Turner (1987) have suggested that information from other group members may be more influential because of the value placed by the individual on membership of that group and the regard shown as a result to regular members.

Roles

As a group develops by setting up consistent patterns of interaction and organizing its task activities, social roles will emerge. To a psychologist, roles are models for behaviour, although they are somewhat differently described in the sociological literature, where they are seen as points in a social structure, as for instance the role of 'mother' in the structure of the 'family'. These behaviours can themselves be divided into compulsory behaviours, forbidden behaviours and optional behaviours. The more precisely specified a given role is in a particular society, the higher the proportion of compulsory and forbidden behaviours in relation to optional ones. Goffman (1961) has also suggested that roles are reciprocal and occur in groups or 'role-sets' such as doctor–nurse, doctor–patient, doctor–hospital porter. In each of these cases the doctor is still a doctor, but different facets of the role are brought into play.

The role of the leader has been studied in considerable detail and is seen as embodying the management of both the task and the social and emotional activities of the group. Leaders are unlikely to be equally gifted in both these respects and one aspect of the role may therefore be delegated to another group member. Fiedler (1964) has suggested that in assessing leadership effectiveness one must take into account not only the leader's personal style, but also the degree of hierarchy in the group structure and the nature of the task to be completed. Thus a directive and task-orientated leadership style which is valuable for handling an emergency being dealt with in a hospital casualty department might be less appropriate in the management of a therapeutic community.

Roles are more institutionalized in some organizations than others. Military and bureaucratic contexts may require a high degree of specificity, while family roles in Western cultures may be more idiosyncratic and influenced by the personalities of their incumbents. Technological and social change require flexibility in roles and their frequent modification. A lack of awareness of this may result in leaders imposing archaic and maladaptive role expectations on group members.

Polarization of Opinion in Groups

In 1961, Stonner carried out a study in which groups were asked to put themselves in the place of an individual who had to make a risky decision, as for instance a man who had to choose between his poorly paid but secure job and a better paid job with a new and unknown company. Measures of members' decisions taken initially and after group discussion showed a 'shift to risk'. Subsequently research demonstrated that in some circumstances a shift to caution may also occur as a result of group discussions, partly depending on the content of the issue to discussed. Lamm and Myers (1978) have evaluated this research and there seems to be no single factor behind these shifts, although their occurrence has been widely documented.

Communication in Groups

Early work on communication in groups originated in the need of military investigators to find the most efficient forms of communication networks for the performance of particular types of task. Such experiments, carried out by Leavitt

(1951) and his successors, allowed subjects either to write messages to each other or to communicate by using a limited number of words over a telephone system. Such an experimental situation mimics well communication systems used in military-type organizations, but the results are not so easily generalizable to small groups interacting in a face-to-face situation. However, a survey of these studies carried out by Glanzer and Glazer (1961) indicated that highly centralized networks in which all information has to be channelled through a central person were quick and efficient in solving simple tasks, but tended not to detect their errors and became less effective over a longer period and when working on more complex problems. Flexible interchange of information, repetition and opportunities for correction of errors seem to be important, not only for avoiding faulty decision-making, but also for maintaining group morale and motivation. These studies demonstrate the need for both involvement by more peripheral group members and also the avoidance of saturating the leader with information overload.

The evidence suggests that not all types of problem are best dealt with in a group situation. In particular, problems which require specialized information or skills which not all group members possess may be better solved by individuals working alone. A common basis of information is essential if groups are to work productively together in most settings.

Therapeutic Groups and Group Processes

It is not the purpose of this chapter to refer in any great detail to the literature on therapeutic groups. It suffices to say that even when well-controlled studies are considered, it is far from clear whether such group methods are consistently effective as a form of treatment, and if so whether they are superior in effectiveness and use of resources compared with other possible forms of treatment such as behaviour therapy or individual psychotherapy.

It should be possible to understand therapeutic groups better by the application to them of the principles outlined above. In view of the very extensive nature of the empirical literature now available on normal groups, it is highly likely that some of the findings which have been consistently observed in a variety of other contexts apply in therapeutic groups also and such issues have been discussed by other authors. The formation and maintenance of group norms and the development of roles exemplify this type of generalization.

Verbal and Non-verbal Communication and Interaction

All aspects of group process have to be mediated by the interaction of those involved. This is partly a matter of the group's communication structure, as has been indicated, but it is also reflected in the meaning of the words and grammatical phrases selected and in the various forms of non-verbal communication which occur. This last facet of social interaction will now be considered in more detail.

What is non-verbal communication?

In discussing definitions of non-verbal communication, Harper, Wiens and Matarazzo (1978) refer to the wide variety of definitions that occur in the literature. For practical purposes a useful definition was, however, provided by Knapp (1972). He said that 'nonverbal communication designates all those human responses which are *not* described as overtly manifested words (either spoken or written)'. Siegman and Feldstein (1987) note that scientists from a whole range of disciplines have contributed to its study with valuable results.

One way of considering non-verbal communication is to categorize it by the modality in which particular cues are perceived. Thus visual cues include facial expression, gesture, posture, the orientation with which one person faces another, their degree of proximity, eye contact and who is looking at whom. Auditory cues include speech rate, interruptions, pauses and the pitch and loudness of the voice. Finally, for some interactions in some cultures, touch and smell may be important.

Harper, Wiens and Matarazzo also discuss the issue of whether all non-verbal cues constitute non-verbal communication or whether some are only accidentally communicative and can be described more properly as non-verbal signs. An example of this would be a cry of pain by someone who has burned his arm. For these types of behaviour to be communicative there probably needs to be an intention to communicate, or encode, some message which is then decoded by an observer or listener. In other words there has to be a shared signalling system. The whole question of conscious intention to communicate is, however, a hazardous one in this area, since much non-verbal behaviour seems to be below the awareness of the interactors, who are frequently unable to introspect what they were doing.

The functions of non-verbal communication

Non-verbal communication, as has been said already, is part of a collection of interactive behaviours which make up the regular interchange in a group. Its functions therefore have to do with keeping the interaction running smoothly as well as with expressing the feelings, attitudes and personalities of the members. These multiple functions of non-verbal communication have been described in a rather different way by Trower, Bryant and Argyle (1978) as contributing to control and rewardingness in social interaction. Both of these dimensions are important for maintaining interaction in small groups and non-verbal communication acts as a carrier for them.

Any given non-verbal sign may serve more than one communicative function, as was noted by Ekman and Friesen (1969). They described these functions as follows:

1. Emblems—signs which are complete in themselves, such as the 'thumbs up' sign.
2. Illustrators—signs which supplement speech, for example, pointing while explaining a direction.

3. Regulators—behaviours which control the interaction, such as using eye contact to indicate who should speak.
4. Affect displays—the expression of emotion, as for instance by facial expression.
5. Adaptors—attempts to maintain self-control, such as fidgeting or scratching.

An understanding of regulators and affect displays is particularly important for interpreting group process.

Regulation and expression in small groups

Some examples of how non-verbal communication operates in small groups are worthy of consideration. Kendon (1967) analysed films of two-person conversations in great detail and found that for utterances of five seconds and over, speakers would start looking away and then look back at the end to signal to the listener that it was his turn to speak. Listeners tend to look at the speaker and were able to pick up the signal to take over the conversation. Kendon also pointed out that looking has two functions. It allows the speaker to monitor what is going on, so that he can adjust his behaviour accordingly and it can also be used to express his feelings about the other people present. This latter point has been dealt with by Argyle and Dean (1965), who put forward an affiliative–conflict theory of looking. According to these investigators, looking, proximity and the intimacy of the relationship are interrelated, so that while looking occurs more often between people who know and like each other, this will be reduced if they have to sit or stand excessively close to each other as might be the case in a crowded party. Later studies have indicated that the way in which this works is complex and probably moderated by other factors such as the sex and personality of the participants. In addition, looking may decrease significantly in certain types of mental illness. Rutter and Stephenson (1972) demonstrated that schizophrenics and depressives looked less at an interviewer than did controls. Since similar results were not found for patients suffering from anxiety states or alcoholism, this is presumably not a function of hospitalization. Lack of looking may be interpreted by other members as rejection and may have social consequences in relation to the individual's position in the group. It exemplifies very clearly the role of rewardingness in group interaction. Another way of approaching the problem has been suggested by Fehr and Exline (1987). Visual behaviour may be used to 'tell' about involvement with others. In doing so it may also be used to 'lie'.

Emotional expression is signalled by a complex range of visual and auditory behaviours in group situations. Facial expression is particularly important in the expression of emotion, because of the many fine changes in the facial muscles which are possible. It has been known since the work of Woodworth (1938) that there is a continuum of emotional expression from fear through to love and that errors in decoding are less severe if they involve emotions close together on the scale. So, for example, confusing fear and joy is a serious mistake, but confusing fear and anger is less so. After evaluating a variety of previous studies, Ekman,

Friesen and Ellsworth (1972) identified seven main categories of emotional expression, namely happiness, surprise, fear, sadness, anger, disgust/contempt and interest. These categories have formed the basis of a number of subsequent investigations.

The effect of culture on emotional expression has been a matter for debate since the time of Charles Darwin. Ekman and Friesen (1971) have proposed that while the meaning of particular facial expressions remains constant across cultures, when they are elicited and how they are modified is likely to be culturally determined. So, for example, although sadness can be recognized universally, it is not an inevitable response to attending a funeral in all cultures. What Ekman calls 'display rules' can result in the intensification of expression, or its reduction or elimination. Alternatively, in some cultures, people may be required to mask one emotion such as envy with another such as pleasure. Cultural modifications of emotional expression are of considerable significance for group work in psychiatry, particularly in contexts where patients (and staff members) come from a variety of widely different cultural background. Scherer, Wallbott and Summerfield (1986) found that even within Europe significant variations exist which may result in misunderstandings.

Conclusion

There is inevitably a gap between any academic understanding of how groups function and its application to professional life. Empirical findings in psychology, as in other sciences, tend to be largely overtaken by more recent work within a few years of their publication. What remains, however, is an increasingly stable and coherent construct system of thinking about how individuals react. It is this construct system which is of value in any consideration of groups within the psychiatrist's working environment.

References

Argyle, M. and Dean, J. (1965). Eye-contact, distance and affiliation. *Sociometry* **28**, 289–304.

Asch, G.E. (1952). *Social Psychology*. Englewood Cliffs, NJ: Prentice-Hall.

Berkowitz, L. (1980). *A Survey of Social Psychology*. New York: Holt, Rinehart & Winston.

Berne, E. (1963). *The Structure and Dynamics of Organizations and Groups*. New York: Grove.

Deutsch, M. and Gerard, H.B. (1955). A study of normative and informational influence upon individual judgement. *J. Abnorm. Social Psychol.* **51**, 629–636.

Ekman, P. and Friesen, W.V. (1969). The repertoire of nonverbal behavior—categories, origins, usage and coding. *Semiotica* **1**, 49–98.

Ekman, P. and Friesen, W.V. (1971). Constants across cultures in the face and emotion. *J. Personal. Social Psychol.* **29**, 288–298.

Ekman, P., Friesen, W.V. and Ellsworth, P. (1972). *Emotion in the Human Face*. New York: Pergamon Press.

Ellemers, N., van Knippenber, A. and Wilker, H. (1990). The influence of permeability of group boundaries and stability of group status on strategies of individual mobility and social change. *Br. J. Social Psychol.* **29**, 233–246.

Fehr, B.J. and Exline, R.V. (1987). Social visual interaction: A conceptual and literature review. In: A.W. Siegman and S. Feldstein (eds) *Nonverbal Behavior and Communication*. Hillsdale, NJ: Lawrence Erlbaum.

Fiedler, F.E. (1964). A contingency model of leadership effectiveness. In: L. Berkowitz (ed.) *Advances in Experimental Social Psychology*, Vol 1. New York: Academic Press.

Glanzer, M. and Glazer, R. (1961). Techniques for the study of group structure and behavior II. Empirical studies on the effects of structure in small groups. *Psychol. Bull.* **58**, 1–27.

Goffman, E. (1961). *Encounters*. Harmondsworth, Middx: Penguin.

Harper, R.G., Wiens, A.N. and Matarazzo, J.D. (1978). *Nonverbal Communication: The State of the Art*. New York: Wiley.

Hogg, M.A. and Turner, J.C. (1987). Intergroup behaviour, self-stereotyping and the salience of social categories. *Br. J. Social Psychol.* **26**, 325–340.

Hinkle, S., Taylor, L.A., Fox-Cardamone, D.L. and Crook, K.F. (1990). Intragroup identification and intergroup differentiation: A multicomponent approach. *Br. J. Social Psychol.* **28**, 305–317.

Kelly, C. (1988). Intergroup differentiation in a political context. *Br. J. Social Psychol.* **27**, 319–332.

Kelvin, P. (1970). *The Bases of Social Behaviour*. London: Holt, Rinehart & Winston.

Kendon, A. (1967). Some functions of gaze direction in social interaction. *Acta Psychol.* **26**, 1–47.

Knapp, M.L. (1972). The field of non-verbal communication: an overview. In: C.J. Stewart and B. Kendall (eds) *On Speech Communication: An Anthology of Contemporary Workings and Messages*. New York: Holt, Rinehart & Winston.

Lamm, H. and Myers, D.G. (1978). Group-induced polarization of attitudes and behavior. In: L. Berkowitz (ed.) *Advances in Experimental Social Psychology*, Vol 2. New York: Academic Press.

Leavitt, J.H. (1951). Some effects of certain communication patterns on group performance. *J. Abnorm. Social Psychol.* **46**, 38–50.

Lott, A.J. and Lott, B.E. (1965). Group cohesiveness and interpersonal attraction: a review of relationships with antecedent and consequent variables. *Psychol. Bull.* **64**, 259–309.

Rutter, D.R. and Stephenson, G.M. (1972). Visual interaction in a group of schizophrenic and depressive patients. *Br. J. Social Clin. Psychol.* **11**, 57–65.

Scherer, K.R., Wallbott, H.G. and Summerfield, A.B. (1986). *Experiencing Emotion: A Cross-Cultural Study*. Cambridge: Cambridge University Press.

Siegman, A.W. and Feldstein, S. (1987). *Nonverbal Behavior and Communication*. Hillsdale, NJ: Lawrence Erlbaum.

Stonner, J.A. (1961). *A Comparison of Individual and Group Decisions Involving Risk*. Unpublished Master's thesis. Cambridge, MA: MIT Press.

Tajfel, H. (1974). Social identity and intergroup behaviour. *Social Sci. Inform.* **13**, 65–93.

Trower, P., Bryant, B. and Argyle, M. (1978). *Social Skills and Mental Health*. London: Methuen.

Woodworth, R.S. (1938). *Experimental Psychology*. New York: Holt.

Zajonc, R.B. (1965). Social facilitation. *Science* **149**, 269–274.

Transcultural Psychiatry

J.L. Cox and M.S. Jorsh

We are the makers of manners, Kate.

King Henry V: William Shakespeare

Introduction

The definition of a delusion as a false belief firmly held against all evidence to the contrary and out of keeping with the socio-cultural environment makes explicit that the understanding of culture, or a subculture, is central to the 'good practice' of psychiatry. Indeed it is surprising that two decades ago transcultural psychiatry was regarded as very peripheral to the work of a psychiatrist, and was caricatured as a colonial interest in exotic cultures and their culture-bound syndromes. Only the CIBA symposium on Transcultural Psychiatry (de Reuck and Porter, 1965) chaired by Aubrey Lewis, with chapters by Carstairs, Yap, Leighton, Murphy, Meyer-Fortes, Lambo and Mead, and the text by Kiev (1972) were available for reference. However, the number of books and papers published since then on transcultural psychiatry is very considerable indeed, and they have been recently reviewed (Cox, 1991). The majority of books are from North America where the writings of psychiatrist/anthropologist Arthur Kleinman are particularly impressive (Kleinman, 1980, 1987, 1988). More recently other major research contributions have been summarized in an important British text by Leff (1988), *Psychiatry Around the Globe*, and the subject popularized by Littlewood and Lipsedge (1982) in their second edition of *Aliens and Alienists*. The growth of the Transcultural Psychiatry Section of the World Psychiatric Association is evidence of persistent interest in the subject.

Nevertheless, the reasons for the attempt to marginalize transcultural psychiatry in the United Kingdom are persuasively put forward by Sashidharan (1986) and Fernando (1988); the subject could be regarded as a covert form of racism as it can be ethnocentric and preoccupied only with the culture of black minorities. Those with a broader interest in the educational and clinical issues of cultural psychiatry were construed as having colluded with an unjust discriminatory society and some transcultural research amongst black communities in the United Kingdom was regarded as a 'no go' area for white psychiatrists. Harrison *et al.* (1988), for example, investigated the frequency of first admission with schizophrenia in Afro-Caribbeans living in Nottingham and found a higher rate than in Caucasians, and McGovern and Cope (1987) found that Afro-Caribbeans were more likely than whites to be compulsorily admitted. This research was criticized as perpetuating a stereotype that Afro-Caribbeans were more likely than other black minorities, or the majority 'white' culture, to have mental illness, and to be violent.

Not all psychiatrists, however, have accepted the need to polarize the 'black' from the 'white' community and regard both terms as being too broad to be meaningful except within the political context of race relations.

We regard transcultural psychiatry as a subject which is not confined to studies of black communities only, nor narrowly restricted by those specifically concerned with racial discrimination—however pathogenic such attitudes can be. It has as much to do with the cultural assumptions of the majority, such as the secularization and individualization of Western society, the effect of migration on the mental health of Scandinavians to New York (Ødegaard, 1932) and the adjustment reactions of first generation Southern Europeans to Australia (Krupinski et al., 1973), as with the provision of services for ethnic minorities in the United Kingdom.

Transcultural psychiatry balances an excessive emphasis on understanding the biological causes of mental illness with the need to grasp the cultural context in which a biomedical explanation may operate—for example the reasons for consanguinity and for the particular nexus of family relationships which indirectly may provoke relapse of a major mental illness, or sustain a remission.

Thus, transcultural psychiatry is now recognized as relevant to the establishment of comprehensive mental health services, for the education of Mental Health Act Commissioners, social workers (Triseliotis, 1986), nurses (Leininger, 1978), and for the adequate postgraduate training of psychiatrists in Britain (Cox, 1977; Royal College of Psychiatrists, 1990) as well as in the United States (Foulks, 1980).

Indeed, the success of transcultural psychiatry has been to articulate the need for such education, to provoke clinical research into the optimum provision of services for ethnic minorities and to provide a critique of taken-for-granted aspects of British psychiatry, such as the present popularity of non-directive counselling. A further reason for increased awareness of socio-cultural aspects of psychiatric service provision has been the changes to the National Health Service whereby mental health services are more responsive to consumer demands. Thus the need of ethnic minorities for a more culturally sensitive Mental Health Service will encourage the translation of educational leaflets from English or Urdu into a variety of other languages, as well as taking greater account of the varying food preferences and religious beliefs of ethnic minorities. In this way consumer demand may lead to a greater emphasis on socio-anthropological concepts such as consultation behaviour, causes of stigma, options of a 'sick role', the effect of institutionalization and the need to consider the patient's own 'explanatory model' for misfortune. Transcultural psychiatry provides a balance to an excessively biomedical reductionist approach to the understanding of psychiatric disorder, and is therefore one component of the biopsychosocial model (Engel, 1980) which provides a useful theoretical framework for an holistic approach.

Definitions

Culture has been defined by Walter (1952) as 'learned ways of acting and thinking, which are transmitted by group members to other group members and which will provide for each individual ready made and tested solutions for vital life problems'.

A more prolonged account of culture by Ioan Lewis (1976) underlines specifically its relevance to a full understanding of childhood development and its impact on adult personality:

> For our purposes culture is simply a convenient term to describe the sum of learned knowledge and skills—including religion and language—that distinguishes one community from another and which, subject to the vagaries of innovation and change, passes on in a recognisable form from generation to generation. Culture thus transcends the lives of its living exponents in any one generation; if it did not it could not survive. Its component elements are absorbed in the first few years of life largely unconsciously and later more deliberately by informal and formal learning processes. Socialisation inevitably takes place within and through the medium of a particular cultural tradition. When people do not know how to bring up or what to teach their children their cultural heritage is indeed in jeopardy.

Transcultural psychiatry is concerned particularly with differences between cultures as they relate to the prevention, detection and management of psychiatric disorder, and with maintaining good mental health. This cultural approach to psychiatry is often explicitly or implicitly comparative; a psychiatrist attempts to understand reasons for the similarities and dissimilarities of psychiatric disorder between cultures and subcultures, such as the determinants of contrasting systems of thought which lead to differences in the criteria for the classification of mental disorder. Other comparisons are between the cultural assumptions of patients, or of the patient and the doctor, which are of clinical relevance to a psychiatrist working in a multicultural area.

However, the safeguard provided by the medical anthropologist's approach to this understanding of the nature of mental illness is the principle of *cultural relativism*, which avoids the ethnocentric perspective that the belief of the majority is 'correct', or is the belief against which health practices of minorities are to be compared. The influence of British colonial history on present-day thinking has to be recognized because of a persistent attitude that British tradition and culture is superior, or is the norm to which an ethnic minority must conform.

In contrast to the United States where the ethnography and mental illness beliefs of ethnic minorities are well documented (Wilkinson, 1986), only Alex Henley's (1979) account of Asian patients in hospital and the book by Krausz (1972) have provided factual information about the health beliefs and customs of ethnic minorities in the United Kingdom. Most recent publications have predominantly emphasized the effect of racism on the mental health of majority and minority groups, and have described how discrimination and disadvantage can increase the likelihood of a psychiatric disorder such as depression occurring, can prolong the duration of the disorder, or restrict access to health services (Littlewood and Lipsedge, 1982; Fernando, 1988).

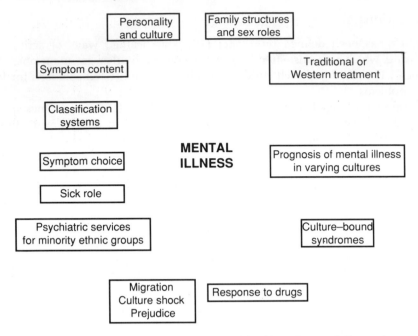

FIG. 27.1   The relationship of culture to mental health and mental illness (from Cox, 1982).

Other aspects of the relationship of culture to mental health and mental illness are shown in Fig. 27.1.

Because of the increasing ethnic diversity of the United Kingdom, and because psychiatrists themselves come from different national and ethnic backgrounds, the sharing of cultural assumptions between doctor and patient cannot be assumed so that a specific effort to empathise across cultures has to be made. The need for racial awareness training by working abroad, experience of, or living with an ethnic minority is more generally recognized. Both authors have worked in Africa and the United Kingdom and this experience has partly determined the content of this chapter.

We believe there is a need for cultural psychiatry to exert a greater influence on psychiatric practice, as without the cultural 'explanatory model' of mental illness, a psychiatrist may justify the 'stereotype' of being preoccupied only with biological causes of illness, or with pharmacological treatments. A complete understanding of schizophrenia depends therefore not only on familiarity with advances in knowledge of its genetics and the impact of earlier obstetric trauma, but also on the nature of the relationship within a family which generate negative emotion and could cause relapse (Leff, 1974). Furthermore, as Lefley (1990) has pointed out, the improved prognosis of schizophrenia in a developing, compared with a developed, country found in the International Pilot Study of Schizophrenia might suggest that chronicity is itself a 'cultural artifact' not solely biologically determined but linked to the cause of stigma, and the Western belief that the loss of self involves a loss of personal autonomy which results in a greater feeling of alienation and despair. The link between the understanding of the relationship of negative 'life-events' to the onset of schizophrenia (Birley and Brown, 1970), and of the association between relapse and critical comments, hostility and emotional over-involvement (Brown *et al.*, 1972; Leff *et al.*, 1987), underlines the need to understand culture, or a subculture, for a full understanding of schizophrenia, or depression.

The DSM-III-R classification of psychiatric disorder (American Psychiatric Association, 1987), which was a partial reaction to the influence of psychoanalysis, emphasized the counting of symptoms and reflected the belief system of that society about the value of a 'medical model' approach. It could commit a 'category fallacy' (Kleinman, 1987) and Kleinman (1988) has questioned whether in DSM-III and DSM-III-R there is a tendency for a spurious numericalized specificity about the psychiatric classification.

Cultural psychiatry is therefore relevant for psychiatrists who are curious about themselves and their subculture and prepared to question taken-for-granted diagnostic assumptions. We do not believe, however, that the medical model is itself an irrelevant cultural artifact, as the diagnostic *approach* is a necessary clinical safeguard for most patients being assessed for the first time, and can inform the mental health professional about the optimum balance of management between contrasting treatment models—biomedical, psychodynamic and socio-cultural.

Migration and Mental Illness

Migration implies a relocation of one's abode; the term suggests that there is either a considerable geographic distance between the two homes, or some other major difference between the two. It may be permanent or temporary and has become increasingly frequent in the twentieth century. It tests an individual's adaptive capacity, especially if the two environments are different. The differences may include climate, language, environmental hazards and diet. Other differences could include the cultural and political attitudes of the new society, and the social role changes demanded of the newcomer. These differences may challenge the migrant's habitual behaviour patterns, beliefs and value systems and even threaten their sense of personal identity (Rack, 1988).

Babiker *et al.* (1980) have devised a Cultural Distance Scale in a study on the adjustment of first year overseas students in Edinburgh. They found that first year examination failure was more likely in overseas than home students, and that November and December were times of particular unhappiness in the first year of the sojourn (Cox *et al.*, 1981). The 'cultural distance' from the home subculture, however, was not related to the experience of a psychiatric disorder, but the conflict between the visitor, student and client roles (Reed *et al.*, 1978) in many individual instances certainly was.

Culture shock

Culture shock is defined by Toffler (1970) as a feeling of profound disorientation experienced by an individual when plunged, with inadequate preparation, into an alien culture. Uprooting disorder is the preferred term of Zwingmann and Gunn (1983) to characterize the adjustment reaction of a student who is a rootless sojourner. The migrant situation therefore demands repeated adaptation to novel conditions and a severe culture shock can occur when the individual is unable to adjust to the new surroundings and people. Events, relationships and objects then become unfamiliar and unpredictable, and usual ways of accomplishing things are no longer appropriate. The individual may acquire a subjective feeling of loss accompanied by isolation and loneliness. Nostalgia and a sense of grief are also components of the disenchantment phase of culture shock which follows the honeymoon phase and which precedes the beginning resolution phase when adjustment is made to the new environment (Gullahorn and Gullahorn, 1963).

The immigrant faces difficulties which render him vulnerable to psychiatric disorder. It is evident from the earliest major transcultural research done by Ødegaard (1932) that immigrants may have a higher incidence of psychiatric morbidity than others in both their countries of origin and their adopted countries. This appears to be a universal trend and although causative theories have been postulated in the many studies since, no one factor appears to have shown prominence. The incidence of psychiatric morbidity appears to be related to the extent of acculturation, the reasons for migration and attitudes within the adopted country.

Motivation for migration

Rack (1988) regards three factors as pertinent for an understanding of immigration: the country of origin; the motivation for the move; and conditions within the country of settlement. The first factor includes aspects of culture such as child-rearing practices and differing epidemiology of mental illness. With respect to the actual move, a distinction should be made between forced and voluntary migration, and in the case of refugees, the varieties of trauma which may have been experienced.

Rack (1986) mentions two theories which were originally believed to account for the increased incidence of psychiatric disorder in migrants. The first, the stress-of-migration hypothesis, postulated that the psychological trauma, isolation, oppression and other vicissitudes experienced in migration and settlement accounted for the increase. The second was the self-selection hypothesis which suggested that individuals who were unable to adapt to their original environment, and were, by implication, mentally unstable, migrated more frequently.

Migrants are not necessarily typical of their culture of origin and Lee (1965) has identified a group of 'high aspirers' with above average enterprise and foresight and a group of 'low achievers' who are unsuccessful, unsettled or deprived. He suggests that the former are influenced by pull factors, while the latter are influenced by push factors. This argument fits in with the one advanced above.

Rack (1986) suggests an alternative categorization and defines three groups of migrants: the Gastarbeiter, the exile and the settler. The Gastarbeiters are usually young males from a rural area who leave their country for economic reasons usually intending to return. Their emotional roots remain in their country of origin. The settlers, on the other hand, migrate with their families to seek better opportunities, with the intention of putting down roots. They are predisposed to take a positive view of the differences they encounter, abandon old customs and learn new ones. Exiles undergo involuntary migration and leave their countries of origin because of some political upheaval or natural disaster. Most have experienced extreme psychological trauma. They have been uprooted and separated from their loved ones and some undergo a bereavement reaction. They may have witnessed or been involved in persecution which may have included extreme violence. They commonly develop psychiatric symptoms and post-traumatic stress disorder after they reach safety. Rack points out that these categories are not comprehensive and frequently overlap.

Adaptation to migration

According to Mavreas and Bebbington (1990), the degree of acculturation depends on the individual's characteristics and how traditional they are. It also depends on the social climate within the host country. These factors will therefore affect psychiatric morbidity according to circumstances pre- and post-migration.

Migration involves separation and loss and one would expect the migrant to experience a grief reaction which usually lessens gradually as the individual adjusts to the new country (Herz, 1988). However, ambivalent feelings for the host country are often retained, especially if the migrant belongs to an ethnic minority which is racially distant from the host society.

Acculturation is defined by Herz (1988) as a 'total adaptive and coping process affecting not only the cultural patterning and value system but also the psychological structure and psychophysiological functions of individuals and families, as adaptations are made to changed conditions created by the impact of people and their environment upon each other'. Difficulties in the process of acculturation contribute to the development of 'culture shock' which, in migrant populations derives from intrapsychic and interpersonal sources. Migrants appear to adjust in three stages. The pre-immigration stage, in which motivation for change is required. Positive expectations of the outcome create the proper emotional atmosphere. Unrealistic expectations increase the risk of later maladjustment. In the honeymoon phase on arrival in the new environment, there are feelings of elation, relief and fulfilment. Reality then creates a rebound reaction, which manifests in feelings of disappointment, often followed by anger and aggressive behaviour or by a depressed mood. There is then a period of increased coping in which language and other communication skills are acquired, familiarity with support systems develops and the group integrates, creating a feeling of security. The final stage is one of settlement. The family identifies with its surroundings and a sense of belonging develops. Reverse culture shock can then occur on return to the native country.

The greater the cohesion of the immigrant group, the better are the chances of successful coping. The family needs to be able to adapt to change and alterations in family relationships—especially in traditional families. Compromise

Questions addressed to immigrants

Is the new culture valued,
and to be adopted?

		Yes	No
Is the old culture valued, and to be retained?	Yes	Integration	Separatism
	No	Assimilation	Marginality

Questions addressed to the host
community

Are newcomers helped and encouraged
to adopt the host culture and rewarded
for doing so?

		Yes	No
Are racial differences and alternative lifestyles respected?	Yes	Integration	Separation
	No	Assimilation	Rejection

FIG. 27.2 Adjustment possibilities for immigrants (Rack, 1986).

will be needed with regard to changes in the status of women, the acceptance of dealing with a different educational system, partner selection for the children and the maintenance of parental authority. Western families who migrate, by contrast, strive for acceptance, search for a feeling of security in the new setting and wish to develop immediate mastery of it. In this case, the maladjusted family presents itself with a sense of emotional and social isolation and concern about the future. Herz points out that migrants from non-democratic countries which have restrictive migration and travel laws may lose the option to make free decisions and are often unable to re-negotiate their original choice. This may compound feelings of isolation and loss.

Integration of migrants depends on a number of personal characteristics. Language and communication may cause difficulties. Frequently, however, the attitudes of the host society to migrants play an extremely important role. If the society tends to be ethnocentric, or if it harbours racist attitudes, the migrants face greater difficulties. Attacks of both a physical or emotional nature may occur, but more frequently, prejudice is encountered. Immigrants may thus be socially and economically disadvantaged and face greater obstacles in gaining education and jobs commensurate with their abilities. Immigration laws may enhance these feelings of insecurity. These problems are generally heightened if the individual is obviously different, for example, in dress or appearance. Rack (1986) has usefully summarized these adjustment possibilities (Fig. 27.2).

Factors which influence adjustment

Mavreas and Bebbington (1990) suggest that the high rates of psychiatric disorders in immigrant populations could be due either to the fact that they make greater use of services or to diagnostic bias. Exposure to certain socio-demographic or psychological factors may increase the rate of morbidity. They may have cultural or biological predispositions which render them vulnerable. Migration and acculturation may be precipitating stressors which are modified by circumstances of immigration and acceptance into the host country. These factors may all apply in varying degrees over time to contribute to their psychiatric morbidity.

In their opinion migration may alter the family organization as a social institution and a source of security. People from traditional cultures may have extended families rather than the Western nuclear family. These extended families have different structures and authority figures which may be challenged in a Western environment where the family tends to function as a vehicle for self-fulfilment and socialization. The new demands may alter the functioning of the extended family and cause trans-generational conflicts, particularly when authority figures are challenged and sex status is altered. Members of the family may be acculturated to varying degrees, which may increase conflicts between them. Second generation immigrants have particular difficulties, for example Asian girls who are trapped in conflict between the Western attitudes of their schools and the traditional attitudes about family loyalty and marriage of their homes.

Racism plays an important role in acculturation (Burke, 1986). The migrant may arrive in the new environment expecting to encounter prejudice and will thus be defensive and possibly aggressive which, in turn, may serve to create or enhance racist attitudes. Racist attitudes result in the migrant experiencing a loss of self-esteem. The victims may be excluded from society in various ways. In extreme cases, they may actually be expelled from the society, but are usually more subtly excluded in that they may be integrated into the society, but may not be given jobs commensurate with their abilities, and services provided to them might be of a lower standard. Many of these reactions on the part of the host country are based on fear, but lead to a feeling of isolation and social deprivation in the victim. Burke (1986) cites the example of the young, large, Black male who is feared and who thus faces difficulties acquiring work and being integrated into society. This person, when in contact with mental health services, faces a greater chance of being detained for treatment and faces a greater chance of being treated in a secure unit.

The closer the immigrants' resemblance to the natives in language and culture, particularly if they have skills of use to the host society, the lower will be their stress levels (Mavreas and Bebbington, 1990). If the immediate aftermath of immigration is particularly stressful, the immigrant may be particularly prone to develop psychiatric disorder, even at a later date. A partial acculturation may render the individual more vulnerable than full, or no, acculturation.

Mavreas and Bebbington (1990) studied the Greek Cypriot immigrant community in Camberwell, South London, and found that previous knowledge of English was associated with reduced prevalence of psychiatric disorder. Difficulties in the settling-in period were related to current disorder. In males disorder was most prevalent in the highly acculturated and in females the least acculturated.

Increased psychiatric morbidity is associated with most, but not all, types of migration (Westermeyer, 1988). Migrants at greatest risk of developing psychiatric disorders appear to be those moving from a rural to urban environment, those changing country, students and refugees. Adversive migration is associated with increased rates of schizophrenia, paranoia, depression and substance abuse. Associated problems have included unemployment, divorce and inter-generational conflict.

Herz (1988) suggests that the effects of migration are frequently related to the form and nature of the migration. It may be either legal or illegal and may be voluntary, forced, ideological or political. Other factors, such as age, sex, ethnic origin, socioeconomic status, and personal family and medical background will contribute. The circumstances of leaving the home country and the process of integration must be considered.

The intrapsychic sources are often related to failure in verbal and non-verbal communication with the environment. Language limitation reinforces the sense of emotional and social isolation. However, non-verbal misunderstandings often have a longer lasting effect than verbal ones. There may also be value conflicts when the migrant is confronted with a new culture. Westernized education emphasizes the need for independence, individual growth and maturity. This approach may be confusing and frightening to people from some traditional cultures whose expectations turn more in the opposite direction, seeking dependent and protecting relationships from authority figures.

Interpersonal conflicts are reinforced by cultural misunderstanding or poor estimation of the new environment by the migrant (Herz, 1988). The faulty application of certain social habits, taboos and customs may often precipitate the intensity of such conflicts. Prejudices originating from the cultural background of the migrant group may interfere with the process of acculturation. The migrants may feel that the new cultural, racial or religious group does not understand them and this may lead to attitudes which create further difficulties.

Epidemiology

In order to obtain accurate epidemiological data on the incidence of any illness in a country, standardized clinical assessment and diagnostic techniques must be used in population surveys. This problem is compounded, in the case of psychiatry, by the fact that most of the diagnostic instruments in use have been developed and standardized in the West, and therefore may not include symptoms that are peculiar to non-Western patients. This position is now changing with the development of instruments which are based on the accounts of traditional healers and take account of folk categories of illness. Carstairs and Kapur (1976) have constructed the Indian Psychiatric Interview Schedule (IPIS) in Kannada, a South Indian language, and Verma and Wig (1976) have produced the PGI Health Questionnaire in Hindi.

Because developing countries have sparse psychiatric facilities, case registers cannot be set up. Unlike the West, where people suffering from functional psychiatric illnesses usually present to medical services early on in the condition, patients in developing countries frequently present to other agencies, such as traditional healers, or may even be cared for by their families without support and may recover without ever seeing a Western-style practitioner. They may only present to psychiatric services once their illness and condition become florid. In calculating prevalence rates, it should be also remembered that half the population is under the age of 15 and as certain conditions, like schizophrenia, are rare in this age group, the rates must be expressed in relation to the proportion of the population at risk for the disease. Leff (1986) has pointed out that it is essential to ensure that epidemiological techniques are sound before invoking cultural factors to explain the differences in incidence and prevalence of psychiatric illness. While it is relatively easy to assess the rates of psychotic illness in developed countries, they share assessment problems with developing countries when attempting to assess the rates of neurotic conditions. However, while in the latter the patients may not present for treatment at all, in the former the patients may present to alternative healers for help. Traditionally the population may believe that it is more appropriate to seek help from traditional healers when suffering from psychiatric problems.

Research conducted in Africa initially suggested that the incidence and prevalence of mental illness, especially that of depression, was lower than that in the West (German, 1987). Many of the conclusions were based on prejudiced views, but the research was hampered by many factors. Lack of financial, academic and staffing resources, as well as the fact that large areas with diverse languages and populations had to be assessed, proved to be large obstacles to accurate assessment. Early studies were based on admissions to psychiatric hospitals. As mentioned above, this posed intrinsic problems because patients were only admitted when they became violent or disruptive and the 'quiet psychoses' were therefore not usually included in the studies. The absence of such disorders among the case material led to the mistaken belief that they were exceedingly rare in Africa. Research in recent times suggests that psychiatric morbidity in Africa is comparable with that in the developed world, even for the distribution of diagnoses across the broad categories of psychoses, psychoneuroses and personality disorders. Some studies have suggested that rates of depression in Africa may in fact be higher than those found in the West (Cox, 1979a,b; Orley and Wing, 1979).

The IPSS

The International Pilot Study of Schizophrenia (IPSS) (World Health Organization, 1973) was a major international study of diagnostic habits and practices. It investigated 1202 patients in nine countries: Colombia, Czechoslovakia, Denmark, India, Nigeria, China, the USSR, the United Kingdom and the United States. Its main aim was to assess whether the diagnosis of schizophrenia could be made using the same diagnostic criteria in all these countries. An international group of psychiatrists was trained in the use of the PSE, which was translated into seven languages for the purposes of the study. The psychiatrists were then instructed to continue making diagnoses on the research patients just as they would in their usual clinical work. Only in the USSR, as represented by Moscow, and the United States, as represented by Washington, were discrepancies found which indicated substantial differences in diagnostic procedure. Both of these centres appear to have used a broader definition of schizophrenia and thus made the diagnosis more frequently. However, the patterns of symptoms exhibited by psychotic patients in all the countries were remarkably similar.

The IPSS has been criticized for a number of reasons, although it remains, to date, the most comprehensive survey of the incidence of schizophrenia. Torrey (1987) expresses concern that the countries involved, and the areas within those countries, are not those with reportedly unusual incidence distributions. He cites the cases of Northern Sweden and Western Ireland, which have high incidence figures, and tropical countries, which have low incidence figures. Stevens and Wyatt (1987) point out that a much higher proportion of the cases identified in developing countries were of acute onset and suggest that if DSM-II criteria were used, they may fit into the categories for reactive psychosis, brief reactive psychosis, or schizophreniform psychosis.

Epidemiology of psychiatric illness in Asia

Lin (1953) surveyed the Chinese population in three areas: a small village; a provincial town; and a seaport on the island of Taiwan off the South China coast. He found no significant differences in the overall rate of psychiatric disorders between the three areas surveyed. The lifetime prevalence of schizophrenia was calculated as 2.1 per 1000, of manic-depressive psychosis as 0.7 per 1000, and of neuroses as 1.2 per 1000. The average age of the population studied was much lower than that of a Western country—over half were under 20 and only 5.5% were over 60. This pattern is characteristic of developing countries, resulting from a high mortality rate and low life-expectancy. When recalculated for the population over the age of 15, these figures increased by 72%. Kato (1969) found that the prevalence rate for schizophrenia in Japan was 2.1 per 1000, while that for manic-depressive psychosis was 0.2 per 1000 (this was a six-month prevalence rate). That for neurosis was 2.8 to 3 per 1000. Sethi et al. (1974) found that the rates for schizophrenia in India were 2.5 per 1000, for manic-depressive psychosis 1.1 per 1000 and for neuroses 27.1 per 1000. The increased rates for neuroses may be attributable to differing diagnostic criteria and different screening instruments used. Dube (1970) found very similar rates. In all the studies, the rates for the functional illnesses were remarkably similar, while those for the neuroses differed markedly, ranging from 1.5 per 1000 in some studies (Elnagar et al., 1971) to 43.2 per 1000 in others (Nandi et al., 1980). This may be due to real differences, or may be an artifact of differing diagnostic criteria and differing instruments used to survey the populations.

Epidemiology of psychiatric illness in Africa

There are fewer studies on the incidence of psychiatric illness emanating from Africa. Surveys in these regions suffer from the same difficulties as those performed in other parts of the developing world. Leighton (1959) studied a number of Nigerian villages and found that 22 per 100 men and 20 per 100 women had psychiatric illness, while Gillis *et al.* (1968) found a prevalence of 11.8% in the coloured population of the Cape Peninsula, of these, 59% were socially or economically impaired. The proportion of men to women was approximately 3 to 2 in all age groups. They also found that 93.1 per 10 000 of the population over 15 suffered from neurotic conditions. Orley and Wing (1979), using the PSE (Wing *et al.*, 1974) on a population in Uganda, found that the prevalence for neurotic conditions for the population between 18 and 65 years was 269 per 1000 for women and 174 per 1000 for men. The frequency of post-natal depression (10%) in a controlled study carried out by Cox (1983) showed a similar rate to that reported by Pitt in London, although the African women seemed more disabled by a greater severity of depressive symptoms. Ben-Tovim and Cushnie (1986) found the prevalence of schizophrenia to be 5.3 per 1000.

Epidemiology of psychiatric illness in United Kingdom immigrants

Hemsi (1967) found that the incidence of psychiatric illness in immigrants to the United Kingdom of West Indian origin between the ages of 15 and 54 was 31.9 per 10 000 population compared with an incidence of 10.9 for the native-born. The highest figure found was that for schizophrenia, men showing a rate of 13.1 per 10 000 as compared with 2.7 per 10 000 in the native population. This compares with Royes' (1961) figure for the incidence of psychosis in the West Indies of 3.8 per 10 000 population. Cochrane (1977) found that the overall prevalence of psychiatric illness was very much the same for natives and persons of West Indian origin, but that West Indian women had a much higher rate than natives and that West Indian men had a greater threshold prevalence of schizophrenia. Cochrane and Bal returned to this study in 1987 and found very similar rates. Carpenter and Brockington (1980) also found increased rates for schizophrenia, but for no other condition, as did Dean *et al.* (1981). Littlewood and Lipsedge (1981) suggested that the higher rates were due to misdiagnosis of other conditions and cultural differences, but when they excluded patients who may have fallen into these categories, they still found a higher rate. Harrison *et al.* (1988) applied the WHO case-finding techniques in a study of first onset of schizophrenia in people of Afro-Caribbean origin and found the rate to be increased. Pinto (1970), in a hospital-based survey, also found that the admission rates were higher. Carpenter and Brockington (1980) had similar findings to those of Pinto. Dean *et al.* (1981) separated the Asian populations into those of Pakistani and those of Indian origin. They found that Indians had a three-fold greater incidence of schizophrenia than did natives, while Pakistanis had the same incidence as the latter. The Pakistanis had significantly lower rates for alcoholism, neuroses and personality disorders for men and neuroses for women.

The Culture-bound Syndromes

Culture-bound disorders have traditionally been referred to as disorders restricted to a particular culture, and resulting from a specific socio-cultural conflict or mode of thinking (Yap, 1951). Thus *Susto*, or soul loss, in Latin America is based on a belief that an individual is composed of a body and immaterial substance, an essence, which can wander freely, or become a captive of supernatural forces. Likewise anorexia nervosa is generally more common in Western countries where a concern with dieting and maintaining a slim figure is culturally sanctioned, and where emphasis on adolescent individuation and separation from the parental home is encouraged. Although the study by Rubel *et al.* (1984) found that *Asustados* were more likely than controls to have psychiatric disorder, we believe that to redefine culture-bound disorders within an international classification (e.g. *Latah* as a form of hysteria) may overlook the importance of the folk explanation. It is imperative to understand this explanation if compliance with Western medicine is to be satisfactory. In Uganda most symptoms of a traditional post-partum mental illness *Amakiro* also occur in Western puerperal psychoses, although the wish to eat the baby is uncommon (Cox, 1979b). Nevertheless, if *Amakiro* is to be treated effectively the African beliefs about causation, its aetiology, promiscuity of the woman or her partner during pregnancy, need to be considered, and the concern with legitimacy understood. Nevertheless Leff has argued that to understand culture-bound syndromes fully there is a need to justify a 'substrate' on which cultural influences operate which could be either physiological or psychological.

Littlewood and Lipsedge (1986) believe that a classic culture-bound reaction follows a triphasic pattern of dislocation of the individual, followed by a behaviour which exaggerates this dislocation, and then finally restitution of the individual back to everyday relationships. They point out that *Sar* possession in Somalia can legitimize 'outrageous behaviour' for women living in an Islamic patriarchal society who have offended, or are neglected by, their husbands. Treatment of *Sar* possession is carried out within women's therapy groups and not surprisingly Lewis (1971) observed that 'the Sar spirits are said to hate men'. Leff (1988) has provided a full account of the culture-bound syndromes in his book—*Psychiatry Around the Globe*—and the following account is based on his writing.

Koro is seen most commonly in South-East Asia where it affects mainly those of Chinese descent. It can occasionally affect females and take on epidemic forms. The affected individual becomes convinced that his genitals are withdrawing into his abdomen and becomes panic-stricken because he is convinced that when they disappear completely, he will die. The remedial action taken is to tether his genitals to a rock or post, or to induce his relatives to hold on to the organ. In Thailand it is known as *Rok joo*. Despite the symptoms appearing to be delusional, the fact that the relatives also share the belief and that this belief is common throughout the region refutes this. It is probably explained by Chinese mythology, which believes that ghosts have no genitals. Yap (1965) states that it is a neurotic condition similar to hypochondriacal conditions, such as cardiac neurosis, commonly seen in the West. Oyebode *et al.* (1986), using plethysmography, found that the penile circumference does shrink in cases of extreme anxiety. Weller (1985) suggests that the penile detumescence is due to vasoconstrictor sympathetic impulses to the arterioles of the penis which occurs in the state of overarousal that accompanies high anxiety. Reassurance and education appear to halt the symptoms unless the patient also suffers from a psychotic or neurotic condition. Ang and Weller (1984) discuss two cases of *Koro* which occurred in the United Kingdom, one in a West Indian immigrant and the other in a Greek Cypriot immigrant. The former patient was diagnosed as suffering from schizophrenia, while the latter was diagnosed as suffering from manic depressive illness. They suggest that it is not specific to a particular category of mental illness.

Wihtigo (*Windigo*) is reported to occur amongst the North American Indians of the Cree, Ojibway and Salteaux tribes who experience very harsh winter conditions, with extreme cold and food shortages. Death from starvation is thus possible and there is a consequent fear of cannibalism. This fear is manifested by a rigid taboo on cannibalism and a belief in the *Wihtigo*, a cannibalistic ice spirit of giant size. Initially the individual affected develops a distaste for ordinary types of food, nausea and possibly vomiting. If these symptoms continue for a time, anxiety develops which reaches a climax if they fail to subside. The individual regards his symptoms as evidence that he is turning into a *Wihtigo*. Sufferers are generally considered to be bewitched and consult a traditional healer. If there is no improvement, the sufferer asks to be killed to prevent the transformation. It is believed to be a form of anxiety state (Leff, 1988).

Amok occurs in the area of the Philippines and Malaysia. Characteristically, a male villager receives a real or imagined insult and then leaves the village and goes into the wilds, where he eats nothing and is socially isolated. He returns to the village in a blind fury and attempts to kill every living thing that he encounters. This only stops when he himself is killed, or caught and securely bound.

Latah has the same geographical distribution as *Amok*, but is also found in Burma (*Yuan*), Thailand (*Bah-tsche*), Philippines (*Mali-mali*), Siberia (*Myriachit*), Lapland (Lapp panic), among the Ainu of Japan (*Imu*), Madagascar (*Ramaninjana*), Malawi (*Misala*) and French Canadians of Maine (*Jumpers*). It affects predominantly women, who develop echolalia and echopraxia. There is an automatic response to commands and occasionally, coprolalia. The behaviour may be set off by a sudden shock. It is believed to be a hysterical state (Nasrallah, 1986).

Piblokto (Arctic hysteria) usually affects Eskimo women. It is regarded as being a short-lived disassociative state during which the person tears off her clothes and runs wildly or throws herself in the snow. The attack is usually followed by amnesia (Nasrallah, 1986).

Possession states occur in many cultures. The subjects are allegedly possessed by a supernatural being and their behaviour changes in accordance with this being. In traditional cultures they almost always occur in the context of a ritual which is designed to induce them. They may be valued and confer status on the possessed and are frequently of short duration. As they are culturally accepted, they are not regarded as being psychotic states despite the resemblance to delusions of control (Leff, 1988).

Eating disorders such as anorexia and bulimia nervosa can be regarded as Western culture-bound conditions linked to preoccupation with dieting and bodily shape. While the prevalence is high in the West, it is seen infrequently in developing countries.

Clinical implications

Psychiatrists need to understand their own cultural assumptions and to appreciate similarities and differences from those of patients. This understanding should then permeate routine clinical methods from a consideration of the method of greeting, the positioning of the seating within the counselling room to the elucidation of abnormalities of the mental state. Only when there is a firm grasp of the patient's subculture (and that of the doctor) can a decision be made for example as to whether or not a patient is deluded. Thus a belief in witchcraft or spirit possession in an African would not necessarily suggest a mental illness (Neki *et al.*, 1986) and a belief that a hex has been put on a patient in Mexico may not indicate paranoid ideation. An overseas African or Asian psychiatrist working in Britain may regard it strange that a depressed native Caucasian talks so little about bodily complaints, and instead complains of feeling worried or sad.

The impact of religious belief which shapes and is determined by culture is also profound in its impact on the presentation of mental illness in some countries. The Christian may lose faith and the feeling of having a personal relationship with God, and may have a heightened sense of sin and guilt when depressed. Whereas for a Muslim the cause of mental illness may be attributed to the will of Allah and daily religiosity is not regarded as excessive.

Understanding the conflict for second generation Asians between loyalty to traditional home values and Western attitudes about courtship behaviour, marriage and filial piety is necessary for a psychiatrist working with an Asian population as Anorexia nervosa and serious suicidal attempts may result. Phillip Rack, who pioneered a clinical service for Asian patients in Bradford, has described *first-order* problems relating to the use of language, diagnostic differences and the adjustment of Asian patients to a hospital routine (Rack, 1977, 1982). The need for an interpreter of language and of cultural values was emphasized, and he points out that to use a relative as interpreter was usually unsatisfactory. Even a doctor from a similar background to the patient may prove to be unsatisfactory as an interpreter because of social class differences. Such communication problems can, however, be overcome by training interpreters to understand the semantic equivalence between languages, and to become familiar with psychiatric concepts. It is nevertheless rarely possible to grasp the subtleties of family relationships adequately to make a psychodynamic formulation, even if an interpreter is used. The interpreter must have a similar code of confidentiality to the doctor. Other factors to consider when treating ethnic minority patients include an awareness of food preferences—the hospital must provide non-beef food for Hindus, and non-pork food for Muslims; the symbolic and religious importance of food and eating behaviours, as well as washing, may be in marked contrast to prevailing attitudes in the majority Caucasian society.

Second-order problems include different attitudes towards consulting behaviour. In some Asian cultures it is unusual to report a symptom other than a physical complaint to the doctor and there may be a greater expectation that the doctor will give advice; a non-directive approach to interviewing or to psychotherapy is less likely to be satisfactory.

Third-order problems are the more personal factors experienced by the psychiatrist who works 'between two cultures'. Rack noticed a tendency for these persons themselves to become marginalized and to identify to an excessive degree with the ethnic minority they were attempting to help.

A sector psychiatrist working with a multicultural population will need to decide how to provide a service for ethnic minorities. It is unlikely that a special clinical service is appropriate as this could be regarded as discriminatory. Nevertheless, a multi-professional team which includes health professionals with a specific knowledge about ethnic groups, their language and customs, is invaluable. Familiarity with the problems of elderly black patients will become increasingly important, especially if support from the extended family breaks down (Ananthanarayanan, 1989; Mays, 1989). Such Asian families are often unfamiliar with the availability of social service provisions such as meals-on-wheels and could therefore become very isolated. A religious expert is also an advantage to a multi-professional team especially when working in a multi-faith city.

Clinicians are assisted in carrying out these clinical tasks if they have an interest in social anthropology. The participant observational methods of this social science, the concept of cultural relativity, the theoretical understanding of family structures, kinship systems and ritual, are all useful in the management of patients. The lack of post-natal rituals within Western society compared with China or India may increase the likelihood of depression after childbirth. Self-esteem is then more uncertain and social support less available; the role of parenting being more ambiguous in Western society than formerly (Cox, 1988).

Research

Although transcultural research in psychiatry is, regrettably, less likely to be funded than biological research, there are nevertheless important research priorities. There is a need to understand and evaluate the 'pathway to care' for ethnic minorities and to ascertain why the Afro-Caribbean community do not use medical services regularly and consult later in the course of an illness. Studies of 'ritual' within a psychotherapy consultation, or the need to ward off misfortune at an ante-natal clinic could be worthwhile.

Murphy, in an unpublished paper, suggested various other priorities at a workshop held in Edinburgh in 1978. He emphasized that these priorities would vary with circumstance and that what was suggested for the United Kingdom would not necessarily be suitable elsewhere. He identified the short- and long-term goals shown in Table 27.1, emphasizing that both types of goal need to be

TABLE 27.1 Suggested priorities for transcultural psychiatrists' research in the United Kingdom (Murphy, unpubl.).

Short-term goals	Long-term goals
1. Improvement of clinical communication across cultures	1. Detailed case study in minorities
(a) Style of communication.	(a) Empirical observations on normal and abnormal thinking.
(b) Preparing glossaries.	(b) Ethno-psychoanalysis.
(c) Semantic differential studies.	(c) Abreaction, dreams, etc.
(d) Exploring concepts of illness, support, deviance, etc.	(d) Inter-disciplinary interviewing.
2. Improvement of diagnosis and prognosis in cultural minorities	2. Improvement of personality theory and psychological models
(a) Reassessing signs and symptoms.	(a) General personality theory.
(b) Mapping limits of normality.	(b) Psychoanalytic theory of psyche.
(c) Course and outcome studies.	(c) Integration of neurophysiological contributions.
(d) Laboratory studies.	
3. Treatment experimentation and evaluation in cultural minorities	3. Understanding cultural influences on mental illness in home society
(a) Variations in drug response.	(a) Subcultural comparisons.
(b) Effectiveness of psychotherapy.	(b) International comparisons.
(c) Assessing folk therapies.	(c) Explaining known variations.
(d) Culture-matched sociotherapy.	(d) Case-studies in depth.
4. Psychosomatic research in cultural minorities	
(a) Studies of somatic and non-verbal communication.	
(b) Differentiation of cultural from genetic.	
(c) Epidemiological studies.	
(d) Cross-cultural testing of psychoanalytic theories regarding psychosomatic disease.	

kept in view, since work serving the one type of goal does not necessarily serve the other.

It is to be hoped that more collaborative research between social anthropologists, social and biological psychiatrists will be carried out and that if the research on black communities by white psychiatrists remains a 'no go' area, black researchers will not hesitate to describe the culture and customs of the majority ethnic community which have to an extent fashioned the classification of psychiatric disorder, determined its symptoms, and influenced profoundly the availability and range of treatments.

References

American Psychiatric Association (1987). *Diagnostic and Statistical Manual of Mental Disorders*, 3rd edn. revised. Washington DC: American Psychiatric Association.

Ananthanarayanan, T.S. (1989). Cultural factors in the organization of a psychogeriatric service for elderly Asians in North Staffordshire. In: J. Cox and S. Bostock (eds) *Racial Discrimination in the Health Service*, pp. 39–50. Penrhos.

Ang, P.C. and Weller, M.P.I. (1984). Koro and psychosis. *Br. J. Psychiat.* **145**, 335.

Babiker, I.E., Cox, J.L. and Miller, P.McC. (1980). The measurement of cultural distance and its relationship to medical consultations, symptomatology and examination performance of overseas students at Edinburgh University. *Social Psychiat.* **15**, 109–116.

Ben-Tovim, D.I. and Cushnie, J.M. (1986). The prevalence of schizophrenia in a remote area of Botswana. *Br. J. Psychiat.* **148**, 576–580.

Birley, J.L.T. and Brown, G. (1970). Crises and life changes preceding the onset or relapse of acute schizophrenia: clinical aspects. *Br. J. Psychiat.* **116**, 327–333.

Brown, G., Birley, J.L.T. and Wing, J.K. (1972). Influence of family life on the course of schizophrenic disorder: a replication. *Br. J. Psychiat.* **121**, 241–258.

Burke, A.W. (1986). Racism, prejudice and mental illness. In: J.L. Cox (ed.) *Transcultural Psychiatry*. London: Croom Helm.

Carpenter, L. and Brockington, I.F. (1980). A study of mental illness in Asians, West Indians and Africans living in Manchester. *Br. J. Psychiat.* **137**, 201–205.

Carstairs, G.M. and Kapur, R.L. (1976). *The Great Universe of Kota*. London: Hogarth Press.

Cochrane, R. (1977). Mental illness in immigrants to England and Wales: an analysis of Mental Hospital Admissions, 1971. *Social Psychiat.* **12**, 25–35.

Cochrane, R. and Bal, S.S. (1977). Migration and schizophrenia: an examination of five hypotheses. *Social Psychiat.* **22**, 181–191.

Cox, J.L. (1977). Aspects of transcultural psychiatry. *Br. J. Psychiat.* **130**, 211–221.

Cox, J.L. (1979a). Psychiatric morbidity and pregnancy: a controlled study of 263 semi rural Ugandan woman. *Br. J. Psychiat.* **134**, 401–405.

Cox, J.L. (1979b). 'Amakiro': a Ugandan puerperal psychosis. *Social Psychiat.* **140**, 111–117.

Cox, J.L. (1982). Medical management culture and mental illness. *Br. J. Hosp. Med.* May, 533–537.

Cox, J.L. (1983). Postnatal depression: a comparison of Scottish and African women. *Social Psychiat.* **18**, 25–28.

Cox, J.L. (1988). The life event of childbirth: Sociocultural aspects of postnatal depression. In: R. Kumar and I.F. Brockington (eds) *Motherhood and Mental Illness. 2: Causes and Consequences*, pp. 64–75. London: Wright.

Cox, J.L. (1991). Readings about transcultural psychiatry. *Br. J. Psychiat.* **158**, 579–582.

Cox, J.L., Babiker, I.E. and Miller, P.McC. (1981). Psychiatric problems and first-year examinations in overseas students at Edinburgh University. *J. Adolescence* **4**, 261–270.

Dean, G., Walsh, D., Downing, H. and Shelley, E. (1981). First admissions of native-born and immigrants to psychiatric hospitals in South-East England 1976. *Br. J. Psychiat.* **139**, 506–512.

de Reuck, A.V.S. and Porter, R. (eds) (1965). CIBA Symposium: *Transcultural Psychiatry*. Boston: Little, Brown and Co.

Dube, K.C. (1970). A study of prevalence and biosocial variables in mental illness in a rural and an urban community in Uttar Pradesh—India. *Acta Psychiat. Scand.* **46**, 327–359.

Elnagar, M.N., Maitra, P. and Rao, M.N. (1971). Mental health in an Indian rural community. *Br. J. Psychiat.* **118**, 499–503.

Engel, G.L. (1980). The clinical application of the biopsychosocial model. *Am. J. Psychiat.* **137**, 223–226.

Fernando, S. (1988). *Race and Culture in Psychiatry*. London: Croom Helm.

Foulks, E.F. (1980). The concept of culture in psychiatric residency education. *Am. J. Psychiat.* **137**, 811–816.

German, G.A. (1987). Mental health in Africa: I. The extent of mental health problems in Africa today. An update of epidemiological knowledge. *Br. J. Psychiat.* **151**, 435–439.

Gillis, L.S., Lewis, J.B. and Slabbert, M. (1968). Psychiatric disorder amongst the coloured people of the Cape Peninsula. *Br. J. Psychiat.* **114**, 1575–1587.

Gullahorn, J.T. and Gullahorn, J.F. (1963). An extension of the U curve hypothesis. *J. Social Issues* **19**, 33–47.

Harrison, G., Owens, D., Holton, A., Neilson, D. and Boot, D. (1988). A prospective study of severe mental disorder in Afro-Caribbean patients. *Psychol. Med.* **18**, 643–657.

Hemsi, L.K. (1967). Psychiatric morbidity of West Indian immigrants. *Social Psychiat.* **2**, 95–100.

Henley, A. (1979). *The Asian Patients in Hospital and at Home.* London: The Kings Fund.

Herz, D.G. (1988). Identity—lost and found: patterns of migration and psychological and psychosocial adjustment of migrants. *Acta Psychiat. Scand.* **78** (Suppl. 344), 159–165.

Kato, M. (1969). Psychiatric epidemiological surveys in Japan: The problem of case finding. In: W. Caudill and T. Lin (eds) *Mental Health Research in Asia and the Pacific.* Hawaii: East–West Center Press.

Kiev, A. (1972). *Transcultural Psychiatry.* Harmondsworth, Middx: Penguin.

Kleinman, A. (1980). *Patients and Healers in the Context of Culture.* Berkeley, CA: University of California Press.

Kleinman, A. (1987). Anthropology and psychiatry. The role of culture in cross-cultural research on illness. *Br. J. Psychiat.* **151**, 447–454.

Kleinman, A. (1988). *Rethinking Psychiatry: from Cultural Category to Personal Experience.* New York. The Free Press.

Krausz, E. (1972). *Ethnic Minorities in Britain.* London: Paladin.

Krupinski, J., Stoller, A. and Wallace, L. (1973). Psychiatric disorder in Eastern European refugees now in Australia. *Social Sci. Med.* **7**, 31.

Lee, E. (1965). A theory of migration. Reprinted in J.A. Jackson (ed.) (1969). *Migration: Sociological Studies.* Cambridge: Cambridge University Press.

Leff, J.P. (1974). Transcultural influences on psychiatrists' rating of verbally expressed emotion. *Br. J. Psychiat.* **125**, 336–340.

Leff, J.P. (1986). The epidemiology of mental illness across cultures. In: J.L. Cox (ed.) *Transcultural Psychiatry.* London: Croom Helm.

Leff, J. (1988). *Psychiatry Around the Globe: A Transcultural View.* London: Gaskell Press.

Leff, J.P., Wig, N.N., Ghosh, A. *et al.* (1987). Expressed emotion and schizophrenia in North India. III. Influence of relatives' expressed emotion on the course of schizophrenia in Chandigarh. *Br. J. Psychiat,* **151**, 156–173.

Lefley, H.P. (1990). Culture and chronic mental illness. *Hosp. and Commun. Psychiat.* **41**, 277–286.

Leighton, A.H. (1959). *My Name is Legion: Foundations for a Theory of Man in Relation to Culture.* New York: Basic Books.

Leininger, M. (1978). *Transcultural Nursing, Concepts, Theories, Practices.* New York: Wiley.

Lewis, I.M. (1976). *Social Anthropology in Perspective.* London: Penguin.

Lin, T. (1953). A study of the incidence of mental disorder in Chinese and other cultures. *Psychiatry* **16**, 313–336.

Littlewood, R. and Lipsedge, M. (1981). Some social phenomenological characteristics of psychotic immigrants. *Psychol. Med.* **11**, 289–302.

Littlewood, R. and Lipsedge, M. (1982). *Aliens and Alienists. Ethnic Minorities and Psychiatry.* London: Penguin.

Littlewood, R. and Lipsedge, M. (1986). The culture-bound syndromes of the dominant culture: culture, psychopathology and biomedicine. In: J.L. Cox (ed.) *Transcultural Psychiatry.* London: Croom Helm.

Mavreas, V. and Bebbington, P. (1990). Acculturation and psychiatric disorder: a study of Greek Cypriot immigrants. *Psychol. Med.* **20**, 941–951.

Mays, N. (1989). Health and social status of elderly Asians in Leicester: a survey. In: J. Cox and S. Bostock (eds) *Racial Discrimination in the Health Service*, pp. 51, 68. Newcastle-under-Lyme: Penrhos.

McGovern, D. and Cope, R. (1987). First psychiatric admission rates of first and second generation Afro-Caribbeans. *Social Psychiat.* **122**, 139–149.

Murphy, H.B.M. (1982). *Comparative Psychiatry.* Berlin: Springer-Verlag.

Nandi, D.N., Mukherjee, S.P., Boral, G.C. *et al.* (1980). Socio-economic status and mental morbidity in certain tribes and castes in India. *Br. J. Psychiat.* **136**, 73–85.

Nasrallah, H.A. (1986). Special and unusual psychiatric syndromes. In: G. Winokur and P. Clayton (eds) *The Medical Basis of Psychiatry.* Philadelphia: W.B. Saunders.

Neki, J.S., Joinet, B., Ndosi, G., Kilonzo, G., Hauli, J.G. and Duvinage, G. (1986). Witchcraft and psychotherapy. *Br. J. Psychiat.* **149**, 145–155.

Ødegaard, Ø. (1932). Emigration and insanity. *Acta Psychiat. Neurol. Scand. (Copenhagen)* **7** (Suppl. 4), 206.

Orley, J.H. and Wing, J.K. (1979). Psychiatric disorders in two African villages. *Arch. Gen. Psychiat.* **36**, 513–520.

Orley, F., Jamieson, R., Mullaney, J. and Davison, K. (1986). Koro—a psychophysiological dysfunction? *Br. J. Psychiat.* **148**, 212–214.

Oyebode, F., Jamieson, R., Mullaney, J. and Davison, K. (1986). Koro—a psychophysiological dysfunction? *Br. J. Psychiat.* **148**, 212–214.

Pinto, R.T. (1970). *A Study of Psychiatric Illness Among Asians in the Camberwell area.* MPhil Thesis, University of London.

Rack, P.H. (1977). Some practical problems in providing a psychiatric service for immigrants. *Mental Hlth Society* **4**, 144–151.

Rack, P.H. (1982). *Race, Culture and Mental Disorder.* London: Tavistock.

Rack, P.H. (1986). Migration and mental illness. In: J.L. Cox (ed.) *Transcultural Psychiatry.* London: Croom Helm.

Rack, P.H. (1988). Psychiatric and social problems among immigrants. *Acta Psychiat. Scand.* **78** (Suppl. 344), 167–173.

Reed, B., Hutton, J. and Bazalgett, J. (1978). *Freedom to Study. Requirements of Overseas Students in the UK.* London: Overseas Students Trust.

Royal College of Psychiatrists (1990). *Report of the Special Committee on Psychiatric Practice and Training in British Multi-Ethnic Society.* London: Royal College of Psychiatrists.

Royes, K. (1961). The incidence and features of psychosis in a Caribbean community. In: *Proceedings of the Third World Congress of Psychiatry*, Montreal 1961, pp. 1121–1125. University of Toronto Press and McGill University Press.

Rubel, A.J., O'Neill, C.W. and Collado-Ardon, R. (1984). *Susto, A Folk Illness.* Berkeley, CA: University of California Press.

Sashidharan, S.P. (1986). Ideology and politics in transcultural psychiatry. In: J.C. Cox (ed.) *Transcultural Psychiatry.* London: Croom Helm.

Sethi, B.B., Gupta, S.C., Mahendru, R.K. and Kumari, R. (1974). Mental health and urban life: a study of 850 families. *Br. J. Psychiat.* **124**, 243–247.

Stevens, J.R. and Wyatt, R.J. (1987). Similar incidence worldwide of schizophrenia: case not proven. *Br. J. Psychiat.* **151**, 131–132.

Toffler, A. (1970). *Future Shock.* London: Corgi.

Torrey, E.F. (1987). Similar incidence worldwide of schizophrenia: case not proven. *Br. J. Psychiat.* **151**, 132–133.

Triseliotis, J. (1986). Transcultural social work. In: J.L. Cox (ed.) *Transcultural Psychiatry.* London: Croom Helm.

Verma, S.K. and Wig, M.M. (1976). PGI Health Questionnaire N-2: construction and initial try outs. *Indian J. Clin. Psychol.* **3**, 135–142.

Walter, P.A.F. (1952). *Race and Culture Relations.* New York: McGraw-Hill Co. Inc.

Weller, M.P.I. (1985). Koro. *Br. J. Psychiat.* **146**, 452.

Westermeyer, J. (1988). National differences in psychiatric morbidity: methodological issues, scientific interpretations and social implications. *Acta Psychiat. Scand.* **78** (Suppl. 344), 23–32.

Wilkinson, C.B. (ed.) (1986). *Ethnic Psychiatry.* London: Plenum Medical Book Co.

Wing, J.K., Cooper, J.E. and Sartorius, N. (1974). *The Measurement and Classification of Psychiatric Symptoms.* London: Cambridge University Press.

World Health Organization (1973). *The International Pilot Study of Schizophrenia*, Vol. 1. Geneva, WHO.

Yap, P.M. (1951). Mental disease peculiar to certain cultures: a survey of comparative psychiatry. *J. Ment. Sci.* **97**, 313–327.

Yap, P.M. (1965). Koro—a culture-bound depersonalization syndrome. *Br. J. Psychiat.* **111**, 43–50.

Zwingmann, C.A.A. and Gunn, A.D.G. (1983). *Uprooting and Health; Psychosocial Problems of Students from Abroad.* Geneva: World Health Organization.

— 28

Life-events

F. Creed

Introduction

Early anectodal reports linking the onset of illness to stressful life-events have been followed by numerous systematic studies examining this relationship. The studies fall into two broad categories. Firstly, single events, such as bereavement or unemployment, have been studied to see whether illness follows more frequently than would be expected by chance. Secondly, the onset of individual disorders has been examined in terms of preceding life-events. Both strategies invite the question 'does the experience of a stressful life-event increase the chance of illness?'. But research in this area has moved on to answer a more sophisticated question: 'which life-events lead to illness, and under what circumstances?'.

It must be appreciated that much life-events research is still at the stage of observing associations. A simple association between life-events and illness onset does not necessarily indicate causality. If a group of patients admitted with pancreatitis are found to have had more contacts with the police over the preceding year compared to a healthy comparison group, this does not necessarily imply that contact with the police causes pancreatitis! It is much more likely that an underlying common factor, alcohol consumption, is responsible for the association between contact with the police and pancreatitis. Similarly, a positive association between admission for depressive illness and work problems over the preceding weeks does not necessarily imply that the work problems cause depression. It is more likely that the insidious onset of depression led to a deterioration in work performance.

In the first example there was a common factor leading to both life-events and disorder; in the second example the life-events were a result of the illness itself. It is necessary to overcome these methodological problems if one is to demonstrate that life-events actually cause illness (Cooke, 1986). A number of strategies have been developed to this end and these will be briefly reviewed. The pattern of life-events in certain disorders will then be considered.

Measurement of Life-events

The problems of obtaining a reliable measure of events has been the subject of many reviews (Brown and Harris, 1978; Paykel, 1983; Brown, 1989). Dohrenwend *et al.* (1987) stated that there were very few case/control life-event studies that 'meet even minimal criteria for adequacy', including use of appropriate controls, assessing which events and circumstances occur independently of the subjects' prior mental state and behaviour, and attempting to date the occurrence of events in relation to episodes of illness.

This statement arises because 90% of studies have used self-administered questionnaires which are unreliable; some have been shown to have a test–retest reliability of as low as 0.2 (Cohen and Wills, 1985). A reliable retrospective interview method has been used only in a minority of studies. These interviews can achieve an inter-rater reliability of 75–92% but are lengthy and expensive in research time. The differences between a self-administered questionnaire and an interview method will be demonstrated by comparing the questionnaire 'Schedule of Recent Experience' (SRE—Holmes and Rahe, 1967) and the lengthy 'Life-Events and Difficulties Schedule' interview (LEDS—Brown and Harris, 1978), as these are the most widely used instruments.

Accurate recall

If events are being collected retrospectively, say for one year prior to the onset of an illness, it is essential to check that respondents can accurately remember life-events over that period of time. Self-administered questionnaires which simply ask respondents to tick life-events on a list make no specific attempt to prompt respondents or check the accuracy of the replies (Jenkins *et al.*, 1979). Later interviews have shown that as many as one-third of events are missed by such questionnaires (Klein and Rubovits, 1987). There is also considerable 'fall-off' of number of events recalled per month with increasing time before interview. This suggests respondents have difficulty recalling events which occurred some months prior to the questionnaire.

Unacceptable rates of fall-off are provided by self-administered questionnaires (about 5% per month) compared with fall-off rates of only 1% per month using the interviews of Paykel (1983), and the LEDS, provided that the interviewer has been adequately trained (Brown and Harris, 1982). For severe events (defined below) the rate of fall-off is even less—0.36% per month for a new German interview method (Wittchen *et al.*, 1989) and as low as 2.9% *per year* with the LEDS over a ten year retrospective study (Neilson *et al.*, 1989). Such a low rate of fall-off is possible because interviews take considerable trouble to prompt the person's memory using probes and reminders (e.g. Brown and Harris, 1978; Wittchen *et al.*, 1989) (Figure 28.1).

Exact dating of illness onset and independence of events

It is not sufficiently appreciated that the life-events research method is only really applicable for illnesses that have a clear dateable onset. Only under these

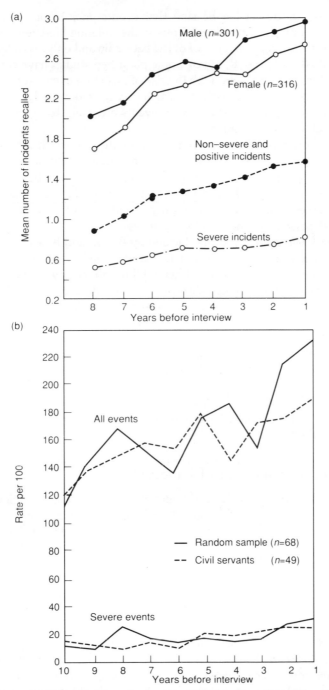

FIG. 28.1 (a) Mean number of events recalled by all male and female subjects and subdivided according to their severity rating (redrawn from Wittchen *et al.*, 1989). (b) Rate of events in ten 1-year periods before interview (redrawn from Neilson *et al.*, 1989). Note low rate of 'fall-off' for severe events.

circumstances can the researcher be sure that events *prior* to onset are being considered in the etiology of the illness. Thus studies relating life-events and back pain must first establish the date of *onset* of the back pain and only consider events prior to that date (Craufurd *et al.*, 1990). Some published studies have considered events prior to the *clinic attendance*, with the risk of including events such as 'being off work' or 'reduction of social contacts' which may have occurred *after* the back pain commenced (Leavitt *et al.*, 1979). Such events are likely to be the result of the back pain rather than its cause.

With many psychiatric illnesses, even when a date of onset has been established, the researcher may be concerned that the patient's behaviour is affected because of the developing illness. This behaviour may bring about such life-events as loss of job or marital separation. As a check on this fact it has become customary to assess the results using only events which can definitely be regarded as independent of the developing illness.

This notion of *independence* was first tackled by Brown and Birley (1968), who interviewed patients and their relatives to ascertain life-events that preceded relapse of schizophrenia. If a patient lost his job through factory closure, this was clearly independent of the ensuing schizophrenic episode. However, job loss for any other reason might mean that the person's declining performance was responsible; this could have been an early symptom of the schizophrenia. The excess of events occurring in the three weeks prior to the relapse was therefore checked using only such independent events—the excess remained.

A self-administered questionnaire has no way of controlling for such independent events. In fact the SRE has been criticized for including many items which might be due to developing psychiatric illness; it also includes a number of actual *symptoms*: loss of sleep or change in eating pattern (Dohrenwend and Dohrenwend, 1978)!

Definition and measurement of life-events

The schizophrenia study involved the development of the interview, now referred to as the 'Life-Events and Difficulties Schedule' (LEDS). This instrument carefully defines each life-event so that a researcher requires training to become familiar with the criteria for inclusion. For example, being off work for the subject has to last four weeks or more to be included; if it is the breadwinner who is off work, the minimum time is eight weeks. These exact definitions are required to ensure accurate measurement and to ensure that identical standards are applied to the experimental and control groups. A depressed person may, because of his or her current mental state, see the past weeks as full of problematic events and record more life-events on a questionnaire than a healthy comparison subject simply because of the depression (Cohen *et al.*, 1988). Such a spurious result is avoided if strict criteria are applied independent of the person's mental state.

The problem is not confined to depression. In an early study mothers who had given birth to a Down's syndrome child were more likely to report that they had experienced 'emotional shocks' during pregnancy than mothers of normal children (Stott, 1958). This reflected their attempt to understand what had happened and were searching after a reason for their abnormal child. This phenomenon, known as 'effort after meaning', applies to all ill subjects and must be prevented from causing bias in any study comparing ill patients compared to a healthy control group.

Scoring events

Once an event has been established it must be scored in some way. All life-events measures pay heed to the notion that the experience of bereavement is different from that of a routine job change. The 'Schedule of Recent Experience' (SRE) used the concept of 'life change units' and gave each life-event a weighted score which was derived empirically using death of spouse as 100 life change units and marriage as 50. Other measures select unpleasant or stressful events and compare the rate of such events in two populations. Such events have been categorized as: undesirable, uncontrollable, exit (from the person's social sphere), major role loss, severe threat.

Other scoring systems have also been devised. The LEDS, for example uses a four-point scale of threat or unpleasantness and applies this rating to both immediate and longer term threat. Thus involvement in an accident may carry high short-term threat (grade 1 for one or two days) but if there are no lasting consequences the long-term threat will be minimal (grade 4 for the ensuing weeks). The latter would be higher if there was serious injury and/or financial consequences extending over weeks or months. Other events, such as diagnosis of cancer in a spouse, marital separation, bereavement or a court appearance when charged with a serious crime, carry high threat both at the time of discovery (short-term) and one week later (long-term threat). Events that carry high long-term threat are known as 'severe events' and are associated with the onset of depression.

The LEDS is especially careful about awarding a degree of threat to a particular event. To avoid bias from the respondent's mental state, the interviewer relays the objective circumstances of the event to a group of experienced researchers *without* stating whether the subject was in the experimental or control group. The group then make a consensus rating, taking into account the circumstances of that individual at that time. This is in contrast to the SRE, which has a standard rating for all individuals for each event. Thus, with the LEDS the theft of a car would be assessed according to an individual's circumstance; it could be very serious for a person who depends on the car to go to work and to keep in touch with friends and family, yet who has no insurance and no possibility of replacing the car. It would be much less serious for a person who has a company car that is immediately replaced. On the SRE both would be awarded the same number of life change units.

The LEDS compares two populations according to the number of subjects in each group who have experienced a particular type of event, e.g. severe event. The SRE scoring system assumes that the effect of events is additive and adds up life change units. However, this may lead to absurd results. Brown and Harris calculated that a young man who had recently been awarded a scholarship

TABLE 28.1   Comparison of 'Schedule of Recent Events' (SRE) with 'Life-events and Difficulties Schedule' (LEDS).

'Schedule of Recent Events'	'Life-events and Difficulties Schedule'
1. Respondent-based: vague items mean that respondent decides on criteria for inclusion as an event.	1. Observer-based: previously defined criteria for inclusion and research group determined rating of severity.
2. Includes symptoms of illness and illness-related events.	2. Excludes symptoms *and* any illness-related events.
3. Standard life change units for each person.	3. Individual meaning of event considered.
4. Severity scale based on 'life change'.	4. Severity scale based on 'threat'.
5. Assumes 'additivity' of events.	5. No additivity assumed and subjects categorized as experiencing a 'severe' event or not.
6. All events over 6 months period counted together.	6. Exact timing of events.
7. Decrease of life change units with time prior to illness assumed to imply life change units related to illness onset.	7. Allows fall-off of reporting to be measured.
8. Events and ongoing difficulties not separated.	8. Events and difficulties rated as separate etiological agents.

at Oxford could gain a total score of 79 life change units (end of formal schooling = 26, outstanding personal achievements = 28, a vacation = 13, Christmas = 12). This score of 79 would be greater than that for a man whose wife has left him, which would produce a score of 65!

The main differences between an interview method and a self-administered questionnaire are demonstrated in Table 28.1.

Life-events in Depression and Schizophrenia

The first LEDS study compared 50 patients following a relapse of schizophrenia with 325 normal subjects, assessing life-events over the preceding three months. There was a clear increase in the number of subjects experiencing an event in the three weeks prior to the relapse of the schizophrenic episode compared to the earlier three weeks and the control group (Table 28.2). This increase was retained if only events of little or no threat were considered; thus relatively minor events, such as promotion or an uncomplicated house move, were associated with the relapse of schizophrenia. The results also held when only independent events were considered, ruling out a spurious result from including events which might have been a consequence of the illness.

The next major study concerned depression; for this purpose 114 in-patients and out-patients at the Maudsley Hospital and 37 women in the community with recent onset of depression were compared with 382 normal women in the

TABLE 28.2   Percentage with at least one event in the four 3-week periods before onset (schizophrenic patients, $n = 50$) and interview general population ($n = 325$) (from Brown and Harris, 1978).

	3-week periods before onset/interview			
	Furthest 4th[b] (%)	3rd[b] (%)	2nd[b] (%)	1st[a] (%)
	Independent events			
1. Schizophrenic patients	14	8	14	46
General population	15	15	14	14
	Possibly independent events			
2. Schizophrenic patients	16	10	6	22
General population	6	5	5	5
	All events			
3. Schizophrenic patients	30	18	20	60
General population	21	20	18	19

[a] $p < 0.001$ in all three groups.
[b] No differences are significant.

community. Life-events were elicited for a full 12 months prior to the onset of the depression or prior to the interview, in the case of healthy comparison women. The results were again clear. During the 38 weeks prior to the onset of depression (or date of interview) 61% of depressed patients (68% of depressed women in the community) had experienced a severe event compared to 20% of controls ($p < 0.001$). This result held for the three weeks prior to onset but did *not* hold for all events, or those of mild or no threat; it was only events with a severe threat which were more common among the depressed group.

This is the first major difference in the life-events preceding the two conditions—events of all magnitudes were related to the onset of schizophrenia, but only severe events were associated with the onset of depression. A similar finding has been reported elsewhere (Jacobs *et al.*, 1974; Dohrenwend *et al.*, 1987). In the Dohrenwend study 'independent fateful events', such as death of a close relative, and serious physical illness and injury affecting the subject, were significantly more frequent in depressed patients than in either schizophrenic patients or healthy controls.

The second difference occurred in the timing. Whereas an increase in the number of subjects experiencing an event occurred in both illnesses during the three week period before onset, in depression the difference was observed as far back as nine months prior to onset. The relative importance of the timing of events prior to the onset of an illness can be understood by reference to the concept of 'brought-forward time'. This mathematical calculation makes an assumption that the episode of schizophrenia or depression would have occurred sooner or later anyway, but the episode is brought-forward by the experience of a life-event. The mathematical calculation explores the difference between the ill population and normal controls. It is very similar to the epidemiological measure of relative risk (Paykel, 1978).

The brought-forward time for schizophrenia was a mere ten weeks. This is a short time and has led to the conclusion that a relapse of schizophrenia was likely to happen fairly soon and that the experience of a life-event has brought this forward only a short period in time. In depression the brought-forward time was nearly two years, leading Brown and Harris to conclude that the experience of a severe life-event is in some way formative rather than simply a trigger, i.e. the episode of depression might well not have occurred were it not for the experience of the severe life-event.

Brown and Harris (1978) calculated the brought-forward time for other studies; in Paykel's depression study (Paykel et al., 1969) it was 2.7 years for exit events, and for Parkes' study of bereavement it was 2.5 years (Parkes, 1964).

It is important to note that the research in schizophrenia was concerned with relapse. However, there have been two subsequent studies which have looked at first onset of schizophrenia; the results were essentially similar. At six centres around the world Day et al. (1987) found a significant increase in the proportion of schizophrenic patients who had experienced an event in the three weeks prior to onset. An advantage of this study was the selection of patients with a clear dateable onset of psychosis. The results held even when 'independent' events were analysed separately. The American study (Dohrenwend et al., 1987) confirmed a similar pattern of events prior to onset and relapse of schizophrenia; the particular category of event associated with schizophrenia was that which disrupted social support.

The results for depression have been repeated many times with similar results to the original study. There have been ten population studies using the LEDS and 11 studies of psychiatric patients using an acceptable methodology (Brown and Harris, 1989a, pp. 55–56). The total results for the population studies indicated that 68% of 312 onset cases of depression in the community had experienced a severe event in the previous 38 weeks compared to 32% of 1745 non-cases in the community. When the figure included major difficulties as well as severe events, the proportion of the cases rose to 84% compared to 32% of controls. A major difficulty is defined as an on-going stress, e.g. nursing a sick relative, which does not take the form of a discrete change during the period of study. Difficulties are scored in an identical way to events.

Vulnerability

Paykel (1978) has clearly demonstrated that most people who experience a severe life-event do not develop depression. Using data from his own research he noted that 25% of depressed patients had experienced an exit event during the previous six months compared to 5% of healthy controls. He extrapolated these figures in a theoretical way to 10 000 subjects in the general population. If 2% of subjects become depressed during a six-month period, then 200 new depressives can be compared with the 9800 non-depressed subjects. Since 25% of the former have experienced an exit event this will have occurred in 50 subjects. In addition, 5%

of the 9800 non-depressed subjects will have experienced an exit event = 490 exit events in the non-depressed group. Thus of 540 exit events only 50 (9%) will lead to the subject becoming depressed. Some authors have tried to argue that this represents a weak effect of life-events in the etiology of depression; others have argued that additional factors must be considered in conjunction with the event experience. Such additional factors are known as vulnerability factors in the model of Brown and Harris (1978).

The original Camberwell study of Brown and Harris demonstrated four vulnerability factors involved in an inner city urban female population. These were:

1. Lack of a close confiding relationship with a husband or cohabitee;
2. Loss of mother before the age of 11 years;
3. Lack of employment outside the home; and
4. Presence of three or more children under 14 living at home.

The presence of one or more of these vulnerability factors increases the chance of depression *if the woman also experiences a severe event or major difficulty*. Thus of the women who had a close confiding relationship with their husband and who also experienced a severe event or major difficulty, only 10% developed depression compared to 41% of women who experienced a severe event but had no such confiding relationship. The more vulnerability factors present the greater the chance of depression if the woman experienced a severe event or major difficulty.

Vulnerability factors were studied in an identical way in a later study in the Outer Hebrides (Brown and Prudo, 1981; Prudo *et al.*, 1981). Two were similar (lack of a confiding relationship, three or more children at home) but the others were different; lack of regular church-going and not living in a croft. The latter indicated the degree of integration into the local community—lack of integration made depression more likely. One other interesting finding emerged from the comparison of the Hebridean and South London women; the prevalence of depression was lower in the Hebrides. This could be attributed to the lower frequency of certain types of severe events: disruptive events, such as broken close relationships, burglaries and marked financial difficulties. Other categories of event, including illnesses and deaths were similar.

Concern has been expressed about the events–vulnerability model because the way of ascribing a threat rating with the LEDS might use data which defines vulnerability; an event might have been rated severe partly because of the woman's unsupported status—i.e. without a confiding relationship (Tennant *et al.*, 1981a). However, later studies have allowed Brown and Harris to test their vulnerability factors prospectively.

The large Islington study of the Bedford College Group (Brown *et al.*, 1986a) assessed 400 women in the community on two occasions one year apart. Of those who experienced a severe event during this time one-fifth developed depression. These women, compared to the remaining four-fifths, were more likely to be without a close confiding relationship at the first interview. The importance of an apparently close relationship reported at the first interview was further tested to see if the support really was forthcoming when a severe event occurred. Those women who enjoyed crisis support at the time of the severe event did indeed enjoy some protection against depression. An additional vulnerability factor emerged from this study—low self-esteem recorded at the first interview was predictive of depression at follow-up.

Again there is a theoretical problem—could low self-esteem be an indicator of pre-existing depression at a subclinical level rather than a true vulnerability factor? Two studies using multiple regression have examined this possibility and demonstrated that even after variance attributed to pre-existing depression is taken into account, there is an additional effect attributable to low self-esteem (Brown et al., 1986b; Miller et al., 1989). Miller and colleagues found the following sequence: first, a life-event occurred which involved severe stress within a close relationship (rows and arguments with someone close to the subject). This led to low self-esteem. A second stressful event of any type would then lead to the onset of major depression.

The Bedford College group have also evolved a model which linked the various vulnerability factors (Bifulco et al., 1987; Harris et al., 1987). Loss of mother as a child was only related to the later development of depression when inadequate parenting was involved. This was reflected in early adult life both in pre-marital pregnancy and an unsatisfactory 'marital' relationship. Thus loss of mother when young, lack of a supportive husband, unemployment and having several young children at home become associated with low self-esteem. These factors are all more common in lower social class women, who experience a higher prevalence of depression than those in the higher social classes.

Life-events and recovery from depression

The longitudinal study of the Bedford group also allowed study of the events and difficulties associated with recovery from depression. Twenty-six women, suffering from chronic depression at the first interview, had recovered by the second interview. They were compared with the women who continued to be depressed; recovery was associated with reduction in chronic difficulties and the experience of 'fresh start' events. The latter usually occurred in the context of considerable hardship, and rehousing, starting a new relationship or similar change represented the opportunity for a fresh start. Others have found that reduction in difficulties or events which 'neutralize' the adverse effects of previous severe life-events (e.g. starting a new close relationship neutralizes the adverse effect of the previous broken one) are associated with improvement in depression (Tennant et al., 1981b; Parker et al., 1986; Miller et al., 1987).

Continued relationship difficulties and/or further threatening events prevent recovery from depression (Paykel and Tanner, 1976; Parker et al., 1985; Miller et al., 1987) and life-events are also as associated with relapse of schizophrenia (Leff et al., 1973).

Vulnerability and unemployment

The role of vulnerability factors has also been demonstrated in recent studies of unemployment: a single life-event, which is increasingly studied. A small but careful retrospective study in London (Eales, 1988) found that depression was more likely to occur following unemployment in those who had experienced pre-existing financial or occupational difficulties, shyness and lack of intimacy with a wife or girlfriend. Others have found financial hardship and the lack of a marital partner/cohabitee predict depression at the time of becoming unemployed (Warr and Jackson, 1985; Jacobson, 1987; Heather et al., 1987).

One study concerned the wives of men made redundant (Penkower et al., 1988); 18.4% of the women with unemployed husbands were highly symptomatic (on the SCL-90) compared to 12.3% of women whose husbands remained employed—a small difference. However, the additional effect of three vulnerability factors—family psychiatric history, financial difficulties and low support from relatives—significantly increased the proportion of variance explained.

Life-Events and Other Conditions

No other condition has been studied as extensively as depression; the main results for several other conditions will be considered in this section.

Anxiety

In order to compare anxiety and depression, Finlay-Jones and Brown (1981) studied life-events in patients presenting to their general practitioner. Similar sized groups of patients with anxiety, depression and mixed symptoms were studied and in each group practically all the subjects had experienced a severe event in the preceding year compared to only one-third of comparison subjects. However, the nature of the severe events differed; loss events preceded depression (such as loss of a valued person through death or separation or loss of the respondent's physical health), whereas danger events preceded anxiety. The latter involved some kind of future threat to the subject, such as being told that a bodily symptom might be cancer or involvement in a love affair, where the consequences of discovery would be disastrous to the subject.

One other study compared the events prior to depression and anxiety (Miller and Ingham, 1985). Events prior to depression involved threat and loss. Those preceding anxiety involved threat or uncertainty of outcome—but not loss.

Faravelli and Pallanti (1989) also found that, compared to control subjects, severe events were more common before the onset of DSM-III panic disorder or agoraphobia with panic attacks. The difference remained significant when only independent events were considered. This study found that loss, rather than danger events, were involved, perhaps reflecting the likeness of panic disorder patients to depressives rather than the 'pure' anxiety seen in the general practice setting of the London study.

Mania

Results concerning mania are conflicting. Although several studies appear to have shown a link between life-events and the onset of mania, most have not used an interview method of assessment or determined the exact date of onset (Sclare and Creed, 1990). Only three studies used an interview method which allowed independent events to be assessed; one found a significant relationship between severe events and the onset of mania (Kennedy *et al.*, 1983) and two did not (Chung *et al.*, 1986; Sclare and Creed, 1990). However, the Kennedy study examined life-events before admission, not onset of symptoms, and there appears to be a considerable delay between onset of first manic symptom and admission (Winokur *et al.*, 1969; Sclare and Creed, 1990). During this time events may well be related to the illness, especially as the most common events involve work and close relationship difficulties, which might arise with early hypomanic irritability.

An interesting example of the study of a single life-event is relevant here. Aronson and Shukla (1987) noted that 14% of lithium clinic attenders relapsed when exposed to the catastrophic effects of a hurricane, whereas 86% remained well. Those authors suggested that there is a subgroup of affective disorder patients who are liable to relapse into mania when exposed to environmental stress.

Self-poisoning patients

It has long been recognized that deliberate self-harm is preceded by adverse life-events; the interest lies in comparing these patients with those included in other life-events studies. Paykel *et al.* (1975) reported twice as many events in the six months prior to a suicide attempt than for a comparable time before the onset of depression. Farmer and Creed (1989) also found an increased rate of severe events for the three week period prior to self-poisoning, and throughout the preceding year. The excess involved events that were not independent— commonly broken relationships and contact with police/court appearance. This, coupled with the finding that the total number of severe events reported for the year correlated with extrapunitive hostility, indicates the importance of underlying personality in relationship to life-events in this group of patients. This finding accords with the observation that loss of mother as a child was associated with suicidal plans or acts among depressed women in the community. The early loss was thought to bring out hostile and attention-seeking behaviours when the woman becomes depressed (Brown *et al.*, 1985).

The Farmer and Creed study (1989) compared two groups of deliberate self-poisoning patients: those with a depressive illness and those without. The pattern of preceding events was similar but the depressed subjects had experienced significantly more chronic difficulties over several months prior to the self-poisoning. It may have been the additional stress of a severe life-event together with an ongoing difficulty that was related to depression. Such 'difficulty-related' events have been shown to be especially potent in causing hopelessness (Brown *et al.*, 1987), which may be related to the self-poisoning. Similarly, Slater and Depue (1981) demonstrated that a high incidence of exit events *after* the onset of depression was associated with parasuicide in depressed patients.

Physical illness

Having established that severely threatening events are related to the onset of depression, anxiety and the act of self-poisoning, and that events of any threat are related to the onset of schizophrenia, we are now in a position to turn to physical illnesses. These have previously been reviewed (Creed, 1985; Brown and Harris, 1989b) and only the studies using the LEDS will be mentioned here.

The measurement of life-events prior to the onset of physical illness is often easier than that of psychiatric illness because a sudden, dateable onset of symptoms often occurs, e.g. in myocardial infarction, appendicitis, cerebro-vascular accident, in contrast to the insidious onset of a depressive or psychotic illness. Comparison groups may be available who have similar symptoms but belong to a different diagnostic group (e.g. appendicectomy—inflamed or normal) so life-events can be measured by an interviewer blind to the eventual diagnosis. It may also be possible to interview the patients within a few days or weeks of the onset of illness.

Two studies of gastrointestinal disorder will illustrate these points. The first study chose patients undergoing appendicectomy as a group of subjects who could be interviewed shortly after the onset of their abdominal pain, but before the pathology (appendicitis or a normal appendix) had been ascertained (Creed, 1981). This meant that the patient, interviewer and event raters were all blind to the eventual diagnosis. There was a striking difference between the groups: 60% of patients whose appendix was categorized as 'not acutely inflamed' had experienced a severely threatening event in the 38 weeks prior to the onset of their abdominal pain, compared to 25% of the appendicitis and 20% of the healthy comparison group. These figures are remarkably similar to those for the original Camberwell study of Brown and Harris (1978) mentioned above.

The experiment was repeated in patients presenting to a gastroenterology clinic (Craig and Brown, 1984). It was necessary to select patients who had a dateable onset of abdominal pain during the six months prior to clinic attendance. Once again the patients could be interviewed to ascertain preceding life-events before it was known whether they had an organic cause for their abdominal pain (e.g. peptic ulcer) or no specific pathology was found: irritable bowel syndrome or functional dyspepsia. The results were similar to the appendicectomy study—67% of the functional abdominal pain group had experienced a severe event or chronic difficulty compared to 23% of the organic and community comparison groups.

These results could indicate that functional abdominal pain (including normal appendix) patients simply had depression and were presenting with abdominal pain. Indeed, there was a higher proportion of psychiatric cases among the functional groups than the organic groups but the majority did not have psychiatric disorder. The proportion of the functional group who had experienced a severe event (approximately two-thirds of patients) was similar whether or not psychiatric disorder was present. This was not so for those with organic disorder. Whereas 50% of patients with peptic ulcer and psychiatric disorder had experienced a severe event, for patients with organic disease and *no* psychiatric disorder the proportion was 25%, i.e. similar to healthy controls.

The results so far make it clear that onset of organic disease, in the absence of psychiatric disorder, is not associated with preceding severe life-events, confirming the results of Murphy and Brown in a community study (1980). Examination of other categories of life-events modifies this conclusion. For patients with clear appendicitis or other organic disease, e.g. peptic ulcer, there was a significant excess of events threatening in the short-term but not the long-term. Examples of such events were examinations and short-lived breaks in close relationships.

An even clearer distinction between peptic ulcer and functional pain patients emerged from another category of life-event; goal-frustration events occurred prior to the former. Such events involved persistent striving towards a goal which could not be achieved (Craig and Brown, 1984).

Thus a consensus is emerging in studies using the LEDS that severely threatening events are associated with the onset of 'functional' disorders such as non-organic abdominal pain and mennorrhagia (Harris, 1989). Severe events are also associated with the onset of organic disorders (where tissue damage is involved) only when there is concurrent psychiatric disorder. For the onset of organic disorders in the absence of depression, life-events with lesser degrees of threat appear to be associated with onset in a more subtle way; life-events play a smaller part in etiology, alongside other agents such as vascular, infective and dietary ones.

However, two recent studies challenge this conclusion. One (Andrews and House, 1989) concerned women with functional dysphonia, where no tissue damage is involved, yet severe events were *not* related to onset. Events of lesser degrees of threat were associated with onset if they belonged to a class of event known as 'conflict over speaking out'. Such events involved situations where the woman felt torn between conflicting obligations (e.g. work versus caring for an elderly relative) but could not speak out for fear of the consequences.

The other recent study involved assessing life-events prior to the onset of multiple sclerosis (MS), which for some patients was several years prior to the interview (Grant *et al.*, 1989). Seventy-seven per cent of the MS patients had experienced a severe event or marked chronic difficulty during the six months prior to onset compared to 35% of the control group ($p < 0.001$). This significant difference remained for those who did and did not know their diagnosis and if those with a first onset and exacerbation were considered separately. Marked marital difficulties and problems with siblings and parents showed the clearest difference between patients and controls. This raises the question whether stressful life-events are related to a change in the immunological status of patients, but it cannot be ascertained in the light of present knowledge whether the life-event precedes or follows an initial change in the immune system.

These two last studies indicate how this area of research holds much promise in increasing our understanding of the relationship between stressful events, physiological change and onset of physical disorders, leading to clarification of 'psychosomatic' relationships.

Conclusion

Life-events research has not been without its critics. However, refinements in life-event measurement, together with carefully selected groups of subjects, has greatly increased our understanding of the etiology of psychiatric and now physical disorders. As vulnerability factors are increasingly understood, the role of environmental and constitutional etiological agents will become clearer—the proportion of each differs in different conditions.

References

Andrews, H. and House, A. (1989). Functional dysphonia. In: G.W. Brown and T.O. Harris (eds) *Life Events and Illness*, pp. 343–360. New York: The Guilford Press.

Aronson, T.A. and Shukla, S. (1987). Life events and relapse in bipolar disorder: the impact of a catastrophic event. *Acta Psychiat. Scand.* **75**, 571–576.

Bifulco, A.T., Brown, G.W. and Harris, T.O. (1987). Childhood loss of parent, lack of adequate parental care and adult depression: a replication. *J. Affect. Dis.* **12**, 115–128.

Brown, G.W. (1989). Life events and measurements. In: G.W. Brown and T.O. Harris (eds) *Life Events and Illness*, pp. 3–45. New York: The Guilford Press.

Brown, G.W. and Birley, J.L.T. (1968). Crises and life changes and the onset of schizophrenia. *J. Hlth Social Behav.* **9**, 203–214.

Brown, G.W. and Harris, T.O. (1978). *Social Origins of Depression: a Study of Psychiatric Disorder in Women*. London: Tavistock.

Brown, G.W. and Harris, T.O. (1982). Fall-off in the reporting life events. *Social Psychiat.* **17**, 23–28.

Brown, G.W. and Harris, T.O. (1989a). Depression. In: G.W. Brown and T.O. Harris (eds) *Life Events and Illness*, pp. 49–93. New York: The Guilford Press.

Brown, G.W. and Harris, T.O. (1989b). The LEDS and physical illness. In: G.W. Brown and T.O. Harris (eds) *Life Events and Illness*, pp. 453–460. New York: The Guilford Press.

Brown, G.W. and Prudo, R. (1981). Psychiatric disorder in a rural and an urban population: 1. Etiology of depression. *Psychol. Med.* **11**, 581–599.

Brown, G.W., Craig, T.K. and Harris, T.O. (1985). Depression: disease or distress? Some epidemiological considerations. *Br. J. Psychiat.* **147**, 612–622.

Brown, G.W., Andrews, B., Harris, T. *et al.* (1986a). Social support, self-esteem and depression. *Psychol. Med.* **16**, 813–832.

Brown, G.W., Bifulco, A.T., Harris, T.O. and Bridge, L. (1986b). Life stress, chronic subclinical symptoms and vulnerability to clinical depression. *J. Affect. Dis.* **11**, 1–20.

Brown, G.W., Bifulco, A. and Harris, T.O. (1987). Life events, vulnerability and onset of depression—some refinements. *Br. J. Psychiat.* **150**, 30–42.

Chung, R.K., Langeluddecke, P. and Tennant, C. (1986). Threatening life events in the onset of schizophrenia, schizophreniform psychosis and hypomania. *Br. J. Psychiat.* **148**, 680–685.

Cohen, L.H., Towbes, L.C. and Flocco, R. (1988). Effects of induced mood on self-reported life events and perceived and received social support. *J. Person Social Psychol.* **55**, 669–674.

Cohen, S. and Wills, T.A. (1985). Stress, social support and the buffering hypothesis. *Psychol. Bull.* **98**, 310–357.

Cooke, D.J. (1986). Inferring causality in life event research. *Stress Med.* **2**, 141–152.

Craig, T.K.J. and Brown, G.W. (1984). Goal frustration and life events in the etiology of painful gastrointestinal disorder. *J. Psychosom. Res.* **28**, 411–421.

Craufurd, D.I.O., Creed, F. and Jayson, M.D. (1990). Life events and psychological disturbance in patients with low-back pain. *Spine* **15**, 490–494.

Creed, F. (1981). Life events and appendicectomy. *Lancet* **i**, 1381–1385.

Creed, F. (1985). Life events and physical illness. *J. Psychosom. Res.* **29**, 113–123.

Day, R., Nielsen, H., Korten, A. *et al.* (1987). Stressful life events preceding the acute onset of schizophrenia: a cross-national study from the World Health Organization. *Culture, Med. Psychiat.* **11**, 1–123.

Dohrenwend, B.P., Levav, I., Shrout, P.E. *et al.* (1987). Life stress and psychopathology: process on research begun with Barbara Snell Dohrenwend. *Am. J. Commun. Psychol.* **15**, 677–715.

Dohrenwend, B.S. and Dohrenwend, B.P. (1978). Some issues in research in stressful life events. *J. Nervous Ment. Disord.* **166**, 17–25.

Eales, M.J. (1988). Depression and anxiety in unemployed men. *Psychol. Med.* **18**, 935–945.

Farmer, R. and Creed, F. (1989). Life events and hostility in self-poisoning. *Br. J. Psychiat.* **154**, 390–395.

Faravelli, C. and Pallanti, S. (1989). Recent life events and panic disorder. *Am. J. Psychiat.* **146**, 622–626.

Finlay-Jones, R.A. and Brown, G.W. (1981). Types of stressful life event and the onset of anxiety and depressive disorders. *Psychol. Med.* **11**, 803–815.

Grant, I., McDonald, W.I., Patterson, T. and Trimble, M.R. (1989). Multiple sclerosis. In: G.W. Brown and T.O. Harris (eds) *Life Events and Illness*, pp. 295–311. New York: The Guilford Press.

Harris, T.O. (1989). Disorders of menstruation. In: G.W. Brown and T.O. Harris (eds) *Life Events and Illness*, pp. 261–294. New York: The Guilford Press.

Harris, T.O., Brown, G.W. and Bifulco, A.T. (1987). Loss of parent in childhood and adult psychiatric disorder: the role of social class position and premarital pregnancy. *Psychol. Med.* **17**, 163–184.

Heather, N., Laybourn, P. and MacPherson, B. (1987). A prospective study of the effects of unemployment on drinking behaviour. *Social Psychiat.* **22**, 226–233.

Holmes, T.H. and Rahe, R.H. (1967). The social readjustment rating scale. *J. Psychosom. Res.* **11**, 213–218.

Jacobs, S., Prusoff, B. and Paykel, G. (1974). Recent life events in schizophrenia and depression. *Psychol. Med.* **4**, 444–453.

Jacobson, D. (1987). Models of stress and meanings of unemployment: reactions to job loss among technical professionals. *Social Sci. Med.* **24**, 13–21.

Jenkins, C.D., Hurst, M.W. and Rose, R.M. (1979). Life changes: do people really remember? *Arch. Gen. Psychiat.* **36**, 379–384.

Kennedy, S., Thompson, R., Stancer, H.C. *et al.* (1983). Life events precipitating mania. *Br. J. Psychiat.* **142**, 398–403.

Klein, D.N. and Rubovits, D.R. (1987). Reliability of subjects' reports on stressful life events inventories—longitudinal studies. *J. Behav. Med.* **10**, 501–512.

Leavitt, F., Garron, D.C. and Bieliauskas, A. (1979). Stressing life events and the experience of low back pain. *J. Psychosom. Res.* **23**, 49–55.

Leff, J., Hirsch, S., Gaind, R., Rohde, P. and Stevens, B. (1973). Life events and maintenance therapy in schizophrenic relapse. *Br. J. Psychiat.* **123**, 659–660.

Miller, P.Mc. and Ingham, J.G. (1985). Dimensions of experience and symptomatology. *J. Psychosom. Res.* **29**, 475–488.

Miller, P.Mc., Ingham, J.G., Kreitman, N.B. *et al.* (1987). Life events and other factors implicated in onset and in remission of psychiatric illness in women. *J. Affect. Dis.* **12**, 73–88.

Miller, P.Mc., Kreitman, N.B., Ingham, J.G. and Sashideran, S.P. (1989). Self esteem, life stress and psychiatric disorder. *J. Affect. Dis.* **17**, 65–75.

Murphy, E. and Brown, G.W. (1980). Life events, psychiatric disturbance and physical illness. *Br. J. Psychiat.* **136**, 326–338.

Neilson, E., Brown, G.W. and Marmot, M. (1989). Myocardial Infarction. In: G.W. Brown and T.O. Harris (eds) *Life Events and Illness*, pp. 313–343. New York: The Guilford Press.

Parker, G., Tennant, C. and Blignault, I. (1985). Predicting improvement in patients with non-endogenous depression. *Br. J. Psychiat.* **146**, 132–139.

Parker, G., Holmes, S. and Manicavasagar, V. (1986). Depression in general practice attenders. 'Caseness', natural history and predictors of outcome. *J. Affect. Dis.* **10**, 27–35.

Parkes, C.M. (1964). Recent bereavement as a cause of mental illness. *Br. J. Psychiat.* **110**, 198–204.

Paykel, E.S. (1978). Contribution of life events to causation of psychiatric illness. *Psychol. Med.* **8**, 245–253.

Paykel, E.S. (1983). Methodological aspects of life events research. *J. Psychosom. Res.* **27**, 341–352.

Paykel, E.S. and Tanner, J. (1976). Life events, depressive relapse and maintenance treatment. *Psychol. Med.* **6**, 481–485.

Paykel, E.S., Myers, J.K., Dienelt, M.N. *et al.* (1969). Life events and depression: a controlled study. *Arch. Gen. Psychiat.* **21**, 753–760.

Paykel, E.S., Prusoff, B.A. and Myers, J.K. (1975). Suicide attempts and recent life events: a controlled comparison. *Arch. Gen. Psychiat.* **32**, 327–333.

Penkower, L., Bromet, E.J. and Dew, M.A. (1988). Husbands' layoff and wives' mental health. *Arch. Gen. Psychiat.* **45**, 994–1000.

Prudo, R., Brown, G.W., Harris, T. and Dowland, J. (1981). Psychiatric disorder in a rural and an urban population: 2. Sensitivity to loss. *Psychol. Med.* **11**, 601–616.

Sclare, P. and Creed, F. (1990). Life events and the onset of mania. *Br. J. Psychiat.* **156**, 508–514.

Slater, J. and Depue, R.A. (1981). The contribution of environment, events and social support to serious suicide attempts in primary depressive disorder. *J. Abnorm. Psychol.* **90**, 275–285.

Stott, D.H. (1958). Some psychosomatic aspects of causality in reproduction. *J. Psychosom. Res.* **3**, 42–55.

Tennant, C., Bebbington, P. and Hurry, J. (1981a). The role of life events in depressive illness: is there a substantial causal relation? *Psychol. Med.* **11**, 379–389.

Tennant, C., Bebbington, P. and Hurry, J. (1981b). The short-term outcome of neurotic disorders in the community: the relation of remission to clinical factors and to 'neutralizing' life events. *Br. J. Psychiat.* **139**, 213–220.

Warr, P. and Jackson, P. (1985). Factors influencing the psychological impact of prolonged unemployment and of re-employment. *Psychol. Med.* **15**, 795–807.

Winokur, G., Clayton, P.J. and Reich, T. (1969). *Manic Depressive Illness.* St. Louis, MO: C.V. Mosby.

Wittchen, H.U., Essau, C.A., Hecht, H., Teder, W. and Pfister, H. (1989). Reliability of life event assessments: test-retest reliability and fall-off effects of the Munich Interview for the assessment of life events and conditions. *J. Affect. Dis.* **16,** 77–92.

Clinical Psychopharmacology and Electroconvulsive Therapy

Anxiolytic and Hypnotic Drugs

J.M. Elliott

Anxiety is an everyday phenomenon of significant survival value in preparing an individual for some anticipated threat. In the pathological situation this emotion becomes inappropriate by virtue of its intensity relative to the cause and subsequently disrupts the social and professional lifestyle of the individual, often leading them to seek medical help. In pharmacological terms, the initial response was to sedate the patient using drugs such as barbiturates. By manipulation of the dose and frequency of administration the degree of sedation could be carefully controlled to achieve, at lower levels, mild reduction in excitability and anxiety or at higher levels, stupor and sleep. Hence hypnotic and anxiolytic effects became synonymous with sedative drugs acting via generalized depression of the central nervous system (CNS). The development of the benzodiazepines and more recently drugs acting on specific monoamine receptor subtypes has gradually dissociated these two systems. Hypnosis still remains a property of CNS depressants but anxiolysis is increasingly being treated by drugs which directly affect monoamine neurotransmitter function. Consequently this chapter will concentrate on the anxiolytic nature of drug action in terms of the limitations of existing drugs and the prospects for future advances.

Clinical Assessment of Anxiety

According to both DSM-III-R and ICD-10 diagnostic systems, anxiety disorders are classified within four major categories: (1) generalized anxiety disorder; (2) panic disorder; (3) stress reactions and adjustment disorders; and (4) phobias. The anxiety symptoms associated with these four groupings do not differ qualitatively and their major distinguishing feature is the relationship with external stimuli. Identification of the appropriate clinical category is significant since the recommended forms of treatment differ substantially. Generalized anxiety disorder presents as persistent and frequently unfocused anxiety which is unrelated to external stimuli. It represents the major group of anxious patients and is generally treated by psychotherapy together with benzodiazepines, although newer drugs such as buspirone are becoming more common. In the case of benzodiazepines, symptoms are immediately reduced but persistence of this effect after discontinuation of drug in the absence of psychotherapy is poor. Panic disorder indicates the sudden occurrence of paroxysmal anxiety with no apparent cause. Such attacks frequently occur in a foreign environment where there is substantial activity (e.g. in a busy street) and cause the patient to seek the sanctuary of a familiar base. Consequently panic disorder can develop into agoraphobia. Treatment consists of psychotherapy and long-term antidepressant drugs, including tricyclic antidepressants and MAO inhibitors. As with the treatment of depression, little clinical benefit is apparent until 2–4 weeks after commencing treatment. Acute stress reactions can be effectively diminished by benzodiazepines but the side effects of cognitive and psychomotor impairment may preclude their use. In such cases β-blockers may prove sufficient. Chronic stress reactions such as post-traumatic stress disorder show little response to drugs and are generally treated by psychotherapy. Similarly phobic reactions are best treated by appropriate exposure treatment and drugs have little effect.

Although presented as four distinct subtypes, there is considerable overlap of symptoms between these categories and the therapeutic strategies associated with each are not exclusive. Hence antidepressants have demonstrated benefit in generalized anxiety disorder (Kahn et al., 1986) and high-dose benzodiazepine treatment is reported effective in panic disorder (Sheehan, 1987). Consequently a more generalized view of anxiety has re-emerged in which some patients may exhibit one or more of the symptoms of anxiety, panic, phobia or depression during different episodes of their illness. This single disorder has been termed the general neurotic syndrome (Tyrer, 1983). Such patients frequently reveal a positive family history of anxiety disorders, suggesting a significant genetic factor to be present (Leckman et al., 1983). The recommended treatment in such cases consists of psychotherapy and antidepressant drugs, which may be required for months or even years.

In addition to the emotional trauma, anxious patients frequently present with peripheral signs of increased autonomic activity including increased heart rate and blood pressure, disturbed respiration, increased skeletal muscle tone and decreased salivation and gastrointestinal motility. Blockade of sympathetic adrenoceptors will reduce such symptoms and may ameliorate the condition. Such an approach can be useful, as outlined below, but does not address the primary dysfunction and is often of limited value. Decreased quality or quantity of sleep is also frequently experienced by anxious patients which, of itself, may seriously interfere with their normal lifestyle. In such cases a short period of treatment with a hypnotic drug may suffice but prolonged treatment will rarely benefit the patient and is likely to lead to problems of tolerance and withdrawal. Furthermore, sleep disturbance could result from other clinical situations including depression and alcoholism which may be difficult to distinguish from anxiety on initial investigation.

Barbiturates and Other CNS Depressant Drugs

The barbiturates formed the mainstay of hypnotic and anxiolytic drug treatment from the early part of this century until the introduction of the benzodiazepines. At subhypnotic doses the barbiturates exhibit anxiolytic activity but both effects probably derive from the depression of neuronal activity within the CNS. Recent studies demonstrate that their biochemical mode of action is closely allied with the $GABA_A$ receptor, increasing the conductance of chloride ions which is regulated by this receptor and hence decreasing neuronal membrane excitability (Olsen *et al.*, 1986). This is similar to the action of the benzodiazepines, hence it is not suprising that these two groups of compounds display similar pharmacodynamic profiles. At higher doses barbiturates appear to block the effects of excitatory neurotransmitters and disrupt membrane function outside the synapse. This probably accounts for their anaesthetic properties (and greater lethality) which do not occur with benzodiazepines. Barbiturates are now rarely prescribed for the treatment of anxiety or insomnia due to problems of toxicity, dependence and drug interactions and their current usage is restricted to anticonvulsant and anaesthetic roles.

The problem of toxicity is reflected by the low therapeutic ratio; indeed barbiturate overdose became a frequent mode of chemically induced suicide. High doses of barbiturates cause respiratory depression which cannot be reversed by any effective antidote and forced elimination of the drug via the kidney is hindered by its accumulation in fatty tissue. Drug tolerance is commonly observed and generally precedes physical addiction. Consequently withdrawal of the drug becomes a difficult and painful process, frequently associated with recurrence of initial symptoms such as anxiety and insomnia and can extend to fits. Drug interactions occur by virtue of the induction of hepatic metabolic enzymes such as cytochrome P_{450}, leading to an increased rate of metabolism and excretion of accompanying drugs prescribed together with the barbiturates.

In the search for safer compounds, several barbiturate derivatives were introduced including glutethimide and thalidomide and alternatives such as meprobamate, but these compounds displayed similar problems. Following the introduction of the benzodiazepines, however, the use of barbiturates as anxiolytic/hypnotics substantially decreased. Other general CNS depressants do remain in clinical practice, including chloral hydrate and chlormethiazole. These compounds are popular hypnotics in elderly patients, particularly within hospitals or other institutions, but again persistent usage should be discouraged due to the gradual development of tolerance and dependence.

Benzodiazepines

Since the introduction of chlordiazepoxide in the 1960s, more than 3000 benzodiazepine structures have been synthesized and over 25 drugs of this type are currently in clinical use. Their popularity as the mainstay of anxiolytic/hypnotic drug treatment derives from their proven efficacy combined with low acute toxicity. These compounds are weakly basic and therefore mostly absorbed within the duodenum. They are highly lipid soluble and rapidly penetrate into the circulation where they are highly protein bound (80–97%). Even though the free plasma concentration is consequently small they rapidly cross the blood–brain barrier, hence the delay between oral administration and onset of effect is less than one hour. Drug elimination generally occurs in two stages: first metabolism

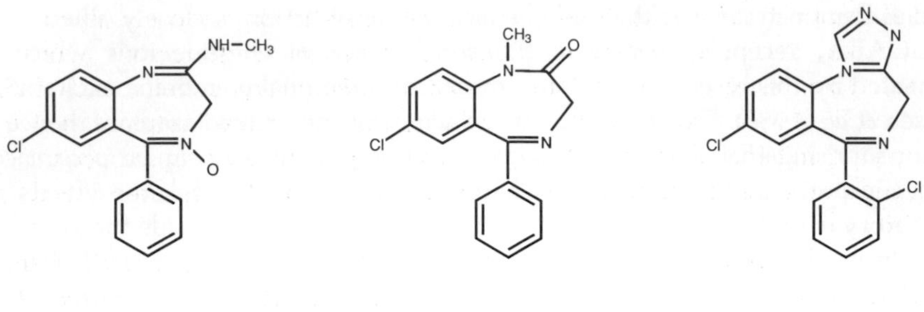

Chlordiazepoxide   Diazepam   Triazolam

FIG. 29.1   Benzodiazepine receptor agonists.

via N-dealkylation or aliphatic hydroxylation; then conjugation via glucuronyl transferases producing water-soluble glucuronides which are excreted by the kidney. However, many of the metabolic intermediates are biologically active and may have much longer half-lives than the parent compound. Consequently the duration of action of some benzodiazepines such as flurazepam, which has a biochemical half-life of 3–6 h, is substantially elongated due to the active nature of the metabolites which exhibit much longer half-lives, in the case of flurazepam being 30–100 h. Benzodiazepines do not induce hepatic microsomal enzyme activity, therefore drug interactions are minimal compared to the barbiturates.

The major differences between existing benzodiazepines relate to their physicochemical properties, which in turn dictate the rate of onset and duration of action. Due to the presence or absence of active metabolites, the biological half-life varies between 2–3 h (triazolam) and 50–150 h (flurazepam). However, the duration of psychotropic action is generally shorter since brain concentration is initially high following drug administration due to efficient brain perfusion but then falls rapidly as the drug is sequestered into fatty tissue. Drugs with shorter effective half-lives are preferred for hypnotic use since little active drug persists the following morning, minimizing the 'morning-after' hangover. Concomitantly drugs with longer half-lives maintain a more even plasma level throughout the day and are preferred for anxiolytic use. However these theoretical principles have been usurped by the findings that tolerance and dependence are established more rapidly to drugs with shorter duration of action.

Spectrum of Effects

Benzodiazepines are primarily used for their anxiolytic and hypnotic properties. Their mode of action as anxiolytics will be considered in greater detail below. Their success as hypnotics depends on a reduction in the latency of sleep onset. However, the balance of sleep phases is modified, producing increased stage 2 non-REM sleep and decreases in REM sleep and slow-wave sleep. The significance of these changes is not clear. Tolerance to the hypnotic effects develops rapidly and withdrawal often corresponds with a rebound increase in the occurrence and duration of REM sleep. Although frequently used as an adjunct to anaesthesia, benzodiazepines themselves will not induce anaesthesia, in contrast to the barbiturates. This may reflect their less generalized depression of neuronal activity. Their ability to prevent the spread of epileptiform activity within the brain is utilized as anticonvulsants, particularly diazepam in the treatment of *status epilepticus*. Similarly their inhibition of polysynaptic reflexes causes centrally mediated relaxation of striated muscle which can be exploited in cases of muscle spasticity.

In terms of undesirable side effects, benzodiazepines may reduce motor coordination causing potential problems for patients whose job involves the operation of heavy machinery or driving vehicles. Benzodiazepine administration is also associated with anterograde amnesia which may be of benefit when used as premedication prior to uncomfortable procedures such as gastroscopy. However it could significantly compromise a patient's performance if the drug was initially prescribed to reduce anxiety associated with the same imminent cognitive assessment, such as an examination. The amnesia appears to result from impairment of the retention rather than the acquisition phase and is reported to be less prominent in respect of 1,5-benzodiazepines such as clobazam than 1,4-benzodiazepines such as diazepam (Koeppen, 1984). A similar differentiation of amnesic effects according to molecular structure has been observed in animal studies (Giurgea *et al.*, 1982). The problem of poor memory while taking benzodiazepines is frequently reported by patients and tolerance to this unwelcome effect does not seem to develop on chronic treatment.

Benzodiazepine Receptors and Ligands

The biochemical site of action of the benzodiazepines remained obscure for several years after their clinical introduction. Early experiments demonstrated their ability to potentiate the presynaptic inhibitory effects of γ-aminobutyric acid (GABA) in the cat spinal cord, since the effects could be inhibited by the GABA antagonist bicuculline. However, depletion of GABA by inhibition of the anabolic enzyme glutamic acid decarboxylase abolished the response to benzodiazepines, indicating that they did not act as intrinsic GABA agonists (Polc and Hafely, 1977). Additional studies indicated that benzodiazepines did not affect the synthesis, release or uptake of GABA, and might therefore operate indirectly via stimulation of a distinct receptor. This hypothesis was confirmed by the identification of a highly specific binding site in neuronal tissue which bound benzodiazepines with much higher affinity than any of the known neurotransmitter compounds, including GABA. Furthermore the clinical anxiolytic potency of a series of benzodiazepines correlated closely with their potency to bind to this novel receptor (Braestrup and Squires, 1978). Although GABA had low affinity itself for the receptor, addition of GABA enhanced the potency of the benzodiazepines at this receptor and vice versa, suggesting a biochemical basis for the functional interactions described previously.

Electrophysiological studies demonstrated that stimulation of the $GABA_A$ receptor reduced membrane excitability by increasing the conductance of chloride ions. In the presence of benzodiazepines, this effect was enhanced due to an increase in the frequency of opening the chloride ion channel (Barker and Owen, 1986). However in the absence of GABA, benzodiazepines themselves did not increase chloride conductance. Hence the effects of stimulating the benzodiazepine receptor must be mediated via the GABA$_A$ receptor, leading to speculation that the two systems might be integrally associated within the membrane. This hypothesis was confirmed when isolation of the benzodiazepine binding protein led to the cloning and sequencing of the GABA$_A$ receptor (Schofield *et al.*, 1987). This receptor comprises at least two (α and β) and probably more (γ, δ, ε) distinct protein subunits which display the properties of the GABA binding site, the benzodiazepine binding site and the chloride ionophore. Subsequent analysis has identified multiple distinct genetic copies of the α, β and γ subunits, leading to the conclusion that many different GABA$_A$ receptor subtypes may exist with differing benzodiazepine sensitivity (Sieghart, 1989). Since the benzodiazepines are known to have multiple effects (as outlined above), this diversity of receptor subtypes introduces the possibility that each effect may be mediated by a separate subtype.

Having identified specific binding sites for the benzodiazepine drugs, attempts were then made to identify the endogenous neurotransmitter which normally acts at these sites. An early candidate isolated from human urine was β-carboline-3-carboxylic acid ethyl ester (β-CCE), a potent inhibitor of [^{3}H]diazepam binding. This compound was specific for the benzodiazepine site, showing much lower affinity at other neurotransmitter receptors including the GABA$_A$ receptor (Braestrup *et al.*, 1980). In terms of biological activity, however, β-CCE produced effects opposite to those of diazepam, enhancing the seizure activity of pentylenetetrazole (a GABA antagonist) and reversing the anxiolytic effects of benzodiazepines in animal models. Biochemical modification of the β-carboline structure produced further compounds such as 6,7-dimethoxy-4-ethyl-β-carboline (DMCM) with even more pronounced anti-benzodiazepine properties, including anxiogenic effects and convulsions at higher dose. However, other β-carboline derivatives, such as the propyl ester β-CCPr, demonstrated benzodiazepine-like properties including anxiolytic and anticonvulsant effects. The diversity of benzodiazepine receptor ligands was further extended with the introduction of the imidodiazepine flumazenil (Ro 15-1788), which blocked the effects of benzodiazepines and benzodiazepine-like β-carbolines and also the effects of anti-benzodiazepine compounds such as DMCM. In order to incorporate these various effects into a theoretical model of benzodiazepine receptor operation, it was proposed that three categories of ligands exist:

(1) benzodiazepine receptor agonists, such as diazepam which initiate the classical benzodiazepine effects including anxiolytic, hypnotic, anticonvulsant, etc;

(2) benzodiazepine receptor inverse agonists, such as DMCM, which demonstrate effects opposite to the therapeutic effects associated with benzodiazepines, including anxiogenic and proconvulsant or even convulsant responses;

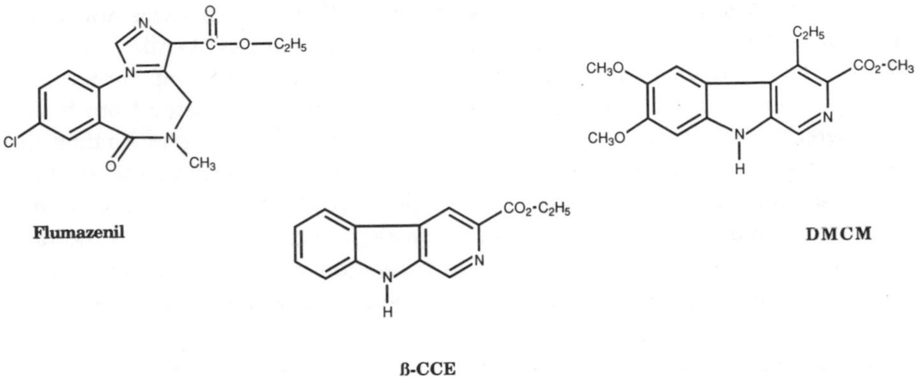

Flumazenil

DMCM

β-CCE

FIG. 29.2   Benzodiazepine receptor antagonist and inverse agonists.

(3) benzodiazepine receptor antagonists, such as flumazenil, which antagonize the effects of both agonists and inverse agonists but have no intrinsic effects.

Although β-CCE was the catalyst which led to this diversification of benzodiazepine receptor effects, attempts to confirm its identity as the endogenous benzodiazepine receptor ligand have foundered due its exceedingly low concentration within brain tissue. Indeed it is now thought that the β-CCE obtained from human urine was formed artifactually during the extraction process, accounting for its anomalously high concentration. However the consequences of isolating β-CCE are substantial, since the debate concerning the identity of the endogenous receptor ligand must now include the possibility that the compound may be an inverse agonist rather than an agonist.

Putative Endogenous Benzodiazepine Receptor Ligands

Several compounds have been proposed as endogenous ligands for the benzodiazepine receptor, generally on the basis of receptor binding activity (identified as the potency to inhibit the binding of [^{3}H]diazepam to the benzodiazepine receptor) or on the basis of electrophysiological or behavioural activity similar to or antagonistic towards effects normally displayed by benzodiazepine drugs. A number of metabolic candidates including inosine, hypoxanthine and nicotinamide competitively inhibit the binding of [^{3}H]diazepam to neuronal membranes. In electrophysiological studies nicotinamide demonstrated effects similar to benzodiazepines and inosine protected against seizures induced by pentylenetetrazole. However, their binding potency is low, affinities being in the millimolar range, and although this may in part be compensated by high intracellular concentrations, they are not currently considered likely endogenous benzodiazepine receptor agonists.

GABA-modulin is a basic protein which was isolated from brain tissue and claimed to inhibit the binding of GABA to GABA$_A$ receptors in a non-competitive manner (Guidotti et al., 1982). Phosphorylation of GABA-modulin abolished this inhibitory activity. Binding of benzodiazepines to their receptor was also proposed to reduce the inhibitory effects of GABA-modulin on GABA binding. However, other workers have been unable to confirm these findings. Diazepam binding inhibitor (DBI) is a somewhat smaller protein also isolated from brain tissue which, as the name implies, competitively inhibits [^{3}H]diazepam binding to benzodiazepine receptors (Costa et al., 1983). Electrophysiological studies in spinal cord neurones indicate that it decreases GABA-induced chloride conductance and in behavioural tests it induces pro-conflict activity in the rat. Hence it would seem to represent an inverse-agonist type ligand. However, evidence for an endogenous role in relation to benzodiazepine receptor activity is lacking.

An alternative approach has been to produce monoclonal antibodies to benzodiazepines by immunizing mice with a benzodiazepine hapten bound to albumin. The resulting antibodies demonstrated high affinity for active benzodiazepines including diazepam and flunitrazepam and also towards an endogenous constituent of rat brain (De Blas and Sangameswaran, 1986). This compound has since been purified and appears to resemble N-des-methyldiazepam, an active benzodiazepine agonist-type ligand. However, the origin of the compound has yet to be determined since it is known that some fungi can synthesize benzodiazepine-like compounds which may then be introduced into the food chain of the animal rather than represent a true endogenous ligand synthesized in situ within the neurones (Medina et al., 1989).

Tolerance and Dependence Associated with Benzodiazepines

Although initially thought to be devoid of the problems of tolerance and dependence which were clearly associated with barbiturates, recent studies have confirmed the potential for benzodiazepines to cause similar, though less severe, effects (Lader and File, 1987). In man tolerance to the various effects of benzodiazepines develops at different rates. The intensity of the sedative and hypnotic effects declines within days of starting treatment whereas the anxiolytic effects persists for several months. To assess tolerance following chronic treatment, patients who had received benzodiazepines for at least six months were challenged with a test dose of diazepam and the responses compared to those obtained in drug-naive control subjects (Petursson and Lader, 1984). Subjective rating of sedation and the increase in plasma level of growth hormone were both substantially less in benzodiazepine-treated patients whereas the EEG fast-wave response showed no difference between the two groups. Similar studies of lorazepam indicated that the degree of tolerance observed was dose-dependent and did not occur in patients receiving a low dose (Aranko et al., 1985).

Sudden termination of treatment, even of short duration, can lead to a rebound syndrome characterized by duplication of the initial symptoms, possibly of greater intensity than before. This effect is dependent on the pharmacokinetic properties of the drug and is most pronounced in benzodiazepines with short duration of action, such as triazolam. Longer term treatment appears to produce dependence as evidenced by withdrawal symptoms which comprise a psychological component (anxiety, insomnia, dysphoria), a physiological component (tremor, palpitations, sweating, muscle spasm) and a perceptual component (hypersensitivity to various stimuli, depersonalization). As with the rebound syndrome, the intensity of these withdrawal effects depends on the rate of elimination of the benzodiazepine and can be minimized by gradual reduction of the dosage. Hence abrupt cessation of treatment with diazepam, which exhibits a relatively long biological half-life due to the persistence of the active metabolite desmethyldiazepam, caused less severe withdrawal effects than the shorter acting drug lorazepam (Tyrer *et al.*, 1981). In those patients receiving diazepam the intensity of the withdrawal syndrome paralleled the rate of elimination of desmethyldiazepam from the plasma. The withdrawal effects could be further minimized by gradually reducing the dose of diazepam over a period of four weeks, again corresponding with a more gradual fall in plasma levels of diazepam and its active metabolites (Tyrer *et al.*, 1983).

Attempts to identify the biochemical mechanisms underlying these changes are based extensively on animal models. As in man, the rate at which tolerance develops varies according to the specific effect, occurring rapidly in relation to sedation and anticonvulsant responses (3–5 days) but more slowly in the case of anxiolytic effects (10–15 days). Treatment of rats with high doses of benzodiazepine over several weeks does not alter the number of benzodiazepine receptors but sudden cessation of the drug precipitates several behavioural changes (File, 1985). Withdrawal effects have also been reported in several other species including primates (Cumin *et al.*, 1982) although usually in response to doses 10–100 times greater than the anxiolytic dose. Withdrawal effects can be elicited at lower doses of benzodiazepine by administration of the benzodiazepine antagonist flumazenil. Conversely, intermittent administration of flumazenil to rats during chronic treatment with a benzodiazepine prevents the appearance of the withdrawal syndrome when treatment with the agonist is suddenly stopped (Gallager *et al.*, 1986). A biochemical model of withdrawal which incorporates these agonist–antagonist interactions proposes that chronic overstimulation by the agonist (benzodiazepine) causes a compensatory increase in the activity of a putative endogenous inverse-agonist (File and Baldwin, 1989). Hence on withdrawal of the exogenous agonist the increased level of endogenous inverse-agonist will initiate a series of behavioural effects opposite to those observed in response to benzodiazepines themselves. The implication of this hypothesis for the treatment of benzodiazepine withdrawal in man is that flumazenil may represent a logical alternative to prolonged, gradual reduction of the benzodiazepine dose. However, chronic benzodiazepine treatment probably causes adaptive changes in neurotransmitter systems other than those related to the $GABA_A$ receptor, particularly noradrenergic, which would require additional therapy.

Novel Drugs Acting at Benzodiazepine Receptors

The diverse nature of effects elicited by benzodiazepine drugs, together with the variable degree of tolerance observed in respect of these effects has stimulated research into the possibility that novel benzodiazepine-like compounds could be created with much greater specificity than those currently used. Biochemical comparison of the inhibition binding profile for [³H]diazepam obtained in the rat cerebellum and hippocampus indicated substantial differences in the potency of several compounds including the β-carboline derivatives (Braestrup and Nielsen, 1981). This led to the proposed existence of benzodiazepine receptor subtypes labelled BZ_1 and BZ_2, corresponding to the cerebellar and hippocampal locations, respectively. Photolabelling studies in which [³H]flunitrazepam covalently bonded to its target receptor(s) on irradiation of the tissue with UV light identified a single peptide in the cerebellum (MW 51 000) but at least four peptides from hippocampal and other brain regions (MW 51 000, 53 000, 55 000, 59 000) (Sieghart and Karobath, 1980). Labelling of the 51 000 MW peptide was selectively inhibited by β-carbolines, suggesting a correspondence with the BZ_1 receptor subtype. Subsequent identification of multiple copies of the $GABA_A$ receptor α and β chains (Sieghart, 1989) has extended the potential for such benzodiazepine receptor subtypes.

Amongst the novel compounds with a potentially selective action at benzodiazepine receptor subtypes, zopiclone is a cyclopyrollone compound which, in animal studies, is more potent as a sedative rather than as an anxiolytic agent. Although not a benzodiazepine structure, the behavioural and electrophysiological effects of zopiclone are blocked by flumazenil. Clinical studies indicate that the hypnotic effect of zopiclone is similar to that of short-acting benzodiazepines but that its anxiolytic properties are weaker than diazepam (Goa and Heel, 1986). Whether this distinction extends to a reduction in the tolerance and dependence potential of zopiclone relative to equivalent short-acting benzodiazepines remains to be demonstrated.

Of greater potential use would be a compound with relatively stronger anxiolytic potency and weaker sedative potency. Premazepam is a pyrollodiazepine which acts as a partial agonist at benzodiazepine receptors in rat cerebral cortex but as an antagonist at receptors in the cerebellum (Barone et al., 1984). Animal behavioural studies indicate significant intrinsic anxiolytic activity but when administered with diazepam it reduced the CNS depressant effects of the benzodiazepine. In man the anxiolytic efficacy of premazepam was confirmed but it proved no different to diazepam in causing dizziness and impaired psychomotor function (Golombok and Lader, 1984). Combined treatment with both premazepam and diazepam produced additive rather than antagonistic effects. Hence it appears that the behavioural distinctions observed between these two compounds in animal models may not translate directly to man.

Alpidem similarly exhibited a selective anxiolytic profile in animal models. Comparison to lorazepam in man demonstrated equivalent anxiolytic efficacy and less initial psychomotor and cognitive impairment, though tolerance to these effects developed rapidly in patients taking lorazepam. Several other novel

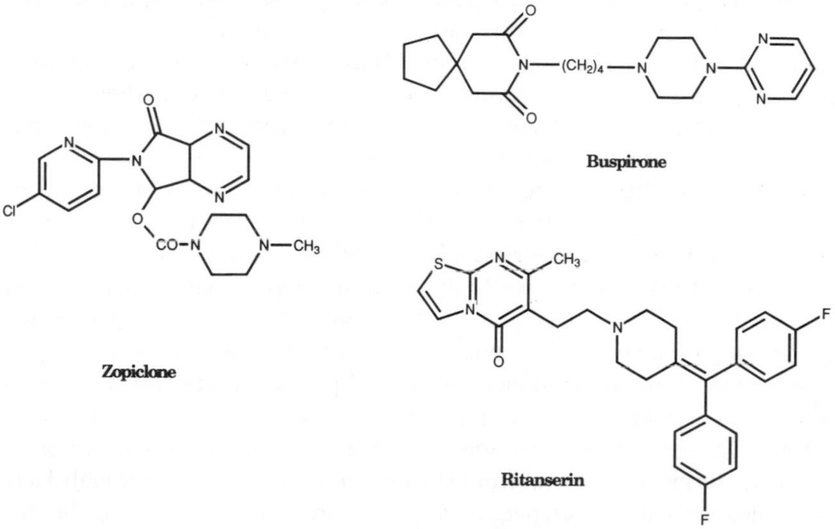

FIG. 29.3 Novel non-benzodiazepine hypnotic and anxiolytic agents.

benzodiazepine and non-benzodiazepine structures which promise selective activity on the basis of animal models now await clinical investigation (Cooper *et al.*, 1987).

Other Neurotransmitter Systems Implicated in Anxiety

The anxiolytic and hypnotic effects of both barbiturates and benzodiazepines result from potentiation of the neuronal depressant effects of GABA, but the neuronal targets of GABA action are still largely unknown. Identification of these 'downstream' neurones could provide alternative sites for anxiolytic drug action. Considerable effort has therefore been directed to this goal either by identifying the modulatory effects of GABA/benzodiazepines on other neurotransmitters or by manipulating the activity of other neurotransmitters (including lesioning and receptor stimulation or blockade) and monitoring the effects on anxiety behaviour. Consequently both noradrenergic and serotoninergic neurones have emerged as potential targets for new anxiolytic drugs.

Role of Noradrenaline in Anxiety

Noradrenergic cell bodies are localized mainly within the locus coeruleus from which axons project to most parts of the brain and spinal cord. In monkeys electrical stimulation of the locus coeruleus induced an intense fear response, whereas lesion of this region abolished fear when the animals were confronted with a threatening situation (Redmond and Huang, 1979). Release of noradrenaline is regulated by presynaptic α_2-adrenergic autoreceptors which can be blocked by yohimbine. In both man and animal models yohimbine administration induced anxiety (Charney et al., 1983; Pellow et al., 1985) together with an increase in sympathetic neuronal activity and increased plasma level of 3-methoxy-4-hydroxy-phenylethylglycol (MHPG), a metabolite of noradrenaline. In man these effects were successfully reversed by subsequent administration of the α_2-adrenoceptor agonist clonidine. Diazepam reversed the anxiogenic but not the autonomic effects of yohimbine.

Several observations suggest that noradrenergic activity is altered following benzodiazepine receptor activation. In the rat benzodiazepines inhibit noradrenaline release and reduce turnover rate but these effects rapidly undergo tolerance and are not observed after chronic drug administration, when anxiolytic effects are still apparent. Conversely administration of the partial inverse agonist N-methyl-β-carboline-3-carboxamide (FG7142) to healthy volunteers caused intense anxiety coupled with increased blood pressure and heart rate, sweating, flushing and tremor (Dorow et al., 1983), suggesting increased noradrenaline release and adrenoceptor activation. Similar autonomic symptoms are observed in patients during withdrawal from chronic benzodiazepine treatment. Hence it appears likely that noradrenergic neurones are 'downstream' of the benzodiazepine receptor and that acute stimulation by either agonists or inverse agonists will alter noradrenergic function. However, their significance in the anxiolytic action of the benzodiazepines remains uncertain.

Attempts to treat anxiety by reducing noradrenaline release centrally using clonidine have not proved successful due largely to the sedative side effects which are apparent in normal use as an antihypertensive drug. However, inhibition of noradrenaline action at postsynaptic receptors using β-blockers is proving increasingly popular as a first-line approach to treatment of mild or transient anxiety associated with significant somatic disturbance. This effect appears to be peripherally mediated since it occurs with compounds such as practolol which do not cross the blood–brain barrier. The effective dose is much lower than that needed for antihypertensive effects and tolerance and dependence do not occur (Turner et al., 1965). No individual β-blocker appears to be preferred in this role. Since both β_1- and β_2-adrenoceptor subtypes are involved, then cardioselective drugs do not convey any advantage bar the acknowledged pulmonary benefits. The major targets of the β-blockers are the cardiovascular system and striated muscle, reducing heart rate, flushing and muscle tremor. This is particularly beneficial in patients facing acute anxiety associated with a public performance or examination where bodily symptoms may reinforce the subjective response to stress leading to the establishment of a positive-feedback loop between the somatic and psychological components of anxiety. Likewise in some chronically anxious patients the use of β-blockers to reduce somatic effects may be sufficient to break the stress–symptom spiral and subsequently lead to improvement in the psychological symptoms (Tyrer, 1982). In severe anxiety, however, β-blockers are generally ineffective.

Disruption of central noradrenergic function has been specifically associated with panic disorder. Challenge with yohimbine in these patients led to increased frequency of panic attacks and enhanced blood pressure response and plasma MHPG level compared to non-anxious control subjects (Charney et al., 1987).

Effective treatment of these patients is achieved by chronic administration of tricyclic antidepressants or MAO-inhibitors, both of which modify adrenoceptor function in animal models, rather than using benzodiazepines.

So it appears that noradrenaline may be primarily concerned with some aspects of anxiety, including panic disorder, where novel drugs designed to reduce adrenoceptor stimulation may be beneficial. In relation to the biochemical mechanism of benzodiazepines, noradrenergic function is altered but this may not be crucial to their anxiolytic action.

Role of 5HT in Anxiety

Cell bodies for the 5HT-containing neurones are distributed between the raphe nuclei of the mesencephalon and project to most regions of the brain and spinal cord. Microinjection of benzodiazepines into the dorsal raphe reduced the firing rate of these neurones and promoted a typical anxiolytic behavioural response (Thiebot and Soubrie, 1983). Other studies demonstrated that benzodiazepines reduced 5HT turnover in several brain regions (Stein et al., 1973). This effect did not show tolerance and corresponded with the development of anxiolytic behaviour. Furthermore, high densities of benzodiazepine receptors were found in the raphe and areas of the limbic system which were also innervated by 5HT neurones. It was therefore proposed that 5HT may play a substantial role in mediating some effects of the benzodiazepines, particularly those associated with anxiety.

Lesion of 5HT pathways from the raphe by administration of the neurotoxin, 5,7-dihydroxytryptamine at the level of the ventral tegmentum resulted in anxiolytic effects in conflict tests similar to those observed following benzodiazepine administration. Similarly reduction of 5HT levels by inhibition of synthesis using p-chlorophenylalanine also caused a decrease in anxiety behaviour, the time-course of behavioural response paralleling the loss of 5HT (Tye et al., 1977). Conversely stimulation of post-synaptic 5HT receptors either by direct agonists such as quipazine or by potentiation of endogenous 5HT, following inhibition of synaptic re-uptake by fluoxetine, induced anxiogenic responses. On this basis, blockade of 5HT receptors would be anticipated to reduce such responses. Although anxiolytic behaviour was observed following some compounds, including ritanserin and cinanserin, others such as metergoline produced the opposite effect (Chopin and Briley, 1987). This initial confusion was dispelled following the identification of several 5HT receptor subtypes and the degree of selectivity (or lack of it) shown by the different antagonists. Currently 5HT receptors are divided into three major groups ($5HT_1$, $5HT_2$, $5HT_3$), although several subtypes of the $5HT_1$ group have been identified and further subdivisions of the other two groups are suspected (Bradley et al., 1986). Clarification of these 5HT receptor subtypes has substantially improved our understanding of the role of 5HT in anxiety and led to the introduction of several novel compounds as potential anxiolytic drugs.

Novel Anxiolytic Drugs Acting at 5HT Receptors

Buspirone is a pyrimidinylpiperazine derivative which demonstrates an anxiolytic action in several animal behavioural models including decreased aggression and increased social interaction. There is some disagreement concerning its effectiveness in conflict tests depending on the precise conditions employed. It is a selective agonist at $5HT_{1A}$ receptors and potently inhibits the firing of target cells in the dorsal raphe and hippocampus following systemic or microiontophoretic application. Although similar in effect to benzodiazepines in some animal models, it is structurally unrelated to the benzodiazepines and does not alter $GABA_A$ receptor function. Furthermore it does not prevent withdrawal symptoms in animals treated chronically with benzodiazepines then switched to buspirone. The sedative and muscle relaxant effects of buspirone itself are much weaker than those of the benzodiazepines and chronic administration of buspirone is not associated with tolerance or withdrawal effects. In some biochemical and behavioural systems buspirone acts as a partial agonist at the $5HT_{1A}$ receptor and can also stimulate dopamine receptors, but these seem unrelated to its anxiolytic effects (Traber and Glaser, 1987).

In a study of patients with generalized anxiety disorder, the anxiolytic effects of buspirone were slow to develop relative to diazepam, but after 4 weeks there was no significant difference between patients treated with either drug (Goa and Ward, 1986). Side effects of sedation, psychomotor and cognitive impairment were reported less frequently for buspirone although fatigue, depression, headache and nausea were more common. A limitation of buspirone, however, is that it proved much less effective in patients who had previously received benzodiazepines than in drug-naive patients (Schweitzer et al., 1986). Consequently it cannot be substituted for benzodiazepines and does not attenuate the withdrawal effects resulting from chronic benzodiazepine use. However, treatment with buspirone for 6 months was not associated with tolerance and abrupt termination of treatment did not induce withdrawal phenomena such as rebound anxiety or recurrence of symptoms. Other $5HT_{1A}$ agonists, including gepirone and ipsapirone, which do not affect dopamine receptor function and display less partial agonist activity, are currently under investigation and also appear to be anxiolytic in man.

Ritanserin is a selective antagonist at $5HT_2$ receptors which exhibits anxiolytic activity in several animal models, although it is generally less effective than diazepam (Colpaert et al., 1985). In man ritanserin is reported to be anxiolytic with little sedative effect compared to lorazepam (Ceulemans et al., 1985). $5HT_3$ receptor antagonists such as ondansetron show anxiolytic activity in several animal species using tests based on social interaction and exploration but not conflict (Jones et al., 1988). As with buspirone, there is no evidence for tolerance or withdrawal problems following chronic administration but ondansetron does attenuate the withdrawal response after chronic benzodiazepine administration when assessed on the basis of social interaction (Oakley et al., 1988). Clinical investigation of ondansetron and similar compounds is still in its early stages.

In summary, several lines of evidence indicate a significant role for 5HT in the mediation and expression of anxiety in both animal models and man. In animals benzodiazepines reduce 5HT activity and drugs acting at 5HT receptors to similar effect can mimic some, but not all, of the behavioural changes associated with the benzodiazepines. In man the initial data indicate that specific 5HT receptor-mediated drugs are anxiolytic and cause less sedation and tolerance/withdrawal problems than benzodiazepines, but are slower in onset and more restricted in their use.

Conclusions

For 30 years the benzodiazepines have been the major pharmacological tool for the treatment of anxiety. Their introduction marked a significant improvement over the barbiturates in terms of both acute and chronic toxicity and their efficacy during short periods of treatment remains unequivocal. However, the problems of tolerance and withdrawal syndrome associated with longer term treatment have accelerated the search for new anxiolytic agents. Current research suggests two particular approaches as offering the greatest potential. The first is the attempt to dissociate the numerous effects of benzodiazepine agonists according to particular subtypes of the benzodiazepine receptor and consequently to identify specific compounds active at each of these subtypes. Biochemical evidence strongly supports the existence of multiple $GABA_A$ receptors and hence potential benzodiazepine receptor subtypes. However, further data are needed to demonstrate an association between the independent functional effects and corresponding receptor subtypes. The second group of compounds modify serotoninergic activity on the basis that 5HT neurones are 'downstream' from the GABA systems which are modulated by benzodiazepines. Agonists for $5HT_{1A}$ receptors such as buspirone exhibit clinical efficacy similar to that of existing benzodiazepines, although their rate of onset is slower and their effectiveness is more limited. This is offset by an apparent lack of tolerance or withdrawal effects. Clinical experience with antagonists at $5HT_2$ and $5HT_3$ receptors is limited but animal models suggest anxiolytic potential. The development of animal models for anxiety has itself seen considerable expansion recently with particular emphasis to identify paradigms for social interaction rather than the pain/conflict models in which benzodiazepines are so effective. The success or failure of these new compounds and the animal models by which they were identified should therefore increase our understanding of the biochemical basis of anxiety and further enhance the efficacy of drugs for its treatment.

References

Aranko, K., Mattila, M.J., Nuutila, A. and Pellinen, J. (1985). Benzodiazepines, but not antidepressants or neuroleptics, induce dose-dependent development of tolerance to lorazepam in psychiatric patients. *Acta Psychiat. Scand.* **72**, 436–446.

Barker, J.L. and Owen, D.G. (1986). Electrophysiological pharmacology of GABA and diazepam in cultured CNS neurons. In: R.W. Olsen and J.C. Venter (eds) *Benzodiazepine/GABA Receptors and Chloride Channels: Structural and Functional Properties*, pp. 135–165. New York: Alan Liss.

Barone, D., Colombo, G., Glasser, A., Luzzani, F. and Mennini, T. (1984) *In vitro* interaction of premazepam with benzodiazepine receptors in rat brain regions. *Life Sci.* **35**, 365–371.

Bradley, P.B., Engel, G., Feniuk, W., Fozard, J.R., Humphrey, P.P.A., Middlemiss, D.N., Mylecharane, E.J., Richardson, B.P. and Saxena, P.R. (1986). Proposals for the classification and nomenclature of functional receptors for 5-hydroxytryptamine. *Neuropharmacology* **25**, 563–576.

Braestrup, C. and Nielsen, M.J. (1981). ^{3}H-Propyl-β-carboline-3-carboxylate as a selective radioligand for the BZ1 benzodiazepine receptor sub-class. *J. Neurochem.* **37**, 333–341.

Braestrup, C. and Squires, R.F. (1978). Brain specific benzodiazepine receptors. *Br. J. Psychiat.* **133**, 249–260.

Braestrup, C., Nielsen, M.J. and Olsen, C.E. (1980). Urinary and brain β-carboline-3-carboxylates as potent inhibitors of brain benzodiazepine receptors. *Proc. Natl. Acad. Sci. USA* **77**, 2288–2292.

Ceulemans, D.L.S., Hoppenbrouwers, M.L.J.A., Gelders, Y.G. and Reyntjeus, A.J.M. (1985). The influence of ritanserin, a serotonin antagonist, in anxiety disorders: a double-blind placebo-controlled study versus lorazepam. *Pharmacopsychiatry* **18**, 303–305.

Charney, D.S., Heninger, G.R. and Redmond, D.E. (1983). Yohimbine induced anxiety and increased noradrenergic function in humans: effects of diazepam and clonidine. *Life Sci.* **33**, 19–29.

Charney, D.S., Woods, S.W., Goodman, W.K. and Heninger, G.R. (1987). Neurobiological mechanisms of panic anxiety: biochemical and behavioural correlates of yohimbine-induced panic attacks. *Am. J. Psychiat.* **144**, 1030–1036.

Chopin, P. and Briley, M. (1987). Animal models of anxiety: the effect of compounds that modify 5HT neurotransmission. *Trends Pharmacol. Sci.* **8**, 383–388.

Colpaert, F.C., Meert, T.J., Niemegeers, C.J.E. and Janssen, P.A.J. (1985). Behavioural and 5-HT antagonistic effects of ritanserin: a pure and selective antagonist of LSD discrimination in rat. *Psychopharmacology* **86**, 45–54.

Cooper, S.J., Kirkham, T.C. and Estell, L.B. (1987). Pyrazoloquinolines: second generation benzodiazepine receptor ligands have heterogeneous effects. *Trends Pharmacol. Sci.* **8**, 180–184.

Costa, E., Corda, M.G. and Guidotti, A. (1983). On a brain polypeptide functioning as putative effector for the recognition sites of benzodiazepine and β-carboline derivatives. *Neuropharmacology* **22**, 1481–1492.

Cumin, R., Bonetti, E.P., Scherschlicht, R. and Hafely, W.E. (1982). Use of the specific benzodiazepine antagonist Ro 15-1788 in studies of physiological dependence on benzodiazepines. *Experientia* **38**, 833–834.

De Blas, A. and Sangameswaran, L. (1986). Current topics: 1. Demonstration and purification of an endogenous benzodiazepine from the mammalian brain with a monoclonal antibody to benzodiazepines. *Life Sci.* **39**, 1927–1936.

Dorow, R., Horowski, R., Paschelke, G., Amin, M. and Braestrup, C. (1983). Severe anxiety induced by FG7142, a β-carboline ligand for benzodiazepine receptors. *Lancet* **ii**, 98–99.

File, S. (1985). Tolerance to the behavioural actions of benzodiazepines. *Neurosci. Behav. Rev.* **9**, 113–121.

File, S.E. and Baldwin, H.A. (1989). Changes in anxiety in rats tolerant to, and withdrawn from benzodiazepines: behavioural and biochemical studies. In: P. Tyrer (ed.) *Psychopharmacology of Anxiety*, pp. 28–51. Oxford: Oxford University Press.

Gallager, D.W., Lakoski, J.M. and Heninger, G. (1986). Periodic benzodiazepine antagonist administration prevents benzodiazepine withdrawal symptoms in primates. *Eur. J. Pharmcol.* **132**, 31–38.

Giurgea, C.E., Greindt, M.G. and Preat, S. (1982). Experimental dysmnesia induced by 1,4- but not by 1,5-benzodiazepines. *Drug Dev. Res.* Suppl. 1, 23–30.

Goa, K.L. and Heel, R.C. (1986). Zopiclone: a review of its pharmacodynamic and pharmacokinetic properties and therapeutic efficacy as an hypnotic. *Drugs* **32**, 48–65.

Goa, K.L. and Ward, A. (1986). Buspirone. A preliminary review of its pharmacological properties and therapeutic efficacy as an anxiolytic. *Drugs* **32**, 114–129.

Golombok, S. and Lader, M. (1984). The psychopharmacological effects of premazepam, diazepam and placebo in healthy human subjects. *Br. J. Clin. Pharmacol.* **18**, 127–133.

Guidotti, A., Konkel, D.R., Ebstein, B. *et al.* (1982). Characterization and purification to homogeneity of a rat brain protein (GABA-modulin). *Proc. Natl. Acad. Sci. USA* **79**, 6084–6088.

Jones, B.J., Costall, B., Domeney, A.M. *et al.* (1988). The potential anxiolytic activity of GR38032F, a 5HT$_3$-receptor antagonist. *Br. J. Pharmacol.* **93**, 985–993.

Kahn, R.J., McNair, D.M., Lipman, R.S. *et al.* (1986). Imipramine and chlordiazepoxide in depressive and anxiety disorders. 2. Efficacy in anxious patients. *Arch. Gen. Psychiat.* **43**, 79–85.

Koeppen, D. (1984). Memory and benzodiazepines: animal and human studies with 1,4-benzodiazepines and clobazam (1,5-benzodiazepine). *Drug Dev. Res.* **4**, 555–563.

Lader, M. and File, S. (1987). The biological basis of benzodiazepine dependence. *Psychol. Med.* **17**, 539–557.

Leckman, J.F., Weissman, M.H., Merikangas, K.R., Pauls, D.L. and Prusoff, B.A. (1983). Panic disorder and major depression: increased risk of depression, alcoholism, panic and phobic disorders in families of depressed probands with panic disorder. *Arch. Gen. Psychiat.* **40**, 1055–1060.

Medina, J.H., Pena, C., Levi de Stein, M., Wolfman, C. and Paladini, A.C. (1989). Benzodiazepine-like molecules, as well as other ligands for the brain benzodiazepine receptors, are relatively common constituents of plants. *Biochem. Biophys. Res. Commun.* **165**, 547–553.

Oakley, N.R., Jones, B.J. and Tyers, M.B. (1988). Tolerance and withdrawal studies with diazepam and GR38032F in the rat. *Br. J. Pharmacol.* **96**, 764P.

Olsen, R.W., Yang, J., King, R.G., Dilber, A., Stauber, G.B. and Ransom, R.W. (1986). Barbiturate and benzodiazepine modulation of GABA receptor binding and function. *Life Sci.* **39**, 1969–1976.

Pellow, S., Chopin, P. and File, S.E. (1985). Are the anxiogenic effects of yohimbine in the social interaction test mediated at benzodiazepine receptors? *Neurosci. Lett.* **55**, 5–9.

Petursson, H. and Lader, M. (1984). *Dependence on Tranquillizers*, Maudsley Monograph No. 28. Oxford: Oxford University Press.

Polc, P. and Hafely, W. (1977). Effects of systemic muscimol and GABA in the spinal cord and superior cervical ganglion in the cat. *Experientia* **33**, 809.

Redmond, D.E. and Huang, Y.H. (1979). New evidence for a locus coeruleus norepinephrine connection with anxiety. *Life Sci.* **25**, 2149–2162.

Schofield, P.R., Darlison, M.G., Fujita, N. *et al.* (1987). Sequence and functional expression of the GABA$_A$ receptor shows a ligand-gated receptor super-family. *Nature* **328**, 221–227.

Schweitzer, E., Rickels, K. and Lucki, I. (1986). Resistance to the anti-anxiety effect of buspirone in patients with a history of benzodiazepine use. *New Engl. J. Med.* **314**, 719–720.

Sheehan, D.V. (1987). Benzodiazepines in panic disorder and agoraphobia. *J. Affect. Disord.* **13**, 169–181.

Sieghart, W. (1989). Multiplicity of GABA$_A$-benzodiazepine receptors. *Trends Pharmacol. Sci.* **10**, 407–411.

Sieghart, W. and Karobath, M. (1980). Molecular heterogeneity of benzodiazepine receptors. *Nature* **286**, 285–287.

Stein, L., Wise, C.D. and Berger, B.D. (1973). Antianxiety action of benzodiazepines: decrease in activity of serotonin neurons in the punishment system. In: S. Garattini, E. Mussini and L.O. Randall (eds) *The Benzodiazepines*, pp. 299–326. New York: Raven Press.

Thiebot, M.-H. and Soubrie, P. (1983). Behavioural pharmacology of the benzodiazepines. In: E. Costa (ed.) *The Benzodiazepines: From Molecular Biology to Clinical Practice*, pp. 67–92. New York: Raven Press.

Traber, J. and Glaser, T. (1987). 5-HT1A receptor-related anxiolytics. *Trends Pharmacol. Sci.* **8**, 432–437.

Turner, P., Granville-Grossman, K.L. and Smart, J.V. (1965). Effect of adrenergic receptor blockade on the tachycardia of thyrotoxicosis and anxiety state. *Lancet* **ii**, 1316–1318.

Tye, N.C., Everitt, B.J. and Iversen, S.D. (1977). 5-Hydroxytryptamine and punishment. *Nature* **268**, 741–743.

Tyrer, P. (1982). The concept of somatic anxiety. *Br. J. Psychiat.* **140**, 325.

Tyrer, P. (1983). Neurosis divisible? *Lancet* **i**, 685–688.

Tyrer, P., Rutherford, D. and Huggett, T. (1981). Benzodiazepine withdrawal symptoms and propranolol. *Lancet* **i**, 520–522.

Tyrer, P., Owen, R. and Dawling, S. (1983). Gradual withdrawal of diazepam after long-term therapy. *Lancet* **i**, 1402–1406.

Depressive Illness and Antidepressant Drugs

M.P.I. Weller

In severe depressive illness, appetites are reduced and social contact minimized. Activities which were previously enjoyable no longer seem interesting. All initiative drains away and each simple task seems daunting, but guilt fuels a sense of duty and sufferers drag themselves through the chores of the day, abandoning their recreations. Despite painful effort, standards slip, reinforcing a pathological sense of worthlessness. Feelings of emptiness, unworthiness and guilt combine with a disbelief that the future holds any prospect of pleasure.

> And I can weep for the state I am in:
> But my laugh has gone for good,
> And gone the charm of tears.
>
> *Suri Purohit Swami*

The unremitting, bleak hopelessness can overwhelm the sufferer and 15% take their lives. Delusions or hallucinations sometimes occur and the condition is then described as a psychotic depression. Such hallucinations can be distinguished from schizophrenic hallucinations in being consonant with mood. They are often of voices addressing the patient (rather than speaking about him) and are characteristically critical and denigratory. Delusions, too, are consonant with mood and are usually of guilt and unworthiness, although paranoid delusions also occur.

Some Nosological Considerations

Depression may alternate with episodes of pathological excitement and euphoric over-optimism. Such a manic-depressive psychosis was recognized by Falret (1854) and Baillarger (1854), who described the condition as 'folie circulaire'. Emil Kraepelin (1856–1926) separated manic-depressive illness from dementia praecox, or what we now call schizophrenia. He regarded psychiatric illness as endogenous or exogenous and observed that 'states of manic-depressive insanity will not be . . . recognized from one isolated symptom . . . but only from the whole clinical picture with cautious weighting of relations which exist between individual features'. Many diseases, such as hypertension and anaemia, have only arbitrary boundaries, with subclinical states and a diversity of causes. Kraepelin recognized this difficulty with manic-depressive illness and acknowledged that it is sometimes difficult to be sure whether or not someone is suffering from it.

Adolf Meyer (1866–1950), a professor at Johns Hopkins University, took a multifactorial view of mental illness and emphasized that environmental stresses interacted with constitutional factors. The wisdom of this approach can be seen in the determinants of pulmonary tuberculosis.

Ernst Kretchmer (1888–1964) portrayed various personality types in vivid and illuminating vignettes. Temperamental characteristics are not illness but may be associated with illness. The cyclothymic personality is more likely to develop manic-depressive psychosis than schizophrenia, whilst the converse is true of borderline and schizotypal personalities. At the very least, the illness is set against a background of personality characteristics. Kretchmer's interest in body build can be seen as a prelude to the continuing quest for biological markers in affective disorders.

Certain symptoms favour particular treatments and controversy has surrounded the question as to whether or not depressive illness can be subdivided on the basis of the presence, or absence, of these symptoms, or whether they are merely indices of severity. Statistical methods provide a powerful tool for determining classes and subgroups. Applying these methods to clinical observations enables us to see relationships that might otherwise elude us. One of the earliest uses of statistical categorization was in psychology, when Spearman used factor analysis to clarify the components of intelligence (see Chapter 19, this volume). Later, Hans Eysenck applied the technique to personality (see Chapter 22, this volume). The first publication applying factor analysis to psychiatric data was that of T.V. Moore, in 1930. Kiloh and Garside applied discriminant function analysis to the classification of depressive disorders in 1963.

There are those who regard all depressive illness as one continuum and others who believe that the illness can be subdivided into two main groups, endogenous and reactive. The dispute between the unitarists and the separatists hinges on the source of the population under study and the statistical procedures used to attempt a separation. Cluster analysis starts with a *tabula rasa*, whilst discriminant function analysis seeks to test a hypothesis. There are many different techniques of cluster analysis which do not yield the same results. Those studies that have shown two separable conditions have generally been based on in-patient populations, in whom the disorder is probably severe. Undoubtedly there is a large group of patients with a mixture of both endogenous and reactive symptoms. Nevertheless, certain symptoms, described as endogenous, character-ize a group of depressive patients whose response to drug treatment, pharmaco-logical challenge and electroconvulsive therapy is different (see Table 30.1 and below).

Based in part on observations in general medical wards, my own view is that endogenous illness, as a constellation of symptoms described in Table 30.1, can be identified independently from the severity of the mood disturbance, and others have found likewise (e.g. van Praag, 1990). A positive family history of affective illness, episodic heavy gambling, or suicide can often be found in such cases. One of the most influential proponents of the unitary model was Sir Aubrey Lewis. It is ironic that analysis of his data, both by discriminant function and by cluster analysis, has yielded two separate groups of patients (Kiloh and Garside, 1977).

TABLE 30.1 Forms of depressive illness.

Endogenous–psychotic	Reactive–neurotic
General	
History of previous discrete episodes	
Somatic	*Somatic*
[a]Early morning waking	Initial insomnia and hypersomnolence
[a]Psychomotor retardation	
Loss of appetite	Hyperphagia
Weight loss of 7 lb or more	
Pyknic habitus	
Psychic	*Psychic*
[a]Qualitative change in mood	
[a]Symptoms worse a.m.	Symptoms worse p.m.
[a]No obvious precipitant	Obvious precipitant and sudden onset
Absence of mood reactivity	Mood variable and responsive to milieu
Poor concentration	
Self-blame	Blaming others and self-pity
Delusions	
Pathological guilt	
Nihilistic	
Somatic	
Paranoid	
Auditory hallucinations	
With derogatory content and in first person	
Pre-morbid personality	*Pre-morbid personality*
Stable or cyclothymic	Vulnerable or neurotic with anxiety
	Hypochondriasis and obsessional
Strong genetic component	Weak genetic component

This table is a composite from several sources including those reviewed by Mayer-Gross *et al.* (1969) and Paykel and Coppen (1979). It does not presuppose a dimension or typological distinction. Only some of the features will be present in any particular case. It is possible to construct a weighted discriminant function for the presence or absence of appropriate symptoms (see Kiloh and Garside, 1977).
[a]Symptoms which are particularly characteristic. The DSM-III-R Melancholic type of Major Depressive Disorder (American Psychiatric Association, 1987) seems to acknowledge that while most depression is mixed there is an endogenous subtype. The criteria include most of the footnoted items and a favourable outcome of previous episode(s) to adequate antidepressant therapy.

Hormonal responses to pharmacological challenges have been used to expose biological features distinguishing between endogenous and non-endogenous illnesses. These include growth hormone response to clonidine, an α-2 agonist (Matussek *et al.*, 1980; Checkley *et al.*, 1984), cortisol response to methyl-amphetamine (Checkley *et al.*, 1984), and prolactin response to the serotonin agonist fenfluramine (Mitchell *et al.*, 1990). On the whole, the results have pointed to a difference in brain neurotransmitter function between the two disorders and supported the clinical distinction. Nevertheless, the term 'endogenous', meaning coming from inside (rather than exogenous), is misleading, since precipitants can often be demonstrated (see Chapter 29, this volume), but the extent, severity and persistence of the symptoms seem disproportionate to the precipitant and the symptoms fall into a distinctive pattern. Some prefer the original term 'melancholia', or vital depression, thus avoiding the implication of lack of precipitation.

Carl Jaspers stressed that a disease process can be inferred when patients have experiences that go beyond our own empathetic understanding. Although he was focusing on schizophrenia, the same concept serves for the unremitting despair of endogenous depression, which could be termed an autochthonous mood state. Neurotic complaints are extensions of our own experiences. The term neurotic implies seemingly inadequate precipitants for the degree of suffering, coupled with maladaptive coping behaviour, whilst reactive implies that the state of mind is understandable as a reaction to events. Unfortunately, in practice the terms are often used interchangeably and, confusingly, reactive is also used descriptively to mean mood reactivity (as distinct from fixity of mood).

Depressive illness is not the same as unhappiness. The distinction is not difficult to make when endogenous features are present; features which will often respond to physical treatment in a predictable way. The character of a person cannot be altered by such treatments, which are ineffective as a cure for dissatisfaction and unhappiness.

The non-endogenous conditions create difficulties in deciding whether or not someone is ill. Severity is the distinguishing feature, but the cut-off may seem arbitrary and the concept of illness, or psychiatric case, therefore, less certain. In fact, despite the concept of a continuum between normality and neurosis, there often seems to be a categorical change in a person when they are neurotically ill (Roth and Kroll, 1986) and at least a subset have disturbed neuroendocrine functioning (Dinan and Barry, 1990). The non-endogenous group frequently had pre-existing neurotic traits before being depressed, and, as a whole, do well when followed up by community nurses. Although endogenous symptoms often occur in combination, non-endogenous symptoms have less tendency to cluster. Some of the variability in treatment and placebo response may be explained by the heterogeneity of this group.

Dysthymia in DSM-III-R differs from major depressive episode in being mild, chronic ('of many years duration') and intertwined with personality disorders. To this author, this classification is unsatisfactory, confounding severity, personality, and outcome with syndromal recognition. These features do not relate to a specific depressive syndrome, but rather vary within that syndrome (van Praag, 1990).

Coexisting anxiety

An intermingling of anxiety and depression is particularly evident in minor depressive disorders, as seen in general practice (Goldberg and Huxley, 1980), and occurs in one-third of cases of manic-depressive psychosis (Cassidy *et al.*,

1957). In the minor, neurotic type disorders it is possible to identify a
depressive syndromes (Roth and Mountjoy, 1982), which could also be se
in a large group of 6317 randomly selected community residents (Huppert *e*
1989). The situation is less clear-cut with respect to severe, endogenous type
illnesses. Some workers, particularly British, including Mapother and Lewis, up
until the present (Johnstone *et al.*, 1980) regard an intermingling of anxiety and
depression as characteristic of affective illness. ICD-10 includes a mixed anxiety
and depressive disorder, but the British term affective illness, widely used in
Europe, has no counterpart in DSM-III-R, which separates mood disorders and
anxious states, as is implicit in the hierarchical model of symptoms* (Foulds,
1978). (Indeed, the hierarchical system of diagnosis with the more serious
disorders taking precedence over the less serious, reified in DSM-III, continues to
resonate throughout in DSM-III-R.) Nevertheless, anxious, agitated depression is
very common in old age and the anxiety that often accompanies endogenous
type depression, at whatever age, generally improves contemporaneously with
the depression when treatment of the latter is successful.

Depression is separated into unipolar and bipolar forms (see Chapter 13, this
volume). Unipolar means that only depressive episodes have occurred; bipolar
means that at least one hypomanic episode has occurred in addition to depression.
If the hypomania occurs during antidepressant medication or ECT the familial
concordance is improved if the patient is classified as suffering from a bipolar
disorder. (The term mania is seldom used in England, although nearly universal
in Spain and Israel, and the British terminology is attributed by some as typical
British understatement! Mania denotes a complete loss of insight: hypomania is
less severe.) A switch from mania to depression (Lucas *et al.*, 1989), or vice versa
occurs in 20–30% of bipolar episodes, at a median period of 4 months after the
onset of the episode and 7 weeks after hospital admission (Angst, 1987). The
occurrence of depression following mania is associated with a cyclothymic
pre-morbid personality, a family history of affective illness and a previous history
of depression (Lucas *et al.*, 1989). Unipolar illness may be endogenous or reactive,
but it is difficult to emphasize with the pathological euphoria and over-excitement
that sometimes succeeds calamity (e.g. Ambelas, 1987) and the various biochemical
disturbances that have been described in endogenous depression, discussed below,
are generally more severe in hypomanic illness (but, somewhat unexpectedly, are
generally in the same direction, rather than being reciprocally related).

Depression *per se*, or complicating other disorders, is the most common
condition with which general psychiatrists are confronted. Mild depressive
symptoms are particularly common and social factors contribute to the symptoms
and their perpetuation (Chapters 27 and 28, this volume). The prevalence of
depression varies according to severity criteria, but a female preponderance of the
order 2 : 1 is a general finding in unipolar depression, the sex ratio being equal
in bipolar states, which typically have an earlier age of onset and earlier

*British workers, explicitly (Marks, 1987) or implicitly (Tyrer, 1986), question whether anxiety and panic
disorder, which can be successfully treated with tricyclics and MAOIs and which occur in depression, should
properly be distinguished, as they are in DSM-III-R and ICD-10, and Lelliott and Bass (1990) question whether
panic disorder is a uniform illness.

polar cases. Although more women than men meet
pression and report more symptoms in a non-clinical
ses the severity is similar in both sexes, and the clinical
le, excepting that women are significantly more likely to
e and weight gain (Young *et al.*, 1990).
ession is likely to recur or remain chronic, and longitudinal
ingly poor outcome, considering the therapeutic optimism
vails (Kiloh *et al.*, 1988; Lee and Murray, 1988). Many
itients have a severe, recurring disorder (Harrow *et al.*, 1990)
and sub.... rmalities may contribute to the chronicity in bipolar patients
(Dupont *et al.*, 1990). However, chronicity is higher for unipolar disorders.
Adverse factors include being female, particularly if there are pre-morbid neurotic
traits, high familial loading for depression (see Scott, 1988) and physical ill health
and disability in the elderly (Kennedy *et al.*, 1991). Although there is an undoubted
genetic component in affective illness, environmental factors, deriving from a
mother's depression, also seem to have enduring, detrimental influences
(Hammen *et al.*, 1990; see Chapter 21, this volume).

The initial response to treatment is a good guide to the future, good
responders tending to remain so (Small *et al.*, 1981), and early intervention
following previously successful treatment significantly shortens episodes by
about 4 to 5 months (Kupfer *et al.*, 1989). Early detection and vigorous treatment are recommended, including giving ECT to the elderly (Baldwin and Jolley,
1986; Burville *et al.*, 1991). Mixed affective disorders, in which both manic and
depressive features coexist, are slow to respond to treatment, taking three times
longer (median 79 weeks) than pure depressives, and six times longer than pure
manics in the NIMH collaborative study.

Although some studies have shown spontaneous improvement in a high proportion of mild cases of depression (e.g. Beck, 1967; Goldberg and Blackwell, 1970),
Gillis and Stone (1973) found that 56% were ill on reassessment after six years, and
Beiser (1971) found that 52% were ill on annual assessments over five years and
26% were chronic cases over a mammoth 17 years follow-up (Murphy *et al.*, 1986).

The unipolar forms of depression tend to breed true, but the relatives of index
cases of bipolar illness have a high risk for both unipolar and bipolar illness,
overall about twice the risk of unipolar probands (McGuffin and Katz, 1986).
Prolactin levels are lower in bipolar than in unipolar patients (Mitchell *et al.*, 1990)
and different research groups have found genetic loci in bipolar pedigrees, but on
restriction fragment lengths of different chromosomes, Xq and 11p15. Others
have been unable to replicate the original findings in different or extended
pedigrees (see Kelso *et al.*, 1989; Merikangas *et al.*, 1989; Chapter 13, this volume)
but this does not invalidate the original findings in isolated populations.

The Biochemistry of Depression

In their simplest form, the biological theories of depression rest on the proposal
that the illness is a consequence of a reduction in one or more neurotransmitters.

Several lines of evidence suggest this. Drugs that interfere with the synthesis of some of the monoamine neurotransmitters, such as the antihypertensive, α-methyl DOPA, can cause depression, as can drugs, such as reserpine and tetrabenazine, which deplete neurotransmitter stores. The depressive effects of reserpine are largely dose-dependent and, like α-methyl DOPA, occur most frequently in patients with a past history of depression.

Neurotransmitter metabolite studies infer changes in the parent amines. However, the relationship is confusing and the interpretation sometimes contradictory. It is argued that an increase in a metabolite implies an increased turnover, but some uncertainties remain. The origin of the metabolite is not always evident, since it is not obtained directly from the brain. Even cerebrospinal fluid (CSF) may reflect a change in the blood–brain barrier, with peripherally derived metabolites entering the CSF. CSF drawn from a lumbar puncture in considerable measure reflects the biochemistry of the spinal cord.

The metabolite of noradrenaline (NA), 3-methoxy-4-hydroxy-phenylglycol (MHPG), has been measured in the urine of depressed patients, and a group of depressed patients has been identified with low levels. However, the proportion of MHPG actually derived from the brain is small. Other workers have found a depletion of serotonin (or 5-hydroxytyptamine, 5HT) and dopamine (DA) metabolites in the CSF of some depressed patients (Asberg *et al.*, 1984). The technique depends on artificially raising the levels with probenecid, which allows the measurement of the accumulated metabolites. Probenecid might, however, itself confound the results.

MHPG derives from adrenaline as well as NA. Rafaelson's group has found low levels of CSF adrenaline, but not NA in depressed patients, measured directly by an isotope-derivative technique (Gjerris, 1982). Levels increased over four-fold on recovery (Christensen *et al.*, 1980).

Some post-mortem studies have found reduced levels of 5HT metabolites (5HIAA) in the brains of those who have committed suicide, but other studies have not. Whether there is a causal connection between reduced 5HT metabolites and depressive illness is a complicated question. The levels of 5HIAA vary with diet, often altered in depression, and levels of 5HT fluctuate greatly over the 24-hour cycle. Based on seasonality of symptoms and the therapeutic effect of bright light and sleep deprivation in some patients, and the ability of lithium and some antidepressants to lengthen circadian rhythms, there has been speculation that the phase of circadian rhythms may be altered in depressed patients, which may account for some of the findings (see Weller and Jauhar, 1981; Wirtz-Justice, 1987).

The levels of 5HIAA *decrease* in the CSF with the antidepressants amitriptyline and imipramine (Post and Goodwin, 1974). The complexity of the interpretation of metabolite studies is illustrated by it being argued that this implies 5HT reuptake blockade. Only when 5HT is taken up by the proximal synaptic bouton can it be exposed to the intraneuronal monoamine oxidase for degradation to 5HIAA. It will be recalled that 5HT was initially thought to be deficient because 5HIAA was low in the CSF of some depressed patients and patients with endogenous depression (according to the Newcastle rating scale, see Kiloh and

Garside, 1977) had significantly higher CSF 5HT levels than controls (Gjerris *et al.*, 1987). This finding could reflect an actual increase, or may reflect a low level in the rate of metabolism, which would then accord with reduced CSF metabolite studies of 5HT (Asberg *et al.*, 1984). The interpretation of the higher 5HT findings and lower adrenaline findings is contradictory. However, an actual increase in 5HT would accord with the original direct brain stimulation experiments in animals, in which stimulation of the 5HT system seemed to act as an aversive stimulus, whilst stimulation of the noradrenergic pathway was powerfully rewarding (see Olds and Fobes, 1981; Phillips and Fiberger, 1989; Chapter 7, this volume).

Some reconciliation of these apparent inconsistencies may be available in our recent understanding of a multiplicity of 5HT receptors. Three classes, the first subdivided into four divisions, each with their own specific protein structure, have been identified and cloned, and a fourth class has been suggested (see Jones, 1990). Quantitative autoradiographic analysis and membrane binding of postmortem brains from suicide victims and controls have demonstrated increase in $5HT_2$ receptors in the pre-frontal cortex of brains of suicide victims compared to controls (as well as β-adrenergic sites in the temporal cortex) (Arango *et al.*, 1990), a finding which would accord with a known genetic component in suicide (Roy, 1986). ($5HT_2$ receptors are down-regulated by 5HT reuptake inhibitors, but, paradoxically, also by $5HT_2$ receptor antagonists (Blackshear and Sanders-Bush, 1982)).

Precursor substances of 5HT that, unlike 5HT itself, cross the blood–brain barrier, have been found therapeutic in their own right, as well as acting as adjuvants which potentiate the therapeutic effects of other antidepressants (van Praag and Mendlewicz, 1982).

Data suggest that antidepressants enhance the responsiveness of dopaminergic neurons (e.g. Maj *et al.*, 1987; Muscat *et al.*, 1990), which is consistent with the dopaminergic agonism of euphoriant drugs, such as cocaine and amphetamine, and the changes in DA metabolites in the CSF of some depressed patients (Asberg *et al.*, 1984). In accord with these arguments, Cassano has reported an enhancement of tricyclic benefit by abruptly stopping concomitant haloperidol, which had been given to implement this strategy and enhance dopamine receptor sensitivity (see also Marazziti *et al.*, 1991).

It has become apparent that polypeptides modulate neurotransmission and that a disturbance of the hypothalamic pituitary axis occurs in some depressed patients, affecting cortisol secretion. The sensitivity of platelet α_2-adrenoreceptors, which regulate the release of noradrenaline in the CNS, is altered (Smith *et al.*, 1982) and disturbances in the renin–angiotensin system, growth hormone, aldosterone and thyroid function have been reported. Which of these changes is primary and which secondary remains unclear.

A point of great nosological interest is that growth hormone response to clonidine and desimipramine can be used to monitor CNS α-adrenergic sensitivity. Using this method, Matussek and Laakmann (1981) have shown a reduced sensitivity of CNS α-adrenergic receptors in patients suffering from endogenous depression, but not those suffering from neurotic depression.

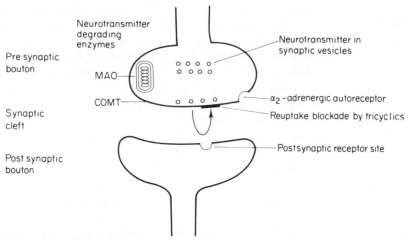

FIG. 30.1 Diagrammatic representation of a synaptosome. MAO, monoamine oxidase; COMT, catechol O-methyl transferase.

The Antidepressant ~~Drugs~~

The immediate euphoriant effects of dextro-amphetamine are dependent on an increase in the pre-synaptic neurotransmitter release. This leads eventually to a reduced receptor sensitivity. Increasing doses must, therefore, be given (tachyphylaxis) and adverse withdrawal effects occur. A further disadvantage is that increasing use can cause psychotic symptoms analogous to schizophrenia. Dextro-amphetamine also blocks the reuptake of NA and DA in the pre-synaptic bouton (see Fig. 30.1). The reuptake effect is exploited specifically by the tricyclic group of drugs.

Tricyclics

After neurotransmitters have been released into the synaptic cleft, they are reabsorbed into the pre-synaptic bouton. Oxidative deamination then degrades a proportion of the neurotransmitter, and the remainder is recycled into vesicles. Originally, tricyclic drugs were thought to work by blocking this reuptake and thereby increasing the amount of neurotransmitter available at the post-synaptic sites. This straightforward explanation of the mechanism of action has been replaced by a confusion of alternatives.

It is not immediately apparent why there should be a delay in the therapeutic effect of between 7 and 21 days when the reuptake blockade is immediate. Another view is that post-synaptic sensitivity is excessive, and reduced by a prolonged increase in neurotransmitter. This is at variance with the immediate beneficial effect of D-amphetamine. Indeed, a favourable response to 10–15 mg of D-amphetamine in a double-blind trial correlated with successful treatment with imipramine and desipramine (Fawcett and Siomopoulos, 1971). The pre-synaptic portion of the α-adrenergic synapse has an autoreceptor, designated the α_2-adrenoreceptor. When this is stimulated, neurotransmitter release is inhibited. Tricyclics modulate sensitivity to the α-adrenoreceptors (Raisman et al., 1979), and several studies have suggested that there is an excess of α_2-adrenoreceptors during depressive illness, which are reduced when the illness is successfully treated with tricyclic drugs, lithium or ECT. The reduction correlates with time of tricyclic treatment, suggesting a time-dependent desensitization of the receptor site (Smith et al., 1982; Garcia-Sevilla, 1989).

Tricyclic antidepressants also act directly on cholinergic and histaminergic sites, and have specific high-affinity binding sites on brain membranes. In addition, they affect the configuration of the 5HT binding sites and modulate post-synaptic sensitivity (Fillion and Fillion, 1981). It could be argued that any of these effects could be responsible for the antidepressant action.

The finding that there are high-affinity imipramine binding sites in the brain is particularly interesting. These sites are concentrated in the hypothalamus and the specific action is subtly modulated by sex hormones (Kendall et al., 1981). This may be one of the mechanisms explaining the increase in depression in females, including pre-menstrual tension, the increase in depression in later life and the shortening interval between episodes (Angst and Grof, 1977; Angst, 1978) (although this last phenomenon may have other explanations, such as electro-physiological 'kindling' in epilepsy and behavioural sensitization (Post et al., 1986; see Chapter 1, this volume)).

Langer et al. (1982) have shown that the imipramine receptors are associated with the reuptake site on 5HT nerve endings. The number is reduced in post-mortem brain samples of people who have committed suicide. Brain binding sites in rats were highly correlated with platelet binding sites, which are low in unmedicated depressed patients.

The basic structure of the tricyclic group is indicated in Fig. 30.2, and the profile of reuptake blockage is indicated in Table 30.2.

The tertiary amines are converted to secondary amines, so that the effect of the derived compound has to be added to the effect of the parent compound.

In practice, the therapeutic difference between the various tricyclics is not very great and down-regulation of noradrenergic receptors and desensitization of the noradrenergic receptor-coupled adenylate cyclase system occur after continuing therapy with a wide variety of antidepressants, irrespective of their main modes of action, and also after ECT (Sulser et al., 1983; Koe and Vinick, 1984). The sedative effect constitutes the main distinguishing feature between one drug and another. This is in part dependent upon the α-adrenergic blockade (U'Prichard et al., 1978) (a characteristic too of neuroleptic drugs, see Chapter 32, this volume) which also contributes to orthostatic hypotension. Clinical impression suggests that imipramine may be particularly successful in anergic, retarded depression, and nortriptyline has also been advocated for this patient group. Amitriptyline is one of the most widely prescribed drugs in the tricyclic group (and also one of the most anticholinergic) and may be particularly appropriate for anxious depression. Doxepin, which is very sedative, may likewise be particularly effective in anxious and restless depression. In a comparison between imipramine and

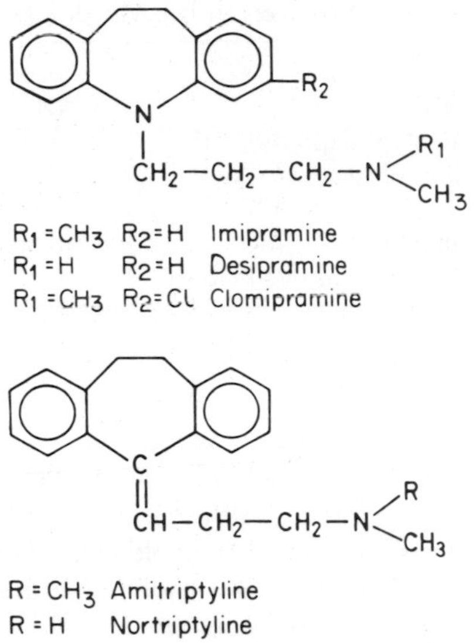

$R_1 = CH_3$ $R_2 = H$ Imipramine
$R_1 = H$ $R_2 = H$ Desipramine
$R_1 = CH_3$ $R_2 = Cl$ Clomipramine

$R = CH_3$ Amitriptyline
$R = H$ Nortriptyline

FIG. 30.2 Structural formulae of some tricyclics.

amitriptyline in the NIMH collaborative study, imipramine was superior for cognitive impairment in bipolar patients. Obsessional features are increased in depressive illness and imipramine, clomipramine, which has a 5HT reuptake emphasis, and the newer, specific 5HT reuptake blocking drugs, have been shown to be beneficial in such cases (e.g. Price *et al.*, 1987). Trimipramine is probably the safest tricyclic for combination with monoamine oxidase inhibitors (MAOIs) and, like doxepin, is particularly helpful for insomnia.

Drugs with a selective effect on the serotoninergic system, such as fluoxetine, fluvoxamine, paroxetine, sertraline and zimelidine, have little sedative effect at

TABLE 30.2 Reuptake profile of some tricyclic drugs.

Amines	Reuptake	Blockade
Tertiary	Serotonin	Noradrenaline
Imipramine	++	++
Amitriptyline	++	+++
Clomipramine	+++	+
Secondary		
Desmethylclomipramine		++
Nortriptyline		++
Desipramine		++

TABLE 30.3   Side-effects of tricyclic drugs.

Cardiac arrhythmias	Anxiety
Tachycardia	Dry mouth
Orthostatic hypotension	Sweating
Aggravation of glaucoma	Weight gain
Epilepsy	Constipation
Urine retention	Blurred vision
Ejaculatory and orgasmic failure	

low doses, and do not tend to cause weight gain, but are associated with insomnia, nausea, agitation, epilepsy and ejaculatory delay. These problems may be overcome by reducing the dosage. Although these compounds are chemically diverse, their clinical effects are similar (Benfield et al., 1986; Benfield and Ward, 1986). The drugs are largely devoid of anticholinergic and cardiovascular effects, which may be particularly advantageous in the elderly. Appetite disorders (Blundell, 1984), as well as obsessive-compulsive neurosis, may be particularly advantaged by this group of drugs.

The increased central 5HT transmission seems to be consequential on two mechanisms, neither of which is strictly dependent on reuptake blockade, although the drugs are often referred to as selective serotonin reuptake blockers: desensitization of somatodendritic 5HT autoreceptors, and desensitization of terminal 5HT autoreceptors. The former leads to an increase in firing activity through the release of powerful negative feedback control, and the latter to larger amounts of 5HT being released per impulse (de Montigny et al., 1990).

Dosage and drug interactions

The half-life of tricyclic drugs is sufficient for single-dose administration and is about 27 h for nortriptyline and 22 h for clomipramine. Divided doses are preferable when side effects are important, since the peak plasma concentrations will not be as high but the sedative side effects are better tolerated with night time administration. Slow-release preparations are an unnecessary expense (Liisberg et al., 1978). The side effects are of particular concern in the elderly and are identified in Table 30.3.

Cardiac arrhythmias are the main hazard. Mental illness can result from physical illness. This is particularly true in the elderly depressed, in whom the cardiovascular system is often disordered (Bergman, 1971). The specific 5HT uptake inhibitors and lofepramine are the least cardiotoxic.

Fear of side effects should be balanced against the morbidity and mortality of depressive illness. Suicide is at least 15% (Sainsbury, 1968), and would be higher but for the success of treatment, and non-suicidal death is increased, particularly from cardiovascular causes, as demonstrated in bereavement studies (see Chapter 28, this volume). Avery and Winokur (1976) found a reduction in non-suicidal mortality, particularly from myocardial infarction, in patients on

150 mg or more per day of typical tricyclics taken for an adequate period. A group given electroconvulsive therapy (ECT) had a significantly lower mortality than groups given either inadequate antidepressant treatment or neither ECT nor antidepressants.

The bioavailability of orally administered imipramine ranged from 29–77% in one study (Gram and Christiansen, 1975), probably as a result of first-pass effects through the liver. Plasma studies overcome these sources of variability, but protein binding is equally variable, ranging between 5 and 24% in 25 consecutively admitted patients (Glassman *et al.*, 1974). Children show less binding, and this, combined with less fatty compartments, in which the lipid soluble drug can penetrate, leads to a greater risk of toxic effects. Phenothiazines (e.g. chlorpromazine) and butyrophenones (e.g. haloperidol) but not flupenthixol, inhibit metabolism. Some anticonvulsants, including barbiturates, reduce plasma concentrations, but benzodiazepines do not and may produce a synergistic effect (King, 1982).

The wide variety of protein binding is a confounding feature of dose–response relationships, even if the plasma levels are studied. In addition, higher doses are likely to produce more side effects. Some workers have suggested that there is an optimal dosage of the drug beyond which the therapeutic effect is progressively lost, but others disagree and the position remains unclear. A difficulty encountered in these studies is that most of the drugs have active metabolites (see Table 30.2). It is not certain whether the plasma level of these should be added to that of the parent compound, and what allowance should be made for their potencies and pharmacological profiles, which differ from the parent compound.

Treatment failures may result from non-compliance, inadequate time on the drug, or inadequate dosage. Manufacturers have been tentative in their dose recommendations and this has been reinforced from other directions, e.g. WHO (1986). The typical tablet size of 25 mg provides a further deterrent to adequate prescribing and patient compliance. Yet a more consistent improvement was noted in patients receiving 300 mg of imipramine daily, when compared to those receiving 150 mg in a double-blind study (Simpson *et al.*, 1976) and up to 700 mg per day has been used successfully (Schuckit and Feighner, 1972). The severity of side effects is probably a clinical index of variations in individual pharmacokinetics. In Schuckit and Feighner's series, patients successfully treated with comparatively high doses suffered few side effects.

Fatalities have been conspicuously low with deliberate clomipramine overdose in attempts at self-harm (deaths per million prescriptions 11.1 as against 80.2 for desipramine, 50.0 for dothiepin and 46.5 for amitryptiline (see Beaumont, 1989)) and high doses have been used for intravenous therapy, making this tricyclic a good choice for higher than conventional oral dose regimes. With the notable exception of the tricyclic lofepramine, the more recent antidepressants, particularly maprotiline (deaths per million prescriptions 77) and mianserin (187), are generally *more* toxic than clomipramine.

There is little evidence that any one antidepressant is more rapid in its action than another and there are methodological problems in assessing such claims (Lydiard *et al.*, 1984).

Hypomania and panic attacks

Tricyclic drugs may convert patients with bipolar illnesses from depression into hypomania. In these patients without a previous hypomanic episode, the pattern of inheritance is clearest if they are classified as suffering from an occult bipolar illness (see Chapter 13, this volume). Paradoxically, tricyclic drugs with pronounced sedative effects can be useful in treating hypomania when combined with antimanic agents, such as chlorpromazine and haloperidol.

Some patients may experience an increase in anxiety and occasionally panic attacks when treated with tricyclics. It is a moot point whether the drug causes the new symptom or uncovers it. Some patients complain of feeling more tense in the first few days of treatment, before the antidepressive benefits occur, favouring the possibility that tricyclics may actually trigger panic attacks in some patients, whilst being successful as a treatment for panic attacks in others. This may explain why there was an increase in symptom rating in the first week on tricyclic drugs in an MRC trial.

Supplements

At the time of writing (July 1991), the commercial preparations Optimax and Pacitron, both drawn from a common source, of the amino acid, L-tryptophan have been withdrawn, except for named patients for whom no alternative therapy is suitable, because of a sometimes fatal, eosinophilia-myalgia reaction. It is believed that an as yet unknown contaminant (possibly the di-tryptophan aminal of acetaldehyde, or DTAA) is responsible. (The issue is casting a cloud over genetic engineering, used in the production.)

L-Tryptophan, in doses of 3–6 g per day, has been shown to potentiate monoamine oxidase inhibitors (e.g. Glassman and Platman, 1969), but inconsistent results have been reported for combination with tricyclics—Walinder et al. (1981) have claimed benefit and Thomson et al. (1982) have not. The recent need to withdraw L-tryptophan has seemingly led to relapse in some patients who appeared to benefit from the supplement (Ferrier et al., 1990). It is suggested that L-tryptophan should not be added to the selective 5HT antidepressants fluoxetine, fluvoxamine, paroxetine, sertraline and zimelidine.

The liver enzyme, tryptophan pyrolase, is induced by L-tryptophan and can be occupied by adding nicotinamide in doses of 1 g per day. (Cortisol, which is elevated in depression, stimulates tryptophan pyrolase, and NA, elevated in stress, inhibits tryptophan hydroxylase, the rate-limiting enzyme for 5HT production.)*

Synthesis of central serotonin is dependent on a cofactor, pyridoxine, which is alternatively utilized with oral contraceptives containing oestrogens.

Lithium, discussed further in the section on prophylaxis, has a potentiating effect on tricyclics in treatment-resistant cases, possibly mediated through a sensitizing effect on post-synaptic 5HT receptors. Early reports suggested a swift

---

*Carcinoid tumour is prone to cause depression by excessive utilization of L-tryptophan for peripheral 5HT synthesis. The condition is of theoretical interest. 5HT does not cross the blood–brain barrier. The addition of L-tryptophan in such cases relieves the depression, but intensifies the hypertensive problems.

response, within 48 hours, but later studies have found a mean time of response of the order of three weeks; about half the cases showing improvement (Price, 1989).

Claims have been made for the success of triiodothyronine (T3) as an adjuvant to tricyclics (e.g. Goodwin *et al.*, 1982), but others have not found it as useful (e.g. Garbutt *et al.*, 1986).

Monoamine Oxidase Inhibitors

Indications

The indication for monoamine oxidase inhibitors (MAOIs) has been stated to be atypical depression (Liebowitz *et al.*, 1988; Stewart *et al.*, 1989) but the term is ambiguous and has been used variously to mean non-endogenous depression, including depression where some of the endogenous features are reversed, depression combined with anxiety, including phobic anxiety, and, idiosyncratically, reactivity of mood with clear depression and one of the following —hyperphagia, hypersomnia, intense lethargy or pathological sensitivity to interpersonal rejection (Stewart *et al.*, 1989), or in other contexts, a schizoaffective disorder. Tyrer has stated that the drugs should be classified as 'delayed psychostimulants', indicated for agoraphobia, anxiety neurosis, anergia and mixed states of anxiety and depression, rather than pure depressions. They often cause insomnia and are therefore commonly prescribed to be taken not later than noon, although they may also have the reverse effect, dictating a corresponding redistribution. Although they are frequently helpful in anxiety, some workers consider that tricyclic drugs are also effective, as they are in reactive depression (Rowan *et al.*, 1981).

No medication will eradicate psychopathic personality features nor change maladaptive behaviour. Yet there is a group of dysphoric, timid, and sometimes seemingly inadequate people who respond well to this class of drugs. Symptoms of hypersomnolence, hyperphagia, rejection sensitivity and reactivity of mood identify the clinical impressions of favourable responsiveness to MAOIs. Unlike tricyclic drugs, patients are often reluctant to stop taking MAOIs. Correspondence in the *British Medical Journal* (1981) and elsewhere has pointed to their dependency potential.

There is contradictory evidence that phenelzine, and stronger evidence that tranylcypromine, are helpful in endogenous illness. More work still needs to be done on the precise indications.

Drugs in common usage and their interactions

MAOIs were discovered by Block and his colleagues, who noticed a mood-elevating effect of isoniazid, used in the treatment of tuberculosis. Because isoniazid and its derivative iproniazid are hepatotoxic (the damage probably being the result of highly reactive acylating and alkylating agents produced from

MONOAMINE OXIDASE INHIBITOR	Avoid
What you need to know	● Chianti wine completely, and drink no more than a little alcohol of any kind.
Drug	● Game, or meat that has not been well preserved.
Name	Other foods cause no problems.
	Do not take other medicines
Carry this card with you always. Show it to any doctor who may treat you; to your dentist if you require dental treatment; and to the pharmacist when you buy any medicine for yourself.	(including tablets, capsules, nose drops, inhalations or suppositories) whether bought by you or previously prescribed by your doctor, without first consulting him.
Please read carefully.	N.B. Cough and cold cures, pain relievers, tonics and laxatives are medicines.
While taking this medicine, and for ten days afterwards, you must follow these instructions.	These drugs are safe if the above precautions are observed:
Do not eat or drink anything which contains:	● You may use plain Aspirin BP or plain Paracetamol BP if necesary.
● Cheese, Bovril, Oxo, Marmite or similar meat or yeast extracts.	● If you need something for constipation, ask your pharmacist for a bulk laxative.
● Pickled herrings.	Report any severe symptoms to your doctor and follow any other advice given by him.
● Broad bean pods (the long green envelope which contains the beans, you can eat the beans themselves).	

FIG. 30.3   Information card for users of monoamine oxidase inhibitors.

the metabolites acetylhydrazine and isopropylhydrazine by oxidation by cytochrome P-450 enzymes in liver microsomes (Nelson *et al.*, 1979)), an effect that might have been increased by the co-administration of the microsome inducing barbiturates, other drugs were developed, of which phenelzine, isocarboxazid and nialamide are current examples of the same hydrazine and hydrazide types. The mechanism of action is blockade of the intracellular enzymes that degrade monoamines. Monoamine oxidase-A (MAO-A) predominantly deaminates serotonin, adrenaline and noradrenaline and the conventional inhibitor drugs are targeted at this enzyme.

The site of action is both nerve terminals and the walls of blood vessels, including those of the blood–brain barrier. The user is rendered vulnerable to tyramine, which binds with pre-synaptic vesicles, causing noradrenaline release (Vaccari, 1986), and to pressor agents. In the altered conditions caused by MAOIs, tyramine and pressor agents cause hypertensive crises. Phentolamine, an α-adrenoceptor blocking drug, is the treatment of choice in these situations. Certain food must be avoided. Many patients comply poorly with medication and the list of forbidden substances can be daunting. The recommendations in Fig. 30.3 attempt to balance prudence with over-caution.

Some overlap between the different classes of drugs is illustrated by the fact that amphetamine has some MAOI activity, and MAOI drugs have some effect on pre-synaptic reuptake.

The risk of hypertension interactions needs to be reconciled with one of the side effects of MAOIs, orthostatic hypertension (see Table 30.4).

TABLE 30.4   Side-effects of MAOIs.

Interactions leading to hypertensive crisis	Urinary retention
Liver damage	Failure of ejaculation
Aggravation of allergic reactions	Dry mouth
Orthostatic hypotension	Blurred vision
Epilepsy	

Consequential on MAOIs, tyramine accumulates in adrenergic neurones. This is converted to octopamine by dopamine-β-hydroxylase, which in turn acts as a false neurotransmitter in the sympathetic nervous system.

Tranylcypromine carries the greatest risk of subarachnoid haemorrhage following interaction with pressor agents. It is structurally very similar to amphetamine (see Fig. 30.4). One of the two isomers has an amphetamine-like action and the commercially available racemic mixture is particularly prone to cause dependency amongst the MAOIs.

Phenelzine is the most extensively tested MAOI. Some trials may have investigated too low a dose over too short a time. Tyrer *et al.* (1973) found

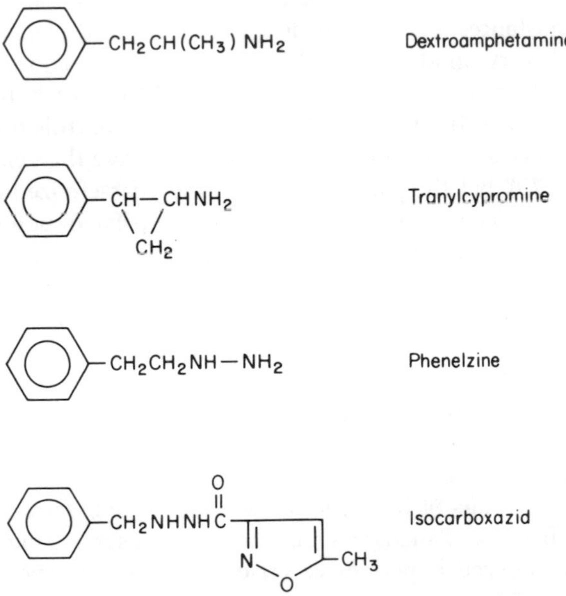

FIG. 30.4   The structure of D-amphetamine compared with some MAOIs.

a superiority over placebo in phobic patients after eight weeks, but not after four. The dose was flexible and there was a significant correlation between dose and improvement. In the Medical Research Council trial (1965), patients who were probably endogenously depressed did less well on phenelzine 60 mg daily for eight days than those patients on placebo tablets. A trend favouring the drug and increasing with time was found after a four-week period on 45 mg per day.

Unlike tranylcypromine, one of the routes of inactivation of phenelzine, a hydrazine drug, is acetylation. Approximately 40% of users acetylate the drug more rapidly than the other 60%. Although some trials have suggested that this is important, others have failed to provide confirmation. In practical terms, the dose is usually increased to 45 mg daily and raised after four weeks if there is an adequate response and absence of side effects.

Isocarboxazid is less therapeutically effective but safer with regard to hypertensive problems. It is more hepatotoxic than tranylcypromine and phenelzine, and anaemia and leucopenia have been reported.

All these drugs inhibit the spontaneous firing of raphé neurones in animals and suppress rapid eye movement (REM) in sleep, whilst increasing slow-wave sleep. The same effect on REM sleep is found with tricyclic drugs. This effect may limit 'incubation' of traumatic experiences (see Chapter 17, this volume).

A wash-out period of at least two weeks is desirable for MAOIs before starting tricyclics. When the change from tricyclics to MAOIs is contemplated, four days wash-out is usually sufficient, but ten days should be given if tranylcypromine is to be used.

Particular caution must be exercised in combining MAOI and tricyclic drugs. In normal circumstances, either both drugs are started in combination and the doses increased very gradually, or MAOIs should be added cautiously, in increasing doses, to an established tricyclic regime. Most experience of combined therapy has been with the tricyclic, trimipramine. A controlled trial on typical out-patients showed the combination to be less effective than either drug alone (Young et al., 1979), but the patients were poorly characterized and there were no specific checks on compliance. Many commentators have suggested it is worth considering the combination in cases that have proved resistant to other treatments, but particular caution is advisable.

Monoamine oxidase-A (MAO-A) predominantly deaminates serotonin, adrenaline and noradrenaline and the conventional inhibitor drugs are targeted at this enzyme. A comparatively new group of monoamine oxidase-B (MAO-B) inhibiting drugs (MAO-BI) have been developed. MAO-B is relatively selective for deaminating phenylethylamine and both MAO-A and MAO-B inhibitors are equal in their effects on tyramine and dopamine.

One of the first drugs of this type to be widely used was L-deprenyl, which has beneficial effects in Parkinson's disease. Low doses ($10 \, \text{mg day}^{-1}$) do not induce tyramine-induced hypertensive crises but lack antidepressant effect. At higher dosage (c. $30 \, \text{mg day}^{-1}$) an antidepressant action is found, but this is accompanied by the same food interactions as occur in MAO-A type inhibitors. This is probably because MAO-A effects are occurring at higher dosage, but other mechanisms are possible such as an inhibition of dopamine reuptake or its metabolism to amphetamine (Mann *et al.*, 1989).

The most effective and best studied reversible MAO-A inhibitor is moclobemide. It is free of anticholinergic effects and is well tolerated. The half-life is 16–20 h. A moderate control of tyramine-containing foods is prudent but the drug can be safely used at the end of a meal containing less than 100 mg of tyramine, a substantial amount (Simpson and De Leon, 1989; see Priest, 1990; Warrington *et al.*, 1991). However, interindividual variation in hypertensive response is considerable, and so too is the tyramine content of even the same type of cheese (Corn, 1990).

Other drugs of this class are cimoxatone and brofaromine, the latter having antidepressant activity and offering some protection from the tyramine pressor effect (see Priest, 1990). Coadministration of sympathomimetic amines is contraindicated (Corn, 1990).

Other antidepressants

The drugs already discussed are well established and have been used as standards against which newer compounds have been tested, often without a placebo control group. The placebo response is generally in the order of 24–30%, even in severely ill patients. (Placebo responders tend to improve abruptly early in treatment, when the improvement tends to be transient, or to improve gradually and evenly, when the improvement may represent spontaneous improvement (Quitkin *et al.*, 1991).) With such a large placebo effect, large numbers are necessary for comparisons to indicate statistically significant differences (see Chapter 5, this volume). The claims for many of the newer compounds are based on a large number of different trials, all of which have totally inadequate numbers. Clinically, the beneficial effects seem less reliable and less complete for many of these agents.

Amoxapine

Amoxapine, a dibenzoxapine tricyclic, primarily inhibits noradrenaline reuptake and weakly inhibits 5HT reuptake. It, and its metabolite 7-hydroxyamoxapine, weakly blocks dopamine receptors. The therapeutic effect is rapid, being detectable in the first week of administration, and the anticholinergic effects are low (Yamhure and Villalobos, 1977; McNair *et al.*, 1986), although dry mouth and constipation were comparable with imipramine in a multicentre trial of 111 patients (Takahashi *et al.*, 1979). Impotence or loss of libido has been reported (Hekimian *et al.*, 1978). Epilepsy and renal failure occur with overdose; rarely neurotoxicity develops.

Mianserin

The drug is less cardiotoxic than tricyclics and used to be popular for treatment of the elderly. However, leucopenia, agranulocytosis and aplastic anaemia were subsequently reported, particularly in the elderly, limiting its use, and blood counts are needed. Agitated states seem to benefit most, but the success of the drug is less well established than that of tricyclics and the indications are less precise. The mechanism of action is undecided, but the drug attaches to different receptors than imipramine (Brunello et al., 1982) and it possesses at least modest potency as an inhibitor of NA. A combination of mianserin and a tricyclic has potential for unresponsive cases but has not been formally investigated.

Maprotiline

This drug is particularly selective at blocking NA reuptake. Epileptic side-effects have been reported, but it seems less cardiotoxic than tricyclics. Users often complain of tiredness and sleepiness.

Flupenthixol

Low doses (1–3 mg in the early part of the day) of this neuroleptic has energizing actions. The paradoxical effect, which may occur with thioridazine also, is probably due to the preferential blockade of the pre-synaptic autoreceptors at low doses. The drug is most successful for mild, neurotic type conditions, in which it can be pleasingly effective. Its potential for abuse is limited by the sedative effects of higher doses and, in the tablet size used for antidepressant purposes, is comparatively safe in overdose.

ECT

ECT is probably the most effective treatment in psychiatry and can be administered together with tricyclics or MAOIs. Recent trials have vindicated the therapeutic benefit of ECT, although in one it was only found effective in deluded patients, the group least advantaged by tricyclic drugs (see Chapter 33, this volume).

Prophylaxis

Lithium exerts a prophylactic effect in bipolar depressive illness. The effect is controversial in unipolar depression, the only prospective, randomized trial finding effective prophylaxis in bipolar but not in unipolar depression (Prien et al., 1984) but other uncontrolled or retrospective studies have often pointed to a beneficial effect (see Souza et al., 1990). It is also probably a weak antidepressant and a stronger antimanic agent, but one which requires persistent dosage because of its slow onset. Because of this it is often combined with neuroleptics. Lithium increases neuroleptic-induced extrapyramidal signs (EPS) (Addonizio et al., 1988) and phenothiazines and thioxanthenes increase lithium red blood cell to plasma levels, suggesting possible generalized raised intracellular levels (Pandey *et al.*, 1979; von Knorring *et al.*, 1982). A particularly severe reaction has occasionally been reported when prescribed with haloperidol and the combination should be avoided.

Lithium potentiates the therapeutic effect of tricyclic drugs (e.g. de Montigny *et al.*, 1983), the process taking about 3 weeks (Price *et al.*, 1983), and has been proposed by Barker and Eccleston (1984) as an adjuvant for MAOIs for treatment-resistant cases.

The conventional plasma level is $0.6–1.2 \, \text{mEq} \, l^{-1}$ 12 h after the last dose. Lower plasma levels have been advocated by some workers. The lower levels are a compromise, balancing reduced therapeutic benefit with the risks of focal interstitial nephropathy and long-term osteoporosis. Divided doses have been advocated to minimize plasma peaks but a one-dose per day schedule is less likely to produce functional or structural kidney changes than when the dose is divided between two or three doses during the day (Plenge *et al.*, 1982). The authors found similar effects in rats given intravenous versus oral schedules (Plenge *et al.*, 1981) and consider that regenerative processes may be inhibited by more consistent plasma concentrations. The evidence in humans is consistent with the animal work (Bowen *et al.*, 1991), and frequency of administration, age, pre-existing renal disease, and intoxication episodes, rather than length of treatment are the variables that adversely affect kidney function (Hetmar *et al.*, 1991).

Intriguingly, nuclear magnetic resonance has demonstrated longer proton T_1 relaxation times in brain tissue of bipolar depressives which was normalized after lithium therapy (Rangel-Guerra *et al.*, 1983) and similar results were found in red blood cells (Rosenthal *et al.*, 1986).

The low therapeutic index of lithium salts, and their tendency to produce toxic effects and side effects that include coarse tremor and weight gain, are serious disadvantages, reducing compliance. Carbamazepine, with a structure resembling imipramine, in doses of 100 mg three times a day to 200 mg twice a day may alter brain 5HT and dopamine functions in humans (Elphick *et al.*, 1990) and has been found to exert significant prophylactic benefit. It is probably less effective than lithium (Watkins *et al.*, 1987) but easier to manage. Blood dyscrasias have occasionally been reported and merit occasional checks.

It is suggested that lithium and carbamezepine should not be combined but this is not an absolute contraindication and is justified in poorly controlled bipolar depressions when the combination may be pleasingly effective. Similarly, the two may be combined successfully in treatment-resistant depression (Kramlinger and Post, 1989). The author has carefully monitored eight patients who benefited from the combined drugs over several years without adverse sequelae.

Recent studies have suggested that carbamazepine significantly lowers plasma haloperidol levels, possibly through enzyme induction (e.g. Arana *et al.*, 1986). Fluoxetine at a dose of 20 mg daily has apparently led to toxic plasma levels of carbamazepine in two previously well maintained cases and levels should be monitored for 6 weeks on combined therapy.

The distress displayed by animals under stressful conditions is reduced by prior exposure to tricyclic drugs (Hrdina *et al.*, 1979; Roche and Leshner, 1979) and relapse of unipolar depression can be reduced by continuing on tricyclic drugs. Relapse after 4 months should be considered as part of the same episode (Angst, 1987) and several studies have shown that continuation of tricyclics provides protection during and beyond this period, up to 8 months on amitriptyline (see Montgomery, 1989). Prophylactic studies of antidepressants have generally contained methodological shortfalls and have been based on small numbers, but have been encouraging. With poorly controlled, recurrent episodes of unipolar depression patients should be encouraged to continue antidepressants for years if necessary. Persistent, dose-related, weight gain often discourages patients from continuing tricyclics, but the serotonin reuptake blocking drugs fluoxetine, fluvoxamine, paroxetine, sertraline and zimelidine do not suffer from this problem. Mianserin does not seem to have prophylactic properties.

It is usual to lower the dose for maintenance therapy. Although this may be successful, published studies have generally been at normal treatment doses and do not warrant this. One study showed favourable results over three years in patients taking an average of 200 mg daily of imipramine (Frank et al., 1990).

Envoi

It is to be expected that this chapter should focus on drugs, but prescribing drugs without support and encouragement can be interpreted as rejection. Chronic cases are associated with persistent social problems (Kedward, 1969) and lack of support (Bullock et al., 1972). Marginalization from the community and lack of a close confidant are risk factors, while integration into the social fabric is protective and therapeutic (Brown and Harris, 1978; Fenig and Levav, 1991) and probably aids recovery. Psychotherapy serves to lengthen the time between episodes (Frank et al., 1990). Despite the caveats in medical education for cautious statements, all patients benefit from kindness and sympathetic understanding and many benefit substantially from practical help if this can be organized (Corney, 1984).

References

Addonizio, G., Roth, S.D., Stokes, P.E. and Stoll, P.M. (1988). Increased extrapyramidal symptoms with addition of lithium to neuroleptics. J. Nervous Mental Dis. **176,** 682–685.

Ambelas, A. (1987). Life-events and mania—a special relationship? Br. J. Psychiat. **150,** 235–240.

American Psychiatric Association (1987). Diagnostic and Statistical Manual of Mental Disorders, 3rd edn., revised. Washington DC: American Psychiatric Association.

Angst, J. (1978). The course of affective disorders II. Typology of bipolar manic-depressive illness. Arch. Psychiat. Nervenkrank. (Berlin) **226,** 65–74.

Angst, J. (1987). Switch from depression to mania, or from mania to depression. J. Pharmacol. **1,** 13–20.

Angst, J. and Grof, P. (1977). The course of unipolar depression and bipolar psychoses. In: A. Villeneuve (ed.) Lithium in Psychiatry: A Symposium. Quebec: Presses de l'Université Laval.

Angst, J., Baastrup, P., Grof, P., Hippius, H., Poldinger, W. and Weis, P. (1973). The course of monopolar depression and bipolar psychoses. *Psychiat. Neurol. Neurochir. (Amst.)* **76**, 489–500.

Arana, G.W., Goff, D.C., Friedman, H., Ornstein, M. and Greenblatt, D.J. (1986). Does carbamazepine-induced reduction of plasma haloperidol worsen psychotic symptoms? *Am. J. Psychiat.* **143**, 650–651.

Arango, V., Ernsberger, P., Marzuk, P.M. *et al.* (1990). Autoradiographic demonstration of increased serotonin 5HT2 and β-adrenergic receptor binding sites in the brain of suicide victims. *Arch. Gen. Psychiat.* **47**, 1038–1047.

Asberg, M., Bertilsson, L., Martensson, B., Scalia-Tomba, G.P., Thorn, P. and Traskman-Bendz, L. (1984). CSF monoamine metabolites in melancholia. *Acta Psychiatr. Scand.* **69**, 201–219.

Avery, D. and Winokur, G. (1976). Mortality in depressed patients treated with electroconvulsive therapy and antidepressants. *Arch. Gen. Psychiat.* **33**, 1029–1037.

Baillarger, J. (1853–54). Note on the type of insanity with attacks characterized by two regular periods, one of depression and one of excitation. *Bull. Acad. Natn. Méd. (Paris)*.

Baldwin, R.C. and Jolley, D.J. (1986). The prognosis of depression. *Br. J. Psychiat.* **149**, 574–583.

Barker, W.A. and Eccleston, D. (1984). The treatment of chronic depression: an illustrative case. *Br. J. Psychiat.* **147**, 317–319.

Beaumont, G. (1989). The toxicity of antidepressants (Comment). *Br. J. Psychiat.* **154**, 454–458.

Beck, A.T. (1967). *Depression: Clinical, Experimental and Theoretical Aspects.* New York: Harper & Row.

Beiser, M. (1971). A psychiatric follow-up study of 'normal' adults. *Am. J. Psychiat.* **127**, 1464–1472.

Benfield, P. and Ward, A. (1986). Fluvoxamine—a review of its pharmacodynamic and pharmacokinetic properties, and therapeutic efficacy in depressive illness. *Drugs* **32**, 313–334.

Benfield, P., Heel, R.C. and Lewis, S.P. (1986). Fluoxetine—a review of its pharmacodynamic and pharmacokinetic properties, and therapeutic efficacy in depressive illness. *Drugs* **32**, 481–508.

Bergman, K. (1971). The neuroses of old age. In: D.W.K. Kay and A. Walk (eds) *Recent Developments in Psychogeriatrics.* (*Br. J. Psychiat.* Special Publication No. 6), pp. 39–50. Ashford, Kent: Medico-Psychological Association.

Blackshear, M.A. and Sanders-Bush, E. (1982). Serotonin receptor sensitivity after acute and chronic treatment with mianserin. *J. Pharmacol. Exp. Ther.* **221**, 303–308.

Blundell, J.E. (1984). Serotonin and appetite. *Neuropharmacology* **23**, 1537–1551.

Bowen, R.C., Grof, P. and Grof, E. (1991). Less frequent lithium administration and lower urine volume. *Am. J. Psychiat.* **148**, 189–192.

Brown, G.W. and Harris, T. (1978). *Social Origins of Depression: A Study of Psychiatric Disorder in Women.* London: Tavistock.

Brunello, N., Chuang, D.M. and Costa, E. (1982). Different synaptic location of mianserin and imipramine binding sites. *Science (NY)* **215**, 1112–1115.

Bullock, R.C., Siegel, R., Weissman, M. and Paykel, E.S. (1972). The weeping wife: marital relations of depressed women. *J. Marriage Family* **34**, 488–495.

Burville, P.W., Hall, W.D., Stampfer, H.G. and Emerson, J.P. (1991). The prognosis of depression in old age. *Br. J. Psychiat.* **158**, 64–71.

Cassidy, W.L., Flanagan, N.B., Spellman, M. and Cohen, M.E. (1957). Manic-depressive patients and 50 medically sick controls. *J. Am. Med. Assoc.* **164**, 1535–1546.

Checkley, S.A., Glass, I.B., Thompson, C. *et al.* (1984). The growth hormone response to clonidine in endogenous as compared to reactive depression. *Psychol. Med.* **14**, 773–774.

Christensen, N.J., Vestergaard, P., Sørensen, T., Jerris, A.G. and Rafaelsen, O.J. (1980). Cerebrospinal fluid adrenaline in endogenous depression (letter). *Lancet* **i**, 722.

Corn, T.H. (1990). Reversible inhibitors of monoamine oxidase A: antidepressants without cheese effect? *Int. Rev. Psychiat.* **2**, 187–192.

Corney, R.H. (1984). The effectiveness of attached social workers in the management of depressed female patients in general practice. *Psychol. Med.* (Monograph Suppl. 6).

Dahl, S.G. (1988). Pharmacokinetics of neuroleptic drugs and the utility of plasma level monitoring. In: D.E. Casey and A.V. Christensen (eds) *Psychopharmacology: Current Trends*, p. 35. Heidelberg: Springer Verlag.

de Montigny, C., Cournoyer, G., Morisette, R., Langlois, R. and Caille, G. (1983). Lithium carbonate addition in tricyclic antidepressant-resistant unipolar depression. *Arch. Gen. Psychiat.* **40**, 1327–1334.

de Montigny, C., Chaput, Y. and Blier, P. (1990). Modification of serotonergic neuron properties by long-term treatment with serotonin reuptake blockers. *J. Clin. Psychiat.* (Suppl.) **51**, 4–8.

Dinan, T.G. and Barry, S. (1990). Response of growth hormone to desipramine in endogenous and non-endogenous depression. *Br. J. Psychiat.* **156**, 680–684.

Dupont, R.M., Jernigan, T.L., Butters, N., Delis, D., Hesselink, J.R., Heindel, W. and Gillin, J.C. (1990). Subcortical abnormalities detected in bipolar affective disorder using magnetic resonance imaging. *Arch. Gen. Psychiat.* **47**, 55–59.

Elphick, M., Yang, J.-D. and Cowen, P.J. (1990). Effects of carbamazepine on dopamine- and serotonin-mediated neuroendocrine responses. *Arch. Gen. Psychiat.* **47**, 135–140.

Falret, J.P. (1853–54). *Clinical Lecture on Mental Medicine. General Symptomatology.* Paris: Baillière.

Fawcett, J. and Siomopoulos, V. (1971). Dextroamphetamine response as a possible predictor of improvement with tricyclic therapy in depression. *Arch. Gen. Psychiat.* **25**, 247–255.

Fenig, S. and Levav, I. (1991). Demoralization and supports among holocaust survivors. *J. Nervous Mental Dis.* **179**, 167–172.

Ferrier, I.N., Eccleston, D., Moore, P.B. *et al.* (1990). Relapse in chronic depressives on withdrawal of L-tryptophan. *Lancet* **336**, 380–381.

Fillion, G. and Fillion, M.P. (1981). Modulation of affinity of postsynaptic serotonin receptors by antidepressant drugs. *Nature (Lond.)* **292**, 349–351.

Foulds, J.A. (1978). *The Hierarchical Nature of Personal Illness.* London: Academic Press.

Frank, E., Kupfer, D.J., Perel, J.M. *et al.* (1990). Three-year outcomes for maintenance therapies in recurrent depression. *Arch. Gen. Psychiat.* **47**, 1093–1099.

Garbutt, J.C., Mayo, J.P., Gillette, G.M., Little, K.Y. and Mason, G.A. (1986). Lithium potentiation of tricyclic antidepressants following lack of T3 potentiation. *Am. J. Psychiat.* **143**, 1038–1039.

Garcia-Sevilla, J.A. (1989). The platelet α_2-adrenoceptor as a potential marker in depression. *Br. J. Psychiat.* **154** (Suppl. 4), 67–72.

Gershon, E.S. (1982). Genetic linkage and vulnerability markers of affective disorders. 13th CINP Congress, Jerusalem, 20–25 June 1982. Abstracts, pp. 262 & 680.

Gillis, L.S. and Stone, G.L. (1973). A follow-up study of psychiatric disturbance in a Cape Coloured Community. *Br. J. Psychiat.* **123**, 279–283.

Gjerris, A. (1982). Adrenaline—a biological marker in depression? 13th CINP Congress, Jerusalem, 20–25 June 1982. Abstracts, p. 271.

Gjerris, A., Werdelin, L., Gjerris, F., Sørensen, P.S., Rafaelsen, O.J. and Alling, C. (1987). CSF-amine metabolites in depression, dementia and in controls. *Acta Psychiat. Scand.* **75**, 619–628.

Glassman, A.H. and Platman, S.R. (1969). Potentiation of a monoamine oxidase inhibitor by tryptophan. *J. Psychiat. Res.* **7**, 83–88.

Glassman, A.H., Hurvic, M.J., Kanler, M., Shostak, M. and Perel, J.M. (1974). Imipramine steady-state studies and plasma binding. In: I.S. Forrest and C.J. Carr (eds) *Advances in Biochemical Psychopharmacology*, Vol. 9, pp. 457–461. New York: Raven Press.

Goldberg, D.P. and Blackwell, B. (1970). Psychiatric illness in general practice. A detailed study using a new method of case identification. *Br. Med. J.* **ii**, 439–443.

Goldberg, D.P. and Huxley, P. (1980). *Mental Illness in the Community: The Pathway to Psychiatric Care*. London: Tavistock.

Goodwin, F.K., Prange, A.J., Post, R.M., Muscettola, G.E. and Lipton, M.A. (1982). Potentiation of antidepressant effects of 1-triiodothyronine in tricyclic non-responders. *Am. J. Psychiat.* **139**, 34–38.

Gram, L.F. and Christiansen, J. (1975). First-pass metabolism of imipramine in man. *Clin. Pharmacol. Ther.* **17**, 555–563.

Hammen, C., Burge, D., Burney, E. and Adrian, C. (1990). Longitudinal study of diagnoses in children of women with unipolar and bipolar affective disorder. *Arch. Gen. Psychiat.* **47**, 1112–1117.

Harrow, M., Goldberg, J.F., Grossman, L.S. and Meltzer, H.Y. (1990). Outcome of manic disorders. *Arch. Gen. Psychiat.* **47**, 665–671.

Hekimian, L.J., Friedhoff, A.J. and Deever, E. (1978). A comparison of the onset of action and therapeutic efficacy of amoxapine and amitriptyline. *J. Clin. Psychiat.* **39**, 633–637.

Hetmar, O., Povlsen, J., Ladefoged, J. and Bolwig, T.G. (1991). Lithium: long-term effects on the kidney. A prospective follow-up study ten years after kidney biopsy. *Arch. Gen. Psychiat.* **158**, 53–58.

Hrdina, P.D., von Kulmiz, P. and Stretch, R. (1979). Pharmacological modification of experimental depression in macaques. *Pharmacologica* **64**, 89–93.

Huppert, F.A., Walters, D.E., Day, N.E. and Elliot, B.J. (1989). The factor structure of the General Health Questionnaire (GHQ-30): a reliability study of 6317 community residents. *Br. J. Psychiat.* **155**, 178–185.

Johnstone, E.C., Cunningham-Owens, D.G., Frith, C.D. *et al.* (1980). Neurotic illness and its response to anxiolytic and antidepressant treatment. *Psychol. Med.* **20**, 321–328.

Jones, B.J. (1990). New possibilities for the drug treatment of schizophrenia. In: M.P.I. Weller (ed.) *International Perspectives in Schizophrenia*, pp. 231–235. London: John Libbey.

Kedward, H. (1969). The outcome of neurotic illness in the community. *Social Psychiat.* **4**, 1–4.

Kelso, J.R., Ginns, E.I., Egland, J.A. *et al.* (1989). Re-evaluation between chromosome 11p loci and the gene for bipolar affective disorder in the Old Order Amish. *Nature* **342**, 238–243.

Kendall, D.A., Stancel, G.M. and Enna, S.J. (1981). Imipramine: effects of ovarian steroids on modifications in serotonin receptor binding. *Science (NY)* **211**, 1183–1185.

Kennedy, G.J., Kelman, H.R. and Thomas, C. (1991). Persistence and remission of depressive symptoms in late life. *Am. J. Psychiat.* **148**, 174–178.

Kiloh, L.G. and Garside, R.F. (1963). The independence of neurotic depression and endogenous depression. *Br. J. Psychiat.* **109**, 451–463.

Kiloh, L.G. and Garside, R.F. (1977). Depression: a multivariate study of Sir Aubrey Lewis's data. *Aust. N.Z. J. Psychiat.* **11**, 149–156.

554   M.P.I. Weller

Kiloh, L.G., Andrews, G. and Neilson, M. (1988). The long term outcome of depressive illness. *Br. J. Psychiat.* **153**, 752–757.

King, L.A. (1982). Synergistic effect of benzodiazepines in fatal amitriptyline poisoning (letter). *Lancet* **ii**, 982–983.

Koe, B.K. and Vinick, F.J. (1984). Adaptive changes in central nervous system receptor systems. *Ann. Rep. Med. Chem.* **19**, 41–47.

Kramlinger, K.G. and Post, R.M. (1989). The addition of lithium to carbamazepine. *Arch. Gen. Psychiat.* **46**, 794–800.

Kupfer, D.J., Frank, E. and Perel, J.M. (1989). The advantage of early treatment intervention in recurrent depression. *Arch. Gen. Psychiat.* **46**, 771–775.

Langer, S.Z., Sechter, D., Raisman, R., Zarifian, E. and Briley, M. (1982). Antidepressant high affinity binding sites in platelets from psychiatric patients. 13th CINP Congress, Jerusalem, 20–25 June 1982. Abstracts Vol. 1, pp. 420–421.

Lee, A.S. and Murray, R.M. (1988). The long term outcome of Maudsley depressives. *Br. J. Psychiat.* **153**, 741–751.

Lelliott, P. and Bass, C. (1990). Symptom specificity in patients with panic. *Br. J. Psychiat.* **157**, 593–597.

Liebowitz, M.R., Quitkin, F.M., Stewart, J.W. *et al.* (1988). Antidepressant specificity in atypical depression. *Arch. Gen. Psychiat.* **45**, 129–138.

Liisberg, P., Rose, H., Amdisen, A., Jørgensen, A. and Petersen, H.E.H. (1978). A clinical trial comparing sustained release amitriptyline (Saroten retard) and conventional amitriptyline tablets (Saroten) in endogenously depressed patients with simultaneous determination of serum levels of amitriptyline and nortriptyline. *Acta Psychiat. Scand.* **57**, 426–435.

Lucas, C.P., Rigby, J.C. and Lucas, S.B. (1989). The occurrence of depression following mania: a method of predicting vulnerable cases. *Br. J. Psychiat.* **154**, 705–708.

Lydiard, R.B., Pottash, A.L.C. and Gould, M.S. (1984). Speed of action of the newer antidepressants. *Psychopharmacology Bull.* **20**, 258–271.

Maj, J., Wedzony, K. and Klimek, V. (1987). Desipramine given repeatedly enhances behavioural effects of dopamine and D-amphetamine injected into the nucleus accumbens. *Eur. J. Pharmacol.* **140**, 179–185.

Mann, J.J., Aaron, S.F., Francis, A.J. *et al.* (1989). A controlled study of the anti-depressant efficacy and side effects of (−) deprenyl: a selective monoamine oxidase inhibitor. *Arch. Gen. Psychiat.* **46**, 45–50.

Marazziti, D., Lenzi, A. and Cassano, G.B. (1991). Biological markers of bipolar disorders. *Biol. Psychiat.* **129**, 320 S.

Marks, I. (1987). Agoraphobia, panic disorder and related conditions in the DSM-IIR and ICD-10. *J. Pharmacol.* **1**, 6–12.

Matussek, N. and Laakmann, G. (1981). Growth hormone response in patients with depression. *Acta Psychiat. Scand.* **63** (Suppl. 290), 122–126.

Matussek, N., Ackenhail, M., Hippius, H. *et al.* (1980). Effect of clonidine on growth hormone release in psychiatric patients and controls. *Psychiat. Res.* **2**, 25–36.

Mayer-Gross, W., Slater, E. and Roth, M. (1969). Clinical psychiatry. In: E. Slater and M. Roth (eds), 3rd edn. London: Baillière Tindall.

McGuffin, P. and Katz, R. (1986). Nature, nurture and affective disorder. In: J.F.W. Deakin (ed.) *Biology of Depression.* London: Gaskell Royal College of Psychiatrists.

McNair, D.M., Rizley, R. and Kahn, R.J. (1986). Amoxapine and speed of onset: new antidepressant faces old methodology. *J. Clin. Psychiat.* (Monograph 4), 18–22.

Medical Research Council (1965). Clinical Psychiatry. Clinical trial of the treatment of depressive illness. *Br. Med. J.* **i**, 881–886.

Merikangas, K.R., Spence, A. and Kupfer, D.J. (1989). Linkage studies of bipolar disorder: methodologic and analytic issues. Report of McArthur Foundation workshop on linkage and clinical features in affective disorders. *Arch. Gen. Psychiat.* **46**, 1137–1141.

Mitchell, P., Smythe, G., Parker, G., Wilhelm, K., Kickie, I., Brodaty, H. and Boyce, P. (1990). Hormonal responses to fenfluramine in depressive subtypes. *Br. J. Psychiat.* **157**, 551–557.

Montgomery, S.A. (1989). Prophylaxis in recurrent unipoar depression: a new indication for treatment studies. Editorial, *J. Pharmacol.* **3**, 47–53.

Moore, T.V. (1930). Empirical determination of certain syndromes underlying praecox and manic-depressive psychoses. *Am. J. Psychiat.* **9**, 719–738.

Murphy, J.M., Olivier, D.C., Sobol, A.M., Monson, R.R. and Leighton, A.H. (1986). Diagnosis and outcome: depression and anxiety in a general population. *Psychol. Med.* **16**, 117–126.

Muscat, R., Sampson, D. and Willner, P. (1990). Dopaminergic mechanism of imipramine action in an animal model of depression. *Biol. Psychiat.* **28**, 223–230.

Nelson, S.D., Mitchell, J.R., Timbrell, J.A., Snodgrass, W.R. and Corcoran, G.B. III (1979). Isoniazid and Iproniazid: activation of metabolites to toxic intermediates in man and rat. *Science* (*NY*) **193**, 901–903.

Olds, M.E. and Fobes, J.L. (1981). The central basis of motivation: intracranial self-stimulation. *Ann. Rev. Psychol.* **32**, 523–574.

Pandey, G.N., Goel, I. and Davis, J.M. (1979). Effect of neuroleptic drugs on lithium uptake by the human erythrocyte. *Clin. Pharmacol. Ther.* **26**, 96–102.

Paykel, E.S. and Coppen, A. (eds) (1979). *Psychopharmacology of Affective Disorders.* London: Oxford University Press.

Phillips, A.G. and Fiberger, H.G. (1989). Neuroanatomical bases of intracranial self-stimulation: untangling the Gordian knot. In: J.M. Liebman and S.J. Cooper (eds) *The Neuropharmacological Basis of Reward*, pp. 66–105. Oxford: Oxford Science Publications.

Plenge, P., Mellerup, E.T. and Nørgaard, T. (1981). Functional and structural rat kidney changes caused by peroral or parenteral lithium treatment. *Acta Psychiat. Scand.* **63**, 303.

Plenge, P., Mellerup, E.T., Bolwig, T.G., Brun, C., Hetmar, O., Ladefoged, J., Larsen, S. and Rafaelsen, O.J. (1982). Lithium treatment: does the kidney prefer one daily dose instead of two? *Acta Psychiat. Scand.* **66**, 121–128.

Post, R.M. and Goodwin, F.K. (1974). Effects of amitriptyline and imipramine on amine metabolites in the cerebrospinal fluid of depressed patients. *Arch. Gen. Psychiat.* **30**, 234–239.

Post, R.M., Rubinow, D.R. and Ballenger, J.C. (1986). Conditioning and sensitization in the longitudinal course of affective illness. *Br. J. Psychiat.* **149**, 191–201.

Price, L.H. (1989). Lithium augmentation of tricyclic antidepressants. In: I. Extein (ed.) *Treatment of Resistant Depression.* Washington DC: American Psychiatric Press.

Price, L.H., Conwell, Y. and Nelson, J.C. (1983). Lithium augmentation of combined neuroleptic–tricyclic treatment in delusional depression. *Am. J. Psychiat.* **140**, 318–322.

Price, L.H., Goodman, W.K., Charney, D.S. *et al.* (1987). Treatment of severe obsessive-compulsive disorder with fluoxamine. *Am. J. Psychiat.* **144**, 1059–1061.

Prien, R.F., Kupfer, D.J., Mansky, P.A. *et al.* (1984). Drug therapy in the prevention of recurrences in unipolar and bipolar affective disorders. *Arch. Gen. Psychiat.* **41**, 1096–1104.

Priest, R.G. (1990). Depression and reversible monoamine oxidase inhibitors—new perspectives. *Br. J. Psychiat.* (Suppl. 6) 155.

Quitkin, F.M., Rabkin, J.G., Stewart, J.W. *et al.* (1991). Heterogeneity of clinical response during placebo treatment. *Am. J. Psychiat.* **148**, 193–196.

Raisman, R., Briley, M. and Langer, S.Z. (1979). Specific tricyclic antidepressant binding sites in rat brain. *Nature (Lond.)* **281**, 148–150.

Rangel-Guerra, R.A., Perez-Payan, H., Minkoff, L. and Todd, L.E. (1983). Nuclear magnetic resonance in bipolar affective disorders. *Am. J. Neuroradiol.* **4**, 229–231.

Roche, K.E. and Leshner, A.I. (1979). ACTH and vasopressin treatments immediately after a defeat increases future submissiveness in male mice. *Science* **204**, 1343–1344.

Rosenthal, J., Strauss, A., Minkoff, L. and Winston, A. (1986). Identifying lithium-responsive bipolar depressed patients using nuclear magnetic resonance. *Am. J. Psychiat.* **143**, 779–780.

Roth, M. and Mountjoy, C.Q. (1982). The distinction between anxiety and depressive disorders. In: E.S. Paykel (ed.) *Handbook of Affective Disorders*, pp. 70–92. Edinburgh: Churchill Livingstone.

Roth, M. and Kroll, J. (1986). *The Reality of Mental Illness.* London, New York, New Rochelle, Melbourne, Sydney: Cambridge University Press.

Rowan, P.R., Paykel, E.S., Parker, R.R., Gatehouse, J.M. and Rao, B.M. (1981). Tricyclic antidepressant and MAO inhibitor: are these differential effects? In: M.B.H. Youdim and E.S. Paykel (eds) *Monoamine Oxidase Inhibitors: The State of the Art*, pp. 125–139. Chichester: Wiley.

Roy, A. (1986). Genetics of suicide. *Ann. NY Acad. Sci.* **487**, 97–105.

Sainsbury, P. (1968). Suicide and depression. In: A. Coppen and A. Walk (eds) *Recent Developments in Affective Disorders*. London: Royal Medico-Psychological Association.

Schuckit, M.A. and Feighner, J.P. (1972). Safety of high-dose tricyclic antidepressant therapy. *Am. J. Psychiat.* **128**, 1456–1459.

Scott, J. (1988). Chronic depression (review article). *Br. J. Psychiat.* **153**, 287–297.

Simpson, G.M. and De Leon, J. (1989). Tyramine and new monoamine oxidase inhibitor drugs. In: R.G. Priest (ed.) Depression and reversible monoamine oxidase inhibitors —new perspectives. *Br. J. Psychiat.* (Suppl. 6) **155**, 32–37.

Simpson, G.M., Lee, J.H., Cuculic, Z. and Kellner, R. (1976). Two dosages of imipramine in hospitalised endogenous and neurotic depressives. *Arch. Gen. Psychiat.* **33**, 1093–1102.

Small, J.G., Milstein, V., Kellams, J.J. and Small, I.F. (1981). Comparative onset of improvement in depressive symptomatology with drug treatment, electroconvulsive therapy, and placebo. *J. Clin. Psychopharmacol.* (Suppl.) **1** (6), 62S–69S.

Smith, C.B., Hollingsworth, P.J., Garcia-Sevilla, J.A. and Zis, A.P. (1982). Platelet alpha-adrenoreceptors are decreased in number during antidepressant therapy. 13th CINP Congress, Jerusalem, 20–25 June 1982. Abstracts, Vol. 2, p. 681.

Souza, F.G.M., Mander, A.J. and Goodwin, G.M. (1990). The efficacy of lithium in prophylaxis of unipolar depression: evidence from its discontinuation. *Br. J. Psychiat.* **157**, 718–722.

Stewart, J.W., McGrath, P.J., Quitkin, F.M. *et al.* (1989). Relevance of DSM-III depressive subtype and chronicity of antidepressant efficacy in atypical depression. *Arch. Gen. Psychiat.* **46**, 1080–1087.

Sulser, F., Vetulani, J. and Mobley, P.L. (1978). Mode of action of antidepressant drugs. *Biochem. Pharmacol.* **27** (3), 257–261.

Sulser, F., Janowsky, A.J., Okada, F. *et al.* (1983). Regulation of recognition and action function of norepinephrine receptor-coupled adenylate cyclase system in brain: implications for the therapy of depression. *Neuropharmacology* **22**, 425–431.

Takahashi, R., Sakuma, A., Hara, T. *et al.* (1979). Comparison of efficacy of amoxapine and imipramine in a multi-clinic double-blind study using the WHO schedule for a standard assessment of patients with depressive disorders. *J. Int. Med. Res.* **7**, 7–18.

Thomson, J., Rankin, H., Ashcroft, G.W., Yates, C.M., McQueen, J.K. and Cummings, S.W. (1982). The treatment of depression in general practice: a comparison of trypto-phan, amitriptyline and a combination L-tryptophan and amitriptyline with placebo. *Psychol. Med.* **12** (4), 741–751.

Tyrer, P. (1986). Classification of anxiety disorders. *J. Affect. Dis.* **11**, 99–104.

Tyrer, P., Candy, J. and Kelly, D. (1973). Phenelzine in phobic anxiety: a controlled trial. *Psychol. Med.* **3**, 120–124.

U'Prichard, D.C., Greenberg, D.A., Sheehan, P.P. and Snyder, S.H. (1978). Tricyclic antidepressants: therapeutic properties and affinity for α-noradrenergic receptor binding sites in the brain. *Science (NY)* **199**, 197–198.

Vaccari, A. (1986). High affinity binding of (^{3}H)-tyramine in the central nervous system. *Br. J. Pharmacol.* **89**, 15–25.

van Praag, H.M. (1990). The DSM-IV (depression) classification: to be or not to be? *J. Nervous Mental Dis.* **178**, 147–149.

van Praag, H.M. and Mendlewicz, J. (eds) (1982). *Management of Depression with Mono-amine Precursors.* New York: Dekker.

von Knorring, L., Smigan, L., Perris, C. and Oreland, L. (1982). Lithium and neuroleptic drugs in combination-effect on lithium RBC/plasma ratio. *Int. Pharmacopsychiat.* **17**, 287–292.

Walinder, J., Carlsson, A. and Persson, R. (1981). 5HT reuptake inhibitors plus tryptophan in endogenous depression. *Acta Psychiat. Scand.* **63** (Suppl. 290), 179–190.

Warrington, S.J., Turner, P., Mant, T.G.K. *et al.* (1991). Clinical pharmacology of moclo-bemide, a new reversible monoamine oxidase inhibitor. *J. Psychopharmacol.* **5**, 82–91.

Watkins, S.E., Callender, K., Thomas, D.R., Tidmarsh, S.F. and Shaw, D.M. (1987). The effect of carbamazepine and lithium on remission from affective illness. *Br. J. Psychiat.* **150**, 180–182.

Weller, M.P.I. and Jauhar, P. (1981). Travel induced disturbances in circadian rhythms as precipitants of affective illness. In: G. Perris, G. Struwe and B. Jansson (eds) *Biological Psychiatry*, pp. 1253–1256. Amsterdam: Elsevier/North-Holland.

WHO (1986). World Health Organisation Collaborative Study Group: Dose effects of antidepressant medication in different populations. *J. Affect. Dis.* **2** (Suppl.), S1–S67.

Wirtz-Justice, A. (1987). Circadian rhythms in mammalian neurotransmitter receptors. *Prog. Neurobiol.* **29**, 219–259.

Yamhure, A. and Villalobos, A. (1977). Amoxapine: a double-blind comparative clinical study of amoxapine and amitriptyline in depressed, hospitalized patients. *Rev. Colomb. Psiquiat* **6** (2), 173–176.

Young, J.P.R., Lader, M.H. and Hughes, W.C. (1979). Controlled trial of trimipramine, monoamine oxidase inhibitors and combined treatment in depressed outpatients. *Br. Med. J.* **ii**, 1315–1317.

Young, M.A., Scheftner, W.A., Fawcett, J. and Klerman, G.L. (1990). Gender differences in the clinical features of unipolar major depressive disorder. *J. Nerv. Mental Dis.* **178** (3), 200–203.

— 31

Neurotransmitters and Schizophrenia

A.V.P. Mackay and L.L. Iversen

Introduction

In his classic description of the 'Schizophrenias', Bleuler (1911) already expressed the view that madness might result from a disorder of brain metabolism. The apparent absence of gross structural brain damage in schizophrenia has stimulated interest in biochemical hypotheses, and attention has focused on chemical neurotransmitter systems in the brain as possibly important elements in the pathophysiology of schizophrenic illness. Such research was greatly stimulated by the discovery that certain drugs, such as mescaline and lysergic acid diethylamide (LSD), can cause hallucinations and other disruptions of normal mental functions, akin to those seen in schizophrenia. This led to a search for naturally occurring 'psychotomimetic' chemicals in schizophrenic patients, a quest that has so far proved singularly unsuccessful.

More progress has been made through a different approach, which seeks to understand the mode of action in the brain of the many drugs known to be valuable in treating the symptoms of acute schizophrenia. The fact that drugs can effectively reverse some of the symptoms of schizophrenic illness itself provides considerable impetus to further research, since it suggests that a modifiable chemical abnormality exists in the brain. Neurotransmitter hypotheses for schizophrenia have been comprehensively reviewed elsewhere (Matthyse and Sugarman, 1979; Owen and Crow, 1987; Reynolds, 1989) and now must be accommodated alongside increasing evidence from post-mortem and *in vivo* imaging studies for localized abnormalities in brain structure.

Inheritance

A compelling case exists for an inherited predisposition to schizophrenic illness (see Sham *et al.*, Chapter 14, this volume). The most robust evidence comes from study of adopted-away offspring and twin studies. Through comparison of the concordance rates in monozygotic and dizygotic twins, recent data suggests an estimated heritability for schizophrenia of 0.87—that is, 87% of the difference in concordance between monozygotic and dizygotic twins can be accounted for genetically. This level of heritability is comparable to that found in anencephaly and in congenital dislocation of the hip (Reveley and Murray, 1980). However, in view of the fact that the monozygotic concordance rate is approximately 50%, it must be emphasized that at least as many monozygotic twins are not concordant for the illness as are, despite being genetically identical, drawing attention to the importance of non-genetic environmental factors.

Molecular genetic studies of schizophrenic illness are currently seeking to define the precise genetic loci for the inherited predisposition. While early studies (Bassett *et al.*, 1988) reported linkage to a site on chromosome 5, later attempts at replication have failed (Owen and Mullan, 1990). As the methodology for linkage analysis becomes more sophisticated the genetic loci will undoubtedly become clearer, raising the exciting possibility of verifying the abnormal genes through study of the predicted phenotypic abnormalities, either in post-mortem brain tissue or through *in vivo* imaging techniques.

All the current evidence points to the conclusion that what is inherited is not the certainty of developing schizophrenic illness, rather a vulnerability to it, upon which some environmental factor(s) operate to increase the probability of breakdown above a threshold level. This has been called the 'two-hit' model (Cannon *et al.*, 1989); the 'first-hit' representing the genetic predisposition, mediated possibly through faulty neuronal wiring and localized vascular fragility in limbic areas of the brain (Murray *et al.*, 1988). The 'second-hit' might derive from peri-natal obstetric complications resulting in ischaemia and anoxia in vulnerable areas. The resultant brain abnormality would then be a complex combination of abnormal neurotransmission and localized, probably subtle, structural abnormality. To take the question of what is inherited down to the neurotransmitter level it may be fruitful to probe further into the neurochemical and neuroanatomical substrates for the stress response which is known to be abnormal in schizophrenia (Parnas *et al.*, 1981). The homeostatic control of physiological stress response (arousal) mechanisms seems particularly vulnerable to perinatal ischaemic damage and from what is known of these central physiological mechanisms it seems likely that the catecholamines dopamine and/noradrenaline would play an important role (see below).

Clinical Clues

The clinical phenomenology of schizophrenic illness has been the subject of an immense amount of literature and yet it has not been possible to relate much of this clinical data to specific brain systems. The neuroanatomy and neurochemistry underlying phenomena such as passivity feelings, delusions or formal thought disorder are essentially as obscure as when the phenomena were first described systematically nearly 100 years ago. However, for some phenomena such as Schneiderian first-rank symptoms, catatonic motor disorder, autonomic hyperactivity (hyperarousal) and laterality imbalance, there appears to be evidence sufficient to justify tentative suggestions.

Auditory hallucinations

Early studies by Penfield in the 1960s showed that complex auditory hallucinations could be evoked by direct electrical stimulation in the vicinity of the primary auditory cortex on the medial surface of the temporal lobe—particularly the superior and lateral surfaces of the first temporal convolutions. It has also been known for some time that stimulation of deep sylvian peri-insular regions of the temporal lobe in patients suffering from epilepsy can cause auditory hallucinations. Horowitz and Adams (1970) found that in epileptic patients, formed hallucinations (but visual rather than auditory) could be provoked by stimulation of the hippocampus, amygdala and globus pallidus. In this study there was associated thought disorder (such as neologisms, thought blocking and semantic distortion) and subjects experienced the phenomena as involuntary intrusions into their awareness. Thus allocortical, rather than neocortical, structures have traditionally been linked to complex hallucinatory experience.

The full range of schizophrenic experience can be associated with temporal lobe epilepsy (complex partial seizures) and here, unlike acute stimulation in non-psychotic individuals, insight is lost. The psychoses of temporal lobe epilepsy can persist following temporal lobectomy, implying that the temporal lobe itself may not be the most important source of these psychotic phenomena. It may be that the afferent subcortical projection systems contribute significantly and here one must consider noradrenergic, serotoninergic and dopaminergic systems, all of which project to allocortical structures. The fact that important dopaminergic pathways arise from the ventral tegmental area and pass rostrally to the midbrain and orbital frontal cortex, with known links of the latter to medial temporal structures, may be of importance in understanding the subcortical mechanisms that are involved in hallucinatory processes and areas affected by temporal lobe stimulation (Trimble, 1981). Based mainly on evidence from patients with epilepsy who develop a schizophrenia-like illness, it has been argued that the full range of first-rank symptoms of Schneider are closely related to temporal lobe pathology, particularly in the dominant hemisphere (Trimble, 1990).

Catatonic movements

Although nowadays quite rare, bizarre motor disorders are a well-documented facet of severe schizophrenic illness. These range from unusual posturing (waxy flexibility) to repetitive muscular stereotypes and mannerisms. Although strict analogy may not be permissible, there is sufficient similarity between these clinical signs and experimentally-induced posturing and stereotypes in animals to suggest some mechanisms in common. These animal behaviours are associated with manipulation of ventral dopamine systems in areas such as the basal ganglia and nucleus accumbens.

Autonomic dysfunction

One consistent finding in most studies has been that some schizophrenic patients show a highly responsive skin conductance which does not habituate to repeated stimuli and which is associated with severe acute symptoms. This has been interpreted as hyperarousal which may not be labelled by the patient as 'anxiety' (Frith et al., 1979). Fast recovery and hyper-responsiveness of the electrodermal response may be specifically correlated with severe delusions and hallucinations (Parnas *et al.*, 1981). It has been suggested that hyper-responsiveness and fast recovery may lead to unnatural vulnerability to external stimuli and a tendency to learn avoidance responses or 'schizophrenic withdrawal' (Parnas *et al.*, 1981). It has also been shown that particular sorts of social and environmental influences such as 'life-events' or exposure to a relative who is prone to display high 'expressed emotion' will bring about abnormal patterns of autonomic reactivity in schizophrenic subjects (Tarrier *et al.*, 1979).

Although it is impossible to define precisely the central neurochemical correlates of autonomic hyper-reactivity, it seems likely that catecholaminergic arousal systems would play some part.

Cerebral laterality

An association has been observed between schizophreniform psychosis and dominant (usually left) temporal lobe dysfunction. This has prompted the suspicion that the critical brain dysfunction underlying schizophrenic illness might arise in the language dominant hemisphere. Several approaches have been used to test this idea.

Many studies have attempted to show over-representation of abnormal lateralization by testing handedness, but results overall do not show any convincing pattern. Likewise, studies of visual processing by tachistoscopy have failed to reveal clear laterality imbalance or interhemispheric transfer deficits. Tests of auditory processing assume special significance in view of the diagnostic importance of auditory hallucinations and there appears to be a preference for right ear input to the speech comprehension of schizophrenic patients. This could be interpreted as either a left hemisphere inhibitory deficit or a deficient interhemispheric integration (Gruzelier, 1981). Other evidence on auditory processing points to a left-sided deficit and it has been shown that these processing abnormalities are reversible by phenothiazine drugs.

A variety of psychophysiological indices point to an abnormal balance of activity between the hemispheres in schizophrenia. Schizophrenic patients tend to have larger orienting and non-specific skin conductance responses on the right hand, which might signify an abnormal influence from limbic structures on the left side of the brain (Gruzelier, 1981).

It is regrettable that there have been few neurochemical studies of laterality in the post-mortem brain in schizophrenic illness, but the work of Reynolds and colleagues which has demonstrated an interhemispheric asymmetry in dopamine concentrations (see below) is a notable exception.

Also worthy of note is the rapidly increasing body of evidence from neuropathological re-examination of fixed brain tissue which suggests both gross anatomical and cytoarchitectural abnormalities in schizophrenic brain which are remarkably concentrated in the left temporal lobe, medial and deep structures such as parahippocampus and amygdala in particular (Jeste and Lohr, 1989; Kerwin, 1989).

As a further development in the interpretation of structural data, it has been suggested that there is reversed hemispheric asymmetry in schizophrenia; that the faulty gene responsible for schizophrenic illness is the 'cerebral dominance gene' and that this gene is located within the pseudo-autosomal region of the sex chromosome (Crow, 1990).

Neuroimaging studies

Modern imaging techniques have brought the study of brain function and structure to the living patient at a level of sophistication which was previously only possible after death. *In vivo* imaging of neuronal 'work' as reflected either in regional cerebral blood flow or glucose consumption can now be visualized through techniques such as single photon emission computerized tomography (SPECT) or positron emission tomography (PET). The elegant studies of Weinberger and his colleagues with SPECT have demonstrated a localized impairment of function in the dorsolateral pre-frontal cortex in schizophrenic illness (Weinberger, 1988). The regional glucose metabolic rate as assessed by PET in medication-free schizophrenic patients has been shown to be reduced in both frontal cortex and temporo-parietal regions (Buchsbaum et al., 1990). Results such as these indicate localized abnormalities of function in the limbic circuits connecting temporal lobe with pre-frontal cortex.

Further support for a focus on rostral limbic structures comes from recent structural imaging studies using the technique of magnetic resonance imaging (MRI). For example, Andreasen and her colleagues have demonstrated selective enlargement of the anterior (frontal) horns of the lateral ventricles in schizophrenia (Andreasen et al., 1990). While the anatomical address for schizophrenic illness may be narrowing down to fronto-temporal systems, the neurochemical address, or in other words the neurotransmitter systems involved in these areas, is more elusive.

Age of onset

Of the many undisputed epidemiological facts about schizophrenic illness, perhaps the most striking and heuristic is the fact that schizophrenic illness only becomes clinically apparent after well into the second decade of life. This must represent an important clue to the brain processes involved, but it is difficult to reconcile this observation with the conviction that the roots of schizophrenia lie in a combination of genetic vulnerability and peri-natal insult. Several authors have suggested an intriguing explanation, first suggested by Weinberger et al. (1986). The origins of the idea lie in the fact that experimental lesions in the dorso-lateral pre-frontal cortex in young primates cause behavioural problems which are evident only several years later, and the fact that myelination in this region of the frontal cortex continues into the second and third decades of life in higher primates. The suggestion is that the pre-frontal cortex and its connections with temporal limbic structures do not become functionally integrated into brain circuitry until after adolescence. While these parts of the brain may be

TABLE 31.1 The major neurotransmitters.

Transmitter	Chemical family	Synaptic action	Drugs with potent effects on transmission
Noradrenaline	Catecholamine	Inhibitory	Antidepressants
Serotonin	Indolamine	Inhibitory[a]	Antidepressants
Dopamine	Catecholamine	Inhibitory	Neuroleptics
Acetylcholine	Choline ester	Excitatory	Neuroleptics Antidepressants
γ-aminobutyric acid (GABA)	Neutral amino acid	Inhibitory	Anxiolytics Hypnotics
Endorphins	Peptide	Inhibitory[b]	Naloxone
L-glutamic acid	Dicarboxylic amino acid	Excitatory	Phencyclidine

[a] Except limbic cortex.
[b] Except hippocampus.

abnormal from birth, the fault is only revealed when these components come 'on stream' at a later date (Weinberger, 1987; Murray et al., 1988). This suggestion begs the question whether the functions carried out by these areas are absent prior to adolescence, or that the functions are carried out by some other brain structures prior to this time. A rather different suggestion, concerning the neurotransmitter L-glutamic acid, has been made by Etienne and Baudry (1987). They suggest that one of the genes which predisposes to schizophrenia is linked to the functioning or maturation of one subtype of glutamic acid receptor; the NMDA receptor. There are marked developmental changes in the second messenger (phosphatidylinositol) responses to NMDA occupancy, and it is proposed that the genetic abnormality in schizophrenic patients gives rise to a delay or failure in the transition from the juvenile to adult form of the NMDA receptor system. This may result in a disruption of the major synaptic reorganisation which appears to occur during adolescence in human frontal cortex (Huttenlocher, 1979), this in turn contributing to the development of schizophrenic symptoms.

Neurotransmitter Systems

The seven neurotransmitters listed in Table 31.1 are those which, over the past 25 years, have attracted most attention from the psychiatrist. Each has, at some time, been implicated in theories of schizophrenia. Much of our knowledge about distribution and function derives from investigation of the brains of lower mammals, but there is at present no reason to doubt its validity for the human brain.

NORADRENALINE

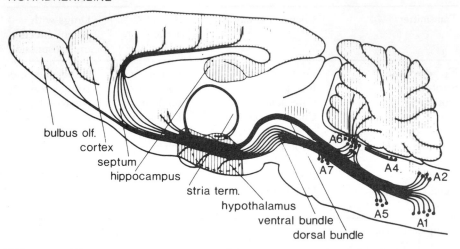

FIG. 31.1   Diagrammatic representation of the arrangement of noradrenaline-containing neuronal pathways in the brain of a rat. The cell groups originating in the brain stem are numbered according to the Swedish histochemical nomenclature (see Iversen, 1980). (Reproduced by courtesy of K. Fuxe.)

Noradrenaline

Distribution. The elegant procedures which render the monoamines (noradrenaline, dopamine and serotonin) fluorescent when thin sections of tissue are viewed under the microscope have been of particular value in determining the distribution of noradrenaline. The most recent refinement, the glyoxylic acid method, has revealed two major noradrenergic systems in the brain. One arises in the pontine locus coeruleus and sends bifurcating axons via the dorsal bundle to innervate the cerebellum, cerebral cortex and hippocampus. The other system innervates the hypothalamopituitary axis by way of the ventral bundle, which receives axons from a number of cell groups throughout the pons and medulla (Fig. 31.1).

Function. The synaptic actions of noradrenaline are mediated by interaction with α- and β-adrenoreceptors, occupation of which leads to inhibition of spontaneous firing of receptive cells.

All noradrenergic projections are diffuse and their function is, therefore, probably general. In addition to participating in the hormonal control of homeostasis through their hypothalamic connections, the noradrenergic systems probably influence arousal through their connections in the cerebral cortex. Noradrenergic innervation of the hippocampus may be concerned in the processes of associative learning and it has been suggested that interaction between noradrenaline and dopamine systems at limbocortical sites may be a vital factor in determining the behavioural consequences of stress-induced arousal (Iversen, 1980).

Serotonin

Distribution. The anatomy of serotoninergic systems in the brain has many similarities to that of noradrenaline. Cell bodies are arranged in eight clusters in the midbrain raphe from which slender, slowly conducting axons fan out to innervate the entire CNS. The nucleus raphe medianus has a selective projection to the limbic system.

Function. Recipient neurones are generally inhibited by serotonin (syn. 5-hydroxytryptamine), but cells of the limbic cortex are unusual in that they respond with increased discharge. Serotonin acts at several different receptor subtypes in brain, termed $5HT_1$, $5HT_2$ and $5HT_3$. Serotoninergic systems have been implicated in diverse physiological roles, many of them homeostatic; for example, the hippocampal/amygdaloid–hypothalamic circuits exert a tonic inhibitory control on adrenocorticotrophin (ACTH) secretion. Serotonin is intimately associated with other primitive functions such as thermal regulation, sleep cycles and pain modulation. More complex social functions such as aggression and sexual behaviour are strongly influenced by serotoninergic inputs to the hippocampus.

The anatomic arrangement of serotoninergic and noradrenergic systems in the brain is generally characterized by enormous divergence, that is by prolific axonal projections derived from small groups of cell bodies. The systems react slowly to exert widespread and long-lasting inhibitory effects. The function suggested by these characteristics is not the rapid transmission of detailed information but rather an overall bias of regional activity which might orchestrate the performance of large segments of brain. It is tempting to picture prevailing mental phenomena such as arousal and mood being determined in this way, providing a tone upon which cognitive aspects of mental state can be superimposed.

Dopamine

Dopamine is a transmitter closely related chemically to noradrenaline but with a significantly different pattern of distribution in the brain.

Distribution. Dopaminergic neurones are arranged in several subsystems with topographically discrete projections. The most dense subsystem is found in the basal ganglia—the nigrostriatal pathway, extending from the substantia nigra (A9 cell group) to the corpus striatum (caudate nucleus, putamen and globus pallidus). The mesolimbic and mesocortical systems arise from cell bodies (A10 cell group) lying medial to the substantia nigra and surrounding the interpeduncular nucleus (Fig. 31.2).

The mesolimbic system includes innervations of the nucleus accumbens, olfactory area, septal nuclei and amygdala, and the mesocortical system includes innervations of the frontal, cingulate and entorhinal cortex (Iversen, 1980). The tubero-infundibular system consists of a short-axon tract coursing along the base of the hypothalamus and releasing dopamine into the pituitary portal veins. Other loci, intrinsic dopaminergic systems are found in the olfactory bulb, medulla oblongata and in the retina. Dopamine is contained in small diameter,

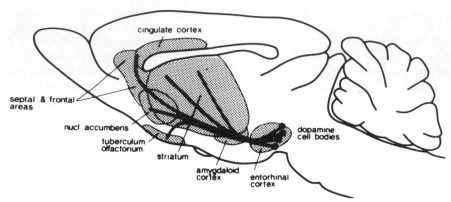

FIG. 31.2 Arrangement of dopamine-containing neuronal pathways in the brain of a rat. Cell bodies in the substantia nigra and in the ventral tegmentum project to the basal ganglia and various limbic forebrain areas (see Iversen, 1980). (Reproduced by courtesy of U. Ungerstedt.)

slowly-conducting fibres and appears to be a predominantly inhibitory neuro-transmitter.

Function. Dopamine interacts specifically with at least two types of receptor in the brain, D1 receptors which are linked to cyclic AMP (in a way analogous to the noradrenergic β-receptors) and D2 receptors, which are not. D2 receptors appear to be involved in the maintenance of normal extrapyramidal function and may mediate the antipsychotic actions of neuroleptic drugs. The functional significance of D1 receptors is not clear (Snyder, 1981).

Dopaminergic neurones are the most numerous central catecholamine-containing neurones and, in contrast to noradrenergic neurones, should probably be considered as components of much broader functional systems which receive connections from several subsystems, each employing a different neurotransmitter. For example, the nigrostriatal tract participates in sensorimotor coordination, the hypothalamopituitary system in the regulation of hormone release, and the retinal system in visual sensory input. The limbic dopamine subsystem seems to have an intimate relationship with noradrenaline in brain mechanisms which focus attention on biologically relevant stimuli and select appropriate behavioural responses to arousal. The nearby cortical subsystem undoubtedly interacts with limbic subsystems and it has been suggested that the abnormally high arousal response of schizophrenic patients to stress may be mediated through cortical dopamine (Eichler and Antelman, 1979). A complete understanding of the role of dopamine in limbic and cortical areas, those traditionally associated with emotional and cognitive disorder, is still tantalizingly out of reach.

Acetylcholine

The mammalian brain contains considerably more acetylcholine than any of the three transmitters already discussed, yet less is known about its distribution and functional significance.

Distribution. With a few exceptions, such as the cholinergic projections from the substantia innominata and medial septum to the cerebral cortex and hippocampus, cholinergic neurones typically have short axons which communicate locally and many can appropriately be considered as 'interneurones'. They are found interspersed among other families of neurones in areas such as the brain stem reticular formation, thalamus and basal ganglia.

Function. Acetylcholine is predominantly an excitatory neurotransmitter, mediating postsynaptic depolarization through nicotinic and muscarinic cholinergic receptors. Cholinergic neurones are commonly found in series with the long-tract catecholamine and serotonin circuits and a functional balance often exists between the excitatory cholinergic and inhibitory catecholaminergic systems. This aspect is well demonstrated in the basal ganglia where normal extrapyramidal function seems to depend upon the functional equilibrium between acetylcholine and dopamine.

The cerebral cortex and hippocampus are innervated by diffuse and highly branched cholinergic ascending inputs, and acetylcholine has been particularly implicated in cognitive processes—the thinking and knowing aspects of mental function.

γ-Aminobutyric acid

In recent years several amino acids have gained recognition as possible major neurotransmitters in the mammalian brain. γ-Aminobutyric acid (GABA), a neutral amino acid, is confined almost exclusively to brain tissue, where concentrations are of the order of μmol g^{-1} (noradrenaline and serotonin concentrations are very much lower).

Distribution. GABA is probably the major inhibitory neurotransmitter in the mammalian central nervous system, being used by as many as one-third of all synaptic junctions. GABA is mainly present in local short-axoned inter-neurones, and the areas with the highest concentrations are the basal ganglia, cerebellum and cerebral cortex.

Function. The pallidonigral tract is popularly considered to form a classical negative feedback loop from the corpus striatum to the substantia nigra and the striatonigral feedback loop plays a role in extrapyramidal function. The role of GABA in cortical function is as the principal inhibitory mediator of local cortical circuits. GABA neurones in the spinal cord are inhibitory components in sensorimotor reflexes.

L-Glutamic acid

A neurotransmitter role at fast excitatory receptors appears probable for glutamate, aspartate and several of their derivatives. Receptors at which glutamate acts have been classified according to their preferred agonist. Thus three major categories of post-synaptic glutamate receptor have been defined; the N-methyl-D-aspartate (NMDA) receptor, the kainate receptor and the quisqualate receptor (Meldrum and Kerwin, 1987).

Distribution. The three major receptor subtypes have distinctive regional distributions. Kainate receptors have their highest density in the mossy fibre system in the hippocampus, but are also prominent in the superficial and deep laminae of the neocortex. NMDA receptors are prominent in the dendritic laminae of the hippocampus and in the cortex. Quisqualate receptors are prominent in hippocampus, cortex and cerebellum.

Function. Activation of these receptors causes depolarization of the neuronal membrane through the opening of cationic channels. Activation of kainate or quisqualate receptor subtypes permits the entry of sodium, activation of NMDA receptors permits the entry of both sodium and calcium. The NMDA receptor has an allosteric site at which glycine acts to increase the frequency of channel opening induced by NMDA (Johnson and Ascher, 1987). There is also a site at which phencyclidine, and other dissociative anaesthetics such as ketamine, and opiates such as cyclazocine and dextrorphan, act to block the conductance change produced by NMDA (Meldrum and Kerwin, 1987). This may relate to the psychotomimetic action of phencyclidine which is discussed below.

Endorphins

The opioid peptides have joined the list of neurotransmitters which have excited psychiatric interest. The collective name 'endorphin' derives from the fact that this family of small endogenous peptides interacts with the same receptors as morphine and shares many of its actions. In 1975 endogenous opiate-like activity in the mammalian brain was attributed to two pentapeptides called Met- and Leu-enkephalin. This discovery was quickly followed by the demonstration of three additional endogenous opioid peptides, of larger molecular size, termed α-, β- and γ-endorphin.

Distribution. The distribution of β-endorphin and of the enkephalins in the brain is beginning to become clear. β-Endorphin-containing neurones exist in the basomedial and basolateral hypothalamus and send axons to the anterior hypothalamus, thalamic nuclei, pons and midbrain. By contrast, enkephalin-containing neurones are more numerous and widely distributed; they are found mainly in intrinsic, short axoned circuits in the corpus striatum, the limbic system and the dorsal horn of the spinal cord. Enkephalinergic interneurones may synapse upon the terminals of other systems in a presumed axo-axonic arrangement such that enkephalin might influence the release of neurotransmitter from the recipient nerve ending. In addition to long-tract systems in the brain, extremely high concentrations of β-endorphin are present in the intermediate and anterior lobes of the pituitary gland.

Function. Electrophysiologically, the enkephalins and endorphins are generally depressant, except in the hippocampus where excitatory actions are so pronounced that hippocampal seizures can be induced in experimental animals. Their actions are mediated through a heterogeneous population of opiate receptors; including μ, δ and κ types. It is the μ receptor which is potently antagonized by naloxone. The physiological function of these opioid peptides which, understandably, first attracted most attention was that of pain perception. Interesting advances have been made which suggest a modulatory role in the transmission of noxious stimuli through primary afferents to the thalamus. The endorphins probably mediate the analgesic effects of acupuncture and even placebo analgesia. However, it was the non-analgesic functions of these peptides, particularly the limbic enkephalin systems, which attracted the interest of psychiatrists and behavioural psychologists.

Other neuropeptides

Other neuropeptides, such as cholecystokinin, somatostatin, substance P and vasoactive intestinal polypeptide are present in the mammalian brain and their topographical distributions and electrophysiological actions qualify them as serious candidates for neurotransmitters, though their roles in brain function have still to be established.

Neurotransmitter Theories

Almost every known neurotransmitter has been proposed, at one time or another, as contributing to the etiology of schizophrenic illness. As new chemical messengers are discovered in the brain (notably in recent years the neuropeptides), so new hypotheses appear. One of the first specific hypotheses was the 'trans-methylation' hypothesis, proposed by Osmond and Smythies (1952). This was based on the fact that the chemical structure of the hallucinogenic drug mescaline (Fig. 31.3) bears some resemblance to naturally occurring catecholamines which function as neurotransmitters in the brain. It was suggested that schizophrenic illness might be related to an excessive production of toxic methylated by-products of catecholamine metabolism. This idea was later extended to encompass the possible formation of other methylated hallucinogenic compounds, such as the indolamines, bufotenin and N-dimethyltryptamine (Rodnight *et al.*, 1977) (Fig. 31.3)

The transmethylation hypothesis appears to be supported by the finding that large doses of the amino acid L-methionine caused an exacerbation of symptoms in many schizophrenic patients, first reported by Pollin *et al.* (1961) and later confirmed by others. L-Methionine can act in the body as a donor of methyl groups for many methylation reactions. However, it is doubtful whether the effects of methionine in schizophrenic patients really represent a worsening of the pre-existing psychosis rather than merely a state of toxic delirium (Pollin *et al.*, 1961).

Furthermore, the psychic phenomena induced by drugs such as mescaline and LSD differ in important ways from schizophrenia, so that the drugs do not represent a very accurate model (Snyder, 1973). Other hallucinogenic drugs,

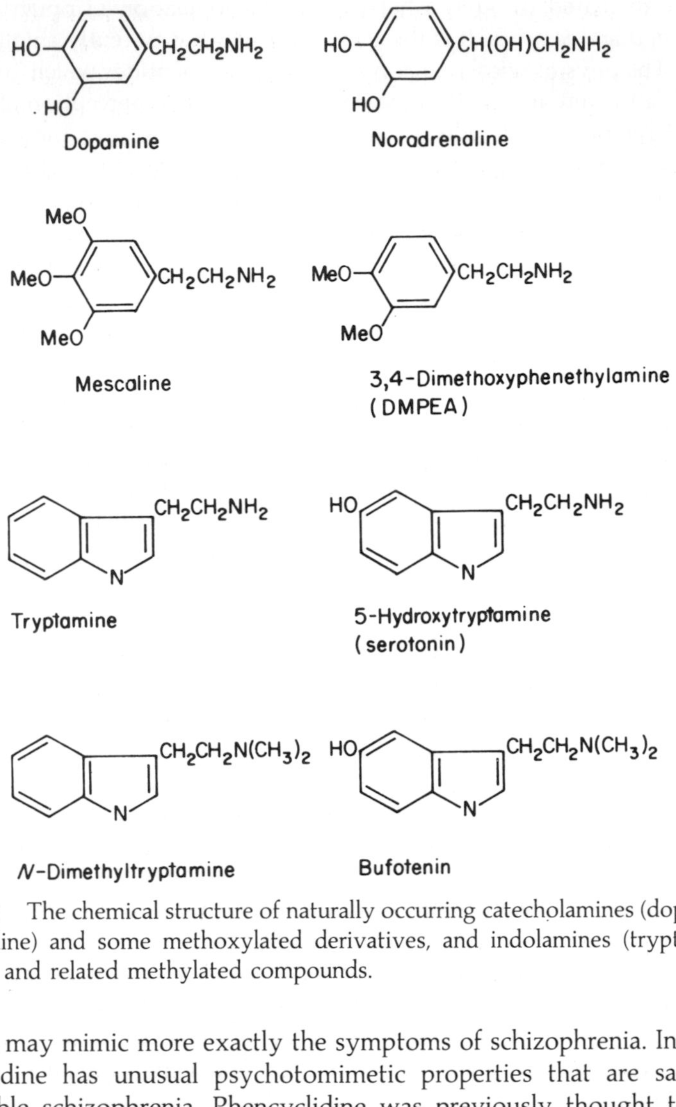

FIG. 31.3 The chemical structure of naturally occurring catecholamines (dopamine and noradrenaline) and some methoxylated derivatives, and indolamines (tryptamine and serotonin) and related methylated compounds.

however, may mimic more exactly the symptoms of schizophrenia. In particular phencyclidine has unusual psychotomimetic properties that are said closely to resemble schizophrenia. Phencyclidine was previously thought to owe its hallucinogenic properties to its anticholinergic effects, but more recent research has revealed other more likely targets. Phencyclidine has a high affinity for sites in brain known as 'σ (sigma) receptors', which are also thought to represent the site of action of pentazocine, cyclazocine and other psychotomimetic opiates. An attractive hypothesis is that σ receptor antagonist drugs may represent a new approach to the treatment of schizophrenic psychosis (Snyder and Largent, 1989). A number of novel antipsychotic agents in development possess affinity for the σ sites in brain (Largent *et al.*, 1988). The σ receptor, however, remains poorly understood and cannot be related to any known neurotransmitter or neuro-peptide system in brain. Matters are further complicated by the observation that phencyclidine and the psychotomimetic benzomorphans also act as antagonists at the NMDA subclass of receptors for glutamic acid in brain. It is not clear whether this contributes importantly to their hallucinogenic and psychostimulant properties, but a major possible role for glutamic acid in psychosis has been considered recently (Olney, 1989), with the suggestion that a hypofunction of excitatory amino acid mechanisms might explain the symptomatology of schizophrenia. This theme has been developed recently by several authors, notably Carlsson, and is the subject of recent reviews (Carlsson and Carlsson, 1990; Wachtel and Turski, 1990). Recent evidence from post-mortem work with brain tissue from schizophrenic patients tends to support the idea of glutamate underactivity, generally finding an increased density of glutamate receptor subtypes, indicating reactive receptor up-regulation. It is of historical interest that the hypoglycaemia accompanying insulin coma therapy is known to produce an increase in cerebral glutamate. The hypothesis currently associated with Carlsson is that glutamate and dopamine operate independently of one another to affect GABA inhibition of the excitatory thalamocortical pathway. In essence, it is proposed that in schizophrenia there is a decreased glutamate excitatory input from cerebral cortex onto inhibitory GABA projections from striatum to thalamus. This leads to a disinhibition of excitatory projections to thalamus, increasing sensory input to the cortex, and thus opening the 'thalamic filter' to cortex. The physiological effect of normal dopamine transmission from substantia nigra and ventral tegmental area tends to facilitate the opening of the filter, and this effect is accentuated when GABA neurones are already underactive due to loss of glutamate input. Thus, in theory, the pathological mechanism underlying schizophrenia might be ameliorated by either potentiating glutamate transmission or blocking dopamine transmission.

Similar theories suggesting a hypofunction of inhibitory (GABAergic) mechanisms, or noradrenaline dysfunction have been proposed but failed to receive any support from detailed post-mortem studies.

Among neuropeptide theories recent interest has focused on the endorphins (see below) and cholecystokinin (CCK). In animal studies CCK acts to dampen the activity of dopamine in limbic forebrain, and in this respect its actions in brain resemble those of neuroleptic drugs. A deficiency of CCK has been proposed as an underlying feature of schizophrenic psychosis and this idea has been supported to some extent by post-mortem findings (see below) (reviewed by Reynolds, 1989).

The Dopamine Hypothesis

Scientific basis

During the past twenty years various lines of evidence have converged to point to the critical role played by dopamine in the actions of antischizophrenic drugs. This conclusion has in turn led to the 'dopamine hypothesis' which proposes that schizophrenia may be associated with an excessive function of dopaminergic pathways in the CNS (for reviews see Snyder *et al.*, 1974; Iversen, 1977; Reynolds, 1989).

Amphetamine psychosis

Amphetamine psychosis, first described by Connell (1958) as a state 'indistinguishable from acute or chronic paranoid schizophrenia', provides one of the closest drug-induced 'model schizophrenias' (Snyder *et al.*, 1974). Numerous patients with amphetamine psychosis have been misdiagnosed as paranoid schizophrenics, and drugs such as the phenothiazines used in the treatment of schizophrenia are also uniquely effective antidotes for amphetamine-induced psychosis. The syndrome is often associated with paranoid delusions, stereotyped compulsive behaviour and auditory and visual hallucinations.

Unlike schizophrenia, however, amphetamine psychosis is also frequently associated with tactile and olfactory hallucinations; thought disorder is rare, agitation and motor overactivity are common, and patients display brisk emotional reactions and anxiety, rather than a blunted effect. A number of studies have shown that psychosis can be consistently produced in volunteer subjects within one to four days of initiating repeated doses of amphetamine. The importance of these observations in the present context is that animal studies have shown that the behavioural stimulant properties of amphetamine are entirely due to its ability to release dopamine from storage sites in the brain (Randrup and Munkvad, 1974; Iversen, 1977, 1980).

Actions of antischizophrenic drugs

Since the discovery of the antipsychotic properties of the phenothiazine, chlorpromazine, many other drugs have been discovered with similar properties, compounds both in the phenothiazine class and in other chemical groups (see Chapter 1, this volume).

There is now compelling evidence that all such drugs owe their unique pharmacological profile to an ability to block receptors for dopamine in the brain. This conclusion is based on various lines of experimental evidence. For example, antischizophrenic drugs have been found to block selectively the stereotyped behaviour and hyperactivity responses induced by amphetamine in experimental animals, phenomena that, as mentioned above, appear to be due to activation of central dopamine mechanisms. Furthermore, the antidopamine effects of these drugs are reflected by their ability to cause an increase in the rate of metabolism of dopamine in the brain, when administered to animals. Such an increase appears to reflect an attempt by brain dopamine mechanisms to compensate for the blockade of receptor actions of the neurotransmitter by increasing the rate of synthesis and release of the monoamine. The most direct evidence for the antidopamine properties of antischizophrenic drugs, however, has come from the demonstration that all clinically effective agents are active in various *in vitro* biochemical model systems for studies of dopamine receptors in the brain. Such models involve demonstrating that antischizophrenic drugs are able to block the

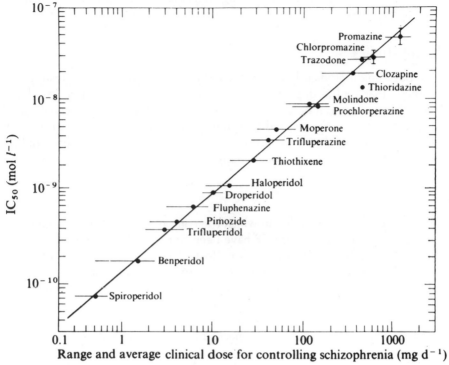

FIG. 31.4 Comparison of the clinical potencies of neuroleptic drugs, measured as the average daily dose in treating schizophrenia, with the potencies of the same drugs in displacing [^{3}H]haloperidol from dopamine receptor binding sites *in vitro* (concentration of drug required to displace 50% of specific haloperidol binding). (From Seeman *et al.*, 1976).

binding of radioactively-labelled dopamine or related drugs to receptor sites in brain membranes *in vitro*. In the latter model in particular, the rank order of potencies of antischizophrenic drugs of different chemical classes is defined by their potency in blocking D2 dopamine receptors, and appears to correlate closely with their known clinical potencies (Seeman *et al.*, 1976) (Fig. 31.4). Further evidence for dopamine receptor blockade by these drugs is provided by their ability to raise plasma prolactin concentrations at doses similar to those needed to obtain beneficial effects on schizophrenic symptoms. The secretion of prolactin from the anterior pituitary gland is normally under a tonic inhibitory control by dopamine, released from the median eminence of the hypothalamus. The dopamine effect is mediated by D2 receptors in anterior pituitary with similar pharmacological properties to those in the brain, which are sensitive to anti-schizophrenic drug actions.

Together these findings strongly support the conclusion that the properties of the antischizophrenic drugs can most likely be attributed to their dopamine-blocking actions at D2 receptors, and this in turn suggests many further questions. Which of the dopamine systems in the brain is crucial for the antipsychotic effect?

Does this mechanism of action of the drugs tell us anything about the biochemical nature of the disease?

Clinical studies

Numerous clinical studies have been conducted with the aim of testing the hypothesis that central dopamine systems are relatively overactive in schizophrenic illness. They can be broadly divided into those which have investigated the concentrations of amines and their metabolites in lumbar CSF, those which have looked for evidence of disordered dopaminergic control of pituitary hormone release, and *in vivo* dopamine receptor imaging studies.

CSF studies

There have been several studies in which the concentrations of monoamines and their metabolites in the lumbar CSF have been compared between schizophrenic patients and controls (for review, see Post *et al.*, 1975) and no consistent abnormality has been shown. Interpretation of lumbar CSF data is, however, limited by the fact that the composition of lumbar fluid is at best a crude and distant reflection of neuronal activity in rostral areas of the brain. An additional limitation of earlier studies was the failure to control the important variable of metabolite removal from CSF. Probenecid blocks the elimination from CSF of the principal dopamine metabolite, homovanillic acid (HVA), and the rate of accumulation of HVA in CSF after probenecid provides a more reliable estimate of overall dopamine release and turnover in the CNS.

Studies using this technique, however, have failed to show increased turnover of dopamine in drug-free schizophrenic patients. Nor has any clear abnormality been detected in the concentrations of MHPG (a noradrenaline metabolite) or 5-HIAA (a serotonin metabolite). Indeed, far from providing evidence for increased dopamine release, findings with drug-free schizophrenic patients suggest that poor prognosis (defined by chronicity of illness, poor premorbid personality, emotional blunting) and severity of illness (number of Schneiderian first-rank phenomena) are associated with decreased accumulation of HVA in the lumbar CSF (Bowers, 1974; Post *et al.*, 1975), indicating, if anything, a decreased rate of central dopamine turnover.

Endocrine data

Dopamine receptor-mediated control of hormone release from the anterior pituitary represents a direct and accessible test system for investigation of dopaminergic function in schizophrenic patients, although it must be remembered that the pituitary gland lies outside the brain and may not provide a faithful analogue of brain dopamine systems.

Prolactin release from the anterior pituitary is under tonic inhibitory control by dopamine released from dopaminergic terminals in the median eminence of the hypothalamus. The released dopamine travels down the pituitary stalk in portal vessels to exert its effect on dopamine receptors on pituitary mammotroph cells. Dopaminergic antagonists such as the neuroleptic drugs disinhibit prolactin release and give rise to hyperprolactinaemia. The dopamine hypothesis for schizophrenia would predict that drug-free schizophrenic patients might normally exhibit hypoprolactinaemia. This is not the case; several studies have found normal basal levels of circulating prolactin in schizophrenic patients (De la Fuente and Rosenbaum, 1981; Rotrosen *et al.*, 1979).

The control of growth hormone release from the anterior pituitary is complex, but enhanced release is seen following administration of dopamine-mimetic agents. Basal levels of plasma growth hormone, like prolactin, have been found to be normal in schizophrenic patients (Rotrosen *et al.*, 1979). These neuro-endocrine studies thus provide no support for the proposal that schizophrenic illness might be associated with generalized dopaminergic overactivity, although it is possible that overactivity might be confined to systems other than the hypothalamopituitary axis.

It has been argued that in the absence of any evidence for increased dopamine release in schizophrenic illness an abnormality might exist in the form of increased 'sensitivity' of postsynaptic dopamine receptors (Crow *et al.*, 1976). The hormone response to provocation with dopamine agonists has provided a way of assessing the characteristics of dopamine receptors on pituitary cells. Findings from a large number of studies seem to agree on the tendency for drug-free chronic schizophrenic patients to have blunted growth hormone and prolactin responses to dopamine agonists. However, it has been suggested that this phenomenon may be a reflection of some lasting effect of chronic neuroleptic medication which persists through a period of acute drug wash-out (Rotrosen *et al.*, 1979). Although more controversial, there is also some agreement on the finding of enhanced growth hormone responses to dopamine agonists in drug-free, acutely ill, schizophrenic patients and this has been taken as evidence for a dopamine receptor supersensitivity in cases of schizophrenic illness uncontaminated by the effects of chronic medication.

Receptor imaging

The advent of non-invasive neuroimaging techniques such as SPECT and PET has enabled the direct investigation in the living patient of various biochemical and pharmacological parameters. In response to the suggestion that schizophrenia may be associated with an excessive density of dopamine receptors in central dopamine synapses, attention has been focused on the measurement of dopamine receptor density and affinity as reflected by binding of isotope-labelled ligands in various brain regions in patients suffering from schizophrenia. Results have varied according to the ligand employed, but results with raclopride, a ligand with a beneficially high degree of specific receptor binding, suggest that the density of dopamine receptors in the brains of drug-free cases is normal (Farde *et al.*, 1990).

Post-mortem biochemistry

The classic studies of Ehringer and Hornykiewicz (1960) 30 years ago were crucial in establishing a dopamine deficiency state in Parkinson's disease. During the past decade a number of studies have been undertaken on monoamines and other neurotransmitters in post-mortem brain samples obtained from patients dying with a diagnosis of schizophrenia. In most such studies particular attention has been given to measurements of dopamine, dopamine metabolites and dopamine receptors, because of the widespread acceptance of the 'dopamine hypothesis' for explaining the mode of action of antischizophrenic drugs, and the hope that this hypothesis could be extrapolated by demonstrating the existence of an abnormality in dopamine systems in the schizophrenic brain.

On the whole, however, this conclusion has not been strongly supported by the experimental findings available so far. Only modest changes in dopamine systems have been observed, with little or no change in any other neurotransmitter mechanisms (Reynolds, 1988, 1989). We did find, however, and others have confirmed, elevations in brain dopamine concentrations in the caudate nucleus, nucleus accumbens and olfactory tubercle region, although these increases were only modest in extent (30–40%) (Bird et al., 1979). The most exciting discovery has been the observation by Reynolds (1983, 1989) of an asymmetric increase in dopamine content in left but not right amygdala, in three series of schizophrenic patients.

Like other laboratories (Lee and Seeman, 1980; Owen et al., 1978), we also observed an increased density of dopamine receptor binding sites in most brain regions, but we believe these changes to be iatrogenic rather than related to the schizophrenic illness (Mackay et al., 1982)—an interpretation supported by the recent PET data mentioned above. Treatment of experimental animals with antischizophrenic drugs is known to lead to a compensatory increase in the number of dopamine receptor binding sites in the brain, and we failed to detect any increase in dopamine receptor densities in brain samples from a small number of schizophrenic patients who were 'drug free' for at least one month prior to death. This conclusion, however, is disputed by other laboratories (Seeman et al., 1987), and the area remains controversial.

Seeman et al. (1984) reported a bimodal distribution of dopamine receptor values in a large post-mortem series, with some schizophrenic patients exhibiting near normal striatal receptor densities, and a subgroup having receptor densities more than double those in normal subjects. The interpretation of this finding, however, remains unclear.

Endorphin Hypotheses

Psychiatric interest in the endorphins began in 1976 when two research groups independently reported striking behavioural effects of endorphin administration in rats. Cerebral administration produced an akinetic syndrome which was variously interpreted as analogous either to cationic schizophrenia or to neuroleptic-induced catalepsy. Diametrically opposite predictions arose from these inferences: schizophrenic illness might be associated with overproduction of a psychotogenic endorphin (capable of inducing 'catatonia'); or the illness might reflect a deficiency of a neuroleptic-like endorphin (normally protecting against psychosis). The literature saw a flurry of claim and counter-claim from clinical studies which could be related to one or other of these premises. If schizophrenic illness were associated with too much endorphin, then blockade of central endorphin receptors should have therapeutic effects. The only clinically acceptable pharmacological tool with which to test this notion has been naloxone and the results to date are scarcely convincing. Early expansive claims for remarkable efficacy of naloxone, particularly in the suppression of auditory hallucinations, have since been modified in the light of a number of double-blind controlled studies. Overall, the clinical effects of naloxone have failed to support the proposal that endorphin overactivity is pathogenic in schizophrenia (Mackay, 1981).

The hypothesis that schizophrenia is associated with underactivity of central endorphin systems has received no real support from carefully conducted trials in which synthetic β-endorphin has been administered intravenously. It has, however, been suggested that schizophrenic illness is due to the lack of a peptide which, while not itself an endorphin, is chemically related to the endorphin family. This peptide, des-tyrosyl-γ-endorphin (DTγE), has been shown to have behavioural actions in rats which are reminiscent of the classical neuroleptics (de Wied *et al.*, 1978). It was proposed that DTγE represents a natural endogenous neuroleptic which is deficient in the schizophrenic brain. Clinical studies of the therapeutic effect of DTγE have demonstrated at best a modest benefit in a small percentage of schizophrenic patients. There is no direct evidence of DTγE deficiency in schizophrenia.

The one hypothesis which has so far withstood experimental test is that no useful relation exists between schizophrenic illness and the endorphins (Mackay, 1981). However it has yet to be rigorously tested—much of the present evidence comes from clinical studies in which endorphin systems have been briefly and crudely manipulated. Much more evidence will have to be heard before the case can be judged.

The endorphins are but one family in an expanding population of neurotransmitter peptides and it would seem not unlikely that some will turn out to play a role in the pathogenesis of psychotic disorder. Evidence which implicates the classical neurotransmitters in schizophrenic illness may well have to be reinterpreted in the light of evidence that neuropeptides and amines coexist in the same neurone and that both may be released to perform discrete transmitter functions (Hökfelt *et al.*, 1980). Progress at the clinical level is still hampered by the relative lack of drugs capable of specific actions on peptide transmission in brain.

Conclusions

A great many hypotheses have come and gone but the biochemical basis of schizophrenia remains an enigma. At present the only internally consistent and robust hypothesis is a pharmacological one—that antischizophrenic drugs exert their therapeutic action by inhibiting central dopamine transmission. Evidence for any primary disturbance in dopamine systems is lacking and it must be concluded that the antischizophrenic action is symptomatic and that dopamine systems represent at most a final common pathway for the expression of various sorts of primary disturbance. Structural and functional imaging studies, and the timely renaissance of neuropathological interest in schizophrenic brain all point to two anatomical areas for the location of the abnormalities; pre-frontal cortex and medial temporal lobe. Many neurotransmitters are represented in these areas, dopamine and glutamate included. For a hypothesis which links neurotransmitter theories to structure, function, and psychotic symptoms the writings of Frith and his colleagues are recommended. Frith suggests that the negative symptoms of schizophrenia are associated with disordered function in pre-frontal cortex, whereas positive symptoms arise out of malfunction of a 'cognitive comparator' or monitor which may lie in or near the hippocampus (Frith and Done, 1989). *In vivo* imaging technology has opened the way for rapid advance in defining those neurotransmitter systems which may play an important role in the malfunction of these areas.

Advances in the chemical treatment of schizophrenia require that these abnormalities are translated into disturbances of neurotransmitter function. In this respect the eventual demonstration of the gene(s) responsible for the schizophrenic liability may turn out to be the quickest and most direct way of defining the most significant neurotransmitter systems. Meanwhile, the existing crude hypotheses which implicate dopamine should not be discarded, but refined in order to accommodate fresh evidence coming from these various directions.

References

Andreasen, N.C., Ehrhardt, J.C., Swayze, V.W., Alliger, R.J., Yuh, W.T.C., Cohen, G. and Ziebell, S. (1990). Magnetic resonance imaging of the brain in schizophrenia: the pathophysiologic significance of structural abnormalities. *Arch. Gen. Psychiat.* **47**, 35–44.
Bassett, A.S., McGillivray, B.C., Jones, B.D. and Pantzar, J.T. (1988). Partial trisomy chromosome 5 cosegrating with schizophrenia. *Lancet* **i**, 799–800.
Bird, E.D., Spokes, E.G.S. and Iversen, L.L. (1979). Increased dopamine concentration in limbic areas of brain from patients dying with schizophrenia. *Brain* **102**, 347–360.
Bleuler, E. (1911). *Dementia Praecox, or the Group of Schizophrenias* (J. Zinkin, trans., 1950). New York: International University Press.
Bowers, M.B. (1974). Central dopamine turnover in schizophrenic syndromes. *Arch. Gen. Psychiat.* **31**, 50–54.
Buchsbaum, M.S., Nuechterlein, K.H., Haier, R.J., Wu, J., Sicotte, N., Hazlett, E., Asarnow, R., Potkin, S. and Guich, S. (1990). Glucose metabolic rate in normals and schizophrenics during the continuous performance test assessed by positron emission tomography. *Br. J. Psychiat.* **156**, 216–227.
Cannon, T.D., Mednick, S.A. and Parnas, J. (1989). Genetic and perinatal determinants of structural brain deficits in schizophrenia. *Arch. Gen. Psychiat.* **46**, 883.
Carlsson, M. and Carlsson, A. (1990). Interactions between glutamatergic and monoaminergic systems within the basal ganglia—implications for schizophrenia and Parkinson's disease. *Trends Neurosci.* **13** (No. 7), 272–276.
Connell, P. (1958). *Amphetamine Psychosis*. London: Chapman and Hall.

Crow, T.J. (1990). The continuum of psychosis and its genetic origins. *Br. J. Psychiat.* **156**, 788.

Crow, T.J., Deakin, J.F.W., Johnstone, E.C. and Longden, A. (1976). Dopamine and schizophrenia. *Lancet* **ii**, 563–566.

De la Fuente, J.R. and Rosenbaum, A.H. (1981). Prolactin in psychiatry. *Am. J. Psychiat.* **138**, 1154–1160.

de Wied, D., Bohus, B., Van Ree, J.M., Kovacs, G.L. and Greven, H.M. (1978). Neuroleptic-like activity of [Des-Tyr^1]-γ-endorphin in rats. *Lancet* **i**, 1046.

Ehringer, H. and Hornykiewicz, O. (1960). Distribution of noradrenaline and dopamine (3-hydroxytyramine) in human brain and their behaviour in diseases of the extrapyramidal system. *Klin. Wschr.* **38**, 1236–1239.

Eichler, A.J. and Antelman, S.M. (1979). Sensitisation to amphetamine and stress may involve nucleus accumbens and medial frontal cortex. *Brain Res.* **176**, 412–416.

Etienne, P. and Baudry, M. (1987). Calcium dependent aspects of synaptic plasticity excitatory amino acid neurotransmission, brain ageing and schizophrenia: a unifying hypothesis. *Neurobiol. Aging* **8**, 367–386.

Farde, L., Wiesel, F.A., Hall, H., Halldin, C., Stone-Elander, S. and Sedvall, G. (1990). D2 dopamine receptors in neuroleptic-naive schizophrenic patients: a Positron Emission Tomography study with (''C)-raclopride). *Arch. Gen. Psychiat.* **47**, 213–220.

Frith, C.D. and Done, D.J. (1989). Experiences of alien control in schizophrenia reflect a disorder in the central monitoring action. *Psychol. Med.* **19**, 359–363.

Frith, C.D., Stevens, M., Johnstone, E.C. and Crow, T.J. (1979). Skin conductance responsivity during acute episodes of schizophrenia as a predictor of symptomatic improvement. *Psychol. Med.* **9**, 100–106.

Gruzelier, J.H. (1981). Cerebral laterality and psychopathology: fact and fiction. *Psychol. Med.* **11**, 219–227.

Hökfelt, T., Johansson, O., Ljungdahl, A., Lundberg, J.M. and Schultzberg, M. (1980). Peptidergic neurones. *Nature (Lond.)* **284**, 515–521.

Horowitz, M.J. and Adams, J.E. (1970). In: W. Kemp (ed.) *Origin and Mechanisms of Hallucinations*, pp. 13–22. New York: Plenum Press.

Huttenlocher, P. (1979). Synaptic density in human frontal cortex: developmental changes and effects of ageing. *Brain Res.* **163**, 195–205.

Iversen, S.D. (1977). Brain dopamine systems and behaviour. In: L.L. Iversen, S.D. Iversen and S.H. Snyder (eds) *Handbook of Psychopharmacology*, Vol. 8, pp. 333–384. New York: Plenum Press.

Iversen, S.D. (1980). Brain chemistry and behaviour. *Psychol. Med.* **10**, 527–539.

Jeste, D.V. and Lohr, J.B. (1989). Hippocampal pathological findings in schizophrenia: A morphometric study. *Arch. Gen. Psychiat.* **46**, 1019–1024.

Johnson, J.W. and Ascher, P. (1987). Glycine potentiates the NMDA response in cultured mouse brain neurons. *Nature* **325**, 529–531.

Kerwin, R.W. (1989). How do the neuropathological changes of schizophrenia relate to pre-existing neurotransmitter and etiological hypotheses? *Psychol. Med.* **19**, 563–567.

Largent, B.L., Wikstrom, H., Snowman, A.M. and Snyder, S.H. (1988). Novel antipsychotic drugs share affinity for sigma receptors. *Eur. J. Pharmacol.* **155**, 345–347.

Lee, T. and Seeman, P. (1980). Elevation of brain neuroleptic/dopamine receptors in schizophrenia. *Am. J. Psychiat.* **137**, 191–197.

Mackay, A.V.P. (1981). Endorphins: implications for psychiatry. In: D.P. Jewell, (ed.) *Advanced Medicine*, Vol. 17, pp. 180–188. London: Pitman Medical.

Mackay, A.V.P., Iversen, L.L., Rossor, M., Spokes, E., Bird, E., Arregui, A., Creese, I. and Snyder, S.H. (1982). Increased brain dopamine and dopamine receptors in schizophrenia. *Arch. Gen. Psychiat.* **39**, 991–997.

Matthyse, S. and Sugarman, J. (1979). Neurotransmitter theories of schizophrenia. In: L.L. Iversen, S.D. Iversen and S.H. Snyder (eds) *Handbook of Psychopharmacology*, Vol. 10, pp. 221–242. New York: Plenum Press.

Meldrum, B.S. and Kerwin, R.W. (1987). Glutamate receptors and schizophrenia. *J. Psychopharmacol.* **1** (No. 4), 217–221.

Murray, R.M., Lewis, S.W., Owen, M.J. and Foerster, A. (1988). The neurodevelopmental origins of dementia praecox. In: P. Bebbington and P. McGuffin (eds) *Schizophrenia —The Major Issue*. Heinemann.

Olney, J.W. (1989). Excitatory amino acids and neuropsychiatric disorders. *Biol. Psychiat.* **25**, 505–525.

Osmond, H. and Smythies, J. (1952). Schizophrenia: a new approach. *J. Ment. Sci.* **98**, 309–315.

Owen, F. and Crow, T.J. (1987). Neurotransmitters and psychosis. *Br. Med. Bull.* **43**, 651–671.

Owen, F., Crow, T.J., Poulter, M., Cross, A.J., Longden, A. and Riley, G.J. (1978). Increased dopamine receptor sensitivity in schizophrenia. *Lancet* **ii**, 223–225.

Owen, M.J. and Mullen, M.J. (1990). Molecular genetic studies of manic-depression and schizophrenia. *Trends Neurosci.* **13** (No. 1), 29–31.

Parnas, J., Mednick, S.A. and Moffitt, T.E. (1981). Perinatal complications and adult schizophrenia. *Trends Neurosci.* **4**, 262–264.

Pollin, W., Cardon, P.V. and Kety, S.S. (1961). Effects of amino acid feedings in schizophrenic patients treated with iproniazid. *Science (NY)* **133**, 104–105.

Post, R.M., Fink, E., Carpenter, W.T. and Goodwin, F.K. (1975). Cerebrospinal fluid amine metabolites in acute schizophrenia. *Arch. Gen. Psychiat.* **32**, 1063–1069.

Randrup, A. and Munkvad, I. (1974). Pharmacology and physiology of stereotyped behaviour. *J. Psychiat. Res.* **11**, 1–10.

Reveley, A. and Murray, R.M. (1980). The genetic contribution to the functional psychoses. *Br. J. Hosp. Med.* (Aug.), 166–171.

Reynolds, G.P. (1983). Increased concentrations and lateral asymmetry of amygdala dopamine in schizophrenia. *Nature* **305**, 527–529.

Reynolds, G.P. (1988). Post-mortem neurochemistry of schizophrenia. *Psychol. Med.* **18**, 793–797.

Reynolds, G.P. (1989). Beyond the dopamine hypothesis. The neurochemical pathology of schizophrenia. *Br. J. Psychiat.* **155**, 305–316.

Rodnight, R., Murray, R.M., Oon, M.G.J., Brockington, I.F., Nicholls, P. and Birley, J.L.T. (1977). Urinary dimethyltryptamine and psychiatric symptomatology and classification. *Psychol. Med.* **6**, 649–657.

Rotrosen, J., Angrist, B., Gershon, S., Paquin, J., Branchey, L., Oleshansky, M., Halpern, F. and Sachar, E.J. (1979). Neuroendocrine effects of apomorphine: characterisation of response patterns and application to schizophrenia research. *Br. J. Psychiat.* **135**, 444–456.

Seeman, P., Lee, T., Cha-Wong, M. and Wong, K. (1976). Antipsychotic drug doses and neuroleptic/dopamine receptors. *Nature (Lond.)* **126**, 717–719.

Seeman, P., Uepian, C., Bergeron, C. *et al.* (1984). Bimodal distribution of dopamine receptor densities in brains of schizophrenics. *Science* **225**, 728–731.

Seeman, P., Bzowej, N.H., Guan, H.C. *et al.* (1987). Human brain D1 and D2 dopamine receptors in schizophrenia, Alzheimer's, Parkinson's and Huntington's disease. *Neuropsychopharmacology* **1**, 5–15.

Snyder, S.H. (1973). Catecholamines as mediators of drug effects in schizophrenia. In: F.O. Schmitt and F.G. Worden (eds) *The Neurosciences, Third Study Program*, pp. 721–732. New York: Rockefeller.

Snyder, S.H. (1981). Dopamine receptors, neuroleptics and schizophrenia. *Am. J. Psychiat.* **138**, 460–464.

Snyder, S.H. and Largent, B.L. (1989). Receptor mechanisms in antipsychotic drug action: focus on sigma receptors. *J. Neuropsychiat.* **1**, 7–15.

Snyder, S.H., Banerjee, S.P., Yamamura, H.O. and Greenberg, D. (1974). Drugs, neurotransmitters and schizophrenia. *Science (NY)* **184**, 1243–1253.

Tarrier, N., Vaughn, C., Lader, M.H. and Leff, J.P. (1979). Bodily reactions to people and events in schizophrenics. *Arch. Gen. Psychiat.* **36**, 311–315.

Trimble, M.R. (1981). Visual and auditory hallucinations. *Trends Neurosci.* **4**, 1–4.

Trimble, M.R. (1990). First-rank symptoms of Schneider. A new perspective? *Br. J. Psychiat.* **156**, 195–200.

Wachtel, H. and Turski, L. (1990). Glutamate: a new target in schizophrenia? *Trends Pharmacol. Sci.* **11**, (No. 6), 219–220.

Weinberger, D.R. (1987). Implications of normal brain development for the pathogenesis of schizophrenia. *Arch. Gen. Psychiat.* **44**, 660–669.

Weinberger, D.R. (1988). Schizophrenia and the frontal lobe. *Trends Neurosci.* **11**, 367–370.

Weinberger, D.R., Berman, K.F. and Zec, R.F. (1986). Physiologic dysfunction of dorsolateral prefrontal cortex in schizophrenia. I. Regional cerebral blood flow evidence. *Arch. Gen. Psychiat.* **43**, 114–124.

— 32

Neuroleptics

M.P.I. Weller

In December 1950, Charpentier synthesized chlorpromazine (CPZ). The drug had been developed as a calming agent, following the earlier beneficial use of the antihistaminic and phenothiazine promethazine in surgical procedures. The impetus had come from the surgeon Laborit, who was far-sighted enough to see the psychiatric potential of the new drug as a calming agent and to persuade Hamon, Paraire and Velluz to use it. These psychiatrists, working at the Val-de-Grace Hospital, were struck by the improvement in psychotic symptoms they obtained with CPZ. Their results were quickly confirmed in 1952 by Jean Delay and Pierre Deniker, working in the nearby St Anne's Psychiatric Hospital (Mackay, 1982).

Delay and Deniker proposed the term 'neuroleptic' for the drug to the French Academy of Medicine in 1955, deriving it from 'psycholepsis', coined by Janet for his concept of reduced psychological tension. The term was intended to describe both the mental and neurological effects. Alternative terms for related agents are antipsychotics, a term that goes to the heart of their use, and major tranquillizers, a term that confuses the laity about the usual purpose of the drugs and sometimes generates unnecessary concern. The early findings were soon confirmed by psychiatrists in many countries. Thus began an effective treatment for schizophrenia that has contributed to a persistent decline in mental hospital populations throughout the world. This is all the more remarkable when judged against the previous persistent increase.

The use of CPZ and its later alternatives has advanced the application of social therapy, each complementing the other. Drugs alone do not help patients to find jobs and accommodation or to adjust to life outside of hospital. Without neuroleptic drugs, social therapy may not aid recovery, but neuroleptics have facilitated personal, family and group psychotherapy, as well as occupational therapy, and they have emphasized the value of community-based services (Weller and Muijen, 1991).

The effectiveness of the neuroleptic drugs for the treatment of the positive symptoms of schizophrenia—hallucinations, delusions and formal thought disorder—is now well established. The class has been found superior to placebos in double-blind controlled trials, whereas phenobarbitone has not (see Davis and Garver, 1978; Mackay, 1982, for reviews). These neuroleptic agents are properly called 'antischizophrenic' or 'antipsychotic' drugs, when used for this purpose.

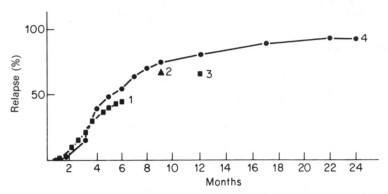

FIG. 32.1 The relapse figures in four neuroleptic withdrawal studies. 1, Prien *et al.* (1968); 2, Hirsch *et al.* (1973); 3, Hogarty *et al.* (1976); 4, Dencker *et al.* (1980).

Their prophylactic benefit in preventing the recurrence of positive symptoms has also been shown (see Fig. 32.1).

Promazine and mepazine have been found inferior to other neuroleptic agents. The remainder are all roughly equal in therapeutic effect, although of differing potencies, CPZ being comparatively weak on a dose equivalence basis, fluphenazine of moderate potency and haloperidol effective in comparatively low doses. Individuals respond better to one than another, perhaps because of differing absorption, metabolism or receptor binding.

When treated with neuroleptics, patients with positive symptoms often show an increase in activity and spontaneity, taking a more active interest in their surroundings. However, when only negative symptoms are evident, such as loss of motivation and volition, and compression of the range of emotional response with loss of rapport, the benefit is less clear, particularly in the later stages of the illness. Apart from the general clinical impression, evidence was obtained in a trial of CPZ, propranolol (see below) and placebo (Peet *et al.*, 1981), in which neither active agent was found to confer discernible benefit on a group of chronically ill patients.

Mechanism of Action

Rauwolfia alkaloids had a reputation in ancient Hindu writings for being antimanic and neuroleptic in action. These effects were redescribed in 1931 by Sen and Bose, and are now believed to be due to their producing a generalized depletion of neurotransmitters in the central nervous system, including a reduction in dopamine (DA). Modern neuroleptic drugs depend on dopamine blockade for their antipsychotic activity, and this has been demonstrated as crucial in an experiment with the two stereoisomers of fluphenthixol. Only the *cis*-form has been shown to have antipsychotic properties and it is over one thousand times more potent than the alternative *trans*-form in blocking dopamine receptors (Johnstone *et al.*, 1978).

The neuroleptic drugs can be divided into three main chemical types: pheno-thiazines, butyrophenones and thioxanthenes. They all show an affinity for dopamine receptors, and the choice between them and the various forms within each category depends, in large measure, on their side effects, the convenience of dosage schedules and routes of administration. Although some have more sedative effects, this is not the same as saying that some have more 'activating' effects, which is sometimes asserted. Until very recently two types of dopamine receptor were known, the D_1 receptor, which when stimulated increases adenyl cyclase activity and D_2 receptors, which when stimulated reduce adenyl cyclase. Both receptor types are widely distributed in all dopaminoceptive areas. Most classical neuroleptics have a high affinity to dopamine D_2 receptors, but a few (e.g. the thioxanthenes) have a high affinity also to D_1 receptors (Hyttel, 1985). The wide difference in the D_1/D_2 affinity ratio, found by assay techniques, is not related to clinical effectiveness, although clozapine, discussed below, has a near equal affinity for the D_1 and D_2 receptors in rodents (Andersson et al., 1986) and man (Farde et al., 1989), a factor suggested as underlying the atypical properties (Farde et al., 1989). This seems unlikely since the same effect could be achieved by judicious mixtures of thioxanthenes, such as flupenthixol, with other classes of neuroleptics. This must be a sufficiently frequent occurrence for the lesson to have been learnt without the risks of catastrophic agranulocytosis associated with clozapine.

An additional dopamine autoreceptor and post-synaptic receptor, D_3, has been characterized with similarities to the D_2 receptor in terms of amino acid sequence and ligand-binding profile. In the rat brain D_3 receptor mRNA is found in highest density in the limbic regions, including the nucleus accumbens and hippocampus, suggesting a role for this receptor in cognitive and emotional CNS functions (Sokoloff et al., 1990). Typical neuroleptics, which commonly induce extra-pyramidal side effects, are 10 to 20-fold more potent at D_2 than D_3 receptors, whereas some atypical neuroleptics which exhibit fewer extra-pyramidal side effects, such as clozapine, are almost equipotent at the two receptors. The identification of selective D_3 antagonists may reveal a novel class of antischizo-phrenic drugs with fewer extra-pyramidal side effects than existing neuroleptics.

It is not immediately clear how so many different types of molecules can all achieve the same effect, nor what common feature they share. Neuroleptics are tertiary amines, or in some cases secondary amines, containing at least one aromatic ring linked to the basic amine portion ($-N<$) (see Fig. 32.2).

It has been claimed that the dose of neuroleptic drugs used in clinical practice (see Table 32.1) correlates well with the potency in animal models, with antagonism of amphetamine-induced stereotopy and displacement of radiolabelled halo-peridol in the caudate nucleus and limbic areas of calf brain (see Fig. 31.4, Chapter 31, this volume).

Nevertheless, this apparently compelling defence of the crucial effect of dopamine blockade begs the question, how do we know the optimal clinical dosages? Indeed, the argument is partially circular since the initial dose levels are often recommended on the basis of dose equivalence in comparative assay techniques, and it is later argued that typical doses may often be excessive (Johnstone et al., 1983; Smith et al., 1984).

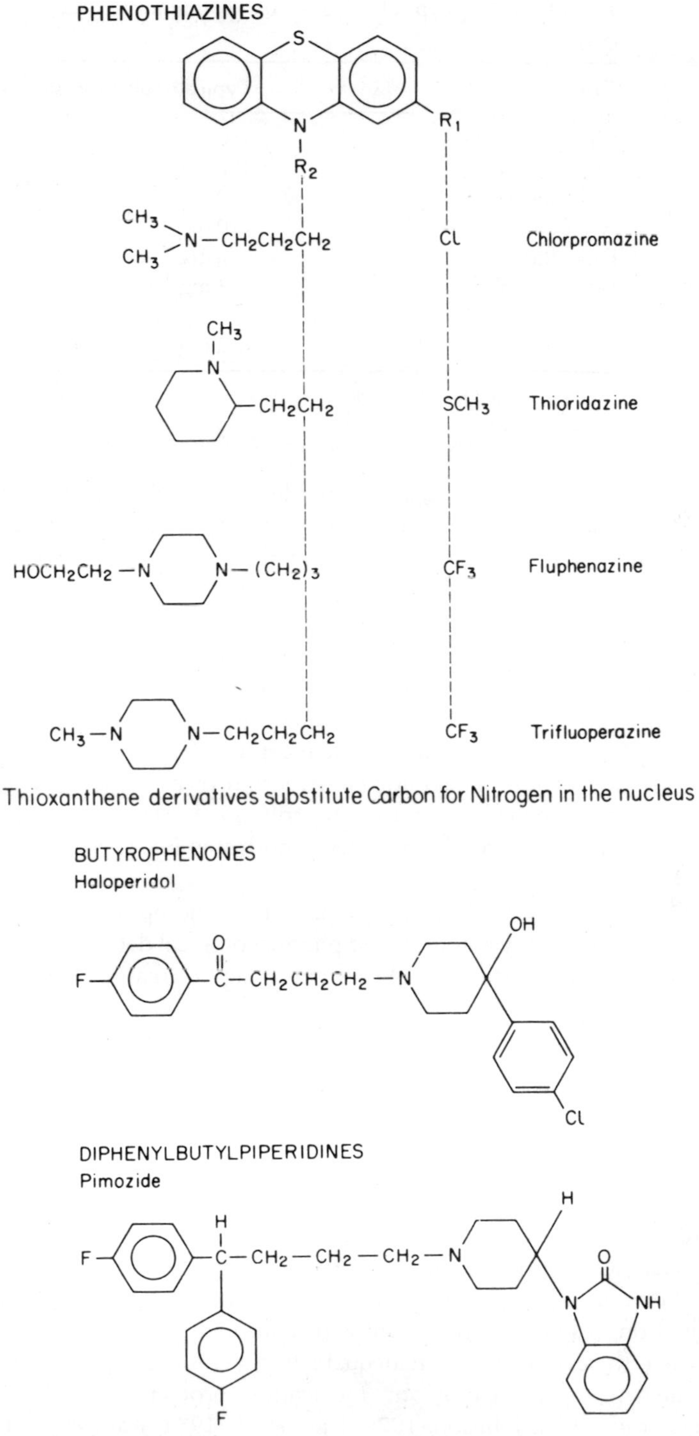

PHENOTHIAZINES

R_2	R_1	
$CH_3$$CH_3$$N-CH_2CH_2CH_2$	Cl	Chlorpromazine
(N-CH₃ piperidine) $-CH_2CH_2$	SCH_3	Thioridazine
$HOCH_2CH_2-N$ $N-(CH_2)_3$	CF_3	Fluphenazine
CH_3-N $N-CH_2CH_2CH_2$	CF_3	Trifluoperazine

Thioxanthene derivatives substitute Carbon for Nitrogen in the nucleus

BUTYROPHENONES
Haloperidol

DIPHENYLBUTYLPIPERIDINES
Pimozide

FIG. 32.2   Some neuroleptic drugs in common usage.

TABLE 32.1 Typical doses of commonly used neuroleptics.

Drug	Typical daily doses
Chlorpromazine	450 mg
Thioridazine[a]	400 mg
Trifluoperazine	10 mg
Haloperidol	10 mg
Pimozide	8 mg
Flupenthixol decanoate	3 mg
Fluphenazine decanoate	2 mg
Fluphenazine enanthate	2 mg

[a]Dosage limited to 600 mg daily for up to four weeks because of risk of retinitis pigmentosa.

The dopamine hypothesis fails to provide a complete understanding of the biochemical nature of schizophrenia (Meltzer, 1979; Crow *et al.*, 1985). Postmortem studies have been inconsistent and the possibility of the confounding effect of previous medication difficult to eliminate. Positron emission tomographic (PET) studies (see Chapter 1, this volume) have failed to substantiate the dopamine hypothesis. Van Kammen *et al.* (1990) argue that noradrenaline activity modulates the pathophysiology. Since many of the neuroleptics, including clozapine, induce significant α-adrenergic blockade (Cohen and Lipinski, 1986) and clozapine has little influence on dopamine receptors (Severson *et al.*, 1984), a case can be made out for the therapeutic contribution of noradrenergic antagonism. A case can similarly be made out for the contribution of serotoninergic (Lerer *et al.*, 1988; Costal *et al.*, 1990; see Jones, 1990) and histaminic (Peroutka and Snyder, 1980) antagonism.

There is an interaction between dopamine (DA) and opioid systems, as shown by anatomical, electrophysiological and pharmacological data and opiate peptides and receptors are modified after chronic neuroleptic treatment (Giardino *et al.*, 1990).

The most disabling long-term problems in schizophrenia are the negative symptoms. Life becomes aimless and drab, the impoverishment of emotions leaving little capacity to feel much more than tension, anxiety and depression. Vitality, animation and the beauty of the personality are replaced by apathy, indifference and self-neglect. These negative symptoms, which can lead to destitution and death, are stubbornly resistant to conventional pharmacotherapy, some 10–20% of hospital-treated patients failing to respond adequately to conventional neuroleptics (Davis *et al.*, 1980). Only one patient of a group of 28 untreated chronic schizophrenic patients, with an average period of 18 years of hospitalization, responded to 9 months of neuroleptics (Letemendia and Harris, 1967). Nevertheless, as far as inadequate information goes, early intervention and maintenance with neuroleptic medication protects against deterioration (Goldberg *et al.*, 1965; Johnson, 1979; May *et al.*, 1981; Kane *et al.*, 1982; Crow *et al.*, 1986).

Atypical neuroleptics

Neuroleptics vary in their relative affinities for nigrostriatal and mesolimbic neurones: clozapine, sulpiride and thioridazine have a high affinity for mesolimbic sites, and haloperidol for the nigrostriatal pathway (Bartolini, 1976; De Belleroche and Neal, 1982; White and Wang, 1983). As an illustration of the differential pathway affinities, the antiemetic metoclopromide seems particularly prone to cause dystonic reactions, yet to have minimal antipsychotic effect (Stanley *et al.*, 1980), acting only on nigral units (Costal *et al.*, 1978; White and Wang, 1983).

In addition to their targeted site of action, clozapine, sulpiride and thioridazine have a different profile of action in animal models, failing to induce catalepsy and the first two have been termed atypical neuroleptics. Clozapine fails to induce the typical neuroleptic effects of dopamine receptor blockade, e.g. catalepsy, and antagonism of apomorphine- and amphetamine-induced stereotypes. It has only mild, transient effects on prolactin in man and DA receptor hypersensitivity does not seem to develop after repeated doses.

Clozapine has been found effective amongst cases refractory to other neuroleptics in double-blind trials (Fischer-Cornelssen and Ferner, 1976; Claghorn *et al.*, 1987; Kane *et al.*, 1988a,b). The drug (8-chloro-11-(methyl-1-piperazinyl)-5H-dibenzo[b,e][1,4]diazepine) is a dibenzodiazepine, similar in structure to loxapine and, as mentioned above, is only weakly active in the dopaminergic system, blocking D_1 and D_2 receptors equally. However it also has serotonin (S_2), adrenergic (α_1) and histaminc (H_1) blocking activity, and is a potent muscarinic acetylcholine antagonist. It is unclear which of these features is responsible for its therapeutic effect but the recent discovery of a D_3 receptor (Sokoloff *et al.*, 1990), discussed above, may provide the key to the distinction between the typical and atypical neuroleptics. The typical neuroleptics, which commonly induce extrapyramidal side effects, are 10 to 20-fold more potent at D_2 than D_3 receptors, whereas clozapine is almost equipotent at the two receptors.

Clozapine first became available for general use in Europe in 1975 but eight deaths from agranulocytosis were recorded the same year in Finland and the drug was withdrawn. There seems to be a 2% cumulative incidence of agranulocytosis after 52 weeks of clozapine treatment (Bablenis *et al.*, 1989). The agranulocytosis potential can be minimized by frequent white blood cell counts and by stopping the drug with non-responding patients before the peak risk period (the second to the sixth month) (Claghorn *et al.*, 1987). With careful monitoring it can be safe over long periods (Lindstrom, 1988).

Before starting this hazardous drug, patients should have failed to respond to adequate doses of at least three conventional neuroleptics from at least two different chemical classes administered for an adequate period. The unique profile of action and the responsiveness of a third to a half of patients to clozapine when other agents have failed (Povlsen *et al.*, 1985), particularly in the areas of emotional withdrawal and blunted affect, is encouraging. Estimations of blood levels is worthwhile, with a target of $< 350 \, \text{ng ml}^{-1}$ in non-responsive cases (Perry *et al.*, 1991). Grand mal seizures have occurred with concentrations of 1313 and 2194 ng ml^{-1} (Kane *et al.*, 1988b), which probably represents the upper limit of plasma level.

Based on the success of chlorpromazine, all the antipsychotic drugs have been selected for their dopamine blocking propensities, and this has obscured the search for alternative antipsychotic agents.

Alternative agents

The serious side effects of conventional neuroleptic agents and their limited potential in many patients motivates a concern to find alternative pharmacological treatments. Such alternatives deepen our understanding of the disease.

Fenfluramine (Kalakowska *et al.*, 1987) and cyproheptadine (Silver *et al.*, 1989), serotonin antagonists, have shown therapeutic benefits in open trials, the former in patients with elevated serum levels.

Recently compounds which selectively block 5HT$_3$ receptors have been shown to mimic the action of neuroleptic drugs in reducing hyperactivity after dopamine agonists have been infused into the nucleus accumbens and amygdala of rodents and primates (marmosets). The effect does not lead to underactivity, as occurs with fluphenazine and sulpiride (Costal *et al.*, 1988, 1990). A similar interaction has been shown in perfused brain slices with 5HT$_3$ receptor-mediated release of dopamine from rat striatal slices (Blandina *et al.*, 1988). In early clinical trials in humans such agents have proved promising as antipsychotic agents, having low toxicity and being free of extrapyramidal side effects.

Neuropeptides are widely distributed within the central nervous system, coexisting with the classical neurotransmitters and other types of messenger molecules, and are particularly concentrated in several hypothalamic nuclei, the central amygdaloid nucleus and the septal area—areas in which malfunction has been postulated to occur in schizophrenia (see Weller, 1990). Cholecystokinin (CCK) coexists with dopamine (DA) and abnormally low levels of CCK have been found in the temporal cortex, hippocampus and amygdala in schizophrenic brains (Roberts, 1990).

Certain opiates are psychotomimetic, such as *N*-allylnormetazocine (SKF 10047) and cyclazocine. The effects are believed to be mediated by the σ-opiate receptor (see Deutsch *et al.*, 1988). Haloperidol, but not other neuroleptics, has a high affinity for σ-receptors. Rimcazole antagonizes the σ-receptor, but does not affect dopamine receptors and showed some promise as a neuroleptic agent, but caused seizures in some patients (Ferris *et al.*, 1986).

The opiate antagonists naloxone and naltrexone have been alleged to confer therapeutic benefit to schizophrenic patients, as have various synthetic enkephalins and endorphins. These therapeutic claims have been fragile, with contradictory findings, particularly when placebo controls have been included in blind comparisons (Montgomery *et al.*, 1990), the beneficial effects of naloxone having the greatest credibility (see Nemroth *et al.*, 1987).

After debate, in which heroic doses were tried with conflicting results, meta-analysis of 34 studies suggest a case for the therapeutic effectiveness of moderately high doses (about 650 mg per day in divided doses) of propranolol (Ratey *et al.*,

1990) and possibly other β-adrenergic blocking drugs. The results are slow to develop, with improvements in thought disorder and non-thought disorder symptoms. Improvement in hostility/aggression and negative symptoms are reported most frequently. The benefits may be slow to develop and a trial of at least two months is desirable. The therapy is probably most successful as an adjuvant and it should be noted that propranolol raises the plasma level of chlorpromazine and a metabolite. The early trials (e.g. Yorkston *et al.*, 1981) may have been confounded by toxic confusional psychoses in some patients. A variety of patients have been selected, including chronic, refractory cases in whom little response is likely. The mechanism is unclear and the dextro-isomer of the lipid soluble propranolol, which has minimal adrenergic blocking action and 5HT antagonism, is also effective (Hirsch *et al.*, 1981). Autoradiographic studies in dogs have shown that the drug is concentrated in limbic structures. Claims have been made for improvement in tardive dyskinesia.

Dosage and Interactions

Wide individual variations have been seen in plasma levels on similar oral doses: up to a 30-fold variation in plasma butaparazine and a 20-fold variation in plasma thioridazine (Davis and Garver, 1978). A closer relationship between oral dose and plasma level is seen with haloperidol. Differences in intestinal mucosal enzymes and dietary interactions are possible sources of variation, as are individual differences in liver metabolism. Antacids, tea, coffee and fruit juices probably retard absorption (Kulhanek and Linde, 1981). Red blood cell levels may be a better indication of clinical response and side effects than plasma levels (Garver *et al.*, 1977).

The variation in gut absorption can be avoided by using intramuscular (i.m.) preparations, which also ensure compliance. An i.m. dose of CPZ, which escapes the first-pass metabolism of intestinal and liver enzymes, will be equivalent, on average, to five times the oral dose. The plasma half-life has been estimated at 10–20 h (Mackay, 1982). Tricyclic drugs elevate plasma neuroleptic levels, propranolol raises the plasma level of CPZ, and anticholinergic agents lower plasma neuroleptic levels.

Davis (1976a) showed that CPZ in oral doses of 600 mg per day was superior to doses between 150 and 300 mg per day. However, provided an adequate dose is given, there is no evidence that higher doses lead to a more rapid recovery in acute episodes (e.g. Rifkin *et al.*, 1991). Indeed, although controversial (e.g. Browne *et al.*, 1988), there may be a therapeutic window, with excessively high doses often being prescribed for optimal antipsychotic effect (Johnstone *et al.*, 1983; Smith *et al.*, 1984), with an increased risk of depressive symptoms (Van Putten, 1988; Johnson, 1980). Factors which may tempt physicians into prescribing doses in excess of those desirable for the treatment of acute psychotic symptoms are agitation, over-activity and insomnia, all of which might be better treated with alternative strategies.

Many trials have failed to show a clear advantage of neuroleptics over placebos before three weeks. The benefits of the ward milieu and the elapse of time are stressed, since both groups improve. Because of considerable individual variability in absorption and metabolism, high doses have been tried with some success in patients who failed to improve on conventional doses (Quitkin *et al.*, 1975). Unless clear benefit is obtained, the practice should be avoided and always reserved for treatment failures on conventional regimes. Fluphenazine enanthate results in lower peak plasma levels than fluphenazine decanoate and is, therefore, preferable when high-dosage depot regimes are employed, but the preparation is no longer available in the United Kingdom. Depot preparations may be directly or indirectly detectable up to six months after administration (Wistedt *et al.*, 1981).

Maintenance

The basis of depot preparations is the slow release of an ester of the active drug from an oil vehicle. Persistent depot prescribing leads to inescapable medication. Despite the assured prophylactic benefit of these agents, drug holidays have been advocated as a means of assessing the need for their continuance. This seems intuitively sensible but is contrary to the evidence. Since prolonged neuroleptic treatment sensitizes DA receptors, this may be one of the factors producing relapse on withdrawal. It is difficult to separate this factor in assessing the prophylactic benefit.

The term drug holiday was used originally for oral medication given only on some days of the week. Since relapse is often secondary to poor compliance, this must be seen as poor preparatory training. Whether neuroleptics are administered orally or parenterally (a term meaning intramuscularly or intravenously, i.e. beside the gut or enteron), it is good practice to try to protect patients on a minimum maintenance dose. However, we do not really know what this is for any individual patient until there has been a treatment failure. Each relapse carries considerable social consequences, which move the patient closer to chronic invalidism, and probably has an adverse effect on the future course of the clinical picture (Johnson, 1979; May *et al.*, 1981; Kane *et al.*, 1982; Crow *et al.*, 1986; see below). The difficulty of dose reduction is emphasized in systematic studies (e.g. Johnson *et al.*, 1987). The balancing of conflicting considerations must be a matter of careful judgement. It should always be borne in mind that a good deal of evidence indicates that a lack of understanding, excessive stimulation and the emotional climate are important determinants of relapse, as well as influencing recovery.

Relapses are probably detrimental to the future course of schizophrenia. Bleuler considered that personality deterioration supervened after the second or third episode. This observation is open to alternative interpretation but is supported by modern studies. Using first-illness schizophrenic cases, the early deployment of neuroleptics led to a better outcome in two studies (May *et al.*, 1981; Crow *et al.*, 1986), and such patients have done better on continuation neuroleptics for at least a year (Johnson, 1979; Kane *et al.*, 1982), which seems to protect against the emergence of new psychotic symptoms (Goldberg *et al.*, 1965). Added to the risk of relapse, in terms of the future progress of the illness, the disruption, perhaps irredeemable, of fragile social networks, and the probability of higher total doses of neuroleptics being administered (Johnson *et al.*, 1983), there is animal evidence that pulsed doses of neuroleptics are more likely to cause receptor supersensitivity than persistent administration (Jeste *et al.*, 1979; see Post, 1980, for review). Receptor supersensitivity is thought to be the source of the most disturbing side effect, late onset or so-called tardive dyskinesia (French *tard* = late).

Side Effects

Prolactin is under tonic DA control in the tubero-infundibular system and blockade of DA receptors releases the storage cells (mammotrophs) in the pituitary from inhibition. All classical neuroleptics cause an increase in prolactin, which may lead to gynaecomastia or galactorrhoea, and reduced male potency or disturb the menstrual cycle. Prolactin can be used to monitor compliance with medication.

Bone-marrow depression can occur and has been associated particularly with clozapine, thioridazine and chlorpromazine; the last two also cause cholestatic jaundice. Patients on maintenance therapy should have differential blood counts every six months, more frequently for clozapine. The possible significance of sore throat as a symptom of leucocytosis should be kept in mind. Contact dermatitis used to be common in nursing staff handling phenothiazine syrups.

Sensitization to the effects of sunlight occurs, particularly with CPZ, and sunscreens are helpful. Long-term exposure to neuroleptics sometimes results in abnormal melanin deposits in skin exposed to sunlight, which make the skin appear metallic blue-grey on naked-eye examination. Opacities occur in the lens and cornea, which seldom interfere with vision, but which can be detected with slit lamp illumination. Some relationship has been observed between the skin and ocular deposits, which are dose/time-related.

. Abnormal T-waves with prolonged ventricular repolarization occur in the ECG, particularly with pimozide and thioridazine. These changes are compatible with the risk of arrhythmias, which will be aggravated by the tachycardia resulting from the vagolytic anticholinergic action. The ECG changes can be reduced with potassium supplements.

Neuroleptics are epileptogenic, particularly the aliphatic phenothiazines, including CPZ. They should be introduced gradually to epileptic patients, with preference being shown for agents such as fluphenazine, and the antiepileptic medication should be maintained. The lowering of blood pressure and some of the sedative effects result from the adrenergic blocking action on central and peripheral receptors (see Creese *et al.*, 1978, for review). CPZ, thioridazine and droperidol are potent blockers of α-receptors and show the greatest tendency to sedation and orthostatic hypotension.

Neuroleptic malignant syndrome is a rare, but life-threatening complication of neuroleptic treatment, characterized by fever, rigidity, altered consciousness and autonomic instability. Confusion may be a useful antecedent (Velamoor et al., 1990). The prevalence has probably been underestimated, because of a failure to identify mild cases (Pope et al., 1980). Men are twice as susceptible as women and younger patients more often affected. Haloperidol is most frequently implicated, but, worldwide, is most often prescribed, and chlorpromazine, fluphenazine, loxapine, thioridazine, thiothixene and trifluoperazine have also been implicated. Prompt discontinuation of neuroleptic medication, cooling blankets and anti-pyretics, and fluid and electrolyte control are indicated. Caution must be exercised in re-introducing neuroleptics.

Dyskinesia

In Parkinson's disease, there is a reduction of DA in the extra-pyramidal pathway and all neuroleptic drugs produce Parkinsonian-like side effects. It is interesting that idiopathic Parkinson's disease and schizophrenia rarely coexist, and when they do, Parkinson's disease tends to succeed the treated schizophrenia. The few cases that have been reported in the converse direction are suspect on various grounds (see Weller, 1981, for review). Drug-induced Parkinsonism is common, particularly in women. There is a suggestion that it may be even more common in patients with a positive family history of Parkinson's disease. The immediate extra-pyramidal effects are dystonic and dyskinetic, including bradykinetic and akathisic.

Dyskinesia is a disorder of movement. Resting tremor is particularly common as an acute reaction. Tardive dyskinesia commonly involves involuntary movements of the tongue, mouth and face, which may present as grimacing or chomping. The patient is often largely unaware of these bucco-lingual-masticatory movements (BLM).

The bradykinetic effects are a reduction in spontaneous movements, which extend to the movements normally associated with purposive activity, such as the swing of the arms whilst walking. There may be difficulty getting out of a chair, and particularly out of a hot bath, as in Parkinson's disease. With a worsening comes a difficulty in initiating movement and a mask-like expressionless face.

Akathisia is an enforced motor restlessness, which prevents the sufferer from sitting still (the literal meaning of the term) for more than a few minutes. The condition is often expressed by a persistent rocking from one foot to the other, or stamping alternate feet, and initially is accompanied by a subjective experience of inner restlessness, which seems to reduce with time. This side effect responds poorly to anticholinergic medication. Benzodiazepines, and sometimes bar-biturates, have been found helpful, and propranolol was effective in double-blind, placebo-controlled trials (e.g. Adler et al., 1985), but a reduction in neuroleptic dosage is the best remedy. The mesocortical DA pathway has been implicated in the mechanism of this uncomfortable side effect (Marsden and Jenner, 1980).

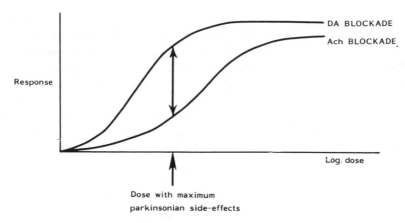

FIG. 32.3 Dose–response relationship for neuroleptic with intrinsic anticholinergic activity. The anticholinergic (Ach) effect continues to increase after the plateau in DA blockade. After the maximal separation of the two effects further dose increases paradoxically ameliorate the drug-induced Parkinsonian symptoms.

Dystonia is a persistent pathological change in muscle tone. Common examples are torticollis, contraction of the tongue, trismus, opisthotonos and occulogyric crises. Extra-pyramidal rigidity is a further problem. Passive movements of the limbs reveal a curious, persistent resistance, the so-called lead-pipe rigidity, or a succession of resistances which are suddenly overcome, known as cogwheel rigidity. When these are only slight, they can be emphasized by asking the patients to move the contralateral limb, for example by making small circling movements with the extended arm.

Many side effects can be attributed to intrinsic antimuscarinic activity in the peripheral nervous system. This is the source of blurred vision, dry mouth, constipation and sometimes difficulty in initiating urination. The variability in extra-pyramidal side effects is largely dependent on the varying degrees of intrinsic anticholinergic activity. Sometimes there is a paradoxical improvement in these side effects with increasing dosage. This can be understood by reference to the lack of parallelism in the dose–response curves to the separate antidopaminergic and anticholinergic effects (see Fig. 32.3).

In addition to the variation in anticholinergic effects, different drugs, at equivalent dosage, have differing propensities to antagonize the neurotransmitter γ-aminobutyric acid (GABA) (Marco *et al.*, 1976), which is known to influence the extra-pyramidal system (Gale, 1980).

Divided doses lessen sharp peaks in plasma levels, but the major dose should be given in the evening. The sedative effects are then advantageous and reduce more rapidly than the antipsychotic benefits. Extra-pyramidal signs are aggravated by anxiety and are less marked during sleep. Initial susceptibility to extra-pyramidal side effects is probably an enduring characteristic (Keepers and Casey, 1991).

Anticholinergic drugs

In animal experiments, prolonged exposure to neuroleptics results in an increase both in the number of receptor sites and in the amount of neurotransmitter which is synthesized. These adaptive responses can be seen in rats after three months' exposure. This is consistent with the period in which tolerance to the extra-pyramidal side effects (EPS) develops in humans (see Weller, 1981). The first few exhibitions of a neuroleptic are most likely to cause acute extra-pyramidal side effects, which are thought to be caused by an over-production of pre-synaptic DA as a result of receptor blockade.

If these initial side effects occur, they can be remedied by the addition of an anticholinergic drug. The additional drug can then often be tailed off after three months and should not be maintained unnecessarily. The antiparkinsonian agent and DA precursor, L-DOPA, is inappropriate, since DA blockade was the intention in prescribing the neuroleptic.

The case for and against anticholinergic medication is complicated and the WHO consensus statement (WHO, 1990) too compressed for an adequate airing of the issues (Abas et al., 1990; Barnes, 1990).

An interaction between the cholinergic system and the dopaminergic system obviously exists, since the effects of DA depletion in Parkinson's disease are partially compensated for by the addition of anticholinergic drugs. There is evidence that anticholinergic drugs exacerbate psychotic symptoms (Johnstone et al., 1983), which may arise, in part, because anticholinergic drugs lower the plasma levels of some neuroleptics, but there may be further adverse factors. Acetylcholine mimetics, such as the anticholinesterase physostigmine and deanol (which is possibly an acetylcholine precursor in the brain), reverse the psychotic effects of DA agonists such as methylphenidate (see Lloyd, 1978, for review). There is a suspicion that anticholinergic drug use predisposes to tardive dyskinesia but the evidence is equivocal and there are potential dangers in their omission, since acute EPS in animals sensitizes them to further EPS. Undoubtedly they cause adverse autonomic effects, detrimentally affect memory, induce toxic confusion, particularly in the elderly, and may be abused as euphoriants. Balancing these caveats, but taking into account the unpleasant dyskinetic side effects of neuro-leptics and the desirability of patient compliance, anticholinergic agents should not be used unnecessarily, and should be discontinued as soon as practicable.

Depression

Emotional display precedes and accompanies goal-directed behaviour. Euphoriant drugs, such as cocaine and amphetamine, and possibly heroin, activate mesolimbic dopaminergic pathways, which provide reward in direct electrical brain stimu-lation in animals (see Phillips and Fiberger, 1989). Appetitive behaviour, such as foraging and hoarding, are dependent on these pathways (e.g. Blackburn et al., 1989). Based on these observations, it might be expected that neuroleptic drugs, which block dopaminergic transmission and reduce emotional responsiveness, are depressing; certainly many patients taking them complain of 'tiredness'. On the other hand, many acute schizophrenic patients gain interest and motivation on neuroleptic medication. Low doses of flupenthixol have an energizing effect, but this is probably by inhibition of autoreceptors, and at least some patients seem to become depressed on neuroleptic medication, which is probably more likely on high doses (Johnson, 1980; Van Putten, 1988), while at appropriate doses there is an improvement in mood in others. Because of the two-way effect, the matter is not resolved by comparative studies of maintenance neuroleptic versus placebo which have shown equal incidence of depression in both groups.

Some of the side effects of neuroleptic medication, such as lessening of spontaneity and diminished conversation as an aspect of bradykinesia, can be mistaken for depression. An impression of depressed mood is also given by the characteristically Parkinsonian facies and the lack of associated movements, including those normally present in emotive expression. Since tricyclic anti-depressants are anticholinergic, a beneficial response to these agents may be ascribed falsely to the antidepressive action. The time course of improvement can help to resolve this ambiguity, but prior exhibition of anticholinergic drugs will also help to clarify the issue. There is some evidence that antidepressants may retard the rate of resolution of psychotic features without helping the depressive symptoms (e.g. Kramer *et al.*, 1989).

Tardive Dyskinesia

After persistent neuroleptic use, a reduction in dose may lead to a characteristic pattern of repetitive involuntary movements of a choreoathetoid type, particularly of the mouth, lips and tongue (BLM). At a later stage in treatment, these same movements occur without a dose reduction and may be suppressed with an increase in dosage. This tardive dyskinesia (TD) may coexist with features of drug-induced Parkinsonism. It arises from the development of supersensitivity to DA in the extra-pyramidal system. The symptoms are made worse by anticholinergic drugs and arousal. Treatment is difficult.

As we have seen, neuroleptics have differing affinities for nigrostriatal and limbic pathways; the newer, atypical neuroleptics, remoxipride, sulpiride and clozapine, as well as thioridazine, have greater affinity for the mesolimbic pathway, and haloperidol for the nigrostriatal pathway. Sulpiride and thioridazine may be less likely to induce tardive dyskinesia and clozapine may actually assist in developed cases (see Lieberman *et al.*, 1991).

Affective patients are prone to develop TD. Lithium is probably a contributing factor (Dinan and Kohen, 1989) (which aggravates EPS (Addonizio *et al.*, 1988)), as are ECT and intermittent neuroleptics, but the risk is four times higher in those with a positive family history for affective disorders. The elderly, who may develop an identical syndrome spontaneously, without exposure to neuroleptics, and females are also particularly susceptible (Barnes and Weller, 1986) (females may be hospitalized earlier and medicated longer). Schizophrenic patients with prominent negative symptoms, cognitive defects, obstetric complications, alcoholism, epilepsy, low intelligence and direct evidence of brain damage are also at particular risk (Guy et al., 1986; Waddington and Yousseff, 1986; Waddington, 1987; O'Callaghan et al., 1990), suggesting that underlying brain damage may predispose to this outcome.

Acetylcholine precursors have been advocated without conspicuous success. The remedy lies in stopping medication. This is not always practical and reversion of supersensitivity may take from one to three years. Complete reversibility is rare but substantial improvement usual, particularly in the young. The process can be accelerated by the addition of dopamine agonists, but this carries the hazard of increasing psychotic symptoms. However, it has been asserted that both L-dopa and apomorphine in low doses confer antipsychotic benefits, perhaps by their action on pre-synaptic inhibitory (auto) receptors. An alternative strategy is to increase the dose of neuroleptics, but the residual potential for further sensitization is considerable and the manoeuvre deplored (see Weller, 1981, for review). In contrast to the increased prevalence of TD in affective patients and patients with a positive family history for affective disorders, affective or schizo-affective disorders are predictors of improvement following discontinuation of medication (Glazer et al., 1990).

The adaptive response of the nigrostriatal system is paralleled by the meso-limbic system and has called into question the rationale of persistent neuroleptics. Pre-frontal DA pathways arising from the midbrain have been identified, which seems to be devoid of adaptive potential (Bannon et al., 1982). This may be related to the absence of nerve-terminal and cell-body receptors (similar to that in the tubero-infundibular pathway). This pathway might be the site of the therapeutic action of neuroleptics. Against this, there seems to be a reciprocal relationship between dopamine levels in the orbital pre-frontal cortex and sub-cortical dopamine systems in rodents (Blanc et al., 1980; Pycock et al., 1980). The relative affinity of different neuroleptics to different brain sites probably determines their immediate and long-term profile.

Additional Uses

Neuroleptic treatment of schizotypal personality disorder produces a perceptible movement, but is poorly tolerated (Francis, 1985), and also produces modest improvements in borderline disorders (Brinkley et al., 1979; Leone, 1982), as evaluated in double-blind trials (Serban and Siegal, 1984; Soloff et al., 1986). The improvement produced by neuroleptics typically includes improvement in depression and anxiety, and Goldberg et al. (1986) also found improvement in obsessive-compulsive problems, suggesting that these symptoms are component parts of the conditions and not independent features, particularly since the tricyclic antidepressant, amitriptyline, seemed to cause a deterioration in some patients.

The antimanic properties led to the group being described as major tran-quillizers. This term arose out of an early underestimation of the antipsychotic properties and a concept of the group as super tranquillizers. The term is unfortunate, since it suggests that a minor tranquillizer should preferably be tried first.

Neuroleptics have certain advantages, both as sedatives and anxiolytics. They are less likely than benzodiazepines to cause psychological dependence or to cause confusion in the elderly. They are particularly helpful in this group in the management of restlessness, over-activity and wandering. There is a well-known reciprocal relationship between cholinergic and dopaminergic activity in the extra-pyramidal pathway. Since brain acetylcholine is reduced in dementia (see Chapter 9, this volume), the restlessness and tendency to wander may arise out of a relative excess of DA activity, in contrary manner to the way that anti-cholinergic drugs help bradykinesia, thus making neuroleptics the theoretical drugs of choice (see Weller, 1987). (A corresponding sensitivity to both neuro-leptics and anticholinergic drugs should be borne in mind.)

Neuroleptics, particularly CPZ, have antiemetic properties. Metoclopramide and prochlorperazine have been specifically developed for this purpose. It is not widely appreciated that these drugs can produce extra-pyramidal side effects, and metoclopramide seems to have a particular affinity for nigral units (Costal *et al.*, 1978; White and Wang, 1983).

Tics and Gilles de la Tourette's syndrome respond to neuroleptics. There is a trend favouring drugs with a high affinity to striatal D_2 receptors, and haloperidol and pimozide are most often prescribed. Dangerous prolongation of the QT interval in the ECG and the slight superiority of haloperidol in a double-blind placebo-controlled trial (Shapiro *et al.*, 1989) makes haloperidol, successfully used since 1961, the continued choice. Schizophrenic patients with no history of tics may acquire a 'Tardive Tourette Syndrome' with tics and vocalizations (see Fog and Regeur, 1986).

Conclusion

Unfortunately, classical neuroleptics are often ineffective, particularly for the disabling negative symptoms, some 10–20% of hospital-treated patients failing to respond (Davis *et al.*, 1969), and the search for new pharmacological agents continues. With current drugs having such adverse side effects, both short-term and long-term, and having only limited success, much more than mechanistic prescribing and increasing doses requires attention. Kindly understanding, a judicious balance between excessive stimulation and under-stimulation, and protection from obvious or subtle emotional display are important components in treatment (Leff, 1990). Exploration and intervention in family dynamics, social relationships and supportive networks, occupation and living conditions are generally helpful, when we know that apathy, indifference and self-neglect can lead to destitution, imprisonment and death. With such hazards, there are often dangers to the patient, and sometimes to the public in well-intentioned but excessive emphasis on self-determination and civil liberties (Weller, 1989). Careful, individually tailored rehabilitation programmes, on behavioural lines, over two or more years, can produce considerable benefit, slowly overcoming an aimless pattern of life (Weller and Muijen, 1991). It is not widely recognized outside psychiatric circles that such programmes must be sustained indefinitely, since such efforts, as well as neuroleptics, generally ameliorate the symptoms rather than cure the terrible disease process.

References

Abas, M.A., Acuda, S.W., Braodhead, J.C. *et al.* (1990). WHO consensus statement (letter). *Br. J. Psychiat.* **157**, 619–620.

Addonizio, G., Roth, S.D., Stokes, P.E. and Stoll, P.M. (1988). Increased extrapyramidal symptoms with addition of lithium to neuroleptics. *J. Nervous Mental Dis.* **176**, 682–685.

Adler, L., Angrist, B., Peselow, E. *et al.* (1985). Efficacy of propranolol in neuroleptic-induced akathisia. *J. Clin. Psychopharmacol.* **5**, 164–166.

Bablenis, E., Weber, S.S. and Wagner, R. (1989). L-Clozapine: a novel antipsychotic agent. Formulary Forum. *DICP, Ann. Pharmacother.* **23**, 109–115.

Bannon, M.J., Reinhard, J.F. Jr, Bunney, E.B. and Roth, R.H. (1982). Unique response to antipsychotic drugs is due to absence of terminal autoreceptors in mesocortical dopamine neurones. *Nature (Lond.)* **296**, 444–446.

Barnes, T.R.E. (1990). Comment on the WHO Consensus statement. *Br. J. Psychiat.* **156**, 413–414.

Barnes, T.R.E. and Weller, M.P.I. (1986). Movement disorders and neuroleptic medication. In: N.S. Shah and A.G. Donald (eds) *Neurobehavioural Dysfunction Induced by Psychotherapeutic Agents*, Ch. 17, pp. 323–341. New York and London: Plenum.

Bartolini, G. (1976). Differential effect of neuroleptic drugs on dopamine turnover in extrapyramidal and limbic system. *J. Pharm. Pharmcol.* **28**, 429–433.

Blackburn, J.R., Phillips, A.G., Jakubovic, A. and Fibiger, H.C. (1989). Dopamine and preparatory behaviour II. Neurochemical analysis. *Behav. Neurosci.* **113**, 15–23.

Blanc, G., Herve, D., Simon, H., Lisoprawski, A., Glowinski, J. and Tassin, J.P. (1980). Response to stress of mesocortical-frontal dopaminergic neurones in rats after long term isolation. *Nature* **284**, 265–267.

Blandina, P., Goldfarb, J. and Green, J.P. (1988). Activation of a $5HT_3$ receptor releases dopamine from rat striatal slice. *Eur. J. Pharmacol.* **155**, 349.

Brinkley, J.R., Beitman, B.D. and Friedel, R.O. (1979). Low dose neuroleptic regimes in the treatment of borderline patients. *Arch. Gen. Psychiat.* **36**, 319–326.

Browne, F.W.A., Cooper, S.J., Wilson, R. and King, D.J. (1988). Serum haloperidol levels and clinical response in chronic, treatment-resistant schizophrenic patients. *J. Pharmacol.* **2**, 94–103.

Claghorn, J., Honigfeld, G., Abuzzahab, F.S. *et al.* (1987). The risks and benefits of clozapine versus chlorpromazine. *J. Clin. Psychopharmacol.* **7**, 377–384.

Cohen, B.M. and Lipinski, J.F. (1986). *In vivo* potencies of antipsychotic drugs in blocking $alpha_1$ and dopamine D_2 receptors: implications for drug mechanisms of action. *Life Sci.* **39**, 2571–2580.

Costal, B., Funderburk, W.H., Leonard, C.A. and Naylor, R.J. (1978). Assessment of the neuroleptic potential of some novel benzamide, butyrophenone, phenothiazine and indole derivatives. *Pharm. Pharmacol.* **30**, 771–778.

Costal, B., Domenev, A.M., Naylor, R.J. and Tyers, M.B. (1988). Inhibition by $5HT_3$ antagonists of hyperactivity caused by dopamine infusion into rat nucleus accumbens. *Br. J. Pharmacol.* **93**, 194 P.

Costal, B., Domeney, A.M., Kelly, M.E. and Naylor, R.J. (1990). Schizophrenia and its treatment. In: M.P.I. Weller (ed.) *International Perspectives in Schizophrenia*, pp. 237–252. London: John Libbey.

Creese, I., Burt, D.R. and Snyder, S.H. (1978). Biochemical action of neuroleptic drugs: focus on the dopamine receptor. In: L.L. Iversen, S.D. Iversen and S.H. Snyder (eds) *Neuroleptics and Schizophrenia*. Handbook of Psychopharmacology, Vol. 10, pp. 37–84. New York: Plenum.

Crow, T.J., Baker, H.F., Cross, A.J. *et al.* (1985). Monoamine mechanisms in chronic schizophrenia: post-mortem neurochemical findings. *Br. J. Psychiat.* **134**, 249–256.

Crow, T.J., Macmillan, J.F., Johnson, A.L. and Johnstone, E.C. (1986). The Northwick Park Study of first episodes of schizophrenia. *Br. J. Psychiat.* **148**, 120–127.

Davis, D.M. Schaffer, C.B., Killian, G.A., Kinard, C. and Chan, C. (1980). Important issues in the drug treatment of schizophrenia. *Schizophrenia Bull.* **6**, 70–87.

Davis, J.M. (1976a). Recent developments in the drug treatment of schizophrenia. *Am. J. Psychiat.* **133**, 208–214.

Davis, J.M. (1976b). Comparative doses and costs of antipsychotic medication. *Arch. Gen. Psychiat.* **33**, 858–861.

Davis, J.M. and Garver, D.L. (1978). Neuroleptics: clinical use in psychiatry. In: L.L. Iversen, S.D. Iversen and S.H. Snyder (eds) *Neuroleptics and Schizophrenia*. Handbook of Psychopharmacology, Vol. 10, pp. 129–160. New York: Plenum.

De Belleroche, J.S. and Neal, M.J. (1982). The contrasting effects of neuroleptics on transmitter release from the nucleus accumbens and corpus striatum. *Neuropharmacology* **21**, 529–537.

Dencker, S.J., Lepp, M. and Malm, U. (1980). Do schizophrenics well adapted in the community need neuroleptics? A depot neuroleptic withdrawal study. *Acta Psychiat. Scand.* (Suppl. 279), 64–76.

Deutsch, S.I., Weizman, A., Goldman, M.E. and Morihisa, J.M. (1988). The sigma receptor: a novel site implicated in psychosis and antipsychotic drug efficacy. *Clin. Neuropharmacol.* **11**, 105–119.

Dinan, T.G. and Kohen, D. (1989). Tardive dyskinesia in bipolar affective disorder: relationship to lithium therapy. *Br. J. Psychiat.* **155**, 55–57.

Farde, L., Wiesel, F.A., Nordstrom, A.L. and Sedval, G. (1989). D_1 and D_2 dopamine receptor occupancy during treatment with conventional and atypical neuroleptics. *Psychopharmacology* **99** (Suppl.), S28–31.

Ferris, R.M., Tang, F.L.M., Chang, K.J. and Russell, A. (1986). Evidence that the potential antipsychotic agent, Rimcazole (BW 234U) is a specific competitive antagonist of sigma sites in brain. *Life Sci.* **38**, 2329–2337.

Fischer-Cornelssen, K.A. and Ferner, V.J. (1976). An example of European multicenter trials: multispectral analysis of doxapine. *Psychopharmacol. Bull.* **12**, 34–39.

Fog, R. and Regeur, L. (1986). Neuropharmacology of tics. *Rev. Neurol. (Paris)* **124**, 856–859.

Francis, A. (1985). Validating schizotypal personality disorder: Problems with the schizophrenia connection. *Schizophrenia Bull.* **11**, 595–597.

Gale, K. (1980). Chronic blockade of dopamine receptors by antischizophrenic drugs enhances GABA binding in substantia nigra. *Nature (Lond.)* **283**, 569–570.

Garver, D.L., Dekirmenjian, H., Davis, J.M., Casper, R. and Ericksen, S. (1977). Neuroleptic drug levels and therapeutic response: preliminary observations with red blood cell bound butaperazine. *Am. J. Psychiat.* **134**, 304–307.

Giardino, L., Calaza, L., Piazza, P.V., Zanni, M., Sorbera, F. and Amato, G. (1990). Opiate receptor modifications in the rat brain after chronic treatment with haloperidol and sulpiride. *J. Pharmacol.* **4**, 7–12.

Glazer, W.M., Morgenstern, H., Schooler, N., Berkman, C.S. and Moore, D.C. (1990). Predictors of improvement in tardive dyskinesia following discontinuation of neuroleptic medication. *Br. J. Psychiat.* **157**, 585–592.

Goldberg, S.G., Klerman, G.L. and Cole, J.O. (1965). Changes in schizophrenia psychopathology and ward behaviour as a function of phenothiazine treatment. *Br. J. Psychiat.* **111**, 120–133.

Goldberg, S.C., Schulz, S.C., Schultz, P.M., Resnick, R.J., Hamer, R.M. and Friedel, R.O. (1986). Borderline and schizotypal personality disorders treated with low dose thiothixene vs placebo. *Arch. Gen. Psychiat.* **43**, 680–686.

Guy, W., Ban, T.A. and Wilson, W.H. (1986). The prevalence of abnormal involuntary movements among chronic schizophrenics. *Int. Clin. Psychopharmacol.* **1**, 134–144.

Hirsch, S.R., Gaind, R., Rohde, P.D. Stevens, B.I. and Wing, J.K. (1973). Out-patient maintenance of chronic schizophrenic patients with long-acting fluphenazine: a double-blind placebo trial. *Br. Med. J.* **2**, 633–637.

Hirsch, S.R., Manchanda, R. and Weller, M.P.I. (1981). Dextro-propranolol in schizophrenia. *Progr. Neuropsychopharmacol.* **4**, 633–637.

Hogarty, G.E., Ulrich, R.F., Mussare, F. and Aristigueta, N. (1976). Drug discontinuation among long-term successfully maintained schizophrenic out-patients. *Dis. Nerv. Syst.* **37**, 494–500.

Hyttel, J. (1985). Receptor binding profile of neuroleptics. *Psychopharmacology* **85** (Suppl.) 2.

Jeste, D.V., Potkin, S.G., Sinha, S., Feder, S. and Wyatt, R.J. (1979). Tardive dyskinesia—reversible and persistent. *Arch. Gen. Psychiat.* **36**, 585–590.

Johnson, D.A.W. (1979). Further observations on the duration of depot neuroptic maintenance therapy in schizophrenia. *Br. J. Psychiat.* **135**, 524–530.

Johnson, D.A.W. (1980). Studies of depressive symptoms in schizophrenia. 1. The prevalence of depression and its possible causes. *Br. J. Psychiat.* **139**, 89–101.

Johnson, D.A.W., Pasterksi, G., Ludlow, J.M., Street, K. and Taylor, R.D.W. (1983). The discontinuance of maintenance neuroleptic therapy in chronic schizophrenic patients: drug and social consequences. *Acta Psychiat. Scand.* **67**, 339–352.

Johnson, D.A.W., Ludlow, J.M., Street, K. and Taylor, R.D.W. (1987). Double-blind comparison of the half-dose and standard-dose flupenthixol decanoate in the maintenance treatment of stabilised out-patients with schizophrenia. *Br. J. Psychiat.* **151**, 634–638.

Johnstone, E.C., Crow, T.J., Frith, C.D., Carney, M.W.P. and Price, J.S. (1978). Mechanism of the antipsychotic effect in the treatment of acute schizophrenia. *Lancet* **i**, 848–851.

Johnstone, E.C., Crow, T.J., Ferrier, I.N., Frith, C.D., Owens, D.G.C., Bourne, R.C. and Gamble, S.J. (1983). Adverse effects of anticholinergic medication on positive schizophrenic symptoms. *Psychol. Med.* **13**, 513–527.

Jones, B.J. (1990). New possibilities for the drug treatment of schizophrenia. In: M.P.I. Weller (ed.) *International Perspectives in Schizophrenia*, pp. 231–235. London: John Libbey.

Kalakowska, T., Gadhvi, H. and Molyneux, S. (1987). An open trial of fenfluramine in chronic schizophrenia: a pilot study. *Int. Clinics Psychopharmacol.* **2**, 83–88.

Kane, J.M. and Smith, J.M. (1982). Tardive dyskinesia: prevalence and risk factors 1959–1979. *Arch. Gen. Psychiat.* **139**, 329–331.

Kane, J.M., Rifkin, A., Quitkin, F., Nayak, D. and Ramos-Lorenzi (1982). Fluphenazine v́s. placebo in patients with remitted acute first episode schizophrenia. *Arch. Gen. Psychiat.* **39**, 70–73.

Kane, J.M., Honigfeld, G., Singer, J. and Meltzer, H. (1988a). Clozapine in treatment resistant schizophrenics. *Psychopharmacol. Bull.* **24**, 62–67.

Kane, J.M., Honigfeld, G., Singer, J. *et al.* (1988b). Clozapine in treatment resistant schizophrenics: a double-blind comparison with chlorpromazine. *Arch. Gen. Psychiat.* **45**, 489–496.

Keepers, G.A. and Casey, D.E. (1991). Use of neuroleptic-induced extrapyramidal symptoms to predict future vulnerability to side effects. *Am. J. Psychiat.* **148**, 85–89.

Kramer, M.S., Vogel, W.H., DiJohnson, C. *et al.* (1989). Antidepressants in 'depressed' schizophrenic inpatients: a controlled trial. *Arch. Gen. Psychiat.* **46**, 922–928.

Kulhanek, F. and Linde, O.K. (1981). Coffee and tea influence pharmacokinetics of antipsychotic drugs (letter). *Lancet* **ii**, 359–360.

Leff, J. (1990). Autonomic changes and expressed emotions. In: M.P.I. Weller (ed.) *International Perspectives in Schizophrenia.* London: John Libbey.

Leone, N.F. (1982). Response of borderline patients to laxapine and chlorpromazine. *J. Clin. Psychiat.* **43**, 148–150.

Lerer, B., Ran, A., Blacker, M., Silver, H. and Weller, M.P.I. (1988). Neuroendocrine response in chronic schizophrenia: evidence for serotonergic dysfunction. *Schizophrenia Res.* **1**, 405–410.

Letemendia, F.J.J. and Harris, A.D. (1967). Chlorpromazine and the untreated chronic schizophrenic: a long-term trial. *Br. J. Psychiat.* **113**, 950–958.

Lieberman, J.A., Saltz, B.L., Johns, C.A., Pollack, S., Borenstein, M. and Kane, J. (1991). The effects of clozapine on tardive dyskinesia. *Br. J. Psychiat.* **158**, 503–510.

Lindstrom, L.H. (1988). The effect of long term treatment with Clozapine in schizophrenia: a retrospective study in 96 patients treated with Clozapine for up to 13 years. *Acta Psychiat. Scand.* **77** (5), 824–829.

Lloyd, K.G. (1978). Neurotransmitter interactions related to central dopamine neurones. In: M.B.H. Youdim, W. Lovenberg, D.F. Sharman and J.R. Lagnado (eds) *Essays in Neurochemistry and Neuropharmacology,* Vol. 3, pp. 129–208. Chichester: Wiley.

Mackay, A.V.P. (1982). Antischizophrenic drugs. In: P.J. Tyrer (ed.) *Drugs in Psychiatric Practice.* Sevenoaks, Kent: Butterworth.

Marco, E., Mao, C.C., Cheney, D.L., Revuelta, A. and Costa, E. (1976). The effects of antipsychotics on the turnover rate of GABA and acetylcholine in rat brain nuclei. *Nature (Lond.)* **264**, 363–365.

Marsden, C.D. and Jenner, P. (1980). The pathophysiology of extrapyramidal side-effect of neuroleptic drugs. *Psychol. Med.* **10**, 55–72.

May, P.R.A., Tuma, A.H. and Dixon, W.J. (1981). Schizophrenia: a follow-up study of the results of five forms of treatment. *Arch. Gen. Psychiat.* **125**, 12–19.

Meltzer, H.Y. (1979). Studies in schizophrenia. In: L. Bellak (ed.) *Disorders of the Schizophrenic Syndrome.* New York: Basic Books.

Montgomery, S.A., Green, M., Montgomery, D. *et al.* (1990). Desenkephalin γ endorphin and thioridazine in the treatment of schizophrenia: a placebo controlled study (abstract). *J. Pharmacol.* **4**, 252.

Nemroth, C.B., Berger, P.A. and Bissette, G. (1987). Peptides in schizophrenia. In: H.Y. Meltzer (ed.) *Psychopharmacology: The Third Generation of Progress,* pp. 727–743. New York: Raven Press.

O'Callaghan, E., Larkin, C., Kinsella, A. and Waddington, J.L. (1990). Obstetric complications, the putative familial-sporadic distinction, and tardive dyskinesia in schizophrenia. *Br. J. Psychiat.* **157**, 578–584.

Peet, M., Bethell, M.S., Coates, A. *et al.* (1981). Propranolol in schizophrenia: I. Comparison of propranolol, chlorpromazine and placebo. *Brit. J. Psychiat.* **139**, 105–111.

Peroutka, S.J. and Snyder, S.H. (1980). Relationship of neuroleptic drug effects at brain dopamine, serotonin, α-adrenergic and histamine receptors to clinical potency. *Am. J. Psychiat.* **137**, 1518–1522.

Perry, P.J., Miller, D.D., Arndt, S.V. and Cadoret, R.J. (1991). Clozapine and norclozapine plasma concentrations and clinical response of treatment-refractory schizophrenic patients. *Am. J. Psychiat.* **148**, 231–235.

Phillips, A.C. and Fiberger, H.G. (1989). Neuroanatomical bases of intracranial self-stimulation: untangling the Gordian knot. In: J.M. Liebman and S.J. Cooper (eds) *The Neuropharmacological Basis of Reward*, pp. 66–105. Oxford: Oxford Science Publishers.

Pope, H.G., Keck, P.E. and McElroy, ?. (1980). Frequency and presentation of neuroleptic malignant syndrome in a large psychiatric hospital. *Am. J. Psychiat.* **143**, 1227–1233.

Post, R.M. (1980). Intermittent versus continuous stimulation: effect of time interval on the development of sensitization or tolerance. *Life Sci.* **26**, 1275–1282.

Povlsen, U.J., Noring, U., Fog, R. and Gerlach, J. (1985). Tolerability and therapeutic effect of clozapine: a retrospective investigation of 216 patients treated with clozapine for up to 12 years. *Acta Psychiat. Scand.* **71**, 176–185.

Prien, R.F., Cole, J.O. and Belkin, N. (1968). Relapse in chronic schizophrenics following abrupt withdrawal of tranquillising medication. *Br. J. Psychiat.* **115**, 679–686.

Pycock, C.J., Kerwin, R.W. and Carter, C.J. (1980). Effects of lesion of cortical dopamine terminals on sub-cortical dopamine receptors in rats. *Nature* **286**, 74–77.

Quitkin, F., Rifkin, A. and Klein, D.F. (1975). Very high dosage vs. standard dosage fluphenazine in schizophrenia. A double-blind study of nonchronic treatment-refractory patients. *Arch. Gen. Psychiat.* **32**, 1276–1281.

Ratey, J., Daehler, M., O'Driscoll, C., Sorgi, P. and Rosenfeld, B. (1990). Betablockers in schizophrenia: a review of the literature. *Schizophrenia Res.* **3**, 49.

Rifkin, A., Doddi, S., Karajgi, B., Borenstein, M. and Wachspress, M. (1991). Dosage of haloperidol for schizophrenia. *Arch. Gen. Psychiat.* **48**, 166–170.

Roberts, G.W. (1990). Brain development and CCK systems in schizophrenia: a working hypothesis. In: M.P.I. Weller (ed.) *International Perspectives in Schizophrenia*, pp. 51–70. London: John Libbey.

Serban, G. and Siegel, S. (1984). Response of borderline and schizotypal patients to small doses of thiothixene and haloperidol. *Am. J. Psychiat.* **141**, 1455–1458.

Severson, J.A., Robinson, H.E. and Simpson, G.M. (1984). Neuroleptic-induced striatal dopamine receptor supersensitivity in mice: relationship to dose and drug. *Psychopharmacology (Berlin)* **84**, 115–119.

Shapiro, E., Shapiro, A.K., Fulop, G. *et al.* (1989). Controlled study of haloperidol, pimozide, and placebo for the treatment of Gilles de la Tourette's syndrome. *Arch. Gen. Psychiat.* **46**, 722–730.

Silver, H., Blacker, M., Weller, M.P.I. and Lerer, B. (1989). Treatment of chronic schizophrenia with cyproheptadine. *Biol. Psychiat.* **25**, 502–504.

Smith, R.C., Baumgartner, R. and Misra, C.H. (1984). Haloperidol: plasma levels and prolactin response as predictors of clinical improvement in schizophrenia: chemical v. radioceptor plasma level assays. *Arch. Gen. Psychiat.* **41**, 1044–1049.

Sokoloff, P., Giros, B., Martres, M.P., Bouthenet, M.L. and Schwartz, J.C. (1990). Molecular cloning and characterization of a novel dopamine receptor (D₃) as a target for neuroleptics. *Nature* **347**, 146–151.

Soloff, P.H., George, A., Nathan, R.S., Schulz, P.M., Ulrich, R.F. and Perel, J.M. (1986). Progress in pharmacotherapy of borderline disorders. A double-blind study of amitriptyline, haloperidol and placebo. *Arch. Gen. Psychiat.* **43**, 691–697.

Stanley, M., Laution, A., Rotrosen, J., Gershon, S. and Kleinberg, D. (1980). Metoclopramide: antipsychotic efficacy of a drug lacking potency in receptor models. *Psychopharmacology* **71**, 219–225.

Van Kammen, D.P., Peters, J.L., van Kammen, W.B., Neylan, T., Yao, J.K., Shaw, D. and Dougherty, G. (1990). Noradrenaline, state dependency and relapse prediction in schizophrenia: a hypothesis. In: M.P.I. Weller (ed.) *International Perspectives in Schizophrenia*, pp. 253–268. London: John Libbey.

Van Putten, T. (1988). The narrow therapeutic index of HPL: A dose comparison study. *Schizophrenia Res.* **1**, 201–202.

Velamoor, V.R., Fernando, M.L.D. and Williamson, P. (1990). Incipient neuroleptic syndrome? *Br. J. Psychiat.* **156**, 581–584.

Waddington, J.L. (1987). Tardive dyskinesia in schizophrenia and other disorders: associations with ageing, cognitive dysfunction and structural brain pathology in relation to neuroleptic exposure. *Hum. Psychopharmacol.* **2**, 11–22.

Waddington, J. and Yousseff, H.A. (1986). Late onset involuntary movements in chronic schizophrenia: relationship of 'tardive' dyskinesia to intellectual impairment and negative symptoms. *Br. J. Psychiat.* **149**, 616–620.

Weller, M.P.I. (1981). Schizophrenia, neuroleptics and Parkinson's disease. In: F.C.R. Rose and R. Capildeo (eds) *Recent Advances in Neurology*, pp. 67–71. London: Pitman Medical.

Weller, M.P.I. (1987). A biochemical theory of wandering. *Med. Sci. Law* **1**, 40–41.

Weller, M.P.I. (1989). Mental illness—who cares? *Nature* **399**, 249–252.

Weller, M.P.I. (1990). Clear consciousness and the diagnosis of schizophrenia: an irreconcilable problem. In: M.P.I. Weller (ed.) *International Perspectives in Schizophrenia*, pp. 1–18. London: John Libbey.

Weller, M.P.I. and Muijen, M. (eds) (1991). *Dimensions of Community Care*. London: W.B. Saunders (in press).

White, F.J. and Wang, R.Y. (1983). Differential effects of classical and atypical antipsychotic drugs on A9 and A10 dopamine neurons. *Science* **221**, 1054–1057.

WHO (1990). Prophylactic use of anticholinergics to patients on long-term neuroleptic treatment: a consensus statement. *Br. J. Psychiat.* **156**, 412.

Wistedt, B., Wiles, D. and Kolakowska, T. (1981). Slow decline of plasma drug and prolactin levels after discontinuation of chronic treatment with depot neuroleptics. *Lancet* **i**, 1163.

Yorkston, N.J., Zaki, S.A., Weller, M.P.I., Gruzelier, J.H. and Hirsch, S.R. (1981). *dl*-Propranolol and chlorpromazine following admission for schizophrenia: a controlled comparison. *Acta Psychiat. Scand.* **60**, 13–17.

— 33

Electroconvulsive Therapy

B. Shapira, S. Kindler and B. Lerer

More than half a century has elapsed since Laszlo Meduna initiated the use of convulsive therapy for the treatment of psychiatric illness (Meduna, 1935). Seizure induction by electrical means soon replaced the use of chemical convulsant agents (Cerletti and Bini, 1938). Modification of the treatment process by the use of general anaesthesia and muscle relaxation was a further significant advance (Bennet, 1940). Diagnostic indications for ECT have also undergone a significant change, the emphasis shifting from schizophrenia to affective disorders, particularly depression, and more recently to medication-refractory depressive illness (Weiner and Coffey, 1988).

Controversy regarding the use of ECT has recently abated somewhat, but remains active in a number of countries. The undeniably traumatic nature of unmodified ECT combined with indiscriminate as well as insensitive application of the treatment by the psychiatric profession were important factors in generating public concern. Although modern techniques of ECT administration and greater attention to consent issues have radically altered the situation, a negative image remains. In spite of technological advances in the administration of the treatment, memory impairment is still a problematic adverse effect and a focal point for advocacy groups opposed to ECT. Nevertheless, a series of official panels and investigative boards in different countries has consistently endorsed the use of ECT, recognizing its central role in the treatment of depression as well as other medication-refractory disorders (Royal College of Psychiatrists, 1977; American Psychiatric Association, 1978; Consensus Conference, 1985). For the same reason, psychiatrists continue to administer ECT and patients in need of the treatment consent to receive it.

The past decade had been characterized by a remarkable resurgence of research interest in ECT on the clinical and basic levels. These efforts have yielded strong empirical evidence in support of the efficacy of the treatment (particularly in depression) as well as important advances in the technique of ECT administration (Fink, 1979; Abrams, 1988). A definitive delineation of the nature, severity and persistence of the memory impairment which ECT induces as well as practical approaches towards alleviating this problem have also been achieved (Weiner, 1987; Calev et al., 1989). In addition, growing insights into mechanism of therapeutic action have emerged (Lerer, 1987). Focusing on the treatment of depression, this chapter will selectively review some of these areas, stress clinical implications and identify issues which should be given greater priority in future research.

Antidepressant Efficacy of Induced Seizures

For many years it was unclear which aspect of the ECT process is responsible for its therapeutic action. Psychological theories, a relationship to memory impairment and a direct action of the electrical stimulus were considered (Fink, 1979; Abrams, 1988). The fact that seizures induced by non-electrical means (e.g. chemical agents) are therapeutically effective, points to a pivotal role for the seizure component. Strong support was supplied by the work of Ottoson (1960) who demonstrated that chemical attenuation of seizure discharge blocked the antidepressant action of the treatment but not its adverse effects (which were primarily attributable to the electric current). Furthermore, a series of studies comparing ECT and simulated treatments (in which seizure induction did not take place) supported this view (Barton, 1977). These studies were, however, characterized by methodological flaws as well as other limitations and did not provide a conclusive answer.

From 1978, a renewed series of studies was undertaken in the United Kingdom comparing real and simulated ECT (anaesthesia and muscle relaxant only) in the treatment of depression (Lambourn and Gill, 1978; Freeman et al., 1978; Johnstone et al., 1980; West, 1981; Brandon et al., 1984; Gregory et al., 1985). These were generally rigorous in methodology and all but one (Lambourn and Gill, 1978) showed a significant advantage for real over simulated treatment (Table 33.1). The authors of this study which employed ultra-brief unilateral stimulation, subsequently published a further trial in which, with conventional stimulus parameters, both bilateral and unilateral modalities were superior to simulated treatment (Gregory et al., 1985).

The antidepressant efficacy of ECT has thus been conclusively established and related to repeated seizure induction. However, other aspects await further investigation. An important question is the predictability of ECT response and the delineation of factors which define a favourable prognosis. Although ECT is highly effective, 20–30% of medication-refractory depressives may fail to respond to the treatment (Shapira et al., 1988). Significant efforts have been invested in attempts to identify factors predicting response in patients administered ECT. Earlier findings pointed towards a more favourable prognosis in depressives with endogenous features and lacking marked neurotic and anxiety components (Fink, 1979; Abrams, 1988; see also Chapter 32, this volume). Today, however, most patients administered ECT tend to fall within a more homogeneous endogenous category and the degree to which neurotic features are present is less helpful.

One factor which has emerged as highly predictive of ECT response is episode duration. As shown in Fig. 33.1, the number of patients responding to ECT is inversely related to the length of time they have been depressed. It is unclear whether earlier administration of ECT would have led to a more favourable outcome in the poor responders or whether this group is different *ab initio* in terms of likelihood to benefit from the treatment. The dexamethasone suppression test has proved of questionable value in predicting ECT response (Abrams, 1988). However, other biological and psychological factors should be examined

TABLE 33.1 Studies comparing real and simulated ECT[a].

Study	No. of subjects	Stimulus parameters	Anaesthesia	Outcome
Lambourn and Gill (1978)	Real = 16 Simulated = 16	UL Brief pulse 6 treatments	Methohexital Suxamethonium	No difference
Freeman et al. (1978)	Real = 20 2 Simulated + Real = 20	BL Sine wave Treatment no. variable	Pentothal Suxamethonium	Real superior More ECTs in sim. group
Johnstone et al. (1980)	Real = 31 Simulated = 30	BL Sine wave 8 treatments	Methohexital Suxamethonium	Real superior
West (1981)	Real = 11 Simulated = 11	BL Sine wave 6 treatments (with cross-over)	Althesin Suxamethonium	Real superior
Brandon et al. (1984)	Real = 43 Simulated = 34	BL Sine wave 8 treatments	Methohexital Suxamethonium	Real superior
Gregory et al. (1985)	Real (UL) = 23 Real (BL) = 23 Simulated = 23	UL or BL Sine wave 6 treatments	Methohexital Suxamethonium	Real UL and BL superior

[a] All treatments administered twice weekly.
UL, unilateral; BL, bilateral.

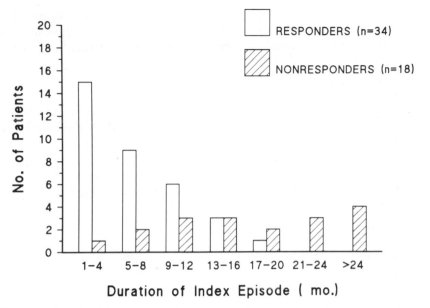

FIG. 33.1 Relationship between duration of index episode and treatment outcome. Significant difference in response as variable of index duration (12 month cut-off) between the two groups ($x^2 = 14.17$, $p = 0.0002$).

in order to determine whether patients with long episode duration and a negative prognosis for ECT can be more specifically characterized.

A related question is the long-term prognosis of depressed patients who are refractory to ECT. Studies on this topic are methodologically problematic because the natural history of depressive illness tends towards ultimate remission. Nevertheless, a report by Shapira *et al.* (1988) suggests that patients who do not respond to ECT may go on to remit when readministered antidepressant agents. In 12 ECT non-responders remission was achieved within 2–3 months of the conclusion of ineffective ECT course. Lithium supplementation of antidepressant medication (tricyclics and monoamine oxidase inhibitors) was found to be particularly effective. These findings suggest that even though an ECT course may be ineffective, it may evoke neurobiological effects which render the patient more likely to respond to a subsequent antidepressant trial.

Optimizing ECT Administration: Stimulus Parameters, Electrode Placement and Schedule

Until relatively recently, ECT was regarded as an 'all or nothing' treatment, the induced seizure being both necessary and sufficient for antidepressant action. This view has been subjected to intense research scrutiny which has indicated that the assumption is incorrect. Seizures which are of inadequate length or are poorly generalized to both hemispheres are associated with a poorer response rate. This work has led to a substantial refinement of the technique of ECT administration. Technical modifications have also been directed at reducing cognitive morbidity induced by the treatment and have been successful in this regard.

Stimulus waveform

The type of waveform traditionally used for ECT was an unmodified sine wave stimulus. Although undoubtedly effective, cognitive morbidity associated with this type of stimulus has been shown to be substantially greater than with modified brief pulse stimulation (Weiner *et al.*, 1983). The latter waveform is now generally accepted and incorporated in most of the new generation ECT devices. The efficacy of ultra-brief pulse stimulation remains questionable (Abrams, 1988).

Stimulus intensity

The question of ECT stimulus intensity has also been carefully examined. Sackeim and colleagues (1987a,b) have developed a technique for defining seizure threshold, i.e. that stimulus intensity required for induction of a therapeutically adequate seizure. This involves the administration of up to a maximum of three subconvulsive stimulations of increasing intensity during the first ECT session until a generalized seizure is induced. The subconvulsive stimulations are not associated with significantly increased cognitive morbidity and the technique is simple to apply. Monitoring of seizure duration is essential since an adequate seizure is defined as one which is 25–30 s in length on the electroencephalogram.

Various levels of stimulation relative to threshold have been examined in terms of efficacy and adverse effects (Sackeim *et al.*, 1987b). The general conclusion emerging from this work is that stimulation at or close to threshold is less effective while markedly suprathreshold stimulation induces an unnecessarily severe level of cognitive impairment. Moderately suprathreshold (100–150% above initial threshold) stimulation is presently the recommended treatment approach. Variations in threshold according to age and sex should be taken into account (Sackeim *et al.*, 1987a) as well as the fact that seizure threshold tends to increase substantially over the course of an ECT series.

Electrode placement

A third element of ECT technique to be considered is electrode placement. The relative merits of unilateral non-dominant (ULND) and bilateral (BL) treatment have been debated for a number of years and a substantial literature on this topic has accumulated. It is clearly established that ULND electrode placement significantly reduces memory impairment (Weiner *et al.*, 1983). However, reports indicating a lesser degree of antidepressant efficacy continue to emerge (Abrams, 1988). It would appear that the efficacy of ULND ECT is more strongly influenced by technique of administration than bilateral treatment. If sufficient care is not taken, inadequate stimulation may result in incomplete generalization of the seizure discharge to the contralateral hemisphere and this could be a factor influencing efficacy (Weiner and Coffey, 1986). Monitoring of seizure duration, by clinical means (in a cuffed limb from which succinylcholine has been excluded) as well as by electroencephalogram should be a regular concomitant of ECT administration but is particularly important in the case of unilateral treatment. A practical clinical approach would be to use ULND ECT unless bilateral treatment is felt to be specifically preferable and to switch to BL ECT if the patient fails to respond.

Schedule of administration

Compared to the above topics, schedule of administration is an aspect of ECT technique which has received relatively little attention (Lerer and Shapira, 1986). The frequency per week of treatment administration and the total number of ECTs in the series are referred to in this regard. Practice varies widely; most psychiatrists in the United States use a three times weekly schedule while their British and European counterparts tend to prefer twice weekly administration and a smaller total number of treatments. The question is not merely procedural since more frequent ECT administration and increased treatment number directly influence cognitive morbidity (Lerer and Shapira, 1986).

An open study by McAllister *et al.* (1987) suggested that twice and three times weekly schedules of ULND ECT are equivalent in efficacy. However, twice weekly treatment involved a lower total number of ECT administrations and a more positive effect on cognitive function. Interim results from a double-blind comparison (using simulated ECT for control purposes) by Lerer *et al.* (1990) confirmed that the two schedules are equivalent in efficacy but suggested that three times weekly treatment induces a significantly more rapid antidepressant effect. Three times weekly treatment was, however, associated with more severe memory impairment. This type of schedule could be considered optimal only if treatment number is held equivalent to that administered in a twice weekly context and cognitive adverse effects thereby reduced, a possibility suggested by the data (Lerer *et al.*, 1990).

Pharmacological Manipulation of Seizure Duration

Over the course of an ECT series, a significant increase in seizure threshold and reduction in seizure duration occurs in most patients. The clinician usually compensates for this development by increasing stimulus intensity. Failure to do so could result in a loss of efficacy as seizure duration drops below the 25–30 s (EEG length) regarded as optimal and there is an increased incidence of missed or incomplete seizures. Increased stimulus intensity is liable to worsen cognitive adverse effects and an alternative strategy for handling this problem is therefore desirable.

Such a strategy has been proposed by Shapira *et al.* (1985, 1987) on the basis of preclinical studies on the effect of electroconvulsive shock (ECS) on adenosine receptors of the A1 subtype in rat cortex. This receptor has been linked

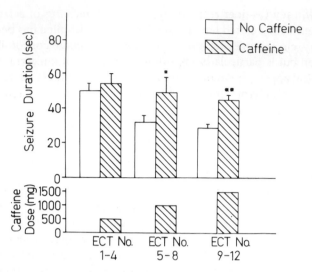

FIG. 33.2   Seizure duration (mean $\pm$ SEM) over an ECT course in the presence or absence of pre-ECT caffeine administration (*$p < 0.05$, **$p < 0.01$).

to an anticonvulsant action and its density is increased by electroconvulsive shock (ECS) administration (Newman *et al.*, 1984). Adenosine antagonists (such as methylxanthines) have been shown to inhibit A1 adenosine receptors and to increase seizure duration in rodents. This finding led Shapira *et al.* (1985, 1987) to propose that administration of an adenosine antagonist such as caffeine prior to ECT administration would result in an increase in seizure duration.

This hypothesis was borne out in a single case study (Shapira *et al.*, 1985) and in a subsequent controlled trial involving eight depressed patients (Shapira *et al.*, 1987). Caffeine sodium benzoate (500–2000 mg) was administered intravenously 10 min before ECT and seizure duration was compared with that of a previous treatment unmodified by caffeine. As shown in Fig. 33.2 seizure duration was significantly increased during ECTs preceded by caffeine. The effect was more prominent later in the ECT course when seizure duration was shorter than at the initial stages of treatment. Administration of caffeine was not associated with significant cardiovascular or other adverse effects.

These observations have been borne out in a number of studies by other authors (Hinkle *et al.*, 1987; Coffey *et al.*, 1990). In a recent controlled comparison, caffeine augmentation emerged as equivalent to increased stimulus intensity in maintaining seizure duration (Coffey *et al.*, 1990). It remains to be clearly established that cognitive impairment is reduced by this intervention. This would be dependent upon the development of an appropriate dosage regimen since seizures extended (as a result of caffeine administration) beyond the optimum length can also contribute to cognitive morbidity.

Mechanism of Action

The mechanism(s) whereby a series of clinically induced grand mal seizures alleviate the most profound depressive symptomatology has intrigued researchers for decades. Since ECT is effective in disorders other than depression (e.g. mania, schizophrenia, Parkinson's disease), theories of ECT action should take into account a spectrum of therapeutic efficacy. Moreover, within the context of depression, ECT is effective in patients who are refractory to antidepressant medication and also in delusional depression in which antidepressants are unhelpful unless supplemented by antipsychotic medication.

Lichtenberg and Lerer (1989) have reviewed the clinical spectrum of ECT and have concluded that the multiple therapeutic actions of ECT are difficult to conceptualize within the context of a unitary mechanism of action. Focusing on neurochemical actions, they have suggested that effects of the treatment on different neurotransmitter systems may underlie its therapeutic action in different syndromes. Thus, enhancement of brain serotoninergic function (Kellar *et al.*, 1981; Vetulani *et al.*, 1981) may, alone or combined with the action of ECT on the noradrenergic (and other) systems, underlie its antidepressant action. Enhancement of dopamine function in the nigro-striatal region (Grahame-Smith *et al.*, 1978) may account for the antiparkinsonian effects of ECT and cholinergic mechanisms (Lerer, 1985) may be implicated in the memory impairment induced by the treatment. A comprehensive review of the data in support of ECT effects on these and other neurotransmitters is beyond the scope of this chapter (see Lerer, 1987).

Another focus of ECT research involves studies in patients administered the treatment as opposed to experiments in rodents and other laboratory animals. Preclinical experiments are obviously limited by phylogenetic considerations and it is important that effects characterized in animal models are also shown to be operative in humans treated with ECT (Lerer and Sitaram, 1983). Neuroendocrine challenge paradigms are important tools in this strategy. For example, enhancement by ECT of serotoninergic responses in rats has also been shown to occur in depressed patients administered ECT. This was demonstrated by Shapira *et al.* (1989) who used the fenfluramine challenge test as an *in vivo* measure of serotoninergic responsivity and showed increased serotoninergically mediated prolactin release following an ECT course compared to pre-treatment values. Enhanced dopaminergic responsivity has also been demonstrated in depressed patients by neuroendocrine challenge (Costain *et al.*, 1982). This parallels findings in rodents and may, as noted previously, explain the antiparkinsonian action of the treatment.

It should be stressed that potential mechanisms of ECT currently under study are not limited to neurochemical aspects. The physiological sequelae of grand mal seizures are numerous, as might be expected of so major a neurometabolic event. It is therefore not surprising that a significant body of data has accumulated regarding ECT effects on neurophysiological parameters such as the permeability of the blood–brain barrier, regional cerebral blood flow and brain electrical activity (see Lerer *et al.*, 1984). These studies have, however, not yielded comprehensive theoretical formulations. It has also been suggested that the anticonvulsant properties of ECT may be related to its antidepressant efficacy and that suppression of neurometabolic activity may underlie both effects (Sackeim *et al.*, 1983). Neuroendocrine theories should also be noted. Depression is associated with significant vegetative symptoms, most of which are hypothalam-ically mediated and reversed by ECT. It has therefore been suggested that ECT may act via a direct effect on the hypothalamus, possibly by the release of specific hypothalamic peptides (Fink and Ottoson, 1980).

Conclusions

Recent advances in ECT research and practice have significantly consolidated the scientific basis of this treatment. Controlled trials of antidepressant efficacy have utilized rigorous methodology and have yielded definitive results which have had a major impact on the field. Optimization of parameters such as stimulus waveform, stimulus intensity and electrode placement have led to a considerable refinement of ECT practice and the definition of an optimum schedule is likely to further advance this process. Pharmacological manipulation of seizure duration is an intriguing example of basic neuroscience findings applied to the clinical context and could substantially influence practice. Finally, studies on mechanism of action hold the key to understanding not only the underlying basis of this unique treatment, but also the pathogenesis of disorders in which it is effective.

Acknowledgement

Supported in part by Grant #MH40734 from the United States National Institute of Mental Health.

References

Abrams, R. (1988). *Electroconvulsive Therapy*. Oxford and New York: Oxford University Press.

American Psychiatric Association (1978). *Electroconvulsive Therapy*, Task force Report 14. Washington DC: American Psychiatric Association.

Barton, J.L. (1977). ECT in depression: The evidence of controlled studies. *Biol. Psychiat.* **12**, 687–695.

Bennett, A.E. (1940). Preventing traumatic complications in convulsive shock therapy by curare. *J. Am. Med. Ass.* **114**, 322–324.

Brandon, S., Cowley, P., McDonald, C., Neville, P. and Wellstood-Eason, S. (1984). Electroconvulsive therapy: Results in depressive illness from the Leicestershire trial. *Br. Med. J.* **228**, 22–25.

Calev, A., Ben-Tzvi, E., Shapira, B., Drexler, H., Carasso, R. and Lerer, B. (1989). Distinct memory impairments following electroconvulsive therapy and imipramine. *Psychol. Med.* **19**, 111–119.

Cerletti, U. and Bini, L. (1938). Un nuevo metodo di shockterapie 'L'elettro-shock'. *Boll. Acad. Med. Roma* **64**, 136–138.

Coffey, C.E., Figiel, G.S., Weiner, R.A. and Saunders, W.B. (1990). Caffeine augmentation of ECT. *Am. J. Psychiat.* **147**, 579–585.

Consensus Conference (1985). Electroconvulsive Therapy. *J. Am. Med. Ass.* **254**, 2103–2108.

Costain, D.W., Cowen, P.J., Gelder, M.G. and Grahame-Smith, D.G. (1982). Electroconvulsive therapy and the brain: evidence for increased dopamine-mediated responses. *Lancet* **ii**, 400–404.

Fink, M. (1979). *Convulsive Therapy: Theory and Practice.* New York: Raven Press.

Fink, M. and Ottoson, J.O. (1980). A theory of convulsive therapy in endogenous depression: significance of hypothalamic functions. *Psychiat. Res.* **2**, 49–61.

Freeman, C.P.L., Basson, J.V. and Crighton, A. (1978). Double blind controlled trial of electroconvulsive therapy (ECT) and simulated ECT in depressive illness. *Lancet* **i**, 738–740.

Grahame-Smith, D.G., Green, A.R. and Costain, D.W. (1978). Mechanism of the antidepressant action of electroconvulsive therapy. *Lancet* **i**, 245–256.

Gregory, S., Shawcross, C.R. and Gill, D. (1985). The Nottingham ECT study. A double-blind comparison of bilateral, unilateral and simulated ECT in depressive illness. *Br. Med. J.* **146**, 520–524.

Hinkle, P.E., Coffey, C.E., Weiner, R.D., Cress, M. and Christison, C. (1987). *Am. J. Psychiat.* **144**, 1143–1148.

Johnstone, E.C., Lawker, P., Stevens, M., Deakin, J.F.W., McPherson, K. and Crow, T.J. (1980). The Northwick Park electroconvulsive therapy trial. *Lancet* **ii**, 1317–1320.

Kellar, K.J., Cascio, C.S., Butler, J.A. and Kurtzke, R.N. (1981). Differential effects of electroconvulsive shock and antidepressant drugs on serotonin-2 receptors in rat brain. *Eur. J. Pharmacol.* **69**, 515–518.

Lambourn, J. and Gill, D. (1978). A controlled comparison of simulated and real ECT. *Br. J. Psychiat.* **133**, 154–159.

Lerer, B. (1985). Studies on the role of brain cholinergic systems in therapeutic mechanisms and adverse effects of ECT and lithium. *Biol. Psychiat.* **20**, 20–40.

Lerer, B. (1987). Neurochemical and other neurobiological consequences of ECT: implications for the pathogenesis and treatment of affective disorders. In H.Y. Meltzer (ed.) *Psychopharmacology: The Third Generation of Progress.* New York: Raven Press.

Lerer, B. and Sitaram, N. (1983). Clinical strategies for evaluating ECT mechanisms: Pharmacological, biochemical and psychophysiological approaches. *Progr. Neuropsychopharmacol. Biol. Psychiat.* **7**, 309–333.

Lerer, B. and Shapira, B. (1986). Optimum frequency of ECT: implications for clinical practice and basic research. *Convulsive Ther.* **2**, 141–144.

Lerer, B., Weiner, R.D. and Belmaker, R.H. (eds) (1984). *ECT: Basic Mechanisms.* London: John Libbey (republished 1986, Washington, DC: American Psychiatric Press).

Lerer, B., Shapira, B. and Calev, A. (1990). Optimising ECT schedule—a double blind study. *Am. Psychiat. Ass. 143rd Annual Meeting,* New York.

Lichtenberg, P. and Lerer, B. (1989). Implications of clinical spectrum for mechanisms of action: ECT and antidepressants reconsidered. *Convulsive Ther.* **5**, 216–226.

McAllister, D.A., Perri, M.G., Jordan, R.C., Rauscher, F.P. and Sattin, A. (1987). Effects of ECT given two vs. three times weekly. *Psychiat. Res.* **21**, 63–69.

Meduna, I.J. (1935). Versuche über die biologische Deeinflussung des abaufes der Schizophrenia: Camphor und Cardiozoldkrampfe. *Ges. Neurol. Psychiatr.* **152**, 235–262.

Newman, M., Zohar, J., Kalian, M. *et al.* (1984). The effects of chronic lithium and ECT on A1 and A2 adenosine receptor systems in rat brain. *Brain Res.* **291**, 188–192.

Ottoson, J.O. (1960). Experimental studies on the mode of action of electroconvulsive therapy. *Acta Psychiat. Neurol. Scand.* (Suppl. 145) **35**, 1–141.

Royal College of Psychiatrists (1977). Memorandum on the use of ECT. *Br. J. Psychiat.* **131**, 261–272.

Sackeim, H.A., Decina, P., Prohovnik, I., Malitz, S. and Resor, S. (1983). Anticonvulsant and antidepressant properties of ECT: a proposed mechanism of action. *Biol. Psychiat.* **18**, 1301–1309.

Sackeim, H.A., Decina, P., Portnoy, S. *et al.* (1987a). Studies of dosage, seizure threshold and seizure duration in ECT. *Biol. Psychiat.* **22**, 249–268.

Sackeim, H.A., Decina, P., Kanzler, M. *et al.* (1987b). Effects of electrode placement on the efficacy of titrated, low-dose ECT. *Am. J. Psychiat.* **144**, 1449–1455.

Shapira, B., Zohar, J., Newman, M. *et al.* (1985). Potentiation of seizure length and clinical response to ECT by caffeine pretreatment. *Convulsive Ther.* **1**, 58–60.

Shapira, B., Lerer, B., Gilboa, D., Drexler, H., Kugelmass, S. and Calev, A. (1987). Facilitation of ECT by caffeine pretreatment. *Am. J. Psychiat.* **144**, 9.

Shapira, B., Kindler, S. and Lerer, B. (1988). Medication outcome in ECT-resistant depression. *Convulsive Ther.* **4**, 192–198.

Shapira, B., Gropp, C. and Lerer, B. (1989). ECT and imipramine enhance prolactin response to fenfluramine challenge. *Soc. Biol. Psychiat., 44th Annual Convention*, San Francisco.

Vetulani, J., Lebrecht, U. and Pilc, A. (1981). Enhancement of responsiveness of the central serotonergic system and serotonin-2 receptor density in rat frontal cortex by electroconvulsive treatment. *Eur. J. Pharmacol.* **76**, 81–85.

Weiner, R.D. (1984). Does electroconvulsive therapy cause brain damage? *Behav. Brain Sci.* **7**, 1–53.

Weiner, R.D. and Coffey, C.E. (1986). Minimizing therapeutic differences between bilateral and unilateral nondominant ECT. *Convulsive Ther.* **2**, 261–265.

Weiner, R.D. and Coffey, C.E. (1988). Indications for use of electroconvulsive therapy. In: A.J. Francis and R.E. Hales (eds) *Review of Psychiatry*, Vol. 7. Washington DC: American Psychiatric Press.

Weiner, R.D., Rogers, H.J., Welch, C.A. *et al.* (1983). ECT parameters and electrode placement. In B. Lerer and R.D. Weiner (eds) *ECT: Basic Mechanisms*. London: John Libbey.

Weiner, R.D., Rogers, H.J., Davidson, J.R. *et al.* (1986). Effects of stimulus parameters on cognitive side effects. *Ann. NY Acad. Sci.* **462**, 315–325.

West, E.D. (1981). Electric convulsive therapy in depression: a double-blind controlled trial. *Br. Med. J.* **282**, 355–357.

Index